1997

YEAR BOOK OF

NEONATAL AND PERINATAL MEDICINE®

Statement of Purpose

The YEAR BOOK Service

The YEAR BOOK series was devised in 1901 by practicing health professionals who observed that the literature of medicine and related disciplines had become so voluminous that no one individual could read and place in perspective every potential advance in a major specialty. In the final decade of the 20th century, this recognition is more acutely true than it was in 1901.

More than merely a series of books, YEAR BOOK volumes are the tangible results of a unique service designed to accomplish the following:

- to *survey* a wide range of journals of proven value
- to *select* from those journals papers representing significant advances and statements of important clinical principles
- to provide *abstracts* of those articles that are readable, convenient summaries of their key points
- to provide *commentary* about those articles to place them in perspective

These publications grow out of a unique process that calls on the talents of outstanding authorities in clinical and fundamental disciplines, trained literature specialists, and professional writers, all supported by the resources of Mosby, the world's preeminent publisher for the health professions.

The Literature Base

Mosby and its editors survey more than 1,000 journals published worldwide, covering the full range of the health professions. On an annual basis, the publisher examines usage patterns and polls its expert authorities to add new journals to the literature base and to delete journals that are no longer useful as potential YEAR BOOK sources.

The Literature Survey

The publisher's team of literature specialists, all of whom are trained and experienced health professionals, examines every original, peer-reviewed article in each journal issue. More than 250,000 articles per year are scanned systematically, including title, text, illustrations, tables, and references. Each scan is compared, article by article, to the search strategies that the publisher has developed in consultation with the 270 outside experts who form the pool of YEAR BOOK editors. A given article may be reviewed by any number of editors, from one to a dozen or more, regardless of the discipline for which the paper was originally published. In turn, each editor who receives the article reviews it to determine whether or not the article should be included in the YEAR BOOK. This decision is based on the article's inherent quality, its probable usefulness to readers of that YEAR BOOK, and the editor's goal to represent a balanced picture of a given field in each volume of the YEAR BOOK. In addition, the editor indicates when to include figures and tables from the article to help the YEAR BOOK reader better understand the information.

Of the quarter million articles scanned each year, only 5% are selected for detailed analysis within the YEAR BOOK series, thereby assuring readers of the high value of every selection.

The Abstract

The publisher's abstracting staff is headed by a seasoned medical professional and includes individuals with training in the life sciences, medicine, and other areas, plus extensive experience in writing for the health professions and related industries. Each selected article is assigned to a specific writer on this abstracting staff. The abstracter, guided in many cases by notations supplied by the expert editor, writes a structured, condensed summary designed so that the reader can rapidly acquire the essential information contained in the article.

The Commentary

The YEAR BOOK editorial boards, sometimes assisted by guest commentators, write comments that place each article in perspective for the reader. This provides the reader with the equivalent of a personal consultation with a leading international authority—an opportunity to better understand the value of the article and to benefit from the authority's thought processes in assessing the article.

Additional Editorial Features

The editorial boards of each YEAR BOOK organize the abstracts and comments to provide a logical and satisfying sequence of information. To enhance the organization, editors also provide introductions to sections or individual chapters, comments linking a number of abstracts, citations to additional literature, and other features.

The published YEAR BOOK contains enhanced bibliographic citations for each selected article, including extended listings of multiple authors and identification of author affiliations. Each YEAR BOOK contains a Table of Contents specific to that year's volume. From year to year, the Table of Contents for a given YEAR BOOK will vary depending on developments within the field.

Every YEAR BOOK contains a list of the journals from which papers have been selected. This list represents a subset of the more than 1,000 journals surveyed by the publisher and occasionally reflects a particularly pertinent article from a journal that is not surveyed on a routine basis.

Finally, each volume contains a comprehensive subject index and an index to authors of each selected paper.

The 1997 Year Book Series

Year Book of Allergy, Asthma, and Clinical Immunology: Drs. Rosenwasser, Borish, Gelfand, Leung, Nelson, and Szefler

Year Book of Anesthesiology and Pain Management®: Drs. Tinker, Abram, Chestnut, Roizen, Rothenberg, and Wood

Year Book of Cardiology®: Drs. Schlant, Collins, Gersh, Graham, Kaplan, and Waldo

Year Book of Chiropractic®: Dr. Lawrence

Year Book of Critical Care Medicine®: Drs. Parrillo, Balk, Calvin, Franklin, and Shapiro

Year Book of Dentistry®: Drs. Meskin, Berry, Kennedy, Leinfelder, Roser, Summitt, and Zakariasen

Year Book of Dermatologic Surgery®: Drs. Greenway, Papadopoulos, and Whitaker

Year Book of Dermatology®: Drs. Sober and Fitzpatrick

Year Book of Diagnostic Radiology®: Drs. Federle, Gross, Dalinka, Maynard, Rebner, Smirniotopolous, and Young

Year Book of Digestive Diseases®: Drs. Greenberger and Moody

Year Book of Drug Therapy®: Drs. Lasagna and Weintraub

Year Book of Emergency Medicine®: Drs. Wagner, Dronen, Davidson, King, Niemann, and Roberts

Year Book of Endocrinology®: Drs. Bagdade, Braverman, Horton, Kannan, Landsberg, Molitch, Morley, Nathan, Odell, Poehlman, Rogol, and Ryan

Year Book of Family Practice®: Drs. Berg, Bowman, Davidson, Dexter, and Scherger

Year Book of Geriatrics and Gerontology®: Drs. Beck, Burton, Ostwald, Rabins, Reuben, Roth, Shapiro, and Whitehouse

Year Book of Hand Surgery®: Drs. Amadio and Hentz

Year Book of Hematology®: Drs. Spivak, Bell, Ness, Quesenberry, Wiernik, and Blume

Year Book of Infectious Diseases®: Drs. Keusch, Barza, Bennish, Poutsiaka, Skolnik, and Snydman

Year Book of Medicine®: Drs. Klahr, Cline, Petty, Frishman, Greenberger, Malawista, Mandell, and Utiger

Year Book of Neonatal and Perinatal Medicine®: Drs. Fanaroff, Maisels, and Stevenson

Year Book of Nephrology, Hypertension, and Mineral Metabolism: Drs. Schwab, Bennett, Emmett, Hostetter, Kumar, and Toto

Year Book of Neurology and Neurosurgery®: Drs. Bradley and Wilkins

Year Book of Nuclear Medicine®: Drs. Gottschalk, Blaufox, Neumann, Strauss, and Zubal

Year Book of Obstetrics, Gynecology, and Women's Health: Drs. Mishell, Herbst, and Kirschbaum

Year Book of Occupational and Environmental Medicine®: Drs. Emmett, Frank, Gochfeld, and Hessl

Year Book of Oncology®: Drs. Ozols, Cohen, Glatstein, Loehrer, Tallman, and Wiersma

Year Book of Ophthalmology®: Drs. Wilson, Augsburger, Cohen, Eagle, Flanagan, Grossman, Laibson, Maguire, Nelson, Penne, Rapuano, Sergott, Spaeth, Tipperman, Ms. Gosfield, and Ms. Salmon

Year Book of Orthopedics®: Drs. Sledge, Poss, Cofield, Dobyns, Griffin, Springfield, Swiontkowski, Wiesel, and Wilson

Year Book of Otolaryngology–Head and Neck Surgery®: Drs. Paparella and Holt

Year Book of Pathology and Laboratory Medicine: Drs. Mills, Bruns, Gaffey, and Stoler

Year Book of Pediatrics®: Dr. Stockman

Year Book of Plastic, Reconstructive, and Aesthetic Surgery®: Drs. Miller, Cohen, McKinney, Robson, Ruberg, Smith, and Whitaker

Year Book of Podiatric Medicine and Surgery®: Dr. Kominsky

Year Book of Psychiatry and Applied Mental Health®: Drs. Talbott, Ballenger, Breier, Frances, Meltzer, Schowalter, and Tasman

Year Book of Pulmonary Disease®: Dr. Petty

Year Book of Rheumatology®: Drs. Sergent, LeRoy, Meenan, Panush, and Reichlin

Year Book of Sports Medicine®: Drs. Shephard, Alexander, Drinkwater, Eichner, George, and Torg

Year Book of Surgery®: Drs. Copeland, Bland, Deitch, Eberlein, Howard, Luce, Seeger, Souba, and Sugarbaker

Year Book of Thoracic and Cardiovascular Surgery®: Drs. Ginsberg, Wechsler, and Williams

Year Book of Urology®: Drs. Andriole and Coplen

Year Book of Vascular Surgery®: Dr. Porter

1997 The Year Book of NEONATAL AND PERINATAL MEDICINE®

Editors

Avroy A. Fanaroff, M.B.B.Ch. (Rand), F.R.C.P.E.

Professor, Department of Pediatrics, Professor of Neonatology, Department of Reproductive Biology, Case Western Reserve University School of Medicine; Director, Division of Neonatology, Rainbow Babies and Children's Hospital, Cleveland, Ohio

M. Jeffrey Maisels, M.B., B.Ch.

Clinical Professor of Pediatrics, Wayne State University School of Medicine, Detroit, and Clinical Professor of Pediatrics, University of Michigan Medical Center, Ann Arbor; Chairman, Department of Pediatrics, William Beaumont Hospital, Royal Oak, Michigan

David K. Stevenson, M.D.

Harold K. Faber Professor of Pediatrics, Associate Chairman, Department of Pediatrics; Chief, Division of Neonatal and Developmental Medicine, Stanford University School of Medicine; Director of Nurseries, Lucile Salter Packard Children's Hospital at Stanford, Palo Alto, California

Mosby

St. Louis Baltimore Boston Carlsbad Chicago Naples New York Philadelphia Portland London Madrid Mexico City Singapore Sydney Tokyo Toronto Wiesbaden

Mosby
Dedicated to Publishing Excellence

A Times Mirror Company

Vice President and Publisher, Continuity Publishing: Kenneth H. Killion
Director, Editorial Development: Gretchen C. Murphy
Acquisitions Editor: Linda Sheehan
Developmental Editor: Bernadette Buchholz
Project Supervisor, Editing: Rebecca Nordbrock
Assistant Project Supervisor, Production: Laura M. Higgins
Freelance Staff Supervisor: Barbara M. Kelly
Illustrations and Permissions Coordinator: Nancy Dunne
Director, Editorial Services: Edith M. Podrazik, B.S.N., R.N.
Information Specialist: Terri Santo, R.N.
Information Specialist: Margery Marble, B.S., R.N.
Circulation Manager: Lynn D. Stevenson

1997 EDITION

Printed in the United States of America
Composition by Reed Technology and Information Services, Inc.
Printing/binding by Maple-Vail

Mosby–Year Book, Inc.
11830 Westline Industrial Drive
St. Louis, MO 63146
Customer Service: customer.support@mosby.com
www.mosby.com/Mosby/CustomerSupport/index.html

Editorial Office:
Mosby–Year Book, Inc.
161 North Clark Street
Chicago, IL 60601
series.editorial@mosby.com

International Standard Serial Number: 8756-5005
International Standard Book Number: 0-8151-9643-1

Table of Contents

Journals Represented

Mosby and its editors survey more than 1,000 journals for its abstract and commentary publications. From these journals, the editors select the articles to be abstracted. Journals represented in this YEAR BOOK are listed below.

ASAIO Journal
Acta Obstetricia et Gynecologica Scandinavica
Acta Paediatrica
American Journal of Clinical Nutrition
American Journal of Obstetrics and Gynecology
American Journal of Perinatology
American Journal of Physiology
American Journal of Public Health
American Journal of Respiratory and Critical Care Medicine
American Surgeon
Annals of Neurology
Annals of Surgery
Annals of Thoracic Surgery
Archives of Disease in Childhood
Archives of Ophthalmology
Archives of Pediatrics and Adolescent Medicine
Australian and New Zealand Journal of Obstetrics and Gynaecology
Biology of the Neonate
British Journal of Obstetrics and Gynaecology
British Journal of Ophthalmology
British Medical Journal
Canadian Journal of Anaesthesia
Canadian Journal of Psychiatry
Canadian Medical Association Journal
Clinical Endocrinology (Oxford)
Clinical Journal of Pain
Clinical Obstetrics and Gynecology
Clinical Pediatrics
Clinical Radiology
Endocrinology
European Journal of Obstetrics, Gynecology and Reproductive Biology
Gastroenterology
Heart
Human Reproduction
Intensive Care Medicine
International Journal of Epidemiology
Israel Journal of Medical Sciences
Journal of Applied Physiology: Respiratory, Environmental and Exercise Physiology
Journal of Bone and Joint Surgery (British Volume)
Journal of Bone and Mineral Research
Journal of Clinical Endocrinology and Metabolism
Journal of Clinical Investigation
Journal of Clinical Pharmacology
Journal of Foot and Ankle Surgery
Journal of Infectious Diseases
Journal of Medical Genetics

Journal of Pediatric Gastroenterology and Nutrition
Journal of Pediatric Ophthalmology and Strabismus
Journal of Pediatric Surgery
Journal of Pediatrics
Journal of Thoracic and Cardiovascular Surgery
Journal of Urology
Journal of the American Medical Association
Lancet
Medical Journal of Australia
Medicine and Science in Sports and Exercise
Nature
New England Journal of Medicine
Obstetrics and Gynecology
Pediatric Infectious Disease Journal
Pediatric Pulmonology
Pediatric Radiology
Pediatric Research
Pediatrics
Prenatal Diagnosis
Radiology
Scandinavian Journal of Work, Environment and Health
Science
Southern Medical Journal
Surgery
Therapeutic Drug Monitoring
Transfusion
Ultrasound in Obstetrics and Gynecology
Western Journal of Medicine

STANDARD ABBREVIATIONS

The following terms are abbreviated in this edition: acquired immunodeficiency syndrome (AIDS), cardiopulmonary resuscitation (CPR), central nervous system (CNS), cerebrospinal fluid (CSF), computed tomography (CT), deoxyribonucleic acid (DNA), electrocardiography (ECG), health maintenance organization (HMO), human immunodeficiency virus (HIV), intensive care unit (ICU), intramuscular (IM), intravenous (IV), magnetic resonance (MR) imaging (MRI), ribonucleic acid (RNA), and ultrasound (US).

NOTE

The YEAR BOOK OF NEONATAL AND PERINATAL MEDICINE is a literature survey service providing abstracts of articles published in the professional literature. Every effort is made to assure the accuracy of the information presented in these pages. Neither the editors nor the publisher of the YEAR BOOK OF NEONATAL AND PERINATAL MEDICINE can be responsible for errors in the original materials. The editors' comments are their own opinions. Mention of specific products within this publication does not constitute endorsement.

To facilitate the use of the YEAR BOOK OF NEONATAL AND PERINATAL MEDICINE as a reference tool, all illustrations and tables included in this publication are now identified as they appear in the original article. This change is meant to help the reader recognize that any illustration or table appearing in the YEAR BOOK OF NEONATAL AND PERINATAL MEDICINE may be only one of many in the original article. For this reason, figure and table numbers will often appear to be out of sequence within the YEAR BOOK OF NEONATAL AND PERINATAL MEDICINE.

Introduction

The YEAR BOOK OF NEONATAL AND PERINATAL MEDICINE, now in its 11th year of publication, is under new stewardship. I am fortunate that my esteemed colleagues, M. Jeffrey Maisels and David K. Stevenson, have readily, and more than ably, filled the void left by the retirement of the founding editor, Marshall H. Klaus. The transition has been smooth, and we look forward to a long and productive collaboration. As editors, we strive to deliver comprehensive and compelling commentaries on contemporary and controversial topics in neonatal and perinatal medicine. There are still gaps in the evidence on which therapy is based; we attempt to provoke the readers to fill these many gaps.

The current YEAR BOOK includes the invited review from Stevenson's group, entitled "Noninvasive Monitoring: The Next Generation," which inadvertently was omitted from the 1996 YEAR BOOK OF NEONATAL AND PERINATAL MEDICINE. As promised, we have included the group B streptococcal guidelines. They are aimed at eradicating morbidity and mortality caused by this organism and, after some remarkable medical diplomacy, have been published in concert by the Centers for Disease Control and Prevention, American College of Obstetricians and Gynecologists, and committees of the American Academy of Pediatrics. William Benitz has developed a model based on the guidelines to determine their prospects for success. His commentary will provide perspective regarding their cost-effectiveness, efficiency, and their chances of succeeding. It will take a major tour de force to apply these guidelines in a uniform manner throughout the United States.

The general format of the 1997 YEAR BOOK OF NEONATAL AND PERINATAL MEDICINE has remained essentially unchanged, with selections covering a wide range of topics and journals. As always, preference is given to randomized, controlled trials, warts and all. An additional feature this year is a section on ethics contributed by our Canadian colleagues, Jonathan Hellman, M.B.B.Ch., and Francoise Baylis, Ph.D. We have been fortunate once again to call on the local and national experts for additional colorful commentaries. They have all given freely and willingly of their time. Indeed, it is gratifying to note that a number of our colleagues volunteer to write commentaries.

As we move deeper into the electronic age, through a service provided by Mosby–Year Book, some commentaries will be available as part of a literature search, prior to the hardcopy publication of the YEAR BOOK. It has been a pleasure once again to work with the wonderful, professional staff at Mosby–Year Book. They make the editorial task as simple as it could be. We would especially like to express our thanks to Bernadette Buchholz, our developmental editor since 1992, and wish her well as she changes careers.

Avroy A. Fanaroff, M.B.B.Ch.

Noninvasive Monitoring: The Next Generation

WILLIAM D. RHINE, M.D.[1]

STEPHEN ASHWAL, M.D.[2]

BARBARA HOLSHOUSER, Ph.D.[3]

HELEN E. D'ARCEUIL, Ph.D.[4]

JOHN P. VAN HOUTEN, M.D.[1]

CHRIS H. CONTAG, Ph.D.[1]

DAVID A. BENARON, M.D.[1]

DAVID K. STEVENSON, M.D.[1]

Departments of Pediatrics[1] and Radiology,[4] Stanford University Medical Center, Stanford, California; and Departments of Pediatrics[2] and Radiology,[3] Loma Linda University School of Medicine, Loma Linda, California

Introduction

Although the engineering foundations of both MR and near-infrared imaging were laid down decades ago, they have more recently been developed into powerful tools to study brain metabolism and injury. The rapid expansion of microprocessor technology has been crucial to providing the computational power needed for these two imaging techniques. These measurement tools are rapidly moving from the bench to the bedside. As a complete review of these technologies would require a whole book of its own, we wish to focus on some of the latest developments as they apply to studies of newborns.

Magnetic Resonance Studies of Neonatal Encephalopathy

Outcome Prediction in Children With Acute CNS Injuries Using ^{1}H-MRS

INTRODUCTION.—Proton MR spectroscopy (^{1}H-MRS) is a clinically useful, noninvasive tool for identifying the biochemical state of the CNS. Metabolites measured with ^{1}H-MRS include: *N*-acetyl aspartate (NA), a neuronal marker; creatine (Cr), comprised of phosphocreatine and its precursor creatine, which are bioenergetic metabolites; choline-containing compounds (Ch), including free choline, phosphoryl, and glycerophosphoryl choline that are released during membrane disruption; lactate (Lac), which accumulates in response to tissue damage; glutamate and immediately formed glutamine (Glx) and myoinositol (mI).[1]

Characteristic ^{1}H-MRS spectra in adults have been described in hepatic encephalopathy, diabetic ketoacidosis, dementia, tumor, stroke, multiple sclerosis, and AIDS-related leukodystrophies.[1–3] In children, abnormalities on ^{1}H-MRS have been observed with ornithine transcarbamylase deficiency, Canavan's and Alexander's diseases, aminoacidopathies, mitochondrial encephalopathies, peroxisomal disorders, neuronal ceroid lipofuscinosis, and other neurodegenerative conditions.[1, 4–18]

Magnetic resonance spectroscopy has also been studied after acute hypoxic-ischemic injury. In adults, hypoxic-ischemic injury has been associated with the presence of lactate and a decrease in NA that correlates with long-term neurologic sequelae.[19–24] Few studies have addressed the metabolic changes in response to acute cerebral injury in children using MRS. The majority of studies have examined neonates and used phosphorus-31–MRS to identify brain injury after hypoxic-ischemic insults. Studies have shown characteristic injury patterns at times earlier than that seen by conventional imaging.[25–34] Investigators have also noted specific alterations of metabolite patterns in periventricular leukomalacia, cerebral infarction, hemorrhage, and disorders of myelination.[29, 31] ^{1}H-MRS has also been used to evaluate the prognosis of pediatric near-drowning victims by correlating outcome with elevations in Glx and Lac in combination with a reduction in NA.[35]

In our recent studies we have shown that ^{1}H-MRS in conjunction with clinical data was useful in predicting outcome after a variety of acute serious CNS injuries.[36] In 30 children (newborn to 180 months studied a mean of 7 days after insult), we found that the NA/Cr and NA/Ch ratios were significantly lower in patients with bad outcomes (severe disability, persistent vegetative state [PVS], death) compared with patients with good outcomes (normal, mild, or moderate disability). In addition, cerebral lactate was present in 80% of bad-outcome patients compared with none of the good-outcome group. We also used a linear discriminant analysis and combined four clinical variables (Glasgow Coma Scale score, initial pH, blood glucose, and number of days unconscious) with the ^{1}H-MRS data and were able to correctly classify outcome in 100% of patients. More recently in a larger series of 98 infants and children we found that ^{1}H-MRS was particularly predictive in children greater than 18 months of age when done 3–5 days after insult.[37]

From the foregoing, it seems likely that any major CNS disease involving either focal neuronal damage or a more generalized hypoxic-ischemic or toxic insult will result in major abnormalities in the proton spectrum. It is also likely that these changes will be best detected at an interval of a few days after the insult. Second, because these quantitative changes have been identified, all of the key metabolites and metabolite ratios are altered depending on the relative reductions of NA, Cr, and Ch that usually result in a reduction in NA/Cr and NA/Ch and an increase in Ch/Cr. With care, nonquantitative ^{1}H-MRS (i.e., using metabolite ratio data) can be a valuable adjunct to clinical criteria, especially in a wide range of acute severe neurologic disturbances in children admitted to ICUs. An important point to remember in evaluating proton spectra from children is that the metabolite concentrations change from birth to approximately 2–3 years of age, making it necessary to compare spectra with those of normal age-matched controls for evaluation.[38–41]

^{1}H-MRS: Principles of Spectral Acquisition.—Certain atomic nuclei such as ^{1}H, ^{31}P and carbon-13 are magnetic and when exposed to a strong magnetic field will align in a particular orientation until equilibrium is reached.[3, 4] If the nuclei are then excited by a radio frequency pulse at their resonant frequency, they will produce detectable signal during relaxation back to equilibrium. During relaxation, because of its local chemical environment, each proton produces a signal at a slightly different frequency, called a chemical shift. After a Fourier transform analysis, the plots of the resulting nuclear MR spectra appear as peaks of signal intensity vs. signal frequency or chemical shift. In in vivo MRS, the frequency axis is usually standardized to the frequency of a strong signal (usually to NA in ^{1}H-MRS) so that the results can be given in parts per million relative to that signal. This allows comparison of data from instruments operating at different magnetic field strengths.

Magnetic resonance imaging uses the strong signals from ^{1}H nuclei of water and their spatial location to reconstruct anatomical images. In contrast, ^{1}H-MRS is interested in the much weaker signals from nonwater protons to obtain quantitative information about biological molecules within tissue. The MRS signal from ^{1}H is inherently stronger than the signal from other nuclei, and until the 1980s, two problems prevented ^{1}H-MRS from being used in humans and in animal experimentation.[3] The first problem relates to the very high water content of tissues, which causes the resulting signal from water protons to be much greater than signal from protons in different tissue metabolites. To overcome this problem, a radio frequency pulse at the water frequency is given just before the signals of interest are acquired. This temporarily disturbs the alignment of the water protons to the magnetic field so that they no longer are capable of producing a signal of sufficient intensity. This brief suppression of the water signal is known as chemical shift selective saturation (CHESS), which can then be used in combination with other sequences such as stimulated echo acquisition mode (STEAM) and allows for the acquisition of the weaker proton signals from different metabolites. The second problem relates to the editing of spectra at the time of acquisition. This is necessary so that different metabolites can be selected and quantitated. This is particularly more complex for ^{1}H signals, which have greater overlap because of the smaller chemical shift dispersions of the proton spectra. The principles underlying this spectral editing are quite complex, and the reader is referred to the reviews by Prichard[3] and Goplerud and Delivoria-Papadopoulos.[4]

^{1}H-MRS: CHANGES WITH DEVELOPMENT.—Several investigators have published developmental curves in normal patients for some of the metabolite ratios, particularly in gray matter.[38–41] It appears that NA increases dramatically from birth until approximately age 2–3 years and becomes more constant after age 6 years. *N*-acetyl aspartate is found primarily in neurons in relatively large concentrations, and although its function remains uncertain, decreased amounts have been demonstrated in a wide variety of pediatric metabolic and degenerative diseases and, as previously noted, after hypoxic-ischemic insults. Creatine, which includes phosphocreatine and creatine, is indicative of cerebral mitochondrial energy function and also increases rapidly during infancy, achieving adult concentrations by age 3 years.[38] Studies with both ^{31}P-MRS and ^{1}H-MRS in neonates have suggested that Cr decreases after asphyxia.[25]

In contrast, the concentration of Ch is highest during infancy and decreases until age 4–6 years as myelination is completed.

Shown in Figure 1 are 4 proton spectra taken in the occipital gray matter from normal children we have studied of different ages. The spectra are drawn on a common scale so the changes in metabolites during human development and maturation can be observed. Although the widths of the peaks are not identical, which may make the peak height seem smaller, one can still observe that NA and (less obviously) Cr increase with age, and that mI and Ch decrease with age. This trend continues until the age of 18–36 months, at which time the child's spectrum appears similar to the adult's.

^{1}H-MRS IN THE NEWBORN.—Although several studies have reported the developmental changes in metabolite ratios during infancy and childhood, there are virtually no normative spectroscopy data on preterm infants and very few data on term infants.[38–41] Comparisons between studies are confounded by numerous technical differences in spectral acquisition as well as the ages of patients and presence of associated diseases. Recently, Hüppi and co-investigators demonstrated regional variations in metabolite distribution as well as subtle age-related increases in NA but not Ch or Cr using in vivo spectroscopic or in vitro chromatographic measurements.[27] Figure 2 shows the occipital and parietal spectra and metabolite ratios of 3 neonates (gestational ages 32, 36 and 40 weeks) who initially had very mild insults with mild abnormalities on neurologic examination and whose 6- to 12-month outcomes were all classified as good. The relation between the

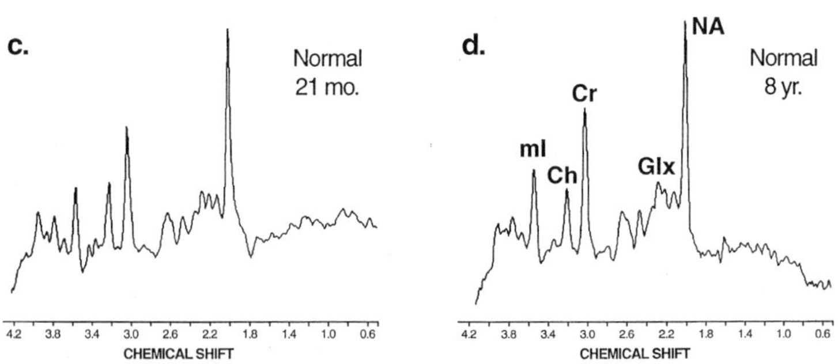

FIGURE 1.—Normal proton MR spectroscopy from children age 1 month, 4 months, 21 months, and 8 years. Note how *N*-acetyl aspartate (*NA*) increases with age as does creatine (*Cr*). In contrast, both choline-containing compounds (*Ch*) and myoinositol (*mI*) decrease during infancy. *Abbreviation: Glx*, glutamine. (Courtesy of Dr. Barbara A. Holshouser, Dept. of Radiology, Loma Linda University Medical Center and Children's Hospital.)

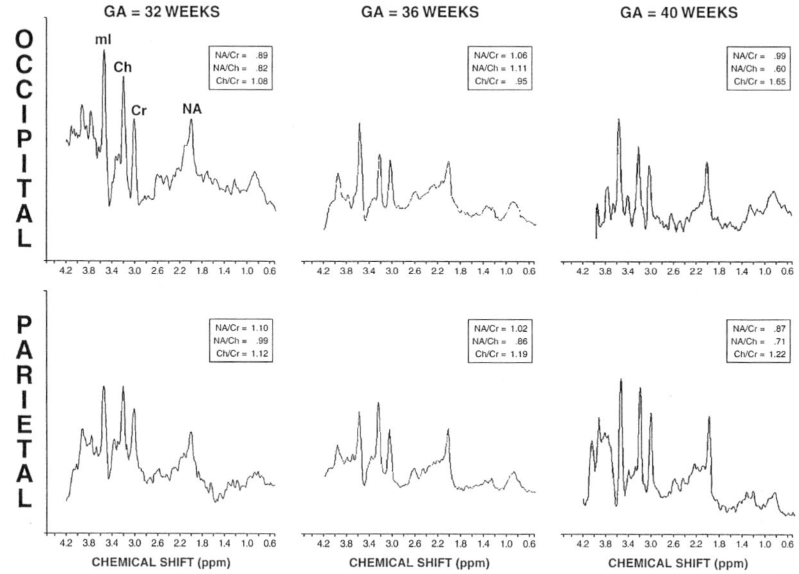

FIGURE 2.—Occipital gray matter (*top*) and parietal white matter (*bottom*) proton spectra taken approximately 2 weeks after birth from 4 infants at 32, 36, and 40 weeks. The relation between *N*-acetyl aspartate (*NA*), creatine (*Cr*), and choline-containing compounds (*Ch*) appears relatively constant from 32 to 40 weeks. The NA and Cr peaks are near equal (NA slightly greater); the Ch peak, which early in gestation appears substantially larger than the Cr peak, is only somewhat larger by 40 weeks. Myoinositol, an important brain osmol, decreases in concentration during gestation and appears greater in gray matter.

3 major metabolites (NA, Cr, Ch) from 32 to 40 weeks appears relatively constant in the occipital gray and parietal white matter. The NA and Cr peaks are near equal (NA slightly greater) and remain so. The Ch peak, which at 32 weeks appears substantially larger than the Cr peak, is only somewhat larger by 40 weeks. Myoinositol, an important brain osmol, decreases in concentration from 32 to 40 weeks and appears greater in gray matter. Although some of our developmental findings are similar to those of Hüppi and colleagues, we were surprised by the relatively small degree of change in the NA, Cr, and Ch peaks that we observed in our 4 preterm patients. Our investigations, like several other neonatal studies, have relied primarily on a limited number of control patients and compared infants with similar injuries but with different outcomes.[15, 16] Our data suggest that it might be possible to use relatively few normal or only mildly affected patients as controls when comparing the results of studies to those neonates who have had more severe CNS insults.

During the past decade, MRS studies have been conducted to evaluate the metabolic changes seen with neonatal asphyxia primarily using ^{31}P-MRS.[4, 25–34] The early investigations by Hope and colleagues of 10 asphyxiated infants found that 6 infants, studied within the first 24 hours, had normal ^{31}P-MRS, but by 5 days all showed reduced PCr/Pi ratios, suggesting that impairment of energy metabolism occurred late rather than early after asphyxia.[25] In a later ^{31}P-MRS study of 61 asphyxiated infants, a

PCr/Pi ratio below the 95% confidence limit was shown to correlate with poor outcome.[26] Of the 28 of 61 infants meeting this criterion, 7 of 9 survivors had serious neurologic compromise and 19 patients died.

Two recent studies of asphyxiated infants using ^{1}H-MRS found that poor neurodevelopmental outcomes correlated with decreases in the NA/Ch ratio.[33, 34] The presence of cerebral lactate was observed in one of these reports and was also indicative of a poor prognosis.[34] Peden and colleagues studied one normal and 10 severely asphyxiated neonates.[33] They found that reduced NA/Ch and NA/Cr ratios correlated with a poor outcome at 1 year. Another major recent study of ^{1}H-MRS of 21 asphyxiated term infants by Groenendaal et al. found that a reduced NA/Ch ratio correlated with poor outcome.[34] These infants were studied a mean of 7.1 days postnatally and again at 3 months. In addition, the presence of lactate also appeared to correlate with a poor outcome as it was present in the 5 patients with severe encephalopathy.

In the past 2 years, we have had the opportunity to study 35 neonates (28–41 weeks' gestation) at 1–42 days after CNS insult (asphyxia in 20 patients; sepsis/meningitis in 7; metabolic in 2; stroke in 2; trauma in 2; hypoglycemia and Rh-incompatibility in 1 each). The median day of ^{1}H-MRS after insult was 7 days (range, 1 to 42 days). We performed a discriminant analysis to determine which of the following criteria were useful in assessing outcome: (1) clinical (5-minute Apgar score, initial blood glucose, Sarnat score); (2) electroencephalography (normal, mild, moderate, severely abnormal); (3) MRI scanning (normal, mild, moderate, severe abnormalities) and ^{1}H-MRS (NA/Cr, NA/Ch, Ch/Cr ratios and the presence of a lactate doublet). Outcomes were assessed 6–12 months after insult using the Glasgow Outcome Scale and were stratified into 2 groups as follows: good/moderate outcome (good, mild, or moderate disability) or poor outcome (severe disability, persistent vegetative state, death). Our results are summarized in Table 1.

Clinical criteria combined with the MRI score correctly predicted outcome in 84%. ^{1}H-MRS (occipital and parietal) alone correctly predicted outcome in 82%; when combined with the MRI score, ^{1}H-MRS correctly predicted 96% of outcomes. In addition, when ^{1}H-MRS data were combined with clinical criteria and the MRI score, they correctly predicted outcome in 100% of patients. Combination of the clinical, MRI, and MRS data not only allowed us to correctly classify 100% of our patients, but there were no false positive or false negative cases. Thus, there were no patients in whom the discriminant analysis of the combined variables would classify a patient as having a poor neurologic outcome who ultimately had a good outcome.

The presence or absence of lactate on spectroscopy also appeared to be an important determinant of outcome. In our studies, 23 of 26 infants who did not have a lactate peak had a good/moderate outcome. In contrast, 5 of 9 infants with lactate had a poor outcome. Thus, the absence of lactate suggests the potential for a better outcome. As noted, not all patients who had a lactate peak had a poor prognosis, and our

TABLE 1.—Discriminant Analysis of ^{1}H-MRS and Clinical and MRI Variables

	Without ^{1}H-MRS	^{1}H-MRS (occ)	^{1}H-MRS (par)	^{1}H-MRS (occ+par)
No clinical	—	83%	75%	82%
Clinical	74%	80%	88%	95%
MRI	74%	90%	79%	96%
Clinical, MRI	84%	96%	88%	100%

Abbreviations: *^{1}H-MRS*, proton MR spectroscopy; *occ*, occipital; *par*, parietal.

preliminary impression is that the presence of lactate in the neonate may not be as ominous a finding as when it is seen in older children, although the majority of patients with lactate peaks had serious neurologic complications.

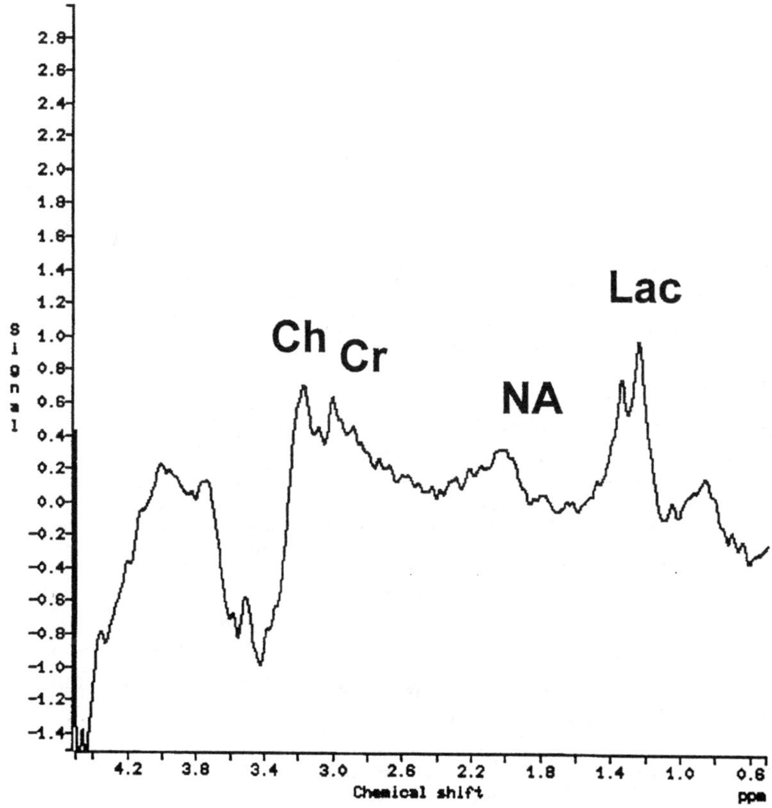

FIGURE 3.—Proton MR spectroscopy (*^{1}H-MRS*) from a 38-week estimated gestational age female who was born by emergency cesarean section because of fetal distress. Apgar scores were 0/0/2/4 (ABG: pH 6.50, pCO_2 92 torr, pO_2 117 torr, BE-39). She had intermittent seizures and her electroencephalogram showed generalized slowing. She was hypotonic and unresponsive to stimuli. Her MRI showed bilateral subacute hemorrhage in the basal ganglia, thalami, and corona radiata. Lactate was found on ^{1}H-MRS, and her *N*-acetyl aspartate (*NA*), creatine (*Cr*), and choline-containing compounds (*Ch*) were reduced. Follow-up examination at 12 months showed severe disability.

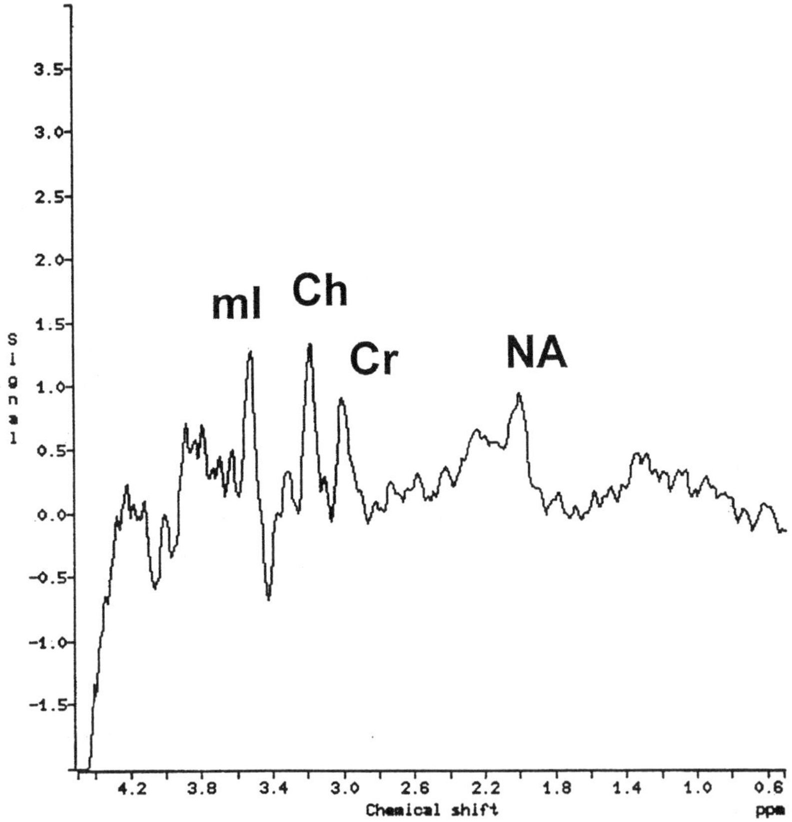

FIGURE 4.—Proton MR spectroscopy (*¹H-MRS*) from a term infant who at 20 hours of life became apneic and asystolic. She was intubated, had a dextrostix of 0 and arterial blood gas with a pH 6.93, pCO_2 87 torr, pO_2 23 torr, BE-14.7. She was hypertonic and inactive; with stimulation, she had clinical seizures. Her electroencephalogram showed generalized slowing and her MRI showed diffuse cerebral edema. ¹H-MRS showed no reduction in her *N*-acetyl aspartate (*NA*) peak, a normal NA/creatine (*Cr*) ratio and no lactate and was interpreted as normal for her age and suggestive of a good outcome. The child was given a diagnosis of dilated cardiomyopathy and was transplanted at 2 months of age. She had mild spasticity and delay at 5 months, and at 10 months was completely normal. *Abbreviations: mI*, myoinositol; *Ch*, choline-containing compounds.

Figures 3 and 4 demonstrate proton spectra from 2 neonates and illustrate the potential clinical usefulness of ¹H-MRS in the evaluation of neonates with acute CNS injuries. Both patients had catastrophic neonatal cerebral insults, yet their spectra and outcomes were different. The patient in Figure 3 with lactate and reduced NA, Cr, and Ch peaks remains severely disabled. The patient in Figure 4 with a normal spectra for age made a good recovery.

These two cases are of interest because they demonstrate the potential usefulness of proton spectroscopy. Metabolite ratio data can be misleading as they do not necessarily reflect decreases in the absolute metabolite concentrations. Because of the difficulties in quantitating in vivo metabolites, ratios have been used to describe changes seen in MR spectra. However, ratios reflect changes in 2 metabolites, so if both metabolites decrease by the same amount, the ratio will remain normal. Thus, reliance on metabolite data alone could lead to misinterpretation of the spectra. Even with this possibility, we have found that if the metabolite ratios, particularly in children older than 18 months of age, are reduced greater than 1 to 2 standard deviations below the normal for age, a poor outcome is likely.[36]

^{1}H-MRS in Infants With Congenital Heart Disease.—Of the approximately 10,000 children who annually undergo cardiac surgery, as many as 25% will experience some form of neurologic morbidity. Although many of these insults result from perioperative cerebral injury, it is also clear that a significant number of patients have either preoperative cerebral ischemia or subtle developmental CNS malformations that contribute to or are responsible for poor neurodevelopmental outcomes. Perioperative cerebral monitoring, particularly with newer techniques such as near-infrared spectroscopy and transcranial Doppler, offer methods to reduce the incidence of such insults. However, for those infants who do have cerebral injury, neurologic evaluation to predict outcome is limited by the lack of specific neurodiagnostic methods.

We recently studied 9 infants and children (ages 1 week to 42 months) with severe acute CNS injuries associated with cardiac disease or corrective surgery with ^{1}H-MRS (Table 2). We were interested in determining whether this technique would be useful in predicting neurologic outcome. Four of our patients experienced cerebral insults prior to surgery, 1 had both a preoperative and perioperative insult, 3 had perioperative insults, and 1 had a prolonged cardiac arrest 2 days after surgery. Outcomes (Glasgow Outcome Scale) were assigned at discharge and 6 to 12 months after injury. Six patients were vegetative or severely impaired at discharge and 2 remained severely impaired at 6- to 12-month follow-up. ^{1}H-MRS showed lactate in these 2 patients, along with markedly reduced NA/Cr and NA/Ch and increased Ch/Cr ratios. The other 4 severely impaired patients recovered to mild disabilities at follow-up. ^{1}H-MRS showed no lactate in these 4 patients; however, 1 patient showed moderately reduced ratios. The 3 patients who were mildly or moderately impaired at discharge showed no lactate and mild or no changes in metabolite ratios, and follow-up revealed normal or mild outcomes. Overall, we found that the presence of lactate and markedly abnormal metabolite ratios were more predictive of severe outcomes at discharge and long-term follow-up, whereas no lactate and mild or no changes in ratios suggested potential for recovery to at least a mild outcome. We are continuing our investigations to determine the optimal selection of candidates and timing of study.

Conclusions.—^{1}H-MRS is an emerging technology that will require careful investigation in selected patient populations to assess its usefulness. ^{1}H-MRS may provide cost-effective information in conjunction with the clinical examination in assessing neurologic outcome in infants and children who experience serious acute CNS injury. Additional studies are necessary to define which populations of patients would be helped by this

TABLE 2.—Summary of ^{1}H-MRS and Outcomes Data of 9 Patients With CNS Injury Associated With Cardiac Disease and/or Surgery

Age (mos)	Etiology of insult	^{1}H-MRS abnormalities	Outcome by ^{1}H-MRS	Discharge outcome	6–12 mos outcome
.25	Pre-op: prolonged cardiac arrest	Normal spectra No lactate	Good outcome	Severe	Normal
.25	Pre-op: prolonged cardiac arrest	Normal spectra No lactate	Good outcome	Moderate	Mild
.5	Pre-op: cardiac and respiratory failure	Mild decrease in NA/Cr in gray matter	Good outcome or mild disability	Mild	Normal
1.25	Pre/peri-op: severe hypoperfusion pre-op;	Normal spectra No lactate	Study suggested potential for recovery	Severe	Mild
1	Peri-op: intraoperative ventricular fibrillation	Lac present; reduced NA/Cr & NA/Ch	Poor outcome	Severe	Severe
10	Pre-op: indeterminable	Normal spectra No lactate	Good outcome	Vegetative state	Mild
14	Peri-op: TCA=69 min; low flow CPB=102 min	Reduced NA/Cr & NA/Ch no lactate	Mixed outcome prediction	Moderate	Mild
42	Peri-op: unknown	Reduced NA/Cr & NA/Ch no lactate	Mixed outcome prediction	Vegetative state	Mild
20	Post-op: late cardiac tamponade and arrest	Lactate present; NA/Cr & NA/Ch reduced	Poor outcome	Severe	Severe

Abbreviations: *^{1}H-MRS*, proton MR spectroscopy; *NA*, *N*-acetyl aspartate; *Cr*, creatine; *Ch*, choline-containing compounds.

technology, the optimal timing and number of studies necessary to obtain valid and reliable data, quantitation of metabolites, and the relation between ^{1}H-MRS and other noninvasive measurements of cerebral function for predicting outcome.

New MR Brain Imaging Techniques

INTRODUCTION.—The development of MRI followed on the footsteps of CT as a powerful method to image the brain. Magnetic resonance imaging is a noninvasive, nonionizing tomographic technique that uses strong magnetic fields and pulsed radio frequency waves to create high-resolution images of human anatomy. This technique depends on slight differences in the magnetic moment of hydrogen atoms in molecules of water and fat (primarily) to provide differentiation of various tissues. Changing the MRI scanner controls can make the images sensitive to a wide variety of tissue properties and can thus generate variable image contrast that is most suited to the particular investigation. T1-weighted MRI yields an image contrast based on the time constant T1 for a magnetic moment of the hydrogen atoms to return to equilibrium orientation after being disturbed by the radio waves (AKA spin-lattice or longitudinal relaxation time). It is often helpful for evaluation of normal brain anatomy and acute injury. T2-weighted MRI examines relaxation time constant T2 of the MRI signal (AKA spin-spin or transverse relaxation time), which is dependent on the mobility of the water molecules. On T2-weighted imaging, myelin appears hypointense.

Magnetic resonance imaging has proven to be extremely valuable in the evaluation of neonatal brain structure and injury.[4, 42–49] It appears to be superior to cranial ultrasonography and CT in the evaluation of hypoxic-ischemic encephalopathy and periventricular leukomalacia. However, the anatomical changes detected by all 3 of these techniques are usually detectable only long after an acute neurologic insult, when therapeutic interventions are no longer effective. Recently developed MR techniques allow imaging based on physiologic processes that precede permanent structural changes. These new applications can detect ongoing neurologic compromise, perhaps even during the "therapeutic window."

DIFFUSION-WEIGHTED IMAGING.—Diffusion-weighted MRI (DWI) is the application of special gradients during MRI signal acquisition upon water protons to measure their diffusivity, calculated as the apparent diffusion coefficient (ADC). This ADC value is dependent on restrictions of water motion in the microcellular environment and has been shown to be very sensitive to the earliest effects of cerebral ischemia. Early cell swelling is thought to be a primary mechanism behind the rapid decrease in ADC (or hyperintensity on DWI) occurring after neuronal compromise. Studies have been done to pinpoint which cellular membrane perturbations most closely correlate to ADC changes.[50–52] In both animal models and human studies, ADC changes occur sooner during stroke and correspond highly to the ultimate area of injury.[53–56] Diffusion-weighted MRI has also been used

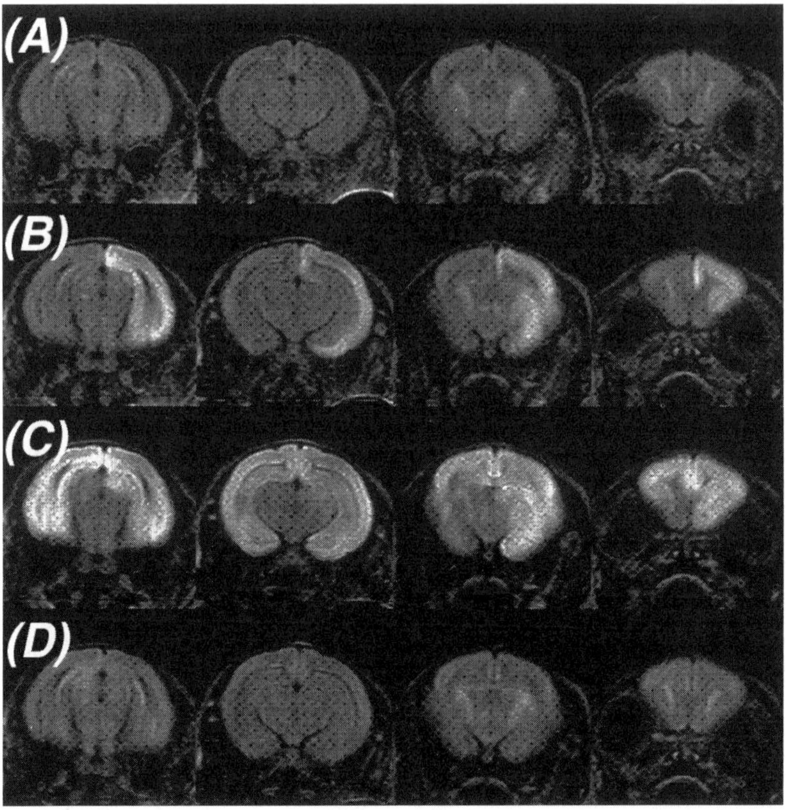

FIGURE 5.—Serial multislice diffusion-weighted images of neonatal rabbit brain after carotid ligation showing the spatial and temporal evolution of ischemic change (bright regions in images). **A**, baseline (pre-hypoxia). **B**, 150 minutes of hypoxia. **C**, 180 minutes of hypoxia. **D**, return to 100% fraction of inspired oxygen. The T2-weighted (b = 0) images showed no signal changes during the protocol.

to study brain injury in seizures,[57] spreading depression,[58] trauma,[59] and multiple sclerosis.[60, 61]

We have studied DWI in a model of neonatal hypoxic-ischemic encephalopathy in newborn rabbits.[62] After unilateral carotid artery ligation, prolonged exposure to hypoxia (fraction of inspired oxygen = 0.10), newborn rabbit pups demonstrated profound DWI changes before any other changes could be seen by conventional T1-weighted and T2-weighted MRI. After 1–3 hours of hypoxia, these ADC changes usually arise in a focal area of the cerebral cortex, and sometimes the adjacent basal ganglia, on the side of ligation (Fig 5). With continuation of hypoxia, DWI changes spread throughout the hemisphere and across to the other side. However, early reversal of hypoxia led to normalization of the DWI. In similar studies of neonatal rats, Rumpel et al. showed significant decrease in ADC ipsilateral to carotid artery ligation after 2 hours of hypoxia in the rat pup.[63] The finding that DWI changes preceded myelin formation in the developing rat pup suggests that DWI may be a means to assess cerebral white matter myelination.[64]

Recent reports of DWI in human neonates who have brain injury suggests that such imaging may be more helpful than conventional MRI in predicting long-term outcome. Cowan et al. found that after infarction and hypoxic-ischemic encephalopathy, DWI better predicted the extent and severity of injury than conventional MRI.[65] Mercuri et al. reported that DWI combined with MRI and ultrasound better helped to show the timing and extent of injury in 16 human newborns evaluated after seizures.[66]

CONTRAST AND PERFUSION IMAGING.—Contrast MRI incorporates the use of injected paramagnetic contrast agents, usually gadolinium-based, to enhance MRI signal, especially of vascular structures and tumors.[67–70] Supraparamagnetic iron oxide can also be used as a contrast agent.[71, 72] Contrast MRI is also useful for detecting brain tumors and blood-brain barrier integrity.[68, 73–76] Perfusion MRI entails high-speed imaging of specific MRI slices serially over time, usually during very rapid contrast bolus injection, to measure relative blood perfusion in the brain, heart, and kidneys.

Perfusion MRI has given insight into the physiology of cerebral perfusion as well as into numerous models of brain injury, especially in studies of stroke.[53, 55, 56, 72] Perfusion MRI studies showed decreased cerebral perfusion and blood-brain barrier alteration in elderly patients with Down's syndrome, similar to those changes seen in dementia.[77] In rats, perfusion MRI was capable of detecting regional increases in cerebral perfusion after amphetamine administration.[78]

We have found that in the neonatal rabbit model of hypoxic-ischemic encephalopathy described above that perfusion deficits closely correlated over time and space with the ADC changes seen in an individual animal

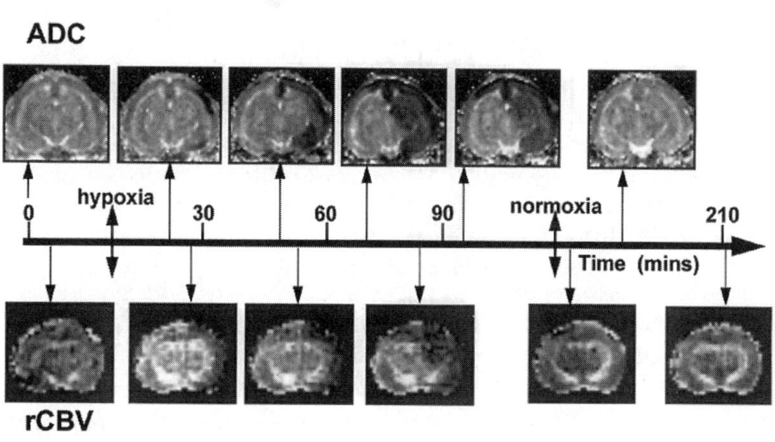

FIGURE 6.—Apparent diffusion coefficient (*ADC*) and regional cerebral blood volume (*rCBV*) maps of neonatal rabbit brain showing the progressive increase in ischemic injury in the cortex/basal ganglia with hypoxia and the subsequent recovery of these tissues in 100% O_2. The regions of perfusion deficit in the rCBV maps are closely matched by those of low ADC (indicated by dark areas in both images). Both rCBV and ADC recover spontaneously on return to normoxia.

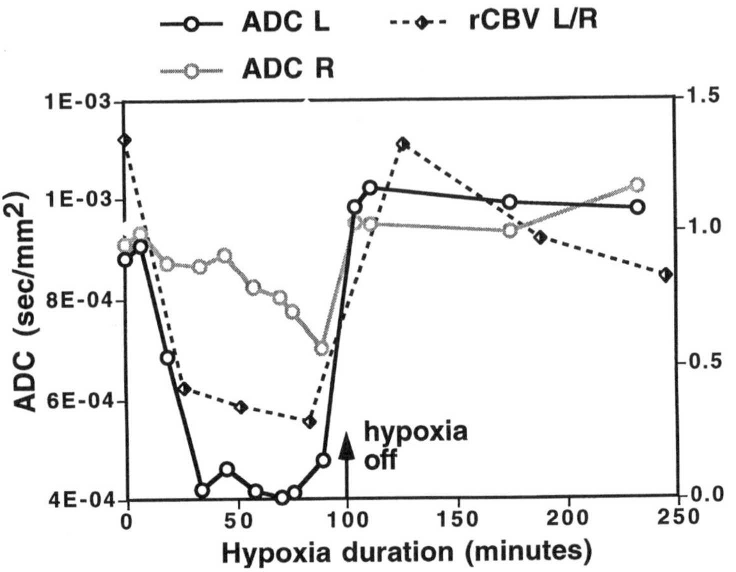

FIGURE 7.—Plots of apparent diffusion coefficient (*ADC*) for the left (*L*) and right (*R*) cortex compared with relative perfusion indices (ratio of left to right cortex). The ADC values in the ipsilateral cortex values decrease rapidly after 19 minutes of hypoxia. Toward the end of the hypoxic interval, the ischemic region had spread to the contralateral hemisphere, so that an ADC decrease was also observed in the right hemispheric region of interest. The change in perfusion is similar to the ADC trace. The ADC and regional cerebral blood volume (*rCBV*) recover spontaneously on the return to normoxia.

(Figs 6 and 7). Our original studies used gadolinium-based contrast injected immediately before obtaining perfusion MRI data at any given time.[62] More recently, we have been able to use a single iron dextran injection that stays in the circulation, allowing for repeat perfusion scans over several hours. Similarly, iron-based contrast has also been useful as a contrast agent in the rat stroke model.[72]

FUNCTIONAL IMAGING.—Functional MRI measures changes in deoxyhemoglobin concentration in brain tissue as a result of local blood flow changes during cortical activation.[79–83] It entails high-speed MRI techniques sensitive to the small magnetic susceptibility changes caused by the paramagnetic deoxyhemoglobin molecules to map out areas of brain activity during localized stimuli. These stimuli usually are repetitive motor or speech tasks or visual or auditory simulation. Functional MRI has also been used to detect changes in cerebral blood oxygenation in hydrocephalus[84] and after drug administration.[85] With further refinement of this technique, it may provide diagnostic insight into neonatal brain functions such as respiratory control.

CONCLUSIONS.—Advances in MRI now allow this technology to give insight into brain function and structure. Further studies using diffusion, perfusion, and functional MRI should yield insight into the relationship between these physiologic changes and the nature and extent of brain injury. Other techniques such as MRS of cellular lipids, which has been shown to correlate with apoptosis of tumor cells,[86] may also turn out to be earlier markers of CNS injury than conventional MRI. Magnetic resonance imaging of critically ill newborns may be limited by difficulties in transportation to, and stabilization and monitoring within, the MRI scanner. Nevertheless, when available in the clinical setting, MRI can yield more than structural information by the addition of diffusion, perfusion, and functional studies.

Near-Infrared Spectroscopy and Optical Imaging*

Introduction

Medical optical imaging uses light emitted into opaque tissues to determine interior structure and chemical content.[87] These optical techniques have been developed in an attempt to prospectively identify impending brain injuries before they become irreversible, thus allowing injury to be avoided or minimized. Optical imaging and spectroscopy center around the simple idea that light passes through the body in small amounts and emerges containing information about the chemical composition (e.g., oxygenation) and physical structure (e.g., histology) of the tissues in the light path as a result of light absorbance and scattering, respectively. Images can then be reconstructed from either absorbance or scattering data using CT. During the past few years, systems have been developed to allow construction of images from such optical data at the bedside. We have used a time-of-flight system to monitor oxygenation and image hemorrhage in the neonatal brain. This section summarizes the problems that we believe can be addressed by such techniques and reports on some of our early results.

Characteristics of Optical Imaging

LIMITATIONS OF CURRENT IMAGING METHODS.—Infants who are critically ill or undergoing major surgery are at risk for brain injury. Such injury is not always predictable. For example, 2 infants may experience perinatal asphyxia; 1 may recover without sequelae, whereas the other may incur major injury leading to permanent brain injury, the development of retardation or cerebral palsy, or even death. How one avoids such brain injuries becomes a question, in part, of detection. To prevent death and minimize long-term injury, early detection of brain injury *before* it becomes irreversible is essential. In addition, monitoring the brain while such injuries are evolving may lead to more effective treatments.

Currently, no bedside imaging or monitoring methods excel at either detecting incipient injury or predicting neurologic outcome. Despite recent advances in noninvasive monitoring, such as in the development of chemically weighted MRI,[1] most imaging techniques remain limited in at least 1 of 4 fundamental ways:

Invasive—Many imaging techniques require exposure to noxious agents and thus involve a degree of risk that increases with exposure. Computed

---

*This section reproduced in part with permission from Benaron DA, van Houten JP, Cheong WF, et al: Early results of clinical optical tomography in a neonatal intensive care unit. *SPIE,* in press.

tomographic scanners, which emit carcinogenic ionizing radiation, cannot be used in a continuous fashion, preventing use as operating room or ICU monitors. Positron emission tomography (PET) scans require a cyclotron and IV injection of radiation emitters. Prolonged ultrasound exposure is suspected of causing at least some degree of thermal or structural cellular injury, particularly in developing tissues.

Not portable—Critically ill infants and those undergoing surgery cannot easily be transported, as such movement may adversely affect their care. Many established techniques, such as MRI, CT, and PET, are not portable and may not be available in the very clinical situations for which such imaging information is crucial. Ironically, the more likely a patient is to require a scan, the more likely it is that the patient will be unable to tolerate transport to an imaging facility.

Not continuous—Critically ill infants tend to have illnesses that are actively changing processes. Thus, an intermittent test (e.g., daily head ultrasound exam) may miss the early signs of physiologic changes that precede the development of irreversible structural injury. Rapidly changing physiologic states require near-continuous monitoring to identify those patients most likely to have physical brain injury develop.

Function not measured—Neonatal brain injury often results from perturbations of tissue *function,* such as altered cerebral blood flow or oxygen delivery, rather than from a structural problem. Although the long-term results of such injury (e.g., periventricular leukomalacia, secondary cerebral ischemia) are relatively easy to detect using conventional imaging modalities, such information often comes too late to prevent the primary injury from occurring in the first place. Most imaging technologies have been designed to measure a static physical structure rather than a cellular state, so that whereas conventional images may reflect tissue structure, they reveal nothing about tissue *function.* Computed tomography, for example, does not distinguish between healthy and dying tissue, and by the time a brain lesion is visible on CT, the damage is often irreversibly far advanced.

OPTICAL IMAGING MAY OVERCOME THESE LIMITATIONS.—Medical optical imaging and spectroscopy use light emitted into scattering media such as human tissue to determine interior structure and chemical content, and they have broad medical application to the continuous, noninvasive bedside monitoring of tissue structure, oxygenation, blood flow, and metabolite concentration. Optical techniques rely on the relationship that variations in the concentration of light-absorbing oxygen-carrying pigments (such as hemoglobin and cytochrome aa_3) produce proportional changes in the way these proteins absorb light, and that such variations in concentration, as well as variations in tissue structure, affect the path of light through tissue. Near-infrared spectroscopy has already been shown to be a nonionizing, relatively safe form of radiation that functions well as a medical probe[88–99] with red and near-infrared light passing easily through structures such as the skull,[89] penetrating deeply into many tissues such as the brain and breast[90–92] and well tolerated in large doses and for prolonged periods of time.[93]

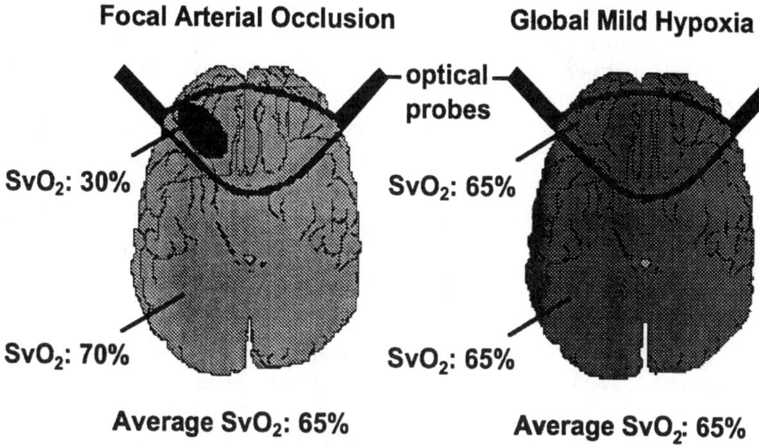

FIGURE 8.—Global vs. regional oxygenation measures. A measurement of cerebral oxygenation may need to be in the form of an image to provide useful information. A focal, acute arterial occlusion (**left**), such as during an embolic event, and a slight but generalized drop in oxygenation (**right**), such as during a drop in cardiac output, both yield a similar drop in overall brain oxygenation figures. However, each requires a different clinical response, and whereas the former constitutes a medical emergency, the latter does not. (Reproduced with permission from Benaron DA, van Houten JP, Cheong WF, et al: Early results of clinical optical tomography in a neonatal intensive care unit. *SPIE,* in press.)

Spectroscopy in vivo is complicated by the scattering of light by tissue, which results in poor spatial localization. However, just as the absorbance of light provides information about the chemical composition (e.g., oxygenation) of the tissue in the light path, scattering provides information about the physical structure (e.g., histology) of the tissue. Resolving the transit time of light travel through tissue allows separation of the combined effects of absorbance and scattering. Using CT, optical images of brain structure or function can be formed using either scattering or absorbance data.

The ability to image multiple parameters such as oxygenation (from absorbance data) and histology (from scattering data) may be beneficial for a number of reasons. First, there are many causes of brain injury, and the appearance of the various measured parameters (oxygenation, scattering) may be very different at different stages of disease. For example, in an asphyxiated infant in whom oxygenation has recovered, brain tissue may nevertheless be committed to a cell death pathway. An oxygenation monitor may provide the clinician with false reassurance and he or she may fail to recognize impending neuronal cell death. However, as cell death progresses, the scattering of light by tissue may be expected to change with the failure of cellular water and ion transport or changes in the stored calcium status of the cell. Therefore, a scattering monitor may be more sensitive in detecting certain stages of brain injury. Second, injury may be the result of small cumulative insults, such that no one particular insult is large enough to be detectable using changes in oxygenation, yet the sum total injury over time is great. Such a cumulative loss of neurons, as a result of many small insults over a long period, may be detectable using a change in the scattering of the tissue. Finally, the usefulness of a nonimaged parameter may be limited. For example, the average brain oxygenation would be the same if a small region of the brain were to be severely hypoxic, such as during an acute arterial obstruction, or if the brain oxygenation of the entire brain dropped in general by a small amount, such as during a drop in cardiac output (Fig 8). Whereas the first situation is an emergency, requiring immediate intervention to prevent irreversible brain injury, the second is not. Furthermore, treatment in the two cases would be very different. Thus, imaging may be essential in determining the proper course of medical treatment of an observed oxygenation change.

Medical Optical Imaging

To produce optical images, we used a portable time-of-flight and absorbance system (TOFA) that emits a pulse of light into tissue at one position and detects the photons that are transmitted through the tissue to other positions. The transit time through the tissue for each photon is measured in picoseconds (10^{-12} s). All photons are collected and a TOFA curve is generated. Absorbance and scattering at each position are determined from the shape and slope of the TOFA. This process is repeated at subsequent positions until a complete circumferential scan of the tissue is obtained. An image is then reconstructed mathematically with custom-written software using either the absorbance or scattering estimates. This system, which has been described in detail elsewhere,[101] uses up to 3 diode lasers from which a pulse of very low intensity light (peak power 1W for 100 psec, or an average power 100 μW) is fed into a flexible fiberoptic emitter cable and directed into the tissue to be imaged. Transmitted light is collected by detector fibers and passed to a photo counter that accumulates time-of-flight curves.

Imaging of Brain Structure

DETECTION OF BRAIN HEMORRHAGE.—In critically ill infants, injury producing maldistributions of heme in the brain were studied for detectability. After Human Subjects Committee approval and informed parental consent were obtained, we studied infants with intraventricular hemorrhage, measuring at multiple skull locations to see whether the bleeding could be identified. Using a comparison of path length on one side of the head vs. that on the contralateral side, we found that superficial bleeding (subdural hematomas, cephalohematomas) could be easily identified, and some instances of intraventricular bleed were detectable as well.[101]

IMAGING OF BRAIN HEMORRHAGE.—We then imaged the brains of infants who had died of problems related to prematurity. Optical images of these postmortem brain specimens correlated well with autopsy results and showed that pathology such as intraventricular hemorrhage and subependymal hemorrhage could be identified and localized based on changes in light absorbance and scattering (Fig 9).[102]

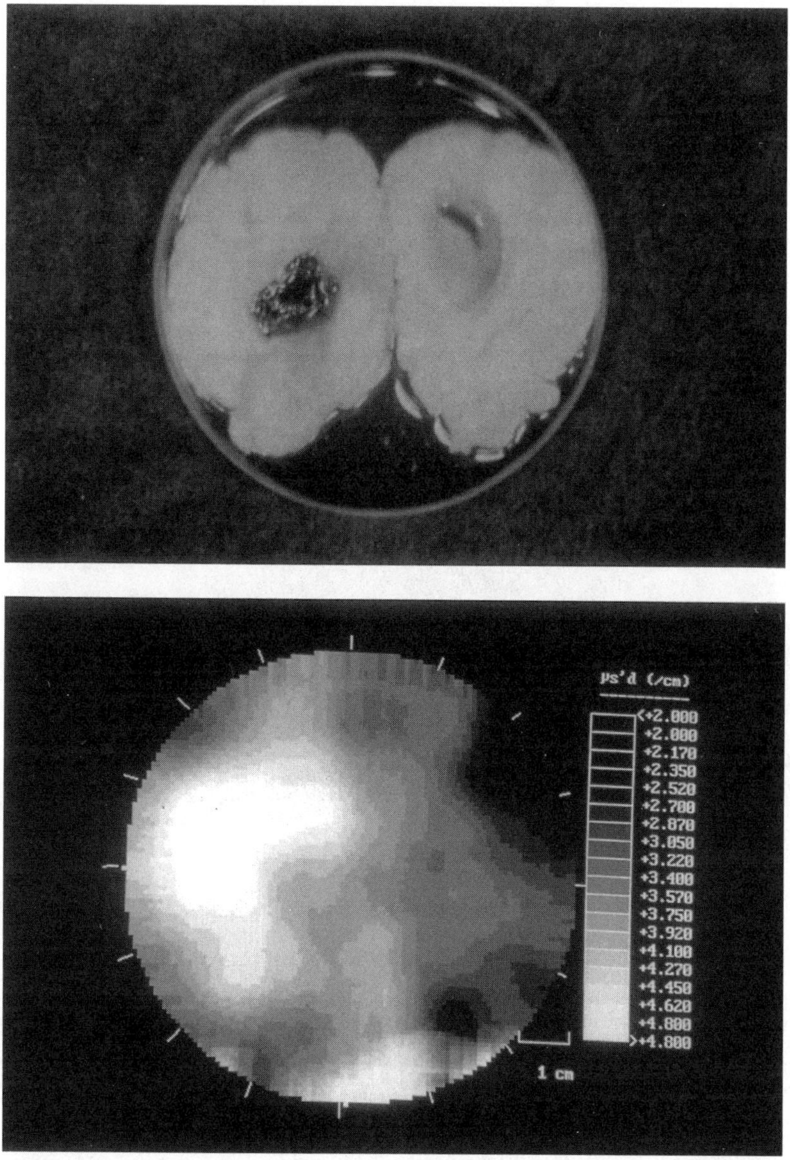

FIGURE 9.—A, photograph of a coronal section of infant brain with left grade III intraventricular hemorrhage. **B,** the optical tomographic image obtained using scattering shows a large area of increased scattering (white area) in the region of the left ventricular blood clot. (Reproduced with permission from Benaron DA, van Houten JP, Cheong WF, et al: Early results of clinical optical tomography in a neonatal intensive care unit. *SPIE,* in press.)

To use the device in a clinical setting, a fiberoptic headband was constructed. This headband consists of an array of multiple emitter/detector fiberoptic pairs (optodes) embedded in a soft rubber backing and placed circumferentially around the head (Fig 10). This device

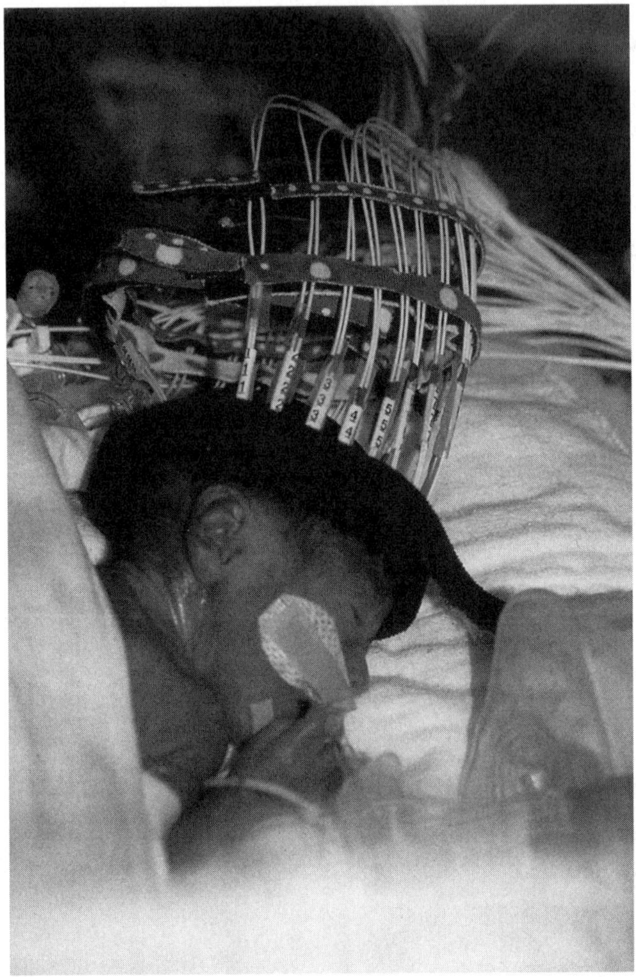

FIGURE 10.—A time-resolved optical imaging headband in place on an infant. Low-level light enters the head through the multiple emitter/detector fiberoptic pairs and the transmitted light is measured at various other points around the head. This headband allows for normal head movement and can be used for prolonged periods. (Reproduced with permission from Benaron DA, van Houten JP, Cheong WF, et al: Early results of clinical optical tomography in a neonatal intensive care unit. *SPIE,* in press.)

allows light to enter the infant's head from all sides, as needed, without the need for mechanical translation.[100, 103–105] The headband itself weighs less than 50 g. The complete imaging device is about the size of a standard ultrasound cart and fits easily at the bedside of an ill infant. Tomographic reconstruction algorithms performed in the on-board computer were also further refined to allow calculation of an image in seconds to minutes. After obtaining human studies approval and parental informed consent, infants at high risk for structural disease (such as bleeding) were studied using optical methods and must have had an additional standard imaging study before the optical scan. The staff performing the optical scans, and those reading the optical scan results, were blinded to the results of the ultrasound examinations. We found that the optical image prediction of the presence and location of bleed agreed with the formal reading of the ultrasound examinations in 6 of 8 cases. One of the incorrect optical diagnoses occurred in an infant with a right grade IV intraventricular hemorrhage detected by ultrasound on day of life 5. In this case, the initial optical scan done on day of life 7 correctly showed a large right-sided bleed. A follow-up scan on day of life 12 showed no bleed despite a repeat ultrasound 2 days earlier showing persistent parenchymal hemorrhage. The second occurred in an infant studied on day of life 32, 9 days after the previous ultrasound showed an evolving unilateral grade I intraventricular hemorrhage. Our findings suggest that the optical representation of a brain hemorrhage changes as the bleed ages, and this may be caused in part by the degradation of the heme component of the blood over time. Thus, optical scanning may not only be able to detect brain hemorrhages but may also serve as a method for dating such bleeds.[106]

Other images have been obtained for infants with other sites of brain hemorrhage and other types of brain injury. We are in the process of analyzing these images more fully. Using updated imaging algorithms, our images can now be processed in less than 2 minutes using a desktop computer once the data are collected, with a fast version of the program in theory being able to process the images in less than 10 seconds. Such images show both substantial distortion of structure and significant error in estimation of absorbance and scattering characteristics, probably as a result of imaging algorithms assuming additivity of the measured phenomena. However, images are both recognizable and agree with ultrasound examinations as to the presence or absence of bleeding. Such a device could have immediate application in the monitoring of infants on heart-lung bypass such as extracorporeal membrane oxygenation, in which serial ultrasound examinations are performed to detect bleeding, but such scans are intermittent and may miss the onset of life-threatening intracranial bleeding.

Imaging of Brain Function

The strength of optical imaging comes from its ability to separate scattering and absorbance and thus allow physicians to look at images of brain function. Such separation makes possible an estimation of chemical content, using absorbance, and histology, using scattering, and allows many different types of brain function to be imaged. Areas that may have importance are listed below.

IMAGING OF OXYGENATION.—Optical images can be processed for oxygenation. For example, we have imaged an infant with a stroke and found an area of low oxygenation on the optical scan that corresponded to the location of the stroke on CT scan.[107] As there is no gold standard for distribution of oxygenation, the oxygenation images had no confirming imaging procedure performed. We have also successfully imaged changes in oxygenation over the intact cerebral motor cortex in adults during regional motor cortical stimulation by sequential finger movements.[107] These findings are being correlated with functional MRI studies.

IMAGING OF CEREBRAL BLOOD VOLUME.—Provided that blood flow through the brain is present, cerebral blood volume can be determined. This requires use of a marker for blood volume, but fortunately a naturally occurring one exists. As the oxygenation of blood changes, such as by altering the inspired oxygen concentration, the blood will change color. The total change in color can be used to determine cerebral blood volume, given that only the starting and ending arterial saturation of the blood with oxygen is known. Similarly, the change in absorbance of hemoglobin with changes in oxygenation is known, such that the change in absorbance across the entire head during oxygenation changes allows determination of total blood volume in the head.

IMAGING OF CEREBRAL BLOOD FLOW.—Once the blood volume in the head is known, the same information can be used to determine cerebral blood flow. The approach is analogous to the use of injected dyes to determine cardiac output using a Fick-based determination. In this case, the endogenous dye is hemoglobin, and by changing the inspired oxygen concentration, and thus altering the hemoglobin saturation in the arterial blood, the rate of increase can be determined and translated into cerebral blood flow. Images of blood flow could be combined with images of oxygenation to produce an image of tissue health.

IMAGING OF NON–OXYGENATION-RELATED INJURY.—The brain injury cascade is complex. In some cases, such as if cell death is caused by activation of a preprogrammed pathway, the initial causes of the activation may have long since disappeared. For example, oxygenation may have returned to normal, but the cells have already been committed to die at some point in the near future. Thus, markers of the impending cell death need to be detected. Of course, detection of a loss of cytochrome oxidation may be used, but this may be a late sign. We believe that cellular swelling that occurs during edema or cellular injury will result in a dilution of the intracellular components as well as a change in intracellular storage components such as calcium or changes in the cell packaging apparatus, all of which are responsible for light scattering. These changes should be detectable using a device that images and quantifies scattering.

Comparison of Structural and Functional Imaging

The separation of structural and functional imaging has clinical importance. The equations that allow imaging using light can be tuned to give the best structural resolution, or the most accurate determination of quantitative values, but not both at the same time. Therefore, different clinical situations may call for a different optimization.

Structural imaging focuses on the generation of image with the best physical resolution. The imaged values may not be directly related to known quantitative values, much as is the case with ultrasound, in which the shadows are visible, but these images are not quantitative. This approach would work best if the maximum image resolution is required, such as in the case of identifying and locating hemorrhage, tumors, or other physical lesions. This approach may also prove useful in the identification of margins of disease.

Functional imaging, on the other hand, involves the quantitative determination of body chemistry. The imaged values should thus correlate well with known physical values, but the resolution of such determinations will not be as fine as that using structural imaging approaches. Although the resolution on a physical scale will be inferior to structural imaging, the technique has great power in that many of the problems that this approach addresses have no discernible physical manifestation. Thus, early stroke, which does not show up on structural scans, will show up clearly on a functional scan. The resolution of a functional image should be sufficient to allow detection of a stroke in the cortex or to identify regional differences in brain oxygenation. Therefore, this approach is potentially useful in the identification and mapping of stroke, ischemic disease, and localized and regional maldistributions of blood volume and blood flow. For brain monitoring, it may be that a combination of structural imaging, functional oxygenation, blood volume, blood flow imaging, and scattering monitoring will all be important in determining tissue health and risk of injury.

Conclusions

Measurements of cerebral oxygenation, blood flow, and blood volume are possible using near-infrared optical spectroscopy. Imaging of cerebral structure, such as hemorrhage, has also been demonstrated. Combining images of cerebral structure with measurements of brain oxygenation and blood flow using spectroscopy should allow for continuous bedside monitoring of cerebral function while avoiding harmful exposures. Clinical applications of medical optical imaging include early identification of infants at greatest risk for irreversible brain injury, which may allow elucidation of the timing and mechanism of neonatal brain injury, prompt intervention to prevent further injury, and assessment of therapeutic interventions such as neuroprotective agents. Because of its ability to noninvasively and unintrusively peer inside the body, medical optical imaging represents a fundamentally new tool in the medical armamentarium. Current studies include structural and functional brain monitoring of critically ill infants with hypoxic-ischemic encephalopathy, seizures, and extreme prematurity and in infants undergoing extracorporeal membrane oxygenation, cardiac surgery, and exchange transfusion. The relationship between optical images and outcome measures such as periventricular leukomalacia and cerebral palsy are being examined as well. Finally, current animal studies include correlation of optical imaging with diffusion-weighted MRI in a neonatal rabbit cerebral hypoxic-ischemic model and imaging of cerebral function in newborn piglets during hypothermic total circulatory arrest.

Bioluminescence

In vivo optical monitoring requires that the process or structure to be monitored possess a unique optical feature that can be distinguished above tissue background, in other words, an optical signature. In addition to variation in the absorbance and scattering properties of tissues, certain biological molecules, such as hemoglobin or melanin, possess inherent optical properties. The absorbing characteristics of these proteins can thereby be exploited to study events in living animals. However, only a fraction of all molecules possess unique optical qualities and, as such, much of the biology in a living organism is not accessible optically. As with other imaging modalities, a solution to this problem is to introduce a contrast agent or other chemical that preferentially enhances the optical properties of the structure or process to be monitored. Bioluminescent proteins have been used as optical tags in small, nearly transparent animals such as fish for real-time analysis of biological events.[108] Given that photons are also transmitted through absorbing and scattering media, such as mammalian tissue, and have been used, noninvasively, to generate images of internal structures in animals[109] and human beings,[110] it seemed reasonable that an internal bioluminescent source of light should be visible externally if the depth of tissue was not too great. Laboratory rodents serve as models for human development and disease and are of a size that should permit transmission of low-intensity photons from a variety of tissue locations. Therefore, we evaluated expression of luciferase as a bioluminescent marker for infectious disease and gene regulation in mouse models for human typhoid and expression from a viral genetic element.

"Glow-in-the-dark" strains of *Salmonella typhimurium,* generated through transformation with a plasmid that encodes a bacterial luciferase and accessory enzymes,[111] were used to infect susceptible strains of mice, and photons transmitted through the tissues were used to monitor infection.[112] Low-light imaging systems (Hamamatsu Corporation) were used to quantify the transmitted photons. In these studies, abortive infections were distinguished from persistent or progressive infections, and the cecum was identified as a primary site of persistence with a likely role in disseminated systemic disease. Efficacy of the antibiotic ciprofloxacin was tested with this approach, and the results indicated rapid cessation of bioluminescence as an indicator of the presence of bacteria in intestinal epithelial cells over a period of several hours after treatment (see Fig 9). These results indicated that a low-intensity bioluminescent light source could be used to follow infections, and possibly other types of biological processes, over time in a living mammal. The advantages of this real-time monitoring system over conventional methods include rapid analyses at multiple sites under natural conditions and survival of animal subjects leading to reductions in numbers of animals used in biomedical research and subsequently lowering the cost of conducting research.

The success of using bioluminescent markers in the infectious disease model suggested that gene expression could also be evaluated using a similar approach. In a transgenic mouse model[113] in which the expression

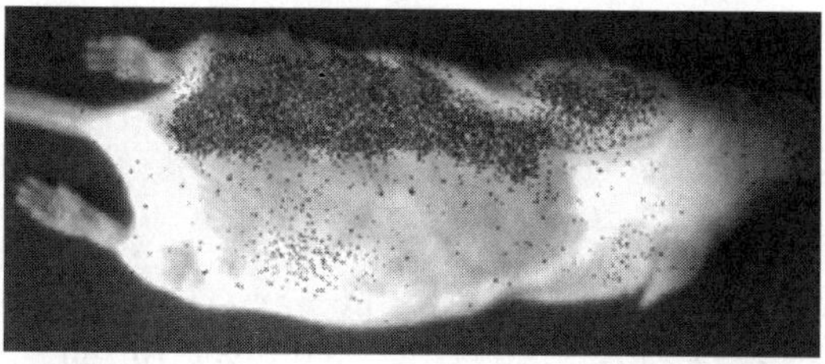

FIGURE 11.—The left half of the shaved dorsal surface of animals and the left ear were treated twice daily for 2 days with DMSO to activate expression of the HIV-1 promoter. Luciferin was applied topically over the entire surface of the back and both ears, and animals were imaged immediately after addition of substrate. Unilateral emission of bioluminescence corresponding to the induced region was observed.

of firefly luciferase is directed by the promoter from HIV-1, the virus that causes AIDS, the activity of the promoter, as indicated by photon emission, was temporally and spatial evaluated in living adult and neonatal mice. Expression from the HIV-1 promoter can be controlled with various agents,[114] including dimethyl sulfoxide, which appears to activate expres-

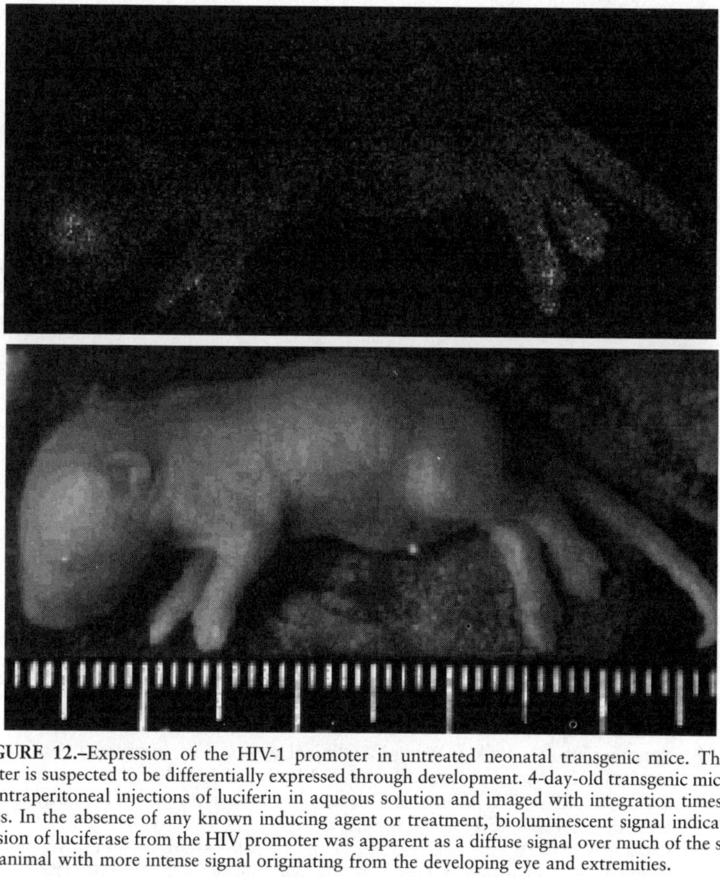

FIGURE 12.–Expression of the HIV-1 promoter in untreated neonatal transgenic mice. The HIV promoter is suspected to be differentially expressed through development. 4-day-old transgenic mice were given intraperitoneal injections of luciferin in aqueous solution and imaged with integration times of 20 minutes. In the absence of any known inducing agent or treatment, bioluminescent signal indicative of expression of luciferase from the HIV promoter was apparent as a diffuse signal over much of the surface of the animal with more intense signal originating from the developing eye and extremities.

sion in adult animal (Fig 11). In neonatal mice, the basal level of expression from the transgene was apparent in the eye and limbs (Fig 12). Infants with HIV often demonstrate rapid progression to AIDS, in contrast to the slow progression (many months to years) usually observed in infected adults. High basal levels of promoter activity in infected infants, represented by the detectable expression in neonatal mice, may in part account for the observed rapid progression in infants. The use of bioluminescent reporters opens a window into living mammals through which we can view biological processes with the contextual influences of an integrated biological system.

Summary

We have reviewed the recent developments in emerging technologies, MR and near-infrared optical imaging, that have been applied to the study of brain metabolism and injury. Data from these instruments have started to contribute to the understanding of animal models of encephalopathy as well as human clinical disease. With further refinement and understanding of these technologies, it is anticipated that they will be added to the repertoire of tools available to assist the clinician in the evaluation of the neurologic state of newborns and older children. These tools will be increasingly important to help guide the introduction of new neuroprotective and neuroreparative therapies. They should also prove useful in helping to predict the long-term outcome of neonates who may have experienced a neurologic insult.

Acknowledgements

Portions of this report have been published or presented earlier. We thank the NIH (RR-00081, M01-RR-00070-30/1, N43-NS-4-2313, N43-NS-4-2315), the Berry Fellowship Grant, The Hess Research Fund, The Mary L. Johnson Research Fund, and the Office of Naval Research (N-00014-91-C-0170) for their partial support of the above projects.

References

1. Ross BD, Kreis R, Ernst T: Clinical tools for the 90s: Magnetic resonance spectroscopy and metabolite imaging. *Eur J Radiol* 14:128–140, 1992.
2. Gadian DG, Williams SR, Bates TE, et al: NMR spectroscopy: Current status and future possibilities. *Acta Neurochir Suppl (Wien)* 57:1–8, 1993.
3. Prichard JW: Magnetic resonance spectroscopy of cerebral metabolism *in vivo*, in Asbury AK, McKhann GM, McDonald WI (eds): *Diseases of the Nervous System Clinical Neurobiology*, vol 2, WB Saunders, New York, 1993, pp 1589–1605.
4. Goplerud JM, Papadopoulos MD: Nuclear magnetic resonance imaging and spectroscopy following asphyxia. *Clin Perinatol* 20:345–367, 1993.
5. van der Knapp MS, van der Grond J, Luyten PR, et al: ^{1}H and ^{31}P magnetic resonance spectroscopy of the brain in degenerative cerebral disorders. *Ann Neurol* 31:202–211, 1992.
6. Zimmerman RA, Valk J, Wang Z: Clinical proton MR spectroscopy of neurodegenerative disease in childhood. *AJNR* 14:1282–1284, 1993.
7. Tzika AA, Ball WS, Vigneron DB, et al: Clinical proton MR spectroscopy of neurodegenerative disease in childhood. *AJNR* 14:1267–1281, 1993.
8. Tzika AA, Ball WS, Vigneron DB, et al: Childhood adrenoleukodystrophy: Assessment with proton MR spectroscopy. *Radiology* 189:467–480, 1993.

9. Bruhn H, Kruse B, Korenke GC, et al: Proton MNR spectroscopy of cerebral metabolic alterations in infantile peroxisomal disorders. *J Comput Assist Tomogr* 16:335–344, 1992.
10. Confort-Gouny S, Chabrol B, Vizon-Dury J, et al: MRI and localized proton MRS in early infantile form of neuronal ceroid lipofuscinosis. *Pediatr Neurol* 9:57–60, 1993.
11. Barkovich AJ, Good WV, Koch TK, et al: Mitochondrial disorders: Analysis of their clinical and imaging characteristics. *AJNR* 14:1119–1137, 1993.
12. Grodd W, Krageloh-Mann I, Klose U, et al: Metabolic and destructive brain disorders in children: Findings with localized proton MR spectroscopy. *Radiology* 181:173–181, 1991.
13. Cross JH, Gadian DG, Connelly A, et al: Proton magnetic resonance spectroscopy studies in lactic acidosis and mitochondrial disorders. *J Inherit Metab Dis* 16:800–811, 1993.
14. Detre JA, Wang ZY, Bogdan AR, et al: Regional variation in brain lactate in Leigh syndrome by localized ^{1}H magnetic resonance spectroscopy: *Ann Neurol* 29:218–221, 1991.
15. Austin SJ, Connelly A, Gadian DG, et al: Localized ^{1}H NMR in Canavan's disease: A report of two cases. *Magn Reson Med* 19:439–445, 1991.
16. Felber SR, Sperl W, Chemelli A, et al: Maple syrup urine disease: Metabolic decompensation monitored by proton magnetic resonance imaging and spectroscopy. *Ann Neurol* 33:396–401, 1993.
17. Bruhn H, Frahm J, Merboldt KD, et al: Multiple sclerosis in children: Cerebral metabolic alterations monitored by localized proton magnetic resonance spectroscopy *in vivo*. *Ann Neurol* 23:140–150, 1992.
18. Schiffmann R, Moller JR, Trapp BD, et al: Childhood ataxia with diffuse central nervous system hypomyelination. *Ann Neurol* 35:331–340, 1994.
19. Bruhn H, Frahm J, Gyngell ML, et al: Cerebral metabolism in man after acute stroke: New observations using localized proton NMR spectroscopy. *Magn Reson Med* 9:126–131, 1989.
20. Felber SR, Aichner FT, Sauter R, et al: Combined magnetic resonance imaging and proton MR spectroscopy of patients with acute stroke. *Stroke* 23:1106–1110, 1992.
21. Ford CC, Grifey RH, Matwiyoff NA, et al: Multivoxel ^{1}H-MRS of stroke. *Neurology* 42:1408–1412, 1992.
22. Gideon P, Hennriksen O, Sperling B, et al: Early time course of N-acetylaspartate, creatine and phosphocreatine, and compounds containing choline in the brain after acute stroke. *Stroke* 23:1566–1572, 1992.
23. Graham GD, Blamire AM, Howseman AM, et al: Proton magnetic resonance spectroscopy of cerebral lactate and other metabolites in stroke patients. *Stroke* 23:333–340, 1992.
24. Graham SH, Meyerhoff DJ, Nat DR, et al: Magnetic resonance spectroscopy of N-acetyl aspartate in hypoxic-ischemic encephalopathy. *Ann Neurol* 35:490–494, 1994.
25. Hope PL, del Costello AM, Cady EB, et al: Cerebral energy metabolism studied with phosphorus NMR spectroscopy in normal and birth-asphyxiated infants. *Lancet* 2:366–370, 1984.
26. Azzopardi D, Wyatt JS, Cady EB, et al: Prognosis of newborn infants with hypoxic-ischemic brain injury assessed by phosphorus magnetic resonance spectroscopy. *Pediatr Res* 25:445–451, 1989.
27. Hüppi PS, Fusch C, Boesch C, et al: Regional metabolic assessment of human brain during development by proton magnetic resonance spectroscopy *in vivo* and by high-performance liquid chromatography/gas chromatography in autopsy tissue. *Pediatr Res* 37:145–150, 1995.
28. Moorcraft J, Bolas NM, Ives NK, et al: Global and depth resolved phosphorus magnetic resonance spectroscopy to predict outcome after birth asphyxia. *Arch Dis Child* 66:1119–1123, 1991.

29. Reynolds EO, McCormick DC, Roth SC, et al: New non-invasive methods for the investigation of cerebral oxidative metabolism and haemodynamics in newborn infants. *Ann Med* 23:681–686, 1991.
30. Hope PL, Moorcraft J: Magnetic resonance spectroscopy. *Clin Perinatol* 18:535–548, 1991.
31. Goplerud JM, Delivoria-Papadopoulos M: Nuclear magnetic resonance imaging and spectroscopy following asphyxia. *Clin Perinatol* 20:345–367, 1993.
32. Radda GK: Spatially localized magnetic resonance spectroscopy of the brains of normal and asphyxiated newborns. *Pediatrics* 87:273–282, 1991.
33. Peden CJ, Rutherford MA, Sargentoni J, et al: Proton spectroscopy of the neonatal brain following hypoxic-ischemic injury. *Dev Med Child Neurol* 35:502–510, 1993.
34. Groenendaal F, Veenhoven RH, van der Grond J, et al: Cerebral lactate and N-acetyl-aspartate/choline ratios in asphyxiated full-term neonates demonstrated *in vivo* using proton magnetic resonance spectroscopy. *Pediatr Res* 1994; 35:148–151, 1994.
35. Kreis R, Arcinue E, Ernst T, et al: Hypoxic encephalopathy after near-drowning studied by quantitative ^{1}H-magnetic resonance spectroscopy. Metabolic changes and their prognostic value. *J Clin Invest* 97:1142–1154, 1996.
36. Auld KL, Ashwal S, Holshouser BA, et al: Proton magnetic resonance spectroscopy in children with acute central nervous system injury. *Pediatr Neurol* 12:323–334, 1995.
37. Ashwal S, Holshouser B, Perkin R, et al: ^{1}H-MRS obtained 3 to 5 days after acute CNS injury predicts outcome in children 18 months or older. *Ann Neurol* 38:552, 1995.
38. Kreis R, Ernst T, Ross BD: Development of the human brain: *In vivo* quantification of metabolite and water content with proton magnetic resonance spectroscopy. *Magn Reson Med* 30:424–437, 1993.
39. Kimura H, Fujii Y, Itoh S, et al: Metabolic alterations in the neonate and infant brain during development: Evaluation with proton MR spectroscopy. *Radiology* 194:483–489, 1995.
40. van der Knapp MS, van der Grond J, van Rijen PC, et al: Age dependent changes in localized proton and phosphorus MR spectroscopy of the brain. *Radiology* 176:509–515, 1990.
41. Hashimoto T, Tayama M, Miyazaki M, et al: Developmental changes in proton MR spectroscopy of the brain. *No To Hattatsu* 26:26–31, 1994.
42. Barkovich AJ, Westmark K, Partridge C, et al: Perinatal asphyxia: MR findings in the first 10 days. *AJNR* 16:427–438, 1995.
43. Martin E, Barkovich AJ: Magnetic resonance imaging in perinatal asphyxia. *Arch Dis Child* 72:F62–70, 1995.
44. Barkovich AJ, Maroldo TV: Magnetic resonance imaging of normal and abnormal brain development. *Top Magn Reson Imaging* 5:96–122, 1993.
45. Cioni G, Bartalena L, Biagioni E, et al: Neuroimaging and functional outcome of neonatal leukomalacia. *Behav Brain Res* 49:7–19, 1992.
46. Barkovich AJ: MR and CT evaluation of profound neonatal and infantile asphyxia. *AJNR* 13:959–972, 1992.
47. Keeney SE, Adcock EW, McArdle CB: Prospective observations of 100 high-risk neonates by high-field (1.5 Tesla) magnetic resonance imaging of the central nervous system: I. Intraventricular and extracerebral lesions. *Pediatrics* 87:421–430, 1991.
48. Keeney SE, Adcock EW, McArdle CB: Prospective observations of 100 high-risk neonates by high-field (1.5 Tesla) magnetic resonance imaging of the central nervous system. II. Lesions associated with hypoxic-ischemic encephalopathy. *Pediatrics* 87:431–438, 1991.
49. Byrne P, Welch R, Johnson MA, et al: Serial magnetic resonance imaging in neonatal hypoxic-ischemic encephalopathy. *J Pediatr* 117:694–700, 1990.

50. Mintorovitch J, Yang GY, Shimizu H, et al: Diffusion-weighted magnetic resonance imaging of acute focal cerebral ischemia: Comparison of signal intensity with changes in brain water and Na+,K(+)-ATPase activity. *J Cereb Blood Flow Metab* 14:332–336, 1994.
51. Back T, Hoehn-Berlage M, Kohno K, et al: Diffusion nuclear magnetic resonance imaging in experimental stroke: Correlation with cerebral metabolites. *Stroke* 25:494–500, 1994.
52. Pierpaoli C, Righini A, Linfante I, et al: Histopathologic correlates of abnormal water diffusion in cerebral ischemia: Diffusion-weighted MR imaging and light and electron microscopic study. *Radiology* 189:439–448, 1993.
53. Warach S, Dashe JF, Edelman RR: Clinical outcome in ischemic stroke predicted by early diffusion-weighted and perfusion magnetic resonance imaging: A preliminary analysis. *J Cereb Blood Flow Metab* 61:53–59, 1996.
54. Welch KM, Windham J, Knight RA, et al: A model to predict the histopathology of human stroke using diffusion and T2-weighted magnetic resonance imaging. *Stroke* 26:1983–1989, 1995.
55. Fisher M, Prichard JW, Warach S: New magnetic resonance techniques for acute ischemic stroke. *JAMA* 274:908–911, 1995.
56. Minematsu K, Fisher M, Li L, et al: Diffusion and perfusion magnetic resonance imaging studies to evaluate a noncompetitive *N*-methyl-D-aspartate antagonist and reperfusion in experimental stroke in rats. *Stroke* 24:2074–2081, 1993.
57. Zhong J, Petroff OA, Prichard JW, et al: Changes in water diffusion and relaxation properties of rat cerebrum during status epilepticus. *Magn Reson Med* 30:241–246, 1993.
58. Latour LL, Hasegawa Y, Formato JE, et al: Spreading waves of decreased diffusion coefficient after cortical stimulation in the rat brain. *Magn Reson Med* 32:189–198, 1994.
59. Hanstock CC, Faden AI, Bendall MR, et al: Diffusion-weighted imaging differentiates ischemic tissue from traumatized tissue. *Stroke* 25:843–848, 1994.
60. Pelletier J, Habib M, Lyon-Caen O, et al: Functional and magnetic resonance imaging correlates of callosal involvement in multiple sclerosis. *Arch Neurol* 50:1077–1182, 1993.
61. Heide AC, Richards TL, Alvord EC Jr, et al: Diffusion imaging of experimental allergic encephalomyelitis. *Magn Reson Med* 29:478–484, 1993.
62. Rhine WD, deCrespigny A, Pelc LR, et al: Magnetic resonance studies of immature rabbit hypoxic-ischemic encephalopathy. *Pediatr Res* 35:386A, 1994.
63. Rumpel H, Buchli R, Gehrrmann J, et al: Magnetic resonance imaging of brain edema in the neonatal rat: A comparison of short and long term hypoxia-ischemia. *Pediatr Res* 38:113–118, 1995.
64. Wimberger DM, Roberts TP, Barkovich AJ, et al: Identification of "premyelination" by diffusion-weighted MRI. *J Comput Assist Tomogr* 19:28–33, 1995.
65. Cowan FM, Pennock JM, Hanrahan JD, et al: Early detection of cerebral infarction and hypoxic ischemic encephalopathy in neonates using diffusion-weighted magnetic resonance. *Neuropediatrics* 25:172–175, 1994.
66. Mercuri E, Cowan F, Rutherford M, et al: Ischaemic and haemorrhagic brain lesions in newborns with seizures and normal Apgar scores. *Arch Dis Child* 73:F67–F74, 1995.
67. Mathur-De Vre R, Lemort M: Invited review: Biophysical properties and clinical applications of magnetic resonance imaging contrast agents. *Br J Radiol* 68:225–247, 1995.
68. Muroff LR, Runge VM: The use of MR contrast in neoplastic disease of the brain. *Top Magn Reson Imaging* 7:137–157, 1995.
69. Runge VM, Wells JW: Update: Safety, new applications, new MR agents. *Top Magn Reson Imaging* 7:181–195, 1995.
70. Eggli KD: The newer radiographic contrast media. *Clin Pediatr* 31:554–558, 1992.
71. Reimer P, Schuierer G, Balzer T, et al: Application of a superparamagnetic iron oxide (Resovist) for MR imaging of human cerebral blood volume. *Magn Reson Med* 34:694–697, 1995.

72. Forsting M, Reith W, Dorfler A, et al: MRI in acute cerebral ischaemia: Perfusion imaging with superparamagnetic iron oxide in a rat model. *Neuroradiology* 36:23–26, 1994.
73. Oppenheimer SM, Bryan RN, Conturo TE, et al: Proton magnetic resonance spectroscopy and gadolinium-DTPA perfusion imaging of asymptomatic MRI white matter lesions. *Magn Reson Med* 33:61–68, 1995.
74. Steen RG, Kromhout-Schiro S, Graham MM: Relationship of perfusion to edema in the 9L gliosarcoma. *J Neurooncol* 16:81–87, 1993.
75. Rhine WD, Benaron DA, Enzmann DR, et al: Gd-DTPA MR detection of blood-brain barrier opening in rats after hyperosmotic shock. *J Comput Assist Tomogr* 17:563–566, 1993.
76. Rubin P, Gash DM, Hansen JT, et al: Disruption of the blood-brain barrier as the primary effect of CNS irradiation. *Radiother Oncol* 31:51–60, 1994.
77. Emerson J, Kesslak JP, Chen PC, et al: Magnetic resonance imaging of the aging brain in Down syndrome. *Prog Clin Biol Res* 393:123–138, 1995.
78. Silva AC, Zhang W, Williams DS, et al: Multi-slice MRI of rat brain perfusion during amphetamine stimulation using arterial spin labeling. *Magn Reson Med* 33:209–214, 1995.
79. Aine CJ: A conceptual overview and critique of functional neuroimaging techniques in humans: I. MRI/FMRI and PET. *Crit Rev Neurobiol* 9:229–309, 1995.
80. Puce A: Comparative assessment of sensorimotor function using functional magnetic resonance imaging and electrophysiological methods. *J Clin Neurophysiol* 12:450–459, 1995.
81. Kwong KK: Functional magnetic resonance imaging with echo planar imaging. *Magn Reson Quarterly* 11(1):1–20, 1995.
82. Le Bihan D, Jezzard P, Haxby J, et al: Functional magnetic resonance imaging of the brain. *Ann Intern Med* 122:296–303, 1995.
83. Turner R: Magnetic resonance imaging of brain function. *Am J Physiol Imaging* 7:136–145, 1992.
84. Kang JK: Neuroimaging and functional examination in hydrocephalus: A comment. *Childs Nerv Sys* 11:478–482, 1995.
85. Bruhn H, Kleinschmidt A, Boecker H, et al: The effect of acetazolamide on regional cerebral blood oxygenation at rest and under stimulation as assessed by MRI. *J Cereb Blood Flow Metab* 14:742–748, 1994.
86. Blankenberg FG, Storss RW, Naumovski L, et al: Detection of apoptotic cell death by proton nuclear magnetic resonance spectroscopy. *Blood* 87:1951–1956, 1996.
87. A review of the field, Optical Tomography, is available from *SPIE* (Bellingham, WA). Other excellent collections of topical related articles can be found in *SPIE* publications 1431 (1991), 1641 (1992), 1888 (1993), 2135 (1994), and 2389 (1995).
88. Jöbsis FF: Noninvasive infrared monitoring of cerebral and myocardial oxygen sufficiency and circulatory parameters. *Science* 198:1264–1266, 1977.
89. McCormick PW, Stewart M, Lewis G, et al: Intracerebral penetration of infrared light. *J Neurosurg* 76:315–318, 1992.
90. Chance B: Comparison of time-resolved and -unresolved measurements of deoxyhemoglobin in brain. *Proc Natl Acad Sci* 85:4971–4975, 1988.
91. Delpy DT, Cope M, van der Zee P, et al: Estimation of optical pathlength through tissue from direct time of flight measurement. *Phys Med Biol* 33:1433–1442, 1988.
92. Svaasand LO, Ellingsen R: Optical properties of human brain. *J Cereb Blood Flow Metab* 3:293–299, 1983.
93. Hebden JC, Kruger RA: Transillumination imaging performance: A time-of-flight imaging system. *Med Phys* 17:351–356, 1990.
94. Wyatt JS, Cope M, Delpy DT, et al: Measurement of optical pathlength for cerebral near infrared spectroscopy in newborn infants. *Dev Neurosci* 12:140–144, 1990.
95. Benaron DA, Kurth CD, Steven J, et al: Non-invasive estimation of cerebral oxygenation and oxygen consumption using phase-shift spectrophotometry. *Proc IEEE Eng Med Biol* 12:2004–2007, 1990.

96. Benaron DA, Gwiazdowski S, Steven J, et al: Optical path length of 754nm and 816nm light emitted into the heads of infants. *Proc IEEE Eng Med Biol* 12:1117–1119, 1990.
97. Drexler B, Davis JL, Schofield G: Diaphanography in the diagnosis of breast cancer. *Radiology* 157:41–44, 1985.
98. Marshall V, Williams DC, Smith KD: Diaphanography as a means of detecting breast cancer. *Radiology* 150:339–343, 1984.
99. Navarro GA, Profio AE: Contrast in diaphanography of the breasts. *Med Phys* 15:181–187, 1988.
100. Benaron DA, Ho DC, Spilman SD, et al: Tomographic time-of-flight optical imaging scanner for highly scattering media using non-parallel ray geometry. *App Opt,* in press.
101. Benaron DA: Imaging neonatal brain pathology using light. *Pediatr Res* 33:369A, 1993.
102. van Houten JP, Benaron DA, Spilman SD, et al: Imaging brain injury using time-resolved near infrared light scanning. *Pediatr Res* 39:470–476, 1996.
103. Benaron DA, van Houten JP: Results of clinical tomographic imaging using light. *Adv Exp Med Biol,* in press.
104. Benaron DA: Optical imaging of brain injury during cardiac surgery, in Jonas R (ed): *Brain Injury in Cardiac Surgery.* Plenum Press, in press.
105. Benaron DA, van Houten JP, Cheong WF, et al: Early results of clinical optical tomography in a neonatal intensive care unit. *SPIE,* in press.
106. Cheong WF, van Houten JP, Kermit EL, et al: Pilot comparison of light-based optical tomography versus ultrasound for real-time imaging of neonatal intraventricular hemorrhage. *Pediatr Res* 39:201A, 1996.
107. van Houten JP, Cheong WF, Kermit EL, et al: Clinical measurement of brain oxygenation and function using light-based optical tomography. *Pediatr Res* 39:382A, 1996.
108. Mayerhofer R, Araki K, Szalay AA: Monitoring of spatial expression of firefly luciferase in transformed zebrafish. *J Biolumin Chemilumin* 10:271–275, 1995.
109. Benaron DA, Stevenson DK: Optical time-of-flight and absorbance imaging in biological media. *Science* 259:1463–1466, 1993.
110. Benaron DA, Stevenson DK: Resolution of near-infrared time-of-flight brain oxygenation imaging. *Adv Exp Med Biol* 361:609–617, 1994.
111. Frackman S, Anhalt M, Nealson KH: Cloning, organization, and expression of the bioluminescence genes of *Xenorhabdus luminescens. J Bacteriol* 172:5767–5773, 1990.
112. Contag CH, Contag PR, Mullins JI, et al: Photonic detection of bacterial pathogens in a living host. *Mol Microbiol* 18:593–603, 1995.
113. Morrey JD, Bourn SM, Bunch TD, et al: *In vivo* activation of human immunodeficiency virus type 1 long terminal repeat by UV type A (UV-A) light plus psoralen and UV-B light in the skin of transgenic mice. *J Virol* 65:5045–5051, 1991.
114. Morrey JD, Bourn SM, Bunch TD, et al: HIV-1 LTR activation model: Evaluation of various agents in skin of transgenic mice. *J Acquir Immune Defic Syndr* 5:1195–1203, 1992.

Featured Topic: Prevention of Perinatal Group B Streptococcal Disease: A Public Health Perspective

Summary

Group B streptococcus (GBS) is a leading cause of serious neonatal infection. Most neonatal GBS infections can be prevented through the use of intrapartum antimicrobial prophylaxis in women who are at increased risk for transmitting the infection to their newborns. However, despite clinical trials that demonstrate the effectiveness of intrapartum antibiotic prophylaxis, prevention strategies have not been implemented widely or consistently, and the incidence of neonatal GBS disease has not declined. To promote a coordinated approach to prevention among obstetric and pediatric care practitioners and among supporting clinical microbiology laboratory personnel, the Centers for Disease Control and Prevention (CDC) had developed prevention guidelines in conjunction with experts from relevant disciplines and with representatives of the American College of Obstetricians and Gynecologists, the American Academy of Pediatrics (AAP), and other professional organizations.

This report provides the epidemiologic basis for prevention protocols, summarizes results of clinical trials demonstrating the efficacy of intrapartum antimicrobial agents, examines limitations of different approaches to prevention, and presents guidelines for the prevention of GBS disease. The CDC recommends use of one of two prevention strategies. In the first strategy, intrapartum antibiotic prophylaxis is offered to women identified as GBS carriers through prenatal screening cultures collected at 35–37 weeks' gestation and to women who experience premature onset of labor or rupture of membranes at less than 37 weeks' gestation. In the second strategy, intrapartum antibiotic prophylaxis is provided to women who have one or more risk conditions at the time of labor or membrane rupture.

Issues addressed by these prevention guidelines include the following: the appropriate clinical and laboratory methods required for prenatal screening programs designed to identify GBS carriers, risk conditions that indicate the need for intrapartum antibiotics, management of newborns whose mothers receive intrapartum antibiotic prophylaxis for GBS disease, and education of prenatal patients regarding GBS disease and the available prevention policy. These guidelines are intended for the following groups: (1) providers of prenatal, obstetric, and pediatric care; (2) supporting microbiology laboratories, hospital administrators, and managed-care organizations; (3) childbirth educators; (4) public health authorities; (5) expectant parents; and (6) advocacy groups for expectant parents.

Introduction

Since its emergence in the 1970s, GBS disease has been the leading bacterial infection associated with illness and death among newborns in the United States. Newborns at increased risk for GBS disease are those born to women who are colonized with GBS in the genital or rectal areas.

Colonized women who experience either a long duration of membrane rupture, premature delivery, or intrapartum fever are at particularly high risk for transmitting GBS infection to their infants during labor and delivery. Infants who have GBS disease can require prolonged hospitalization and expensive supporting therapy, and survivors may experience permanent disability (e.g., hearing or visual loss or mental retardation).

Many perinatal GBS infections can be prevented through intrapartum antimicrobial prophylaxis. Programs to prevent GBS disease require coordinated efforts among numerous specialties (e.g., providers of prenatal, obstetric, and pediatric care; supporting microbiology laboratories; managed-care organizations; quality assurance personnel; childbirth educators; and public health authorities).

The CDC developed these GBS disease prevention guidelines through clinical analysis of clinical trial data and subsequent review of guidelines by consultants representing numerous disciplines. In December 1994, a draft version of the guidelines was published in the Federal Register. On March 10, 1995, the CDC convened a meeting of clinical experts, public health authorities, representatives from professional organizations, and patient advocates to further consider these guidelines. The guidelines published in this report have been reviewed by both the American College of Obstetricians and Gynecologists and the American Academy of Pediatrics. In addition, this document provides the epidemiologic basis for prevention protocols, summarizes results of clinical trials, examines limitations of various approaches to prevention, and presents prevention guidelines.

Background

Group B streptococcus, or *Streptococcus agalactiae,* is a gram-positive coccus that causes invasive disease primarily in newborns, pregnant women, and adults with underlying medical conditions (e.g., diabetes mellitus). In infants, GBS disease is characterized as either early onset (i.e., occurring in infants younger than 7 days of age) or late onset (i.e., occurring in infants 7 days of age or older). Disease in infants usually occurs as bacteremia, pneumonia, or meningitis.[1] Other syndromes (e.g., cellulitis and osteomyelitis) also can occur. Approximately 25% of the cases of neonatal GBS disease occur in premature infants.[2]

In pregnant women, GBS infection causes urinary tract infection, amnionitis, endometritis, and wound infection; stillbirths and premature delivery also have been attributed to GBS.[1] In nonpregnant adults, skin or soft-tissue infection, bacteremia, genitourinary infection, and pneumonia are the most common manifestations of disease.[2, 3]

The case-fatality rate for GBS disease is estimated to be 5% to 20% for newborns[1, 2, 4] and 15% to 32% for adults.[2, 3, 5] A recent multistate, active surveillance system in a population of 10 million individuals[2] demonstrated that 6% of early-onset GBS infections resulted in death. This case-fatality rate is lower than those reported previously,[1, 6] particularly the rates of 15% to 50% observed in studies from the 1970s.[7–9] This reduction in deaths most likely has resulted from improvements in neonatal care.[10, 11]

Epidemiology

COLONIZATION

The gastrointestinal tract is the most likely human reservoir of GBS, with the genitourinary tract being the most common site of secondary spread.[1] Colonization rates can differ among ethnic groups, geographic locales, and by age; however, rates are similar for pregnant and nonpregnant women.[1, 12–14] In most populations studied, from 10% to 30% of pregnant women were colonized with GBS in the vaginal or rectal area.[12, 13, 15, 16] Of all infants born to colonized parturients, approximately 1% to 2% will develop early-onset invasive disease.[1]

The isolation rate of GBS from clinical specimens depends on several factors. Culturing specimens from both the anorectum and the vaginal introitus increases the likelihood of GBS isolation by 5% to 27% over vaginal culture alone.[15–17] The use of selective media (i.e., broths containing antimicrobial agents to inhibit competing organisms) is essential because they can increase the yield of screening cultures by as much as 50%.[18, 19] Appropriate selective broth media—either SBM broth or Lim broth—are commercially available.

INCIDENCE OF NEONATAL DISEASE

Multistate, population-based methods of case-finding have been used to estimate the incidence of neonatal GBS disease in the United States. Age- and race-adjusted projections from multistate surveillance suggested that, in 1990, 7,600 episodes (i.e., incidence rate of 1.8 per 1,000 live births) and 310 deaths in the United States resulted from GBS disease among infants 90 days of age or younger.[2] Early-onset infections accounted for approximately 80% of neonatal GBS infections.[2] Based on data from early case series, long-term neurologic sequelae have been estimated to occur in 15% to 30% of meningitis survivors[1]; more recent estimates of the incidence and costs of sequelae from neonatal GBS disease are not available.

RISK FACTORS FOR PERINATAL GBS DISEASE

Results of studies indicate that several obstetric, maternal, and neonatal factors increase the likelihood that early-onset GBS disease will occur in a newborn (Table 1). Infants born to women who were identified prenatally as GBS carriers had 29 times the risk of early-onset disease than did infants born to women whose prenatal cultures were negative.[20] In the same study population, deliveries in which prematurity, longer duration of membrane rupture, or intrapartum fever occurred were approximately seven times more likely to be complicated by early-onset GBS disease.[20]

The incidence of GBS disease also is higher among infants born to mothers who are 20 years of age or younger[21, 22] or of black race.[2, 21] Other women with increased likelihood of delivering an infant with invasive GBS disease are those with heavy colonization of GBS in genital cultures[8] or with low levels of anti-GBS capsular antibody[23] and women who previously delivered an infant who had GBS disease.[24–26] Women with GBS bacteriuria during pregnancy usually are heavily colonized with GBS and

TABLE 1.—Risk for Early-onset Group B Streptococcal (GBS) Disease (*20*), by Prenatal Maternal Colonization Status and Intrapartum Risk Factors

Risk status*	No. of episodes of early-onset GBS disease	No. of deliveries	Attack rate (per 1,000 births)	Deliveries (%)	Early-onset GBS cases (%)
Total population	16	5,292	3.0	100.0	100.0
Colonization+	14	1,029	13.6	19.4	87.5
Colonization−	2	4,263	0.5	80.7	12.5
Risk factors+	11	1,311	8.4	24.7	68.8
Risk factors−	5	3,981	1.3	75.2	31.3
Colonization+ Risk factors+	10	245	40.8	4.6	62.5
Colonization+ Risk factors−	4	784	5.1	14.8	25.0
Colonization− Risk factors+	1	1,066	0.9	20.0	6.2
Colonization− Risk factors−	1	3,197	0.3	60.0	6.2

*Colonization assessed by prenatal rectovaginal cultures. Risk factors defined as rupture of membranes greater than 12 hours, less than 37 weeks' gestation, or intrapartum temperature greater than 99.5°F (greater than 37.5°C).

"+" refers to present; "−" refers to absent.

(Reprinted from Centers for Disease Control and Prevention: Prevention of perinatal group B streptococcal disease: A public health perspective. *MMWR* 45(No. RR-7):1–24, 1996.)

appear to be at increased risk for perinatal transmission.[27-30] Although multiple gestation has been suggested as a risk factor for GBS disease,[31, 32] only one study indicated increased risk independent of prematurity.[31] Recent large studies failed to detect increased risk associated with multiple gestation.[21, 22] Risk factors identified for neonates include low birth weight and heavy surface colonization with GBS.[8, 33]

Determinants of late-onset GBS disease are not well documented; however, some evidence suggests that late-onset disease can be acquired through either vertical or nosocomial transmission,[6, 34, 35] although acquisition of disease from community sources also is possible.[14]

The role of GBS colonization in maternal infections was recently investigated.[36] Factors that independently increased the risk for clinical amnionitis included GBS colonization, duration of membrane rupture (i.e., more than 6 hours), duration of internal monitoring (i.e., more than 12 hours), and number of vaginal examinations (i.e., more than 6).[36]

Prevention Strategies

Almost half the cases of invasive GBS disease occur in newborns[2]; therefore, efforts to prevent GBS disease have been concentrated on this group. Research has focused on either inducing protective immunity in the newborn (active and passive immunization) or eradicating colonization from the mother and/or newborn (chemoprophylaxis).

Immunization

Several studies have indicated that susceptibility to neonatal GBS disease is caused by a deficiency of maternal anticapsular antibody.[23, 37] Active maternal immunization may prevent peripartum maternal disease and neonatal disease by transplacental transfer of protective IgG antibodies.[38]

Several vaccines designed to induce antibodies against the polysaccharide capsule of GBS are being developed.[39] These vaccines can potentially be used to prevent GBS disease in nonpregnant adults as well. The potential impact of effective vaccines may be limited because of reduced transplacental transport of protective antibody before 32–34 weeks' gestation and because of possible difficulty in making the vaccine available to pregnant women.

Chemoprophylaxis

Efficacy Studies

Administering antimicrobial agents to pregnant women before the onset of labor or rupture of membranes is not likely to prevent neonatal GBS disease; however, some early studies have indicated that maternal colonization might be reduced by this method.[40, 41] In one study, asymptomatic pregnant women colonized with GBS were given oral antimicrobial drugs for 1 week during the third trimester; more than 30% of those treated were still colonized at delivery, and no substantial difference was observed in carriage of the organism at delivery between treated and untreated groups.[42] Another study indicated that nearly 70% of colonized women who were treated for 12–14 days during the third trimester were colonized 3 weeks later and again at delivery, even when their sex partners also had been treated.[43]

Postnatal chemoprophylaxis with IM penicillin administered to infants just after birth has also been studied. Only one prospective, randomized, controlled study has been published in which blood cultures were collected from all newborns before chemoprophylaxis was conducted.[44] In this study, in which only low–birth weight infants were observed, no differences were observed between treated and untreated groups in either the incidence of early- or late-onset GBS disease or in mortality. Another study suggested that postnatal chemoprophylaxis with penicillin may decrease neonatal illness caused by GBS.[45, 46] However, no significant effect on overall mortality was observed, and mortality associated with penicillin-resistant pathogens was higher in the penicillin-treated group than in the control group (1.0 vs. 0.4 deaths per 1,000 live births, $P = 0.06$).[46] Because the majority of neonatal GBS infections are acquired in utero, antimicrobial agents administered to neonates, although useful for treatment, are unlikely to prevent the majority of GBS disease.

Intrapartum chemoprophylaxis (i.e., the administration of antimicrobial agents after onset of labor or membrane rupture but before delivery) is the most likely method of preventing both early-onset disease and maternal illness resulting from GBS; several antimicrobial regimens have been used for intrapartum chemoprophylaxis (Table 2). Several studies have indicated that intrapartum chemoprophylaxis decreases neonatal colonization[47–51] and early-onset invasive disease[50–53] when administered to unselected pregnant women colonized with GBS (Table 3).

TABLE 2.—Summary of Antimicrobial Regimens Used for Studies of Intrapartum Chemoprophylaxis for Group B Streptococcal (GBS) Disease

Agent	Dose and schedule	Comments
Ampicillin (*47*)	500 mg IV every 6 hrs	30/34 received only one dose before delivery
Ampicillin (*52*)	500 mg IV	Administered every 6 hrs
Benzyl penicillin (*48*)	600 mg IM every 8 hrs	Erythromycin 100 mg IM for women allergic to penicillin
Ampicillin (*50*)	500 mg IV every 6 hrs	46/57 received only one dose before delivery
Penicillin (*53*)	1 mU IV every 6 hrs	
Ampicillin (*54*)	2 g IV load, then 1 g IV every 4 hrs	Mean duration of prophylaxis 5.4 hrs
Penicillin G (*58*)	5 mU IV every 6 hrs	If labor lasted 18 hrs, then penicillin V 1 mU should be administered orally every 8 hrs after initial IV therapy
Ampicillin (*59*)	1 g IV every 6 hrs	
Ampicillin (*57*)	1 g IV every 6 hrs	Ampicillin levels measured in eight mother-infant pairs

Abbreviation: mU, million units.

(Reprinted from Centers for Disease Control and Prevention: Prevention of perinatal group B streptococcal disease: A public health perspective. *MMWR* 45(No. RR-7):1–24, 1996.)

TABLE 3.—Summary of Trials Employing Intrapartum Chemoprophylaxis for Prevention of Neonatal Colonization and Early-onset Group B Streptococcal Disease

Study design, control selection*	Case selection criteria†	Neonatal colonization			Early-onset disease		
		IC§	No IC	P value	IC	No IC	P value
R (*47*) Random	I	0/34	14/24	0.001	0/34	0/24	NA¶
P/R (*52*) Nonrandom	I	4/57	62/136	<0.01	0/57	9/136	0.06
P (*48*) Random	PC	0/38	17/49	0.001	ND	ND	NA
P (*50*) Random	I or PC	2/60	24/65	<0.01	0/60	3/65	0.14
P (*53*) Nonrandom	PC	ND	ND	NA	16/ 30,197	27/ 26,915	0.04
P (*54*) Random	PC and Pre/PROM	8/85	40/79	0.001	0/85	5/79	0.02
P (*54*) Nonrandom	PC and Pre/PROM	5/82	102/233	<0.01	0/82	7/233	0.02
P (*58*) Random	Heavy PC	ND	ND	NA	1/88	10/111	0.03
P/R (*59*) Nonrandom	Light I and PPROM	ND	ND	NA	0/29	6/37	0.03
P/R (*59*) Nonrandom	Heavy I and PPROM	ND	ND	NA	0/7	7/11	0.01
P (*57*) Random	Light PC	0/98	35/98	<0.01	0/98	0/98	NA
	Heavy PC	0/37	24/30	<0.01	0/37	3/30	0.09

**R* indicates retrospective; *P/R*, prospective case selection, retrospective control selection; *P*, prospective.

†*I* indicates intrapartum colonization; *PC*, prenatal colonization; *Pre/PROM*, preterm labor (less than 37 weeks' gestation) or prolonged rupture of membranes (greater than 12 hours); *PPROM*, "preterm premature rupture of membranes" (i.e., rupture of membranes at 34 weeks' gestation or less and more than 12 hours before onset of labor).

§*IC* indicates intrapartum chemoprophylaxis; *ND*, not done.

¶*NA* indicates not applicable.

(Reprinted from Centers for Disease Control and Prevention: Prevention of perinatal group B streptococcal disease: A public health perspective. *MMWR* 45(No. RR-7):1–24, 1996.)

Other studies have examined the use of intrapartum chemoprophylaxis for selected women colonized with GBS who were at increased risk for delivering an infant who had GBS disease. The only prospective, randomized, controlled clinical trial in which this approach was used focused on pregnant women colonized with GBS who experienced either preterm labor or membrane rupture (at less than 37 weeks' gestation) or prolonged rupture of membranes (more than 12 hours before delivery).[54] In a preliminary study of the obstetric population in the same community, the incidence of early-onset GBS disease in this high-risk group was eightfold greater than that among colonized women without any of these risk factors and 45-fold greater than that among women with these risk factors who were not colonized (see Table 1).[20, 55, 56]

In the intrapartum chemoprophylaxis trial, colonized mothers with preterm labor or whose membranes ruptured more than 12 hours before delivery were randomly selected to receive either IV ampicillin or no chemoprophylaxis. Infants born to mothers in the treatment (85 infants) and control groups (79 infants) differed substantially with respect to neonatal colonization (9% vs. 51%, $P < 0.001$) and early-onset invasive disease (0% vs. 6%, $P < 0.02$). Postpartum maternal febrile illness also was substantially reduced in the treatment group ($P < 0.04$). Researchers estimated that this strategy could prevent at least 50% of the early-onset GBS infections in their patient population.

Other studies also have documented the protective efficacy of intrapartum chemoprophylaxis administered to GBS carriers in certain high-risk groups (e.g., women with heavy genital colonization[57, 58] and with rupture of membranes at 34 weeks' gestation or less and more than 12 hours before labor onset.[59] The published studies of the efficacy of intrapartum chemoprophylaxis are summarized (see Table 3). A recent meta-analysis of seven trials, which included studies of carriers with and without risk factors, estimated a 30-fold reduction in early-onset GBS disease with intrapartum chemoprophylaxis.[60] Other investigators have argued that, because of the heterogeneity of therapeutic interventions and flaws in trial methods, combining results of GBS chemoprophylaxis trials is inappropriate.[61]

Identification of Carriers

Most of the studies of intrapartum chemoprophylaxis have been used to evaluate its impact on subsets of women who had not been identified as GBS carriers. Although the GBS carriage rate in pregnancy does not change with trimester,[12, 14] the duration of carriage is unpredictable,[14] and prenatal screening cultures will not correctly identify all women with intrapartum GBS carriage. The later in pregnancy that cultures are performed, the closer the correlation with intrapartum culture results. However, scheduling routine cultures late in pregnancy means that some women who deliver prematurely will not be screened for GBS. In one study, when sedative (antimicrobial-containing) broth medium was used and cultures were obtained from both the vagina and anorectum, only 7.4% of women with a negative culture at 26–28 weeks were found to carry GBS at delivery.[16] The same study indicated that a single positive GBS culture during pregnancy was 67% predictive of a positive culture at delivery; the estimated sensitivity and specificity were 70.0% and 90.4%, respectively.[16] Among 26 women whose prenatal cultures were obtained 5 or fewer weeks before delivery, there was 100% concordance with intrapartum culture status (i.e., no false negative or false positive prenatal cultures).[16] Data from follow-up of more than 5,000 deliveries by women who had had prenatal cultures for GBS indicated that 14 (88%) of the 16 infants who had early-onset GBS disease develop were born to mothers who were detected prenatally as carriers.[56]

Optimal identification of GBS carriers is dependent on technique. The correlation of prenatal culture results with intrapartum GBS carriage is likely to be reduced substantially when screening does not incorporate appropriate culture sites (i.e., rectum and vaginal introitus), timing (as close to delivery as feasible), and culture medium (selective broth). Because cultures of specimens from the vagina and rectum are more sensitive than specimens from the cervix,[13] pelvic examination or visualization of the cervix by speculum examination should not be performed for collection of screening cultures. Appropriate broth media are commercially available (e.g., SBM broth or Lim broth). When a transport medium (e.g., Amies' medium) is used, group B streptococci from rectovaginal swabs will survive at room temperatures for up to 96 hours, permitting shipment from satellite clinics to a central microbiology laboratory.

Selection Criteria

Because of the findings of a randomized clinical trial, investigators recommended intrapartum chemoprophylaxis for women identified through prenatal cultures as GBS carriers who subsequently had one of the following signs: rupture of membranes more than 12 hours before delivery, onset of labor or membrane rupture at less than 37 weeks' gestation, or intrapartum fever (temperature greater than 99.5°F [37.5°C]).[54] The AAP supports the use of this strategy and added the following indications for intrapartum chemoprophylaxis: previous delivery of an infant with GBS disease and multiple-gestation pregnancy in a GBS carrier.[62]

In another report, investigators proposed an approach to GBS prevention that focused on prevention of disease associated with premature birth.[63] That proposal suggested administering intrapartum antimicrobial agents to women with preterm labor or preterm rupture of membranes who were either colonized with GBS or whose colonization status was unknown. However, strategies designed to prevent infection only in preterm deliveries would have limited impact nationwide because fewer than 30% of all infants with GBS disease are preterm.[2]

A pragmatic approach to determining the need for antimicrobial prophylaxis was advocated by the American College of Obstetricians and Gynecologists.[64, 65] This strategy consists of using intrapartum antimicrobial agents for all women with one or more of the following conditions: preterm labor (at less than 37 weeks' gestation), premature rupture of membranes (at less than 37 weeks' gestation), prolonged rupture of membranes (i.e., more than 18 hours before delivery), previous child affected by symptomatic GBS infection, or maternal fever during labor.[65] This approach is less complex than protocols requiring either prenatal or intrapartal identification of GBS carriage; however, its efficacy against disease has not been evaluated in the controlled clinical trial setting, nor has the impact of the strategy on disease been measured in routine clinical practice.

In Australia, researchers evaluated a strategy that recommended intrapartum penicillin prophylaxis for all women identified as GBS carriers through prenatal cultures collected at 32 weeks' gestation.[53] Although the study was not a randomized trial, data from the study indicated a substantially lower incidence of early-onset GBS disease among the 30,197 women in the screened population compared with the 26,915 deliveries in the population that had no prenatal screening ($P = 0.04$).[53]

Clinical trials have not been conducted that directly compare the efficacy of the suggested prevention strategies. Conducting a study designed to find a statistically significant difference in efficacy may not be feasible; a recent article estimated that 100,000 women would be required for each study group of a randomized, prospective trial comparing the efficacy of universal screening and selective intrapartum chemoprophylaxis with treatment based on risk factors alone.[66] This limitation is reflected in a recent national consensus statement by the Society of Obstetricians and Gynaecologists of Canada and the Canadian Paediatric Society, which recommend use of either universal screening and selective intrapartum chemoprophylaxis or prophylaxis based on risk factors alone; the statement underscored the need for further prevention research.[67]

A combination of the features of a screening-based strategy and a strategy focused on prematurity offers a comprehensive approach to perinatal GBS prevention. This combination strategy relies on detection of GBS by rectovaginal cultures collected at 35–37 weeks' gestation; because some preterm deliveries will occur before culture results are available, the strategy also provides for intrapartum chemoprophylaxis for women who begin labor and/or membrane rupture before 37 completed weeks of gestation (unless results of the GBS culture are already available and are negative). Antibiotics would be offered intra partum to all GBS carriers and to women at less than 37 weeks' gestation whose culture status is unknown. For women with rupture of membranes at less than 37 weeks who are not in labor, obstetric care providers may choose either to begin antimicrobial prophylaxis until cultures are completed and negative or to delay beginning antimicrobial prophylaxis until a positive culture is identified. Data regarding which of these approaches is the most effective are not available.

For women at 37 or more weeks' gestation, if antenatal GBS culture status is unknown, antibiotics would be given if the intrapartum fever is present or if membrane rupture has been greater than 18 hours. This precise strategy had not been directly evaluated in clinical trials, although treatment of all GBS carriers identified through screening at 32 weeks' gestation was evaluated in a trial in Australia.[53] Data from another study

TABLE 4.—Estimated Impact of Several Strategies for the Use of Intrapartum Antimicrobial Prophylaxis (IAP) Against Early-onset Group B Streptococcal (GBS) Disease in a Hypothetical Population (*68*)

Prevention strategy	Proportion of early-onset GBS disease prevented (%)	Proportion of deliveries receiving IAP (%)
Prenatal culture at 35–37 weeks' gestation; IAP for preterm deliveries and all GBS carriers*	86.0	26.7
Prenatal culture at 26–28 weeks' gestation; IAP for GBS carriers who develop intrapartum risk factors (e.g., fever, prolonged rupture of membranes, <37 weeks' gestation) (*54*)	50.7	3.4†
No prenatal cultures; IAP for all women with intrapartum risk factors (e.g., fever, prolonged rupture of membranes, <37 weeks' gestation)¶	68.8	18.3§

*Combination strategy; refer to Figure 1.

†Percentage was estimated for a hypothetical population (*68*); actual proportion of deliveries among women who had prenatal screening cultures positive for GBS and who also developed intrapartum risk factors was 4.6% (*20*).

§Percentage was estimated for a hypothetical population (*68*); actual proportion of deliveries among women who had intrapartum risk factors was 24.7% (*20*).

¶Empiric strategy suggested by the American College of Obstetricians and Gynecologists in 1993 (*64,65*); refer to Figure 2.

(Reprinted from Centers for Disease Control and Prevention: Prevention of perinatal group B streptococcal disease: A public health perspective. *MMWR* 45(No. RR-7):1–24, 1996.)

demonstrated that the closer to delivery screening cultures are collected, the higher the test's predictive value will be.[16] In addition, this combination strategy and 18 other strategies have been evaluated by decision analysis[68]; results indicate that the combination strategy would require intrapartum antimicrobial prophylaxis in 26.7% of deliveries and would prevent approximately 86% of the cases of early-onset disease. Comparative estimates for other strategies also are provided (Table 4).

Adverse Effects

Because a substantial proportion of pregnant women are colonized with GBS, administration of intrapartum chemoprophylaxis to all GBS carriers may cause an unacceptably high number of adverse reactions. Administering intrapartum antimicrobial agents to all women who are GBS carriers could result in approximately 10 deaths per year from anaphylaxis, assuming a GBS colonization rate of 25%, 4 million deliveries in the United States annually, and a rate of fatal anaphylaxis to penicillin of 0.001%.[69] Another 0.7% to 10% of women to whom prophylaxis is administered are expected to have less severe reactions.[70] Severe complications can occur in the fetus even when maternal anaphylaxis is not life threatening.[71]

Widespread antimicrobial use also increases the risk for emergence of antimicrobial-resistant organisms. Infections with penicillin-tolerant GBS have been described,[72–74] but GBS isolates have not developed clinically important resistance to penicillin. Development of antimicrobial resistance in other peripartum pathogens is a greater threat. In one study, investigators reported four episodes of adverse perinatal outcome caused by antimicrobial-resistant Enterobacteriaceae among women treated with ampicillin or amoxicillin for premature rupture of membranes.[75]

Restricting antimicrobial agents to selected populations at increased risk for delivering a newborn with GBS disease would decrease the likelihood of adverse reactions and antimicrobial-resistant infections. The administration of intrapartum ampicillin to women identified prenatally as GBS carriers who have rupture of membranes for longer than 12 hours, labor or membrane rupture at less than 37 weeks' gestation, or intrapartum fever (temperature greater than 99.5°F [37.5°C]) would have required the administration of antimicrobial agents to 4.6% of the obstetric population served by one urban hospital.[54] In another approach, administering antimicrobial agents to women with either labor or membrane rupture at less than 37 weeks' gestation who were intrapartum carriers of GBS or whose GBS status was unknown was estimated to require prophylaxis for 8.9% of parturients.[63] Strategies that treat all GBS carriers[53] or all women with obstetric risk factors (e.g., prolonged membrane rupture and prematurity)[64] are estimated to require administering antimicrobial agents in a substantially higher proportion of deliveries.

Penicillin G may be preferable to ampicillin for routine prophylaxis.[76] Ampicillin and penicillin G have similar activity against GBS, and both cross the placenta and achieve bactericidal levels in fetal tissues. However, ampicillin had a broader spectrum of antimicrobial activity than penicillin; thus, widespread prophylaxis with ampicillin may be more likely to lead to selection of resistant organisms than would widespread use of penicillin.[76]

Implementation of Chemoprophylaxis

Despite the encouraging results of efficacy studies, routine GBS screening and selective intrapartum chemoprophylaxis have not been widely adopted in the obstetric community.[65, 77] Practical problems include logistic concerns related to screening for GBS colonization and concern about the cost-effectiveness of implementing chemoprophylaxis.

A strategy based on detecting colonization by prenatal screening and using these results to guide selective intrapartum chemoprophylaxis would not be effective for women who are not receiving prenatal care or whose prenatal records are not available to health care providers at the time of delivery. Ideally, GBS carriage would be determined at the time of labor onset or at rupture of membranes. However, because identification of GBS by culture takes 24–48 hours, intrapartum culture results would not be available in time for intervention in most deliveries. Rapid detection of GBS antigen from vaginal specimens may identify GBS carriers when prenatal screening is not available.[78] Although rapid tests for detection of GBS are specific and many recently developed tests can be performed in less than 1 hour, the sensitivity of rapid-detection tests has been variable and, often, unacceptably low (15% to 74%).[78] Some rapid-detection kits are sensitive for detecting women who are heavily colonized. Three studies have confirmed the efficacy of intrapartum chemoprophylaxis administered to women identified as GBS carriers by rapid-detection techniques.[57–59] However, because many infants with neonatal GBS disease are born to women who are lightly colonized,[59, 79] using currently available rapid-detection techniques to identify women for prophylaxis would probably prevent only a minority of GBS cases.

The cost-effectiveness of selective intrapartum chemoprophylaxis for the prevention of GBS disease has been studied by using population-based rates of disease.[80] The approach evaluated by two investigators[54] and later endorsed by the AAP[62] was demonstrated to be cost-effective at the current rates of disease.[80] The cost per case prevented (less than $35,000) was similar to that associated with maternal screening and intervention programs for other perinatal diseases (e.g., congenital syphilis).[81] Data from four other studies also have suggested that selective intrapartum chemoprophylaxis is cost-effective for the prevention of neonatal GBS disease.[56, 68, 82, 83] In particular, one study evaluated the combination strategy (i.e., prophylaxis for all women with preterm membrane rupture or labor whose culture status is unknown and for all GBS carriers identified through cultures obtained late in the pregnancy); this combination strategy was cost saving and was among the least expensive of 18 potential preventive strategies.[68]

Implementation of chemoprophylaxis is limited by two additional problems. First, clinicians have been concerned about adopting a strategy that inevitably will have failures.[64] This concern may be influenced by the complexity of communicating risk information regarding GBS to women during pregnancy or by medicolegal considerations. Previous efforts to promote use of intrapartum chemoprophylaxis for only those GBS carriers who experience intrapartum complications (e.g., longer duration of membrane rupture, fever, or less than 37 weeks' gestation) appear to have been poorly accepted by both clinicians and patients. Some clinicians and patient groups have advocated informed consent for women who are GBS carriers. For example, women colonized with GBS would be informed of their risk for early-onset GBS disease (approximately 1 in 200). Also, the potential risks of intrapartum penicillin would be described (mild allergic reaction: approximately 1 in 10; anaphylaxis: approximately 1 in 10,000; and fatal anaphylaxis: approximately 1 in 100,000). Thus, patients could make an informed decision regarding intrapartum antibiotics. In instances in which this approach has been applied, few women choose not to receive antibiotics during labor.

A second problem is that increasing intrapartum antimicrobial use may have a substantial impact on clinical management of the newborn.[84, 85] Some pediatricians routinely perform additional diagnostic tests on all infants whose mothers received intrapartum antimicrobial agents or observe these infants longer, leading to prolonged hospital stays for many newborns who are at low risk for GBS disease.[84] The decision of how to manage newborns whose mothers received intrapartum antimicrobial agents can be based on clinical manifestations, the infant's estimated gestational age, and the adequacy of intrapartum antibiotics.[62] An algorithm for evaluating and managing infants after administration of maternal antibiotics has been developed as an empiric guide; however, clinical evaluation of alternative approaches remains appropriate at this time.

Some of the challenges of instituting a prevention strategy are illustrated in two recent reports. In the first report, investigators initiated selective intrapartum chemoprophylaxis in their hospital in response to an increased rate of early-onset GBS disease.[85] They enrolled 2,040 women, 332 (16.3%) of whom were colonized with GBS. Among women colonized at delivery, 122 (37%) had at least one obstetric risk factor and, according to the hospital's protocol, should have received intrapartum chemoprophylaxis. The circumstances of 16 (14%) women who did not receive intrapartum chemoprophylaxis illustrate some limitations of this strategy; these women did not receive intrapartum antimicrobial drugs because they either delivered less than 1 hour after arriving at the hospital ($n = 9$), had had no prenatal care ($n = 3$), or had had a negative prenatal culture but had a positive culture at delivery ($n = 4$). Intrapartum chemoprophylaxis was not administered to an additional 17 (14%) women because protocol was not followed. Eleven infants had early-onset GBS disease, two had received one dose of intrapartum chemoprophylaxis and were asymptomatic, and nine were born to carriers with risk factors who did not receive intrapartum chemoprophylaxis. No affected infants were born to colonized women without risk factors or to women whose prenatal screening cultures were negative for GBS. One woman who received intrapartum chemoprophylaxis experienced a rash and transient hypotension and was delivered by cesarean section because of transient fetal bradycardia. The study suggested that selective intrapartum chemoprophylaxis was effective in preventing early-onset GBS disease, that the infants of colonized women without labor complications are at low risk for disease, and that administering intrapartum antimicrobial agents is not without risks.

The second report illustrates that a prevention strategy using selective intrapartum chemoprophylaxis is not easily implemented.[86] In this study, which was conducted in an academic setting, 114 (80.3%) of 142 women who had positive GBS screening cultures and who had risk factors at delivery received intrapartum antimicrobial drugs. Reasons for failing to receive appropriate treatment included failure to follow protocol, marginal indications for chemoprophylaxis, or patient refusal. Early results of the study suggest that institution of the protocol was associated with a downward trend in the rate of disease.

Discussion

Group B streptococcal disease continues to be a major cause of illness and death among newborns despite clinical advances in the past two decades. Major risk factors for early-onset neonatal GBS disease include maternal GBS colonization, longer duration of membrane rupture, intrapartum fever, less than 37 weeks' gestation, GBS bacteriuria during pregnancy, and previous delivery of an infant who had GBS disease.[6, 21, 25, 27] A substantial number of cases of early-onset neonatal GBS disease can be prevented by administering prophylactic antimicrobial agents during labor.[56] Furthermore, obtaining specimens from the lower vagina and rectum during the third trimester for culture in selective broth media will identify the vast majority of women who are colonized with GBS at delivery. Increasing evidence suggests that treating GBS-infected newborns is more costly than preventing the infection and that well-implemented prevention programs can substantially reduce illness and death resulting from GBS disease.[56, 68, 80, 82, 83] Any prevention program for GBS must be implemented carefully. For example, failure to use optimal culture methods can compromise the effectiveness of screening strategies. A recent survey of obstetric care providers in Georgia identified several barriers to effective prevention activities. For example, only 9% of providers who obtained screening cultures followed recommended procedures, and 32% administered antimicrobial agents prenatally when carriage was detected, even though 93% of providers stated they knew such treatment to be ineffective.[87]

An optimal prevention strategy currently is a combination of routine prenatal screening for GBS colonization late in pregnancy and empiric management of those preterm deliveries that occur before the GBS culture is available. This approach includes collecting rectovaginal cultures at 35–37 weeks' gestation and offering intrapartum treatment to all carriers. Because some preterm deliveries occur before culture results are available, the strategy also provides for intrapartum chemoprophylaxis for women who begin labor and/or membrane rupture before 37 completed weeks of gestation (unless results of the GBS culture are already available and are negative).

Criticism of previous screening-based strategies has included concerns regarding the predictive value of prenatal cultures, the ethical and legal difficulties inherent in withholding intrapartum antibiotics from GBS carriers without risk factors, and the pressure experienced by clinicians to respond to antenatal GBS carriage results by treating with oral antimicrobial agents remote from delivery. Critics of empiric approaches have been concerned that despite use of intrapartum antimicrobial prophylaxis in a substantial proportion of deliveries, the strategy does not prevent the 25% of all early-onset GBS cases that occur in GBS carriers without risk factors. Further, empiric approaches do not address the strong preference of some patients and providers for prenatal screening cultures.

Rationale for Screening-based Approach to Prevention

The combination of late prenatal screening cultures and empiric management offers several potential advantages over exclusive reliance on either a screening-based approach or an empiric approach. Because the combination strategy schedules collection of a GBS culture at 35–37 weeks' gestation, the concordance of prenatal and intrapartum GBS carriage status will be high. Thus, false negative prenatal culture results will be minimized (i.e., few women with negative cultures at 35–37 weeks' gestation will become colonized with GBS by the time of delivery), and nearly all women identified antenatally as carriers will still be carrying the organism at delivery, potentially justifying exposure of this group to adverse effects associated with antibiotics. Even women who begin prenatal care late in gestation should be eligible for late screening. By avoiding collection of cultures earlier in gestation, this strategy should reduce pressure on clinicians to treat GBS carriage antenatally. Because all GBS carriers will be offered intrapartum chemoprophylaxis, clinicians will not need to wait for the development of intrapartum risk factors in a GBS carrier (e.g., duration of membrane rupture more than 18 hours or intrapartum fever). Intrapartum prophylaxis for most women can therefore begin earlier, so that most GBS carriers will be administered antimicrobial agents more than 4 hours before delivery or in time for adequate antibiotic levels to be reached in amniotic fluid. In one analysis, the combination of late prenatal screening and intrapartum prophylaxis of carriers and preterm deliveries was estimated to prevent approximately 86% of early-onset disease, was cost saving compared with no intervention, and was among the least expensive of 18 potential preventive strategies.[68]

Large-scale clinical experience with the combination approach previously described is not yet available, although the strategy has been applied in several institutions. The theoretical advantages of this approach address most concerns that have been raised regarding the prevention strategies previously considered. Although antimicrobial prophylaxis will be used in a high proportion of deliveries, some clinicians and patients have found selective approaches (e.g., treating only carriers with risk factors) unacceptable, because treatment is withheld from a group of women with moderately increased risk of GBS disease—GBS carriers without intrapartum risk factors. Assessment of the current situation suggests that any prevention program that is acceptable to both clinicians and their patients will involve using antimicrobial prophylaxis in a substantial proportion of deliveries; thus, the strategy that directs use of these antimicrobial agents to women at the highest risk for GBS disease seems reasonable. Communication mechanisms and information systems should be developed and monitored to ensure that prenatal culture results are available at the time and place of delivery.

RESEARCH INTO ENHANCING PREVENTION

A program combining late prenatal screening for GBS with empiric treatment of women with preterm deliveries is not a permanent solution to the problem of neonatal GBS disease, although it may be a reasonable option that is available now. A more sensitive rapid screening test for GBS that could accurately detect women who carry GBS at the time of delivery would obviate the need for prenatal screening. Sensitive intrapartum testing also would permit detection of GBS carriage among women who did not receive adequate prenatal care. Because an intrapartum test might detect a higher proportion of women who carry the organism at delivery and will not detect women who only carry the organism earlier in the prenancy, intrapartum use of a sensitive rapid-detection test could make a prevention program simpler and more efficient. An adequate rapid-detection test must be sensitive (e.g., 85% to 90% compared with culture in a selective broth media); rapid (results available to clinicians in time for antibiotics to be given before delivery); and convenient (for integration into routine laboratory use). Even a highly sensitive rapid-detection test would not be adequate if results were not available to clinicians 24 hours per day, 7 days per week. Development of a vaccine against GBS that is highly immunogenic in women and permits transplacental transfer of protection to the fetus also would eliminate the need for prenatal screening and could potentially address the problem of late-onset GBS disease, which intrapartum antimicrobial agents do not prevent.

SURVEILLANCE AND EVALUATION

Because incidence may vary widely, state or local health departments or groups of affiliated hospitals should consider either establishing surveillance systems for neonatal GBS disease or reviewing data from existing systems to identify the current magnitude of disease and gain further information for evaluating the effectiveness of prevention measures. In hospital settings, prevention programs should monitor the occurrence of adverse reactions to chemoprophylaxis, the emergence of perinatal infections caused by antimicrobial-resistant organisms, and the impact of obstetric antimicrobial use on pediatric management protocols.

Recommendations

Enhanced communication among personnel in multiple disciplines is needed to ensure that programs for prevention of GBS disease succeed. Open communication between clinicians and patients is a critical component of GBS disease prevention. An informational brochure on GBS for pregnant women is available through CDC (Childhood and Respiratory Diseases Branch, Division of Bacterial and Mycotic Disease, National Center for Infectious Diseases, Mailstop C09, Atlanta, GA 30333; Internet address: http://www.cdc.gov/ncidod/diseases/bacter/strep-b.htm. The following recommendations for the prevention of GBS disease will need periodic reappraisal to incorporate advances in technology or other refinements in prevention strategies:

1. Obstetric care practitioners, in conjunction with supporting laboratories and labor and delivery facilities, should adopt a strategy for the prevention of early-onset GBS disease. Patients should be informed regarding the GBS prevention strategy.
2. Regardless of which preventive strategy is used, women with symptomatic or asymptomatic GBS bacteriuria detected during pregnancy should be treated at the time of diagnosis; because such women are usually heavily colonized with GBS, they should also receive intrapartum chemoprophylaxis. Also, women who previously have given birth to an infant with GBS disease should receive intrapartum chemoprophylaxis; prenatal screening is not necessary for these women.
3. Until further data become available to define the most effective strategy, the following two approaches are appropriate:

Screening-based Approach—All pregnant women should be screened at 35–37 weeks' gestation for anogenital GBS colonization (Fig 1). Patients

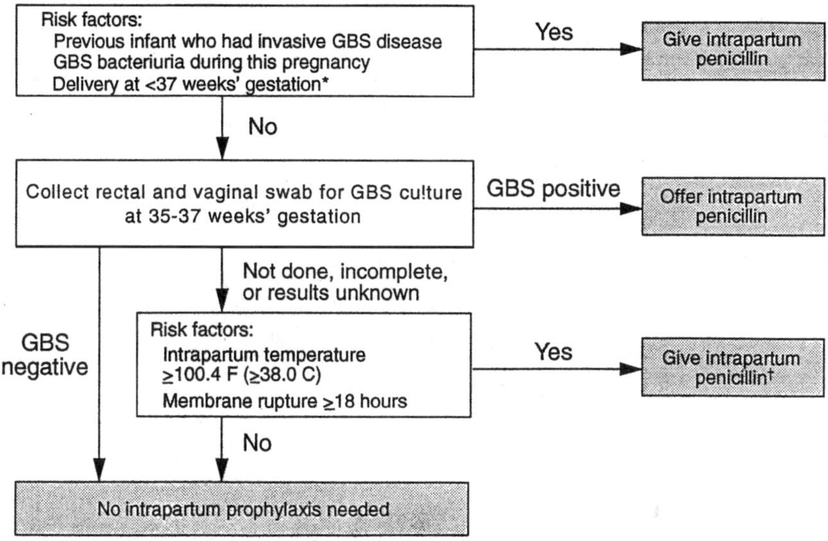

FIGURE 1.—Algorithm for prevention of early-onset group B streptococcal (*GBS*) disease in neonates, using prenatal screening at 35–37 weeks' gestation. *If membranes rupture at less than 37 weeks' gestation, and the mother has not begun labor, the GBS culture should be collected and either antibiotics should be administered until cultures are completed and the results are negative or antibiotics should be begun only when positive cultures are available. No prophylaxis is needed if culture obtained at 35–37 weeks' gestation was negative. †Broader spectrum antibiotics may be considered at the physician's discretion, based on clinical indications. (Reprinted from Centers for Disease Control and Prevention: Prevention of perinatal group B streptococcal disease: A public health perspective. *MMWR* 45(No. RR-7):1–24, 1996.)

should be informed of screening results and of potential benefits and risks of intrapartum antimicrobial prophylaxis for GBS carriers. Information systems should be developed and monitored to ensure that prenatal culture results are available at the time and place of delivery. Intrapartum chemoprophylaxis should be offered to all pregnant women identified as GBS carriers by culture at 35–37 weeks' gestation.

If the result of GBS culture is not known at the time of labor, intrapartum antimicrobial prophylaxis should be administered if one of the following risk factors is present: fewer than 37 weeks' gestation, duration of membrane rupture of 18 hours or more, or temperature of 100.4°F (38.0°C) or greater.

Culture techniques that maximize the likelihood of GBS recovery should be used. Because lower vaginal and rectal cultures are recommended, cultures should not be collected by speculum examination. The optimal method for GBS screening is collection of a single standard culture swab or two separate swabs of the distal vagina and anorectum. Swabs may be placed in a transport medium (e.g., Amies') if the microbiology laboratory is offsite. The sample should be identified for the laboratory as specifically for GBS culture. Specimens should be inoculated into selective broth medium (either SBM broth or Lim broth), followed by overnight incubation and then subcultured onto solid blood agar medium. In this screening

BOX 1. Procedure for Collecting and Processing Clinical Specimens for Culture of Group B Streptococcus

1. Obtain one or two swabs of the vaginal introitus and anorectum. Cervical cultures are not acceptable; a speculum should not be used for culture collection.
2. Place the swabs into a transport medium. The swabs in a transport medium will maintain GBS viability for up to 4 days at room temperature or under refrigeration. Appropriate nonnutritive moist swab transport systems (e.g., Amies') are commercially available.
3. Remove the swabs from the transport medium and inoculate both swabs together into selective broth medium. Todd-Hewitt broth supplemented with either colistin (10 g/mL) and nalidixic acid (15 g/mL) or with gentamicin (8 g/mL) and nalidixic acid (15 g/mL) may be used; appropriate commercially available options include Lim or SBM broth.
4. Incubate selective broth for 18–24 hrs. Subculture the broth to sheep blood agar plate.
5. Inspect and identify organisms suggestive of GBS (beta hemolytic or nonhemolytic, gram-positive and catalase negative). If GBS is not identified after incubation for 18–24 hrs on sheep blood agar plate, reincubate and inspect at 48 hrs to identify suspected organisms.
6. Various slide agglutination tests or other tests for GBS antigen detection (e.g., genetic probe or fluorescent antibody) may be used for specific identification, or the CAMP test may be employed for presumptive identification.

(Reprinted from Centers for Disease Control and Prevention: Prevention of perinatal group B streptococcal disease: A public health perspective. *MMWR* 45(No. RR-7):1–24, 1996.)

culture, there is no need for the laboratory to culture for other organisms. A laboratory procedure to maximize recovery is detailed (Box 1).

Laboratories should report results (positive and negative) to both the anticipated site of delivery and the health care provider who ordered the test. Ideally, laboratories that perform GBS cultures will ensure that clinicians have continuous access (i.e., 24 hours per day, 7 days per week) to culture results.

Oral antimicrobial agents should not be used to treat women who are found to be colonized with GBS during prenatal screening. Such treatment is not effective in eliminating carriage or preventing neonatal disease.

Risk Factor Approach—A prophylaxis strategy based on the presence of intrapartum risk factors alone (e.g., less than 37 weeks' gestation, duration of membrane rupture of 18 hours or more, or temperature of 100.4°F [38.0°C] or more) is an acceptable alternative (Fig 2).

For intrapartum chemoprophylaxis, IV penicillin G (5 mU initially and then 2.5 mU every 4 hours) should be administered until delivery (Box 2). Intravenous ampicillin (2 g initially and then 1 g every 4 hours until delivery) is an acceptable alternative to penicillin G, but penicillin G is preferred because it has a narrow spectrum and thus is less likely to select for antibiotic resistant organisms. Clindamycin or erythromycin may be used for women who are allergic to penicillin, although the efficacy of these drugs for GBS disease prevention has not been measured in controlled trials. (Note: Penicillin G does not need to be administered to women who have clinical diagnoses of amnionitis and who are receiving other treatment regimens that include agents active against streptococci [e.g., ampicillin or clindamycin].)

Routine use of prophylactic antimicrobial agents for infants born to mothers who received intrapartum prophylaxis is not recommended. However, therapeutic use of these agents is appropriate for those infants suspected clinically of having sepsis. Additional research is needed to

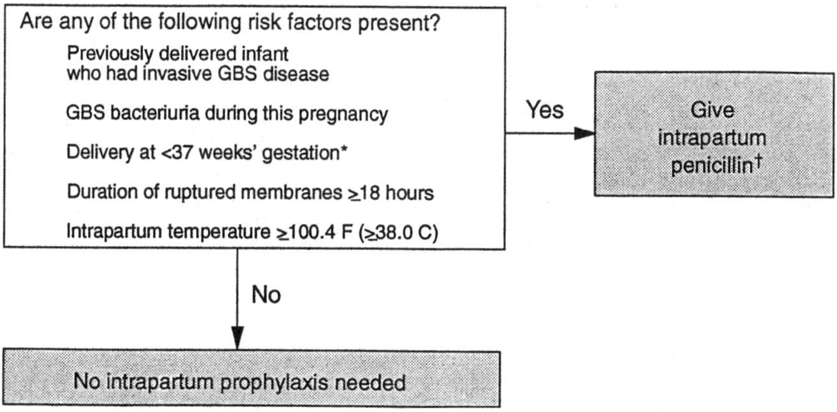

FIGURE 2.—Algorithm for prevention of early-onset group B streptococcal (*GBS*) disease in neonates, using risk factors. *If membranes rupture at less than 37 weeks' gestation, and the mother has not begun labor, the GBS culture should be collected and either antibiotics should be administered until cultures are completed and the results are negative or antibiotics should be begun only when positive cultures are available. No prophylaxis is needed if culture obtained at 35–37 weeks' gestation was negative. †Broader spectrum antibiotics may be considered at the physician's discretion, based on clinical indications. (Reprinted from Centers for Disease Control and Prevention: Prevention of perinatal group B streptococcal disease: A public health perspective. *MMWR* 45(No. RR-7):1–24, 1996.)

determine algorithms for management of infants born to mothers who receive intrapartum antimicrobial prophylaxis. One algorithm for empiric management of these newborns is provided (Fig 3). Other management approaches, developed by individual physicians or institutions, may be appropriate alternatives.

Local and state public health agencies, in conjunction with appropriate groups of hospitals, should consider establishing surveillance to monitor the incidence of neonatal GBS disease, occurrence of adverse reaction to antimicrobial prophylaxis, and the emergence of perinatal infections caused by penicillin-resistant organisms.

BOX 2. Recommended Regimens for Intrapartum Antimicrobial Prophylaxis for Perinatal Group B Streptococcal Disease

Recommended	Penicillin G, 5 mU IV load, then 2.5 mUs IV every 4 hrs until delivery
Alternative	Ampicillin, 2 g IV load, then 1 g IV every 4 hrs until delivery
If penicillin-allergic	
Recommended	Clindamycin, 900 mg IV every 8 hrs until delivery
Alternative	Erythromycin, 500 mg IV every 6 hrs until delivery

*If patient is receiving treatment for amnionitis with an antimicrobial agent active against group B streptococci (e.g., ampicillin, penicillin, clindamycin, or erythromycin), additional prophylactic antibiotics are not needed.

(Reprinted from Centers for Disease Control and Prevention: Prevention of perinatal group B streptococcal disease: A public health perspective. *MMWR* 45(No. RR-7):1–24, 1996.)

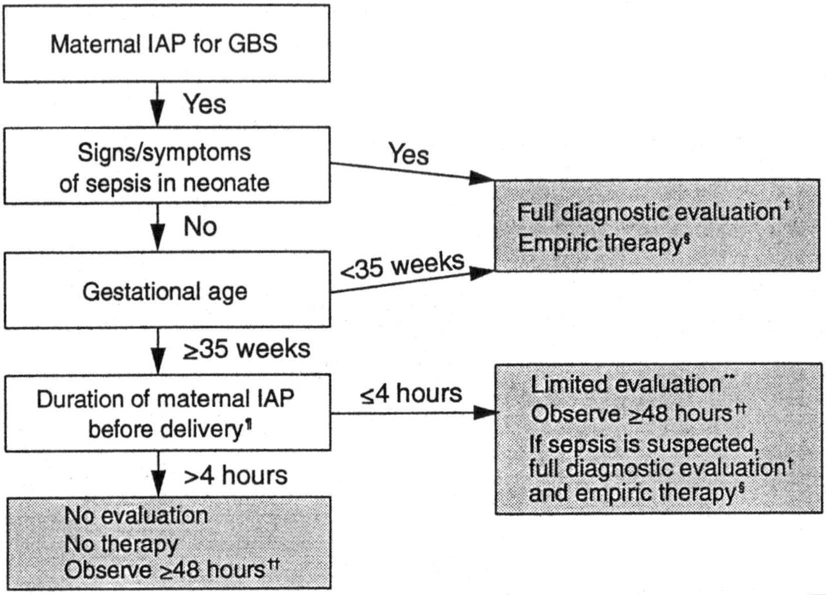

FIGURE 3.—Algorithm* for management of a neonate born to a mother who received intrapartum antimicrobial prophylaxis (*IAP*) for prevention of early-onset group B streptococcal (*GBS*) disease. *This algorithm is not an exclusive course of management. Variations that incorporate individual circumstances or institutional preferences may be appropriate. †Includes a complete blood count (*CBC*) and differential, blood culture, and chest radiograph if neonate has respiratory symptoms. Lumbar puncture is performed at the discretion of the physician. §Duration of therapy will vary depending on blood culture and cerebrospinal fluid (*CSF*) results and the clincial course of the infant. If laboratory results and clinical course are unremarkable, duration of therapy may be as short as 48–72 hours. ¶Duration of penicillin or ampicillin chemoprophylaxis. **CBC and differential and a blood culture. ††Does not allow early discharge. (Reprinted from Centers for Disease Control and Prevention: Prevention of perinatal group B streptococcal disease: A public health perspective. *MMWR* 45(No. RR-7):1–24, 1996.)

Investigations designed to evaluate and compare these two strategies and others are needed. Such studies will require the participation of multiple institutions and should evaluate multiple outcomes (e.g., perinatal GBS infections, adverse reactions to antimicrobial prophylaxis, and perinatal infections caused by penicillin-resistant organisms). Characterization of protocol failures may contribute to improvement of future prevention strategies.

References

1. Baker CJ, Edwards MS: Group B streptococcal infection, in Remington J, Klein JO (eds): *Infectious Diseases of the Fetus and Newborn Infant*, ed 4. Philadelphia, WB Saunders, 1995, pp 980–1054.
2. Zangwill KM, Schuchat A, Wenger JD: Group B streptococcal disease in the United States, 1990: Report from a multistate active surveillance system. *MMWR CDC Surveill Summ* 41(6):25–32, 1992.
3. Farley MM, Harvey RC, Stull T, et al: A population-based assessment of invasive disease due to group B streptococcus in nonpregnant adults. *N Engl J Med* 328:1807–1811, 1993.

4. Weisman LE, Stoll BJ, Cruess DF, et al: Early-onset group B streptococcal sepsis: A current assessment. *J Pediatr* 121:428–433, 1992.
5. Schwartz B, Schuchat A, Oxtoby MJ, et al: Invasive group B streptococcal disease in adults: A population-based study in metropolitan Atlanta. *JAMA* 266:1112–1114, 1991.
6. Dillon HC, Khare S, Gray BM: Group B streptococcal carriage and disease: A 6-year prospective study. *J Pediatr* 110:31–36, 1987.
7. Opal SM, Cross A, Palmer M, et al: Group B streptococcal sepsis in adults and infants: Contrasts and comparisons. *Arch Intern Med* 148:641–645, 1988.
8. Pass MA, Gray BM, Khare S, et al: Prospective studies of group B streptococcal infections in infants. *J Pediatr* 95:431–433, 1979.
9. Ancona RJ, Ferrieri P, Williams PP: Maternal factors that enhance the acquisition of group B streptococci by newborn infants. *J Med Microbiol* 3:273–280, 1980.
10. Lannering B, Larsson LE, Rojas J, et al: Early onset group B streptococcal disease: Seven year experience and clinical scoring system. *Acta Paediatr Scand* 72:597–602, 1983.
11. Gladstone IM, Ehrenkranz RA, Edberg SC, et al: A ten-year review of neonatal sepsis and comparison with the previous fifty-year experience. *Pediatr Infect Dis J* 9:819–825, 1990.
12. Anthony BF, Okada DM, Hobel CJ: Epidemiology of group B Streptococcus: Longitudinal observations during pregnancy. *J Infect Dis* 137:524–530, 1978.
13. Regan JA, Klebanoff MA, Nugent RP: Vaginal infections and prematurity study group: The epidemiology of group B streptococcal colonization in pregnancy. *Obstet Gynecol* 77:604–610, 1991.
14. Yow MD, Leeds LJ, Mason EO, et al: The natural history of group B streptococcal colonization in the pregnant woman and her offspring. I. Colonization studies. *Am J Obstet Gynecol* 137:34–38, 1980.
15. Dillon HC, Gray E, Pass MA, et al: Anorectal and vaginal carriage of group B streptococci during pregnancy. *J Infect Dis* 145:794–799, 1982.
16. Boyer KM, Gadzala CA, Kelly PD, et al: Selective intrapartum chemoprophylaxis of neonatal group B streptococcal early-onset disease. II. Predictive value of prenatal cultures. *J Infect Dis* 148:802–809, 1983.
17. Badri MS, Zawaneh S, Cruz AC, et al: Rectal colonization with group B streptococcus: Relation to vaginal colonization of pregnant women. *J Infect Dis* 135:308–312, 1977.
18. Baker CJ, Goroff DK, Alpert S, et al: Vaginal colonization with group B streptococcus: A study of college women. *J Infect Dis* 135:392–397, 1977.
19. Ferrieri P, Blair LL: Pharyngeal carriage of group B streptococci: Detection by three methods. *J Clin Microbiol* 6:136–139, 1977.
20. Boyer KM, Gotoff SP: Strategies for chemoprophylaxis of GBS early-onset infections. *Antibiot Chemother* 35:267–280, 1985.
21. Schuchat A, Oxtoby M, Cochi S, et al: Population-based risk factors for neonatal group B streptococcal disease: Results of a cohort study in metropolitan Atlanta. *J Infect Dis* 162:672–677, 1990.
22. Schuchat A, Deaver-Robinson K, Plikaytis BD, et al: Multistate case-control study of maternal risk factors for neonatal group B streptococcal disease. *Pediatr Infect Dis J* 13:623–629, 1994.
23. Baker CJ, Kasper DL: Correlation of maternal antibody deficiency with susceptibility to neonatal group B streptococcal infection. *N Engl J Med* 294:753–756, 1976.
24. Carstensen H, Christensen KK, Grennert L, et al: Early-onset neonatal group B streptococcal septicaemia in siblings. *J Infect* 17:201–204, 1988.
25. Faxelius G, Bremme K, Christensen KK, et al: Neonatal septicemia due to group B streptococci: perinatal risk factors and outcome of subsequent pregnancies. *J Perinat Med* 16:423–430, 1988.

26. Christensen KK, Dahlander K, Linden V, et al: Obstetrical care in future pregnancies after fetal loss in group B streptococcal septicemia: A prevention program based on bacteriological and immunological follow-up. *Eur J Obstet Gynecol Reprod Biol* 12:143–150, 1981.
27. Wood EG, Dillon HC: A prospective study of group B streptococcal bacteriuria in pregnancy. *Am J Obstet Gynecol* 140:515–520, 1981.
28. Moller M, Thomsen AC, Borch K, et al: Rupture of fetal membranes and premature delivery associated with group B streptococci in urine of pregnant women. *Lancet* ii:69–70, 1984.
29. Liston TE, Harris RE, Foshee S, et al: Relationship of neonatal pneumonia to maternal urinary and neonatal isolates of group B streptococci. *South Med J* 72:1410–1412, 1979.
30. Persson K, Christensen KK, Christensen P, et al: Asymptomatic bacteriuria during pregnancy with special reference to group B streptococci. *Scand J Infect Dis* 17:195–199, 1985.
31. Pass MA, Khare S, Dillon HC: Twin pregnancies: Incidence of group B streptococcal colonization and disease. *J Pediatr* 97:635–637, 1980.
32. Edwards MS, Jackson CV, Baker CJ: Increased risk of group B streptococcal disease in twins. *JAMA* 245:2044–2046, 1981.
33. Cochi SL, Feldman RA: Estimating national incidence of group B streptococcal disease: The effect of adjusting for birth weight. *Pediatr Infect Dis J* 2:414–415, 1983.
34. Easmon CSF, Hastings MJG, Clare AJ, et al: Nosocomial transmission of group B streptococci. *BMJ* 283:459–461, 1981.
35. Anthony BF, Okada DM, Hobel CJ: Epidemiology of the group B streptococcus: Maternal and nosocomial sources for infant acquisitions. *J Pediatr* 95:431–436, 1979.
36. Yancey MK, Duff P, Clark P, et al: Peripartum infection associated with vaginal group B streptococcal colonization. *Obstet Gynecol* 84:816–819, 1994.
37. Baker CJ, Edwards MS, Kasper DL: Role of antibody to native type III polysaccharide of group B streptococcus in infant infection. *Pediatrics* 68:544–549, 1981.
38. Baker CJ, Rench MA, Edwards MS, et al: Immunization of pregnant women with a polysaccharide vaccine of group B streptococcus. *N Engl J Med* 319:1180–1185, 1988.
39. Schuchat A, Wenger JD: Epidemiology of group B streptococcal disease: Risk factors, prevention strategies and vaccine development. *Epidemiol Rev* 16:374–402, 1994.
40. Lewin EB, Amstey MS: Natural history of group B streptococcus colonization and its therapy during pregnancy. *Am J Obstet Gynecol* 139:512–515, 1981.
41. Merenstein GB, Todd WA, Brown G, et al: Group B beta-hemolytic streptococcus: Randomized controlled treatment study at term. *Obstet Gynecol* 55:315–318, 1980.
42. Hall RT, Barnes W, Krishnan L, et al: Antibiotic treatment of parturient women colonized with group B streptococci. *Am J Obstet Gynecol* 124:630–634, 1976.
43. Gardner SE, Yow MD, Leeds LJ, et al: Failure of penicillin to eradicate group B streptococcal colonization in the pregnant woman: A couple study. *Am J Obstet Gynecol* 135:1062–1065, 1979.
44. Pyati SP, Pildes RS, Jacobs NM, et al: Penicillin in infants weighing two kilograms or less with early-onset group B streptococcal disease. *N Engl J Med* 308:1383–1389, 1983.
45. Siegel JD, McCracken GHJ, Threlkeld N, et al: Single dose penicillin prophylaxis against neonatal group B streptococcal infections: A controlled trial in 18,738 newborn infants. *N Engl J Med* 303:769–775, 1980.
46. Siegel JD, McCracken GHJ, Threlkeld N, et al: Single-dose penicillin prophylaxis of neonatal group B streptococcal disease. *Lancet* i:1426–1430, 1982.
47. Yow MD, Mason EO, Leeds LJ, et al: Ampicillin prevents intrapartum transmission of group B streptococcus. *JAMA* 241:1245–1247, 1979.

48. Easmon CSF, Hastings MJG, Deeley J, et al: The effect of intrapartum chemoprophylaxis on the vertical transmission of group B streptococci. *Br J Obstet Gynaecol* 90:633–635, 1983.
49. Boyer KM, Gadzala CA, Kelly PD, et al: Selective intrapartum chemoprophylaxis of neonatal group B streptococcal early-onset disease. III. Interruption of mother-to-infant transmission. *J Infect Dis* 148:810–816, 1983.
50. Matorras R, Garcia-Perea A, Omenaca F, et al: Intrapartum chemoprophylaxis of early-onset group B streptococcal disease. *Eur J Obstet Gynecol Reprod Biol* 40:57–62, 1991.
51. Lim DV, Morales WJ, Walsh AF, et al: Reduction of morbidity and mortality rates for neonatal group B streptococcal disease through early diagnosis and chemoprophylaxis. *J Clin Microbiol* 23:489–492, 1986.
52. Allardice JG, Baskett TF, Seshia MMK, et al: Perinatal group B streptococcal colonization and infection. *Ann J Obstet Gynecol* 142:617–620, 1982.
53. Garland SM, Fliegner JR: Group B streptococcus and neonatal infections: The case for intrapartum chemoprophylaxis. *Aust N Z J Obstet Gynaecol* 31:119–122, 1991.
54. Boyer KM, Gotoff SP: Prevention of early-onset neonatal group B streptococcal disease with selective intrapartum chemoprophylaxis. *N Engl J Med* 314:1665–1669, 1986.
55. Boyer KM, Gadzala CA, Burd LI, et al: Selective intrapartum chemoprophylaxis of neonatal group B streptococcal early-onset disease. I. Epidemiologic rationale. *J Infect Dis* 148:795–801, 1983.
56. Boyer KM, Gotoff SP: Antimicrobial prophylaxis of neonatal group B streptococcal sepsis. *Clin Perinatol* 15:831–850, 1988.
57. Morales WJ, Lim DV, Walsh AF: Prevention of neonatal group B streptococcal sepsis by the use of a rapid screening test and selective intrapartum chemoprophylaxis. *Am J Obstet Gynecol* 155:979–983, 1986.
58. Tuppurainen N, Hallman M: Prevention of neonatal group B streptococcal disease: Intrapartum detection and chemoprophylaxis of heavily colonized parturients. *Obstet Gynecol* 73:583–587, 1989.
59. Morales WJ, Lim D: Reduction of group B streptococcal maternal and neonatal infections in preterm pregnancies with premature rupture of membranes through a rapid identification test. *Am J Obstet Gynecol* 157:13–16, 1987.
60. Allen UD, Navas L, King SM: Effectiveness of intrapartum penicillin prophylaxis in preventing early-onset group B streptococcal infection: Results of a meta-analysis. *Can Med Assoc J* 149:1659–1665, 1993.
61. Ohlsson A, Myhr TL: Intrapartum chemoprophylaxis of perinatal group B streptococcal infections: A critical review of randomized controlled trials. *Am J Obstet Gynecol* 170:910–917, 1994.
62. American Academy of Pediatrics: Guidelines for prevention of group B streptococcal infection by chemoprophylaxis. *Pediatrics* 90:775–778, 1992.
63. Minkoff H, Mead P: An obstetric approach to the prevention of early-onset group B beta-hemolytic streptococcal sepsis. *Am J Obstet Gynecol* 154:973–977, 1986.
64. Hankins GV, Chalas E: Group B streptococcal infections in pregnancy: ACOG's recommendations. *ACOG Newsletter* 37:2, 1993.
65. American College of Obstetricians and Gynecologists: Survey shows continued confusion over management of GBS in pregnancy. *ACOG Newsletter* 38:1, 10, 1994.
66. Landon MB, Harger J, McNellis D, et al: Prevention of neonatal group B streptococcal infection. *Obstet Gynecol* 84:460–462, 1994.
67. Society of Obstetricians and Gynaecologists of Canada and Canadian Pediatric Society: National consensus statement on the prevention of early-onset group B streptococcal infections in the newborn. *J Soc Obstetricians Gynaecologists Canada Can Pediatr Soc* 16:2271–2278, 1994.
68. Rouse DJ, Goldenberg RL, Cliver SP, et al: Strategies for the prevention of early-onset neonatal group B streptococcal sepsis: A decision analysis. *Obstet Gynecol* 83:483–494, 1994.

69. Schwartz B, Jackson L: Invasive group B streptococcal disease in adults. *JAMA* 266:3284, 1991.
70. Goodman LS, Gilman A, Gilman AG (eds): *Goodman and Gilman's The Pharmacologic Basis of Therapeutics*, ed 8. New York, Pergamon Press, 1990.
71. Hein K, Alge A, Marth C: Anaphylactic reaction to ampicillin and severe complication in the fetus. *Lancet* 337:859–860, 1991.
72. Cunningham R, Walker C, Ridgway E: Prosthetic hip-joint infection associated with a penicillin-tolerant group B streptococcus. *J Infect* 25:77–81, 1992.
73. Steinbrecher UP: Serious infection in an adult due to penicillin-tolerant group B streptococcus. *Arch Intern Med* 141:1714–1715, 1981.
74. Severin MJ, Wiley JL: Change in susceptibility of group B streptococci to penicillin G from 1968 through 1975. *Antimicrob Agents Chemother* 10:380–381, 1976.
75. McDuffie RS, McGregor JA, Gibbs RS: Adverse perinatal outcome and resistant *Enterobacteriaceae* after antibiotic usage for premature rupture of the membranes and group B streptococcus carriage. *Obstet Gynecol* 82:487–489, 1993.
76. Amstey MS, Gibbs RS: Is penicillin G a better choice than ampicillin for prophylaxis of neonatal group B streptococcal infections? *Obstet Gynecol* 84:1058–1059, 1994.
77. Gibbs RS, McGregor JA, Mead PB, et al: A survey of practices in infectious diseases by obstetrician-gynecologists. *Obstet Gynecol* 83:631–636, 1994.
78. Yancey MK, Armer T, Clark P, et al: Assessment of rapid identification tests for genital carriage of group B streptococci. *Obstet Gynecol* 80:1038–1047, 1992.
79. Towers CV, Garite TJ, Friedman WW, et al: Comparison of a rapid enzyme-linked immunosorbent assay test and the Gram stain for detection of group B streptococcus in high-risk antepartum patients. *Am J Obstet Gynecol* 163:965–967, 1990.
80. Mole-Boetani J, Schuchat A, Plikaytis BD, et al: Comparison of prevention strategies for neonatal group B streptococcal infection: A population-based economic analysis. *JAMA* 270:1442–1448, 1993.
81. Stray-Pederson B: Economic evaluation of maternal screening to prevent congenital syphilis. *Sex Transm Dis* 10:167–172, 1983.
82. Strickland DM, Yeomans ER, Hankins GDV: Cost effectiveness of intrapartum screening and treatment for maternal group B streptococcal colonization. *Am J Obstet Gynecol* 163:4–8, 1990.
83. Yancey MK, Duff P: An analysis of the cost-effectiveness of selected protocols for the prevention of neonatal group B streptococcal infection. *Obstet Gynecol* 83:367–371, 1994.
84. Wiswell TE, Stoll BJ, Tuggle JM: Management of asymptomatic, term gestation neonates born to mothers treated with intrapartum antibiotics. *Pediatr Infect Dis J* 9:826–831, 1990.
85. Pylipow M, Gaddis M, Kinney JS: Selective intrapartum prophylaxis for group B streptococcus colonization: Management and outcome of newborns. *Pediatrics* 93:631–635, 1994.
86. Gibbs RS, McDuffie RS, McNabb F, et al: Neonatal group B streptococcal sepsis during two years of a universal screening program. *Obstet Gynecol* 84:496–500, 1994.
87. Jafari HS, Schuchat A, Hilsdon R, et al: Barriers to prevention of perinatal group B streptococcal disease. *Pediatr Infect Dis J* 14:662–667, 1995.

Commentary

These recommendations from the CDC, prepared in collaboration with the American College of Obstetrics and Gynecology and the AAP, create a clear mandate for every institution with an obstetric service to adopt a strategy for prevention of early-onset neonatal sepsis caused by GBS. However, it is not clear that the two strategies proposed for management of pregnant women or the strategy suggested for management of neonates are the most effective, least expensive, most efficient, most easily implemented, or are "the best" by any other criteria.

Widespread implementation of antepartum screening is improbable, because of the logistical difficulty of ensuring that screening culture results are available at the time of delivery and the untenable medicolegal risk associated with even an occasional failure. Intrapartum prophylaxis based on risk factors alone is relatively inexpensive and logistically straightforward but is much less effective. Because of inaccurate assumptions and procedural errors in the analysis, the reductions in attack rates estimated by the CDC (86% and 79%, respectively) are excessive; we have estimated efficacies of 75% and 54%, respectively. Strategies other than those recommended in the consensus statement may be more effective and less costly. An alternative strategy based on intrapartum screening with a rapid diagnostic test, intrapartum prophylaxis of women who deliver before 31 weeks' gestation or have prolonged rupture of membranes, intrapartum fever, or GBS colonization, and postpartum prophylaxis of selected high-risk infants, is estimated to reduce the attack rate by 79%, at a cost more than 25% below that of the more effective of the CDC strategies.

This consensus statement should not be the last word on the subject, but it should prompt a renewal of vigorous debate of strategies for prevention of early-onset GBS disease. Each center should develop a systematic approach to management of this problem, which may differ from the options presented by the CDC. Recommendations for management of neonates should be integral components of these strategies. Failure to implement the CDC-approved protocols should not be considered to constitute substandard care, because other alternatives may be equivalent or even superior. Finally, it must be recognized that *no* strategy—even prophylactic treatment of all mothers and infants—will completely eradicate this devastating disease.

William E. Benitz, M.D.

1 The Fetus

A United States National Reference for Fetal Growth
Alexander GR, Himes JH, Kaufman RB, et al (Univ of Alabama, Birmingham; Univ of Minnesota, Minneapolis; Univ of Hawaii, Honolulu; et al)
Obstet Gynecol 87:163–168, 1996 1–1

Background.—Previous fetal growth curves defining small-for-gestational-age (SGA) infants have not been geographically or ethnically inclusive of the whole U.S. population. A national reference fetal growth curve was developed from 1991 U.S. resident live birth data, and sex-specific SGA criteria were developed. The new curve was compared with 4 curves developed earlier.

Methods.—The 1991 U.S. Live Birth File, from the National Center for Health Statistics, provided 3,808,689 cases of single, live birth weight for gestational age. After statistical removal of spurious-appearing data, 3,134,879 cases remained, from which fetal growth curves were con-

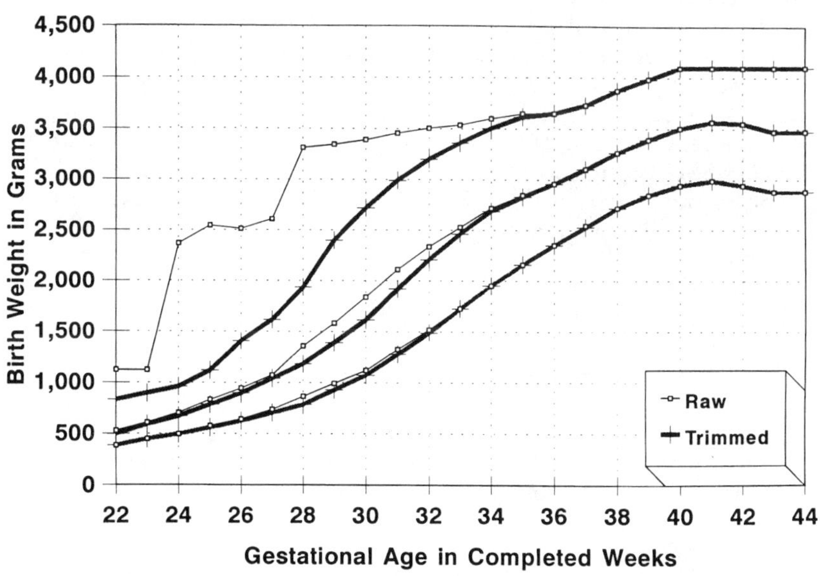

FIGURE 1.—Fetal growth curves for trimmed and raw data. (Courtesy of Alexander GR, Himes JH, Kaufman RB, et al: A United States national reference for fetal growth. *Obstet Gynecol* 87:163–168, 1996. Reprinted with permission of the American College of Obstetricians and Gynecologists.)

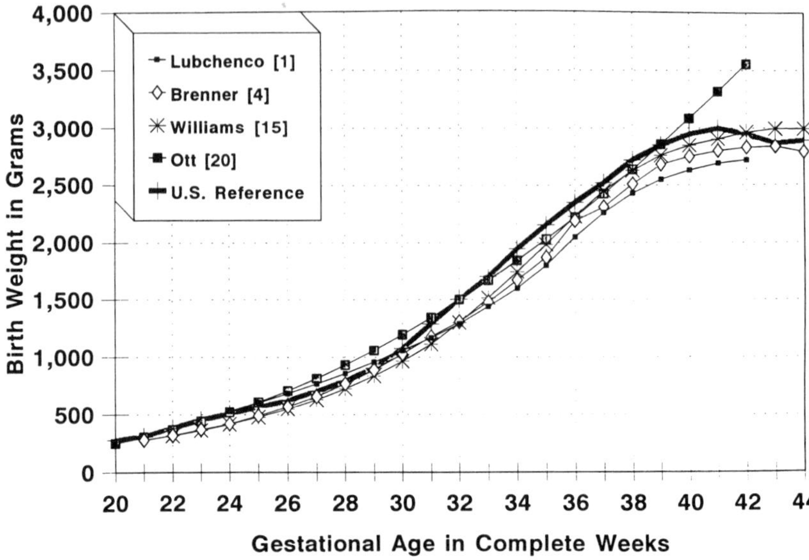

FIGURE 2.—Fetal growth by selected references. (Courtesy of Alexander GR, Himes JH, Kaufman RB, et al: A United States national reference for fetal growth. *Obstet Gynecol* 87:163–168, 1996. Reprinted with permission of the American College of Obstetricians and Gynecologists.)

structed and birth weight percentiles were calculated. They were compared to the prior growth charts of Lubchenco and colleagues, Brenner and associates, Williams, and Ott.

Results.—Because the raw data for the 90th percentile appeared to include many instances of inaccurately underestimated gestational age, the curves for the 10th, 50th, and 90th percentiles of fetal growth were trimmed statistically (Fig 1). Three of the 4 reference curves, when compared with the resulting 10th-percentile curve, tended to underestimate the number of SGA births, but Ott's curve tended to overestimate SGA births except for moderately preterm infants (Fig 2). After 32 weeks' gestation, male fetal weights for gestational age exceeded those of females at the 10th percentile.

Conclusions.—A new reference fetal growth curve was presented from current data compiled from the entire United States. Compared with this nationally inclusive fetal growth curve, previously developed curves generally tended to underestimate the number of SGA births.

► Patience supports purpose. The purpose of this U.S. national reference for fetal growth is to provide clinicians and investigators with the framework to define fetal growth restriction. Patience is paramount in sorting and manipulating more than 3 million data sets. The manuscript should serve as an excellent reference for readers interested in fetal growth. In addition to the curves it presents, there are smoothed tables of birth weight for gestational age from 20 to 44 weeks presented in percentiles from 5 to 95 and by sex.

The authors are to be congratulated on condensing this vast database into a presentable form. After resolution of implausible birth weight/gestational age combinations, or out-of-range and missing birth weight or gestational age values, the fetal growth curves were developed from 3,134,879 cases, yet the data are presented humbly as a national reference, not a standard. "Standards of growth assume an established rate of optimal development that can be applied widely to assess clinically relevant growth deviations that entail morbid consequences. At present limitations to our data preclude proposing standards." We accept the explanation, even if the distinction between national reference and standards flutters over our heads.

A.A. Fanaroff, M.B.B.Ch.

Antenatal Management of Alloimmune Thrombocytopenia With Intravenous γ-Globulin: A Randomized Trial of the Addition of Low-dose Steroid to Intravenous γ-Globulin

Bussel JB, Berkowitz RL, Lynch L, et al (Cornell Univ, New York; Mount Sinai School of Medicine; Tufts Med Ctr, Boston; et al)
Am J Obstet Gynecol 174:1414–1423, 1996 1–2

Purpose.—Fetal and neonatal thrombocytopenia occurring when a maternal IgG antibody against a paternal platelet antigen crosses the placenta is known as alloimmune thrombocytopenia. The condition recurs in nearly all platelet antigen–positive siblings; it is often more severe in subsequent siblings, and intracranial hemorrhage may occur in utero. In a pilot study, the authors found that IV γ-globulin, with or without concomitant steroids, can significantly increase the platelet count in most fetuses with alloimmune thrombocytopenia while reducing the risk of intracranial hemorrhage. The use of IV γ-globulin for antenatal treatment of alloimmune thrombocytopenia was evaluated in a prospective, randomized study.

Methods.—The study included 54 pregnant women with alloimmune thrombocytopenia and thrombocytopenic fetuses. The patients were randomized to receive maternal infusions of IV γ-globulin, 1 g/kg per week, with or without dexamethasone, 1.5 mg/day. For patients who did not respond by 4–6 weeks, IV γ-globulin therapy continued with the addition of prednisone, 60 mg/day. The analysis sought to determine whether the γ-globulin infusions could increase the platelet count and prevent intracranial hemorrhage in the fetuses with alloimmune thrombocytopenia, and to assess the additive effects of dexamethasone and prednisone.

Results.—Dexamethasone had no effects beyond those of IV γ-globulin. The mean fetal platelet count increased by 36,000/μL from the first to the second sampling, and by 69,000/μL from the first sampling to birth. The fetal response rate was 62% to 85%, and none had intracranial hemorrhage. "Salvage" therapy with prednisone increased the platelet count in 5 of 10 nonresponding fetuses.

Conclusion.—Maternal infusions of IV γ-globulin appear to be effective in increasing the platelet count and preventing intracranial hemorrhage in fetuses with alloimmune thrombocytopenia. This treatment should be tried before beginning weekly in utero platelet transfusions, even for fetuses with severe thrombocytopenia. The best approach to treating alloimmune thrombocytopenia remains to be determined; some noninvasive technique of predicting severe thrombocytopenia would be helpful.

▶ This comment has been co-authored by Daniel S. Seidman, M.D., The Sheba Medical Center, Tel-Hashomer, Israel:

▶ Fetal and neonatal alloimmune thrombocytopenia (analogous to Rhesus hemolytic disease of the newborn) arises from maternal-fetal platelet antigen incompatibility, which stimulates the production of maternal IgG platelet-specific antibodies. These antibodies cross the placenta, leading to fetal thrombocytopenia, which results in intracranial hemorrhage in 10% to 30% of affected fetuses and newborns. Alloimmune thrombocytopenia, the most frequent cause of severe thrombocytopenia in term newborns, is one of the few potentially catastrophic fetal conditions that can be effectively managed in utero.

The treatment of alloimmune thrombocytopenia has been based, in severely affected cases, on serial fetal blood sampling with transfusion of compatible platelets. This treatment demands high physician expertise and is associated with iatrogenic fetal loss, as fetuses affected with alloimmune thrombocytopenia are at increased risk for fatal exsanguination associated with cordocentesis.[1] The prenatal identification of fetal compatibility using fetal DNA derived from amniotic fluid may limit the need for percutaneous umbilical blood sampling.[2] However, no antenatal universal screening is currently available for detecting the 50% of cases with intracranial hemorrhage occurring in the first pregnancy.

Better techniques are being developed to allow large-scale screening by phenotyping platelets in whole blood samples.[3] The role of steroids and IV gamma globulin in the antenatal management of fetomaternal alloimmune thrombocytopenia is a controversial issue, especially in severely affected cases. The study abstracted here further supports the effectiveness of IV gamma globulin treatment for thrombocytopenic fetuses, although this has not been shown in other recent studies.[4] However, the most important contribution of this randomized study is the evidence that there is no benefit gained from adding dexamethasone to the gamma globulin regimen.

D. Seidman, M.D.
D.K. Stevenson, M.D.

References

1. Paidas MJ, Berkowitz RL, Lynch L, et al: Alloimmune thrombocytopenia: Fetal and neonatal losses related to cordocentesis. *Am J Obstet Gynecol* 172:475–479, 1995.

2. Denomme GA, Waye JS, Burrows RF, et al: The prenatal identification of fetal compatibility in neonatal alloimmune thrombocytopenia using amniotic fluid and variable number of tandem repeat (VNTR) analysis. *Br J Haematol* 91:742–746, 1995.
3. Bessos H, Mirza S, McGill A, et al: A whole blood assay for platelet HPA1 (PLA1) phenotyping applicable to large-scale screening. *Br J Haematol* 92:221–225, 1996.
4. Giers G, Hoch J, Bauer H, et al: Therapy with intravenous immunoglobulin G (iv IgG) during pregnancy for fetal alloimmune (HPA-1a) (Zw) thrombocytopenic purpura. *Prenat Diagn* 16:495–502, 1996.

The Effects of Antenatal Steroid Use in Premature Rupture of Membranes

Tucker L, Hoff C, Peevy K, et al (Univ of South Alabama, Mobile)
Aust N Z J Obstet Gynaecol 35:390–392, 1995 1–3

Background.—The use of antenatal steroids in the treatment of patients with premature rupture of the membranes (PROM) is one of the most controversial topics in obstetrics and gynecology. The value of such treatment was further investigated.

Methods.—One hundred forty-five mothers and neonates were included. Forty-five women with PROM were given steroids during gestational weeks 24–35. The remaining 100 women were given no antenatal steroids. The groups were identical in gestational age at membrane rupture, gravity, parity, race, fetal sex, socioeconomic status, smoking status, and preterm labor risk factors.

Findings.—The incidence of bronchopulmonary dysplasia was 0 in the neonates of the mothers who received steroids and 9% in the neonates of mothers not given steroids. This difference was significant. Maternal chorioamnionitis developed in 35.6% of those given steroids, compared with 67% of those not given steroids. The incidence of endometritis was not increased in the steroid group. The 2 groups did not differ significantly in preterm delivery rate, necrotizing enterocolitis, respiratory distress syndrome, intraventricular hemorrhage rate or hemorrhage severity, length of hospital stay, latency to delivery, or number of days on the ventilator.

Conclusions.—Bronchopulmonary dysplasia is a significant cause of morbidity in premature infants. The administration of steroids in women with PROM, which reduces the incidence of this process, therefore seems justified. Antenatal steroids were not associated with an increased risk of chorioamnionitis or endometriosis in this series.

▶ Commenting on this article is Louis P. Halamek, M.D., Professor of Pediatrics, Division of Neonatal and Developmental Medicine, Stanford University Medical Center, Palo Alto, California:

▶ Although this study suffers from the limitations of one that is retrospective in nature, it examines the important question of the maternal and fetal risks of steroid use in PROM. The authors confirmed the benefit to the fetus/neonate of a decreased risk of bronchopulmonary dysplasia. Surprisingly, they also found a maternal benefit in a *decreased* risk of maternal chorioamnionitis. This study adds to the growing body of literature that supports the liberal use of steroids in preterm labor; it appears that with few exceptions (e.g., maternal insulin-dependent diabetes mellitus) the benefits of prenatal steroids far outweigh the risks.

L.P. Halamek, M.D.

Trends and Variations in Use of Antenatal Corticosteroids to Prevent Neonatal Respiratory Distress Syndrome: Recommendations for National and International Comparative Audit

Tarnow-Mordi W, for the Scottish Neonatal Consultants' Collaborative Study Group, International Neonatal Network (Univ of Dundee, Scotland)

Br J Obstet Gynaecol 103:534–540, 1996 1–4

Introduction.—Respiratory distress syndrome and neonatal mortality were reduced by about 50% in infants delivered before 34 weeks' gestation of women who had received a course of antenatal corticosteroids given between 24 hours and 1 week before birth. There also was a reduction in neurologic abnormalities in childhood, necrotizing enterocolitis, and periventricular hemorrhage. A meta-analysis of 11 randomized, controlled trials confirmed these findings in 1990. A retrospective study was conducted to test the hypothesis that the use of antenatal corticosteroids in very preterm infants had increased since 1990 and to document variations in their use by hospital of birth.

Methods.—A total of 1,601 infants in 9 neonatal units were studied to determine whether corticosteroids had been administered for 24 hours or more before delivery on a more consistent basis. These infants were at 31 weeks' gestation. The infants were considered to have been exposed to antenatal corticosteroid therapy if their mothers had received a course of steroids, corticosteroids, glucocorticoids, glucocorticosteroids, betamethasone, dexamethasone, or hydrocortisone parenterally or orally before birth.

Results.—From 1988 to 1989, the proportion of infants in each hospital whose mothers had received antenatal corticosteroids for 24 hours or more before delivery was 16%. Between 1990 and 1993, the proportion was 29%. In district hospitals, 20% of infants had been treated for 24 hours or more, whereas in teaching hospitals, 28% had been treated. There were significant differences between individual hospitals in the proportions of infants who had been treated with antenatal corticosteroids, with a range of 0% to 36%.

Conclusions.—The use of antenatal corticosteroid therapy had increased in these hospitals. Further research should be done to evaluate the use of corticosteroid therapy in women at risk for preterm delivery, but this is complicated by difficulties in standardizing risks and indications for delivery. The benefits of antenatal corticosteroids will be denied to some infants unless permanent, systematic efforts are made to ensure their routine use. There should be a target for performance in which 90% of women whose infants are delivered 48 hours or more after hospital admission should have been treated with antenatal corticosteroids, and at least 70% should have been treated for 24 hours or more.

► It took a long time for the evidence that antenatal steroids were the most potent single strategy for reducing the consequences of preterm birth to translate into increased use. Indeed, it was rather remarkable when Sinclair presented a cumulative meta-analysis at the National Institutes of Health Consensus Conference in 1994; there was no deviation from the clinical significance reported in the initial studies by Liggins some 20 years ago.[1] Until the Consensus Conference, however, there was a reluctance to use steroids such that only about 20% of infants in the United States with birth weights of less than 1.5 kg were the beneficiaries of antenatal steroid therapy. Since the conference, there has been a rapid escalation such that almost 65% of these infants are now being treated with apparent success.[2] There has been a substantial decrease in mortality and respiratory distress syndrome as well as severe intracranial hemorrhage. There has been an increase in necrotizing enterocolitis for infants with birth weights of less than 1 kg, attributable to the presence of more survivors in this birth-weight category.[3]

The study of the Scottish Neonatal Consultants Collaborative Study Group is now reported. Essentially these researchers had observed an increase from 16% from 1988 to 1989 to 29% from 1990 to 1993, a far cry from the 70% achieved by Cooke and colleagues in Liverpool or by the Montreal group, who had long ago exceeded the 65% mark.[4] The reasons for the slow acceptance of very hard evidence are not worth delving into at this time. What is important is to set goals, as the Scottish group has done, and then to monitor steroid use. Remember that whereas a complete course (i.e., 24 hours) of therapy is desirable, partial therapy also is effective. The target of 70% for women hospitalized for at least 24 hours before premature birth is reasonable. It is equally important to continue to educate health care providers and the public so that they will request such therapy.

The need for patients on long-term steroid treatment to increase their dose of glucocorticoids when under stress is a principle that rests in one of the most tranquil corners of medical dogma.—Lancet 347:846, 1996.

A.A. Fanaroff, M.B.B.Ch.

References

1. National Institutes of Health Consensus Development Panel: Effect of corticosteroids for fetal maturation on perinatal outcomes. *JAMA* 273:413–418, 1995.
2. 1996 YEAR BOOK OF NEONATAL-PERINATAL MEDICINE. 1–2—1–8, 4–12.
3. Wright L, et al: *Pediatr Res* 41:214a 1997.
4. Cooke RWI, Ryan S, Walkinsaw S: Steroids for babies. *Lancet* 341:569, 1993.

Transabdominal Amnioinfusion in Oligohydramnios at Term Before Induction of Labor With Intact Membranes: A Randomized Clinical Trial

Vergani P, Ceruti P, Strobelt N, et al (Univ of Milan, Italy)

Am J Obstet Gynecol 175:465–470, 1996 1–5

Objective.—Because oligohydramnios increases the rate of perinatal morbidity and mortality, restoration of an adequate amount of amniotic fluid by transcervical amnioinfusion has been used for the past decade and has achieved a 75% reduction in the number of cesarean sections performed. Transabdominal amnioinfusion has been studied retrospectively only. A randomized clinical trial of transabdominal amnioinfusion evaluating the prevention of fetal distress, the rate of cesarean section, and perinatal outcome was performed.

Methods.—Between June 1991 and September 1994, labor was induced with prostaglandin E_2 in 39 amnioinfused and 40 control nonlaboring primiparous women with fetuses of 37 weeks or greater gestational age. The diagnostic criteria for oligohydramnios were a largest amniotic fluid pocket measuring less than 2 × 2 cm and color Doppler imaging demonstrating cord-free amniotic fluid pockets. Maternal and fetal heart rates were monitored continuously. Outcomes were compared statistically.

Results.—All the women assigned to the amnioinfusion group were infused successfully, and no bleeding complications or infections occurred. Significantly more women in the control group underwent cesarean section than in the amnioinfused group (Table 4). The control group also had a significantly higher incidence of fetal heart rate abnormalities than did the amnioinfused group (Table 5). Eight of the amnioinfused group and 6 of the control group showed meconium-stained amniotic fluid. Neonatal Apgar scores were similar. An umbilical artery pH level of 7.10 or less was observed in 1 of 22 neonates in the amnioinfused group and 4 of 22 neonates in the control group.

Conclusion.—Transabdominal amnioinfusion is a safe and effective alternative therapy for preventing fetal distress in nonlaboring women with oligohydramnios.

TABLE 4.—Mode of Delivery

	Amnioinfused group (n = 39)	*Control group (n = 40)*	*Significance*
Spontaneous vaginal delivery	34 (87%)	28 (70%)	
Cesarean deliveries	5 (13%)	12 (30%)	$p = 0.11$, RR 2.3 (0.8–10.9)
Cesarean deliveries for fetal distress	2 (5%)	10 (25%)	$p = 0.031$, RR 4.9 (1.1–32.4)

Note: χ^2 test.
Abbreviation: *RR*, relative risk.
(Courtesy of Vergani P, Ceruti P, Strobelt N, et al: Transabdominal amnioinfusion in oligohydramnios at term before induction of labor with intact membranes: A randomized clinical trial. *Am J Obstet Gynecol* 175:465–470, 1996.)

TABLE 5.—Fetal Heart Rate (FHR) Pattern During First Stage of Labor

FHR pattern	*Amnioinfused group (n = 37)*	*Control group (n = 33)*
Reassuring, nonreassuring	35 (95%)	19 (58%)
Suspicious, omnious	2 (5%)	14 (42%)

Note: $P = 0.0007$, relative risk 10.6 (2.4 to 56.4), χ^2 test.

(Courtesy of Vergani P, Ceruti P, Strobelt N, et al: Transabdominal amnioinfusion in oligohydramnios at term before induction of labor with intact membranes: A randomized clinical trial. *Am J Obstet Gynecol* 175:465–470, 1996.)

► There is a very descriptive title to this trial. It may take a few milliseconds for the significance to sink in, but we are more familiar with the use of amnioinfusion for oligohydramnios when the membranes have ruptured, labor has commenced, and the cervix has started to dilate, or when the amniotic fluid is heavily meconium stained.[1] Prophylactic transabdominal amnioinfusion, to prevent cord problems during labor and decrease the rate of operative deliveries for fetal distress in the presence of oligohydramnios, was the stated primary objective of this study. Oligohydramnios, which complicates about 4% of pregnancies, was defined by a largest amniotic fluid pocket measuring less than 2 × 2 cm. Color Doppler imaging was used to exclude the presence of umbilical cords within amniotic fluid pockets. Transabdominal amnioinfusion, under sonographic guidance by experienced operators, was accomplished successfully for all women assigned to that limb of the study. It resulted in a significant reduction in abnormal fetal heart rate tracings and a lower operative delivery rate. The cesarean section rate for the amnioinfused group equaled 12%, equivalent to that of the general population, a number one can publish proudly when the rate in many units exceeds 25%.

An unanticipated benefit was that transabdominal amnioinfusion appeared to induce labor for some women. Transabdominal amnioinfusion will be suitable for a small and select population of pregnancies with oligohydramnios and intact membranes. It should not be attempted in the presence of placenta previa, abruptio placentae, fetal malpresentations, multiple gestations, or abnormal fetal heart rate patterns before labor.

A.A. Fanaroff, M.B.B.Ch.

Reference

1. Cialone PR, Shere DM, Ryan RM, et al: Amnioinfusion during labor complicated by particulate meconium-stained amniotic fluid decreases neonatal morbidity. *Am J Obstet Gynecol* 170:842–849, 1994.

Chorionic Villus Sampling Safety

Kuliev A, Jackson L, Froster U, et al (World Health Organization Collaborating Ctr, Chicago)

Am J Obstet Gynecol 174:807–811, 1996 1–6

Objective.—In association with the Seventh International Conference on Early Prenatal Diagnosis of Genetic Diseases (1994), a World Health Organization (WHO)/EURO meeting analyzed the prevalence and pattern of limb reduction defects in children born after chorionic villus sampling (CVS). The source of the data was a WHO-sponsored CVS registry containing the accumulated experience of 138,996 cases.

Methods.—The WHO-sponsored CVS registry has been maintained since 1983. Reported cases came from 63 centers, most of which follow up with direct contact of patient or physician. Follow-up was recommended after a few clusters of children born with limb anomalies after CVS were described. A special format for registering cases was published to standardize data collection.

Results.—Chorionic villus sampling usually is performed between 9 and 12 weeks' gestation. The rate of spontaneous pregnancy loss after CVS has averaged 2.5% to 3.0%. At some large-volume centers, loss figures are 2% or lower, a rate comparable to that of amniocentesis. Neither the incidence nor the pattern of limb defects differed from that of the general population. The overall incidence of limb reduction defects after CVS is 5.2 to 5.7 per 10,000, compared with 4.8 to 5.97 per 10,000 in the general population. Transverse limb defects, in particular, showed no increased risk after CVS. Because data for evaluating the effect of sampling in the earliest weeks of pregnancy are lacking, CVS should not be performed before 9 weeks' gestation.

Conclusions.—Analysis of the data from the WHO-sponsored CVS registry confirms the overall safety of this procedure. The fetal loss rate is comparable to that of amniocentesis, and limb defects have not occurred at a rate higher than that of the general population. Reported clusters of limb reduction defects may be related to certain environmental exposures, such as maternal smoking.

▶ This abstract provides further insight into the risks of CVS and serves to justify the continuation of the registry. Despite the fact that the data represent 63 of 146 centers who report on a regular basis, any series that includes more than 100,000 patients, providing the data are collected reliably, will yield important information. The major objective was to analyze the prevalence of limb reduction defects in the registry and make recommendations regarding the use of CVS in practice. There was no increase in the overall incidence of limb reduction defects, and no difference in the pattern of deficiencies compared with the general population. There were too few data to analyze a potential causal relation with early CVS. The manuscript drew my attention to an association between maternal smoking and terminal transverse limb defects.[1]

We also have included the comments of Thomas H. Kirschbaum, M.D., editor of the YEAR BOOK OF OBSTETRICS, GYNECOLOGY AND WOMEN'S HEALTH, on a related article. (See also the 1995 YEAR BOOK OF NEONATAL AND PERINATAL MEDICINE, pp 1–2 and 21–22.)

A.A. Fanaroff, M.B.B.Ch.

Reference

1. Czeizel A, Koda I, Lenz W: Smoking during pregnancy and congenital limb deficiency. *BMJ* 308:1473–1476, 1994.

► This commentary, by Dr. Thomas H. Kirschbaum, Professor of Obstetrics & Gynecology at the Albert Einstein College of Medicine in the Bronx, New York, was taken from the 1997 YEAR BOOK OF OBSTETRICS, GYNECOLOGY, AND WOMEN'S HEALTH, on an article by Nicolaides et al.entitled, "Limb defects and chorionic villus sampling: Results from an international registry, 1992–1994." *Lancet* 347:489–494, 1996.

► This report of limb reduction defects after CVS collected from 63 European and American centers reporting to the WHO CVS Registry established in 1992 helps bring us up to date on this controversy.[1] After 2 initial reports of case incidences of more than 1% among 2 series of 289 and 394 cases of CVS, 2 larger studies, 1 of more than 80,000 cases of CVS[2] and 1 in a population study of 1.2 million births,[3] yielded incidence figures of about 1 in 1,600 (0.06%). In this, the largest collection of reported cases of CVS, the incidence of limb reduction defects ranged from 0.05% to 0.06%, depending on whether simple nail defects alone were counted and whether abortion material was included. Still, occasional reports of limb defects after CVS before 8 weeks' gestational age continue.[4] In this study, almost 25% of cases were excluded for inadequacies in data, and reports from multiple centers increase the chance of differences in data management and diagnostic criteria. It is impossible to prove that CVS does not result in an increased incidence of limb defects, just as it is impossible to prove any negative hypothesis. Nonetheless, the preponderance of data suggests that it does not occur with increased risk. It still seems prudent to avoid CVS before complete limb differentiation at 10 weeks' gestational age.

T.H. Kirschbaum, M.D.

References

1. 1993 YEAR BOOK OF OBSTETRICS AND GYNECOLOGY, pp 185–187.
2. Kuliev AM, Modell B, Jackson L, et al: Limb abnormalities and chorionic villus sampling. *Lancet* 340:668, 1992.
3. Froster-Iskenius UG, Baird PA: Limb reduction in over one million consecutive livebirths. *Teratology* 39:127–135, 1989.
4. Brambati B, Simoni G, Travi M, et al: Genetic diagnosis by chorionic villus sampling before 8 gestational weeks: Efficiency, reliability, and risks on 317 completed pregnancies. *Prenat Diagn* 12:789–799, 1992.

Size Disparity of the Choroid Plexuses of the Lateral Ventricles: Prenatal Diagnosis and Neonatal Outcome

Petrikovsky BM, Kaplan GP (North Shore Univ, Manhasset, NY; New York Univ)

Prenat Diagn 16:670–672, 1996 1–7

Background.—Reports of an association between fetal choroid plexus cysts and aneuploidy have prompted considerable debate. The natural history of another possible variation of choroid plexus structure—size disparity, defined as a marked asymmetry in appearance—was reported.

Methods and Findings.—Five of 1,260 second-trimester ultrasonography studies demonstrated a disparity in choroid plexus size. Monthly fetal brain sonography showed appropriately sized lateral ventricles for gestational age in all fetuses. Disparate choroid plexus appearances were no longer visible at the first follow-up at 20 weeks' gestation in 3 fetuses and at the second follow-up at 24 weeks' gestation in all 5. Perinatal outcomes were normal in 4 newborns, and 1 was delivered at 28 weeks. The karyotype was normal in all infants. No other structural anomalies were associated with the disparate choroid plexuses.

Conclusion.—In these 5 fetuses, the isolated findings of choroid plexus size disparity were rare and benign. Fetal ventriculomegaly did not develop in any of the fetuses. However, further research on size disparity of choroid plexuses is needed.

▶ Commenting on this article is Louis P. Halamek, M.D., Professor of Pediatrics, Division of Neonatal & Developmental Medicine, Stanford University Medical Center, Palo Alto, California:

▶ To paraphrase Yogi Berra, "You can observe a lot just by watching." Certainly, prenatal US has opened a picture window to the womb, and the views are breathtaking. The significance of many of these findings remains to be determined.

L.P. Halamek, M.D.

Antenatal Diagnosis of Cystic Hygroma or Nuchal Pad: Report of 92 Cases With Follow Up of Survivors

Boyd PA, Anthony MY, Manning N, et al (Oxford Radcliffe Women's Centre, England)

Arch Dis Child 74:F38–F42, 1996 1–8

Background.—An increased thickness at the back of the fetal neck has been associated with karyotypic abnormality in numerous studies. The prognosis for patients with a nuchal thickening or cystic hygroma, particularly those with a normal fetal karyotype, was investigated.

Methods.—All fetuses with a nuchal thickness of 6 mm or greater on the antenatal ultrasound during a 5-year period were studied. Outcome was determined with postmortem reports, neonatal records, and reports from the child's physician for children older than 1 year of age.

Results.—Ninety-two patients with nuchal thickening were identified, of whom 43 had a confirmed karyotypic abnormality, 25 had a normal karyotype but an additional abnormality detected on the antenatal US scan, and 24 had a normal karyotype and no other abnormalities. Of the 25 fetuses with normal karyotype but other abnormalities, 10 were liveborn. Of these 10 infants, 7 had a major problem. Of the 24 fetuses with solitary neck lesions and normal karyotype, 5 pregnancies were terminated. Of these 5, 2 had isolated cystic hygroma, 1 had cystic hygroma plus cleft palate, and 2 had no detected abnormality. Two other fetuses died before birth, although no abnormality was identified. There were 17 liveborn infants; all had normal neonatal evaluations. At follow-up, 10 of these infants ranged in age from 1 to 5 years; all were developmentally normal.

Conclusion.—The association between nuchal thickening and karyotypic abnormality was confirmed. There is also a high risk for other abnormalities in fetuses with nuchal thickening but normal karyotype. However, a good outcome is relatively likely when there is no evidence of another abnormality and the karyotype is normal.

▶ Christine Comstock, M.D., Director of Fetal Imaging, William Beaumont Hospital, Royal Oak, Michigan, comments:

▶ Because most infants with trisomy 21 are born to mothers less than 35 years of age (who would, therefore, not be considered at significant enough risk to warrant invasive testing such as amniocentesis or chorionic villus sampling), noninvasive methods of identifying fetuses with trisomy 21 are constantly being sought. Until recently, US has not been more than occasionally helpful in the detection of trisomy 21. However, increased nuchal thickness has proven to be very useful in multiple studies, demonstrating a specificity for abnormal karyotype of up to 50%, depending on the age of the mother and the reason for the initial scan. Nuchal thickness can be measured on antenatal US examinations by measuring from the calvarium to the outer skin line on an axial view of the fetal head. Although the original intent was to detect trisomy 21, almost half of the fetuses with an abnormal karyotype and increased nuchal thickness have trisomy 18 or Turner's syndrome.

In this 5-year study, an age range of 12–24 weeks was used; this is slightly expanded from the usual 16- to 21-week range and, more recently, 11 to 14 or 15 weeks. As the authors state, a nuchal thickness of greater than 3 mm is now used in the 11- to 14-week range, with increased sensitivity but decreased specificity. As other authors have found, there seems to be an increase in specificity if the nuchal pad contains septations vs. those that do not. Half of those fetuses with a thickened nuchal pad but normal karyotype had other anomalies discernible by US. Of these, 25% died in utero and 25% were liveborn but with significant abnormalities. Thus, parents cannot be completely reassured if the karyotype is normal. Measurement of the nuchal pad has gradually become part of the standard antenatal screen from 11–21 weeks. The extension to 24 weeks has not been justified in this or other studies.

C. Comstock, M.D.

Survival Motor Neuron Gene Deletion in the Arthrogryposis Multiplex Congenita–Spinal Muscular Atrophy Association

Bürglen L, Amiel J, Viollet L, et al (Hôpital des Enfants Malades, Paris; Hôpital du Kremlin-Bicêtre, France; Université de Liège, Belgium)

J Clin Invest 98:1130–1132, 1996 1–9

Introduction.—Infants with acute spinal muscular atrophy (SMA type I) have severe, generalized muscle weakness and hypotonia and usually die of respiratory failure within the first 2 years. The survival motor neuron (*SMN*) gene has been identified as the SMA-determining gene. In at least 90% of typical patients with SMA, this gene is absent or interrupted. Deletions of the *SMN* gene also appear in congenital heart disease and were present in 6 of 12 patients described who had the arthrogryposis multiplex congenita (AMC)-SMA association.

Methods.—Included in the study were 12 unrelated patients who were given a diagnosis of AMC-SMA association at birth. All had congenital joint contractures of at least 2 regions of the body, generalized muscle weakness with muscular atrophy and areflexia, electromyographic abnormalities, and a muscle biopsy specimen consistent with denervation. These patients had DNA extracted from peripheral blood leukocytes, lymphoblastoid cell lines, or muscle tissues.

Results.—Decreased fetal movements had been observed in 7 of the 12 patients and 9 had neonatal respiratory distress requiring artificial ventilation. Eight of the infants died of respiratory failure within the first month of life. In only 1 case was there a family history, suggesting an autosomal dominant form of AMC. In 6 of 12 infants *SMN* exons 7 and 8 were lacking on both mutant chromosomes. Three infants had a large, inherited deletion involving both loci on 1 parental allele; the other parental allele carried only 1 locus instead of the expected 2. The other 6 infants had neither point mutation in the *SMN* gene nor evidence for linkage to chromosome 5q13. All 6 infants with *SMN* gene deletions died within the first month of life; 4 of the 6 without the deletion are still alive.

Discussion.—Whereas arthrogryposis has been viewed as an exclusion criterion in SMA, data from this analysis strongly suggest that AMC of neurogenic origin is genetically heterogeneous, with a subgroup allelic to SMA. With *SMN* gene analysis, diagnosis will be easier in the AMC-SMA association and prenatal diagnosis will be possible.

▶ The geneticists are unraveling many of the mysteries of clinical medicine at a frenetic pace. This rapid publication in the prestigious *Journal of Clinical Investigation* sheds further light on the AMC-SMA complex. The international collaboration has accelerated this process as the various disorders have been classified and cases pooled for analysis.[1] The current investigators recently identified deletions of the *SMN* gene associated with SMA and congenital heart disease.[2] In the present report, the *SMN* gene was found in 6 of 12 patients who met strict criteria for AMC associated with SMA. All the patients had congenital joint contractures of at least 2 regions of the body; generalized muscle weakness with muscular atrophy and areflexia, without extraocular involvement; denervation and diminished motor action potential amplitude on electromyography; and muscle biopsy consistent with denervation and no evidence of storage material or other structural abnormalities.[1]

To support my statement about unraveling the mysteries of clinical medicine, the reader should know that this review was written on the day of the announcement of the cloning of the first mammal in history. The technological possibility of cloning mammals, including human beings, now exists. This generates profound moral, social, cultural, and economic questions that we will have to answer. For more information on this topic, see references 3 and 4.

To be what we are and to become what we are capable of becoming, it is the only end of life.—Robert Louis Stevenson

A.A. Fanaroff, M.B.B.Ch.

References

1. Munsat TL: Workshop Report: International SMA Collaboration. *Neuromuscul Disord* 1:81, 1991.
2. Lefebvre S, Burglen L, Reboullet S, et al: Identification and characterization of spinal muscular atrophy–determining gene. *Cell* 80:155–165, 1995.
3. Rodrigues NR, Owen N, Talbot K, et al: Deletions in the survival motor neuron gene on 5q13 in autosomal recessive spinal muscular atrophy. *Hum Mol Genet* 4:631–663, 1995.
4. Bussaglia E, Clermont O, Tizzano E, et al: A frame-shift deletion in the survival motor neuron gene in Spanish spinal muscular atrophy patients. *Nature* 11:335–337, 1995.

Congenital Cystic Adenomatoid Malformation in the Fetus: Natural History and Predictors of Outcome

Miller JA, Corteville JE, Langer JC (Washington Univ, St Louis)
J Pediatr Surg 31:805–808, 1996 1–10

Background.—Congenital cystic adenomatoid malformation (CCAM) is rare but often diagnosed by prenatal US. In some fetuses, nonimmune hydrops fetalis develops, which is fatal. In others, spontaneous resolution occurs and the fetus shows no signs of the lesion at birth. It is important to provide accurate prognostic information to the parents. Most prior studies have not included long-term follow-up information. The natural history of CCAM was studied, and prognostic indicators of this lesion were identified.

Methods.—The medical records of all fetuses with CCAM during a 7-year period were reviewed. The data that were collected and analyzed included gestational age at diagnosis and delivery, size and location of lesion, presence or absence of hydrops fetalis or other anomalies, and degree of mediastinal shift. The lesions were typed according to the Stocker classification. Follow-up data were obtained from hospital records and by telephone interview.

Results.—Congenital cystic adenomatoid malformation was diagnosed in 17 fetuses by prenatal US. Five fetuses died in utero, 4 with hydrops. Of the 12 fetuses carried to term, 1 had a thoracoamniotic shunt placed at 24 weeks. Resection was performed in all 12 infants. Four needed neonatal support. There was no correlation between outcome and CCAM-to-chest ratio, degree of mediastinal shift at diagnosis, location of lesion, or age at diagnosis. There was no correlation between outcome and predicted pathologic type by US or postoperative pathologic diagnosis. Predictors of outcome were the presence of hydrops and a decrease in the size of the malformation during gestation.

Conclusions.—A thoracoamniotic shunt or resection of the lesion in utero should be considered only for a fetus with signs of hydrops. Fetuses with CCAM should be monitored with serial US and delivered at a perinatal center. All CCAMs observed at birth should be resected. Pulmonary resection during infancy has low morbidity and mortality rates, and may prevent infection and occult malignant transformation. Counseling should stress the frequently positive outcome.

▶ Congenital cystic adenomatoid malformation of the lung has been the topic of a recent heated case discussion[1] and subsequent lively correspondence in *The New England Journal of Medicine*.[2, 3] This condition has been attributed to an arrest in lung development at a premature stage. The lesion can be reproduced in mice by overexpression of the gene for keratinocyte growth failure, and there have been concerns that failure of the lung at this immature state may predispose it to neoplastic changes.[4] Indeed, several neoplasms have been reported from unresected CCAMs, sparking the debate about the merits of resection. Adding fuel to the fire concerning the need for operation are the data from Thorpe-Beeston and Nicolaides, who reported a series of 61 liveborn infants, 16 of whom (26%) did not need operation.[5] The issue of diagnosis and treatment in the fetus is clarified by Barret's series from Toronto. In the absence of nonimmune hydrops, the prognosis is excellent and no intervention before birth need be contemplated. It was encouraging to read that if there was no hydrops at the time of diagnosis of the CCAM, hydrops fetalis subsequently developed in only 6% of patients. The presence of hydrops fetalis, however, places the fetus in great jeopardy and selected surgical intervention may be warranted.

A.A. Fanaroff, M.B.B.Ch.

References

1. Case records of the Massachusetts General Hospital (case 20—1996). *N Engl J Med* 334:1726–1732, 1996.

2. Ward SJ: Surgery for congenital cystic adenomatoid malformation of the lung. *N Engl J Med* 335:1689, 1996.
3. Kinane TB: Surgery for congenital cystic adenomatoid malformation of the lung (reply). *N Engl J Med* 335:1689–1690, 1996.
4. Simonet WS, DeRose ML, Bucay N, et al: Pulmonary malformation in transgenic mice expressing human keratinocyte growth factor in the lung. *Proc Natl Acad Sci U S A* 92:12,461–12,465, 1995.
5. Thorpe-Beeston JG, Nicolaides KH: Cystic adenomatoid malformation of the lung: Prenatal diagnosis and outcome. *Prenat Diagn* 14:677–688, 1994.

Outcome of Isolated Congenital Complete Heart Block Diagnosed In Utero

Groves AMM, Allan LD, Rosenthal E (Guy's Hosp, London)
Heart 75:190–194, 1996 1–11

Background.—Recently, cardiac failure and death have been documented in fetuses with isolated congenital complete heart block diagnosed

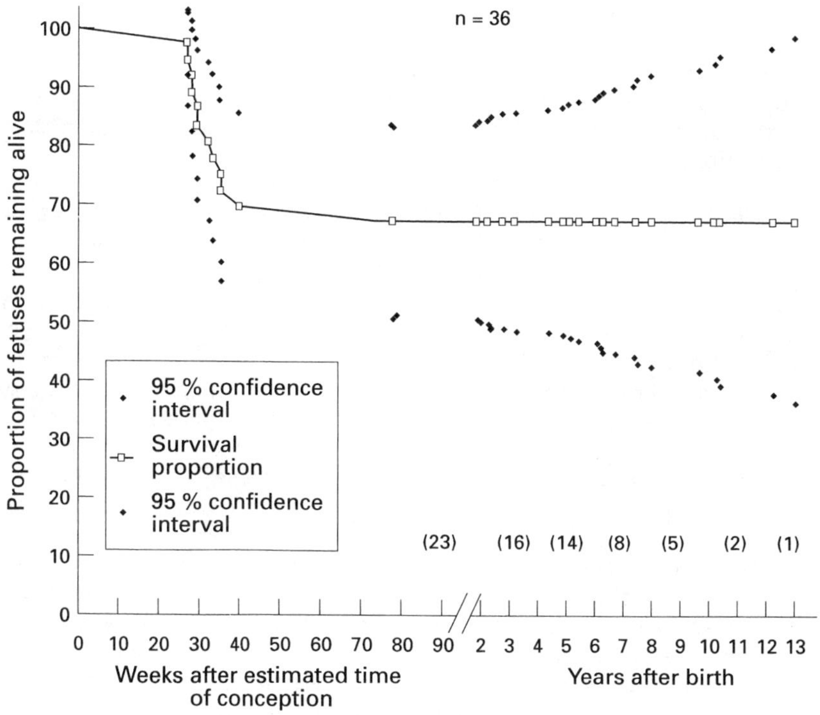

FIGURE 1.—Kaplan-Meier survival curve for congenital complete heart block detected prenatally. This curve shows that the major attrition of patients in the prenatal series is antenatal. The noncardiac death has been excluded. There was no fetal loss before 27 weeks' gestation. *Numbers in parentheses* are the numbers of patients alive at the follow-up interval. (Courtesy of Groves AMM, Allan LD, Rosenthal E: Outcome of isolated congenital complete heart block diagnosed in utero. *Heart* 75:190–194, 1996.)

in utero. Prenatal factors in fetal heart block that might predict death in utero, the need for intervention, and the probability of the need for a pacemaker were identified.

Methods and Findings.—Thirty-six fetuses with congenital complete heart block and structurally normal hearts detected at a tertiary referral unit for fetal echocardiography between 1980 and 1993 were included in the analysis. Twenty-four fetuses survived, 11 with pacemakers. Seven of the nonsurvivors died in utero, and 2 died immediately after birth. Another 2 fetuses were aborted electively because of severe hydrops, and the remaining infant died of unrelated causes. Heart rates tended to decrease in utero and postnatally. Deteriorating cardiac function was not necessarily associated with the lowest heart rates. A poor prognosis was associated with bradycardia of less than 55 beats/min in early pregnancy or a rapid reduction in heart rate prenatally. Hydrops also was an indicator of a poor prognosis, with 83% of the 12 affected fetuses dying. Nine of 10 fetuses with initial heart rates exceeding 60 beats/min survived, 3 of whom needed pacing. Only 3 of 7 fetuses with initial heart rates of 50 beats/min or less survived, 2 of whom required pacing. Two fetuses had negative maternal anti-Ro antibodies. One of these died in utero, and 1 underwent heart transplantation after a pacemaker was inserted (Fig 1).

Conclusions.—The prognosis of isolated complete heart block identified in utero can be poor. Individual heart rates do not accurately predict outcomes in utero or the need for postnatal pacing. Regular, careful prenatal monitoring is required to optimize the timing of necessary interventions.

▶ The etiology of nonimmune hydrops generates an extensive list, in addition to much anxiety for perinatal health care providers. Cardiac disorders of the fetus feature prominently and should be searched for diligently in fetuses with signs of hydrops. Fetal arrhythmias, including heart block, may account for intrauterine cardiac failure, manifested by ascites, pleural or pericardial effusions, and skin edema.

Groves and his colleagues have documented an impressive series of cases of isolated congenital complete heart block diagnosed in utero. In 1988, they reported 16 cases with isolated complete heart block and 21 with structural heart disease, concluding that fetal outcome with isolated heart block was good compared with a mortality rate of 85% with structural heart disease. They have had to revise their opinion on the prognosis of isolated heart block. The advent of fetal hydrops with isolated heart block is tantamount to a death sentence (93% mortality rate). Other poor prognostic signs include bradycardia of less than 55 beats/min in early pregnancy and a rapid decrease in heart rate prenatally. The series included 2 cases with interruption of the bundle of His, 1 of which required cardiac transplantation. In general, neither the administration of steroids nor plasmapheresis were efficacious in this series. One fetus responded to the administration of inotropes, and transabdominal pacing of the fetus was initiated successfully for some hours before fetal death. Endocardial pacing was required in 11 patients, including those who were symptomatic or had low heart rates with either long QT or exit block with pauses.

The group at Guy's Hospital performed fetal echocardiography on more than 10,000 cases referred between 1980 and 1994. We derive the benefit of this extensive experience as it is translated into a logical care pathway for the fetus with bradycardia.

A.A. Fanaroff, M.B.B.Ch.

2 Genetics and Teratology

Birth Outcomes in Pregnant Women Taking Fluoxetine

Chambers CD, Johnson KA, Dick LM, et al (Univ of California–San Diego, La Jolla)

N Engl J Med 335:1010–1015, 1996 2–1

Introduction.—Fluoxetine (Prozac) is the most commonly used antidepressant drug in the United States. Its safety in pregnancy has not been fully determined, despite its widespread use in both sexes and all ages. The effects of treatment with fluoxetine during pregnancy were evaluated.

Methods.—During a 6-year period, 228 pregnant women receiving fluoxetine were prospectively identified. The pregnancy outcomes of these women were compared with those of 254 women who were not taking fluoxetine.

TABLE 4.—Relative Risks of Selected Outcomes in Infants of Women With Late Exposure to Fluoxetine as Compared With Infants of Women With Early Exposure

Outcome	Crude Relative Risk (95% CI)*	Adjusted Relative Risk (95% CI)*†
Prematurity (<37 wk of gestation)‡	3.5 (1.1–10.7)	4.8 (1.1–20.8)§
Admission to special-care nursery	2.7 (1.4–5.0)	2.6 (1.1–6.9)¶
Poor neonatal adaptation‖	5.7 (2.5–13.1)	8.7 (2.9–26.6)**

**Abbreviation: CI,* confidence interval.

†Adjusted relative risks and CIs were approximated from the adjusted odds ratios obtained by logistic regression analysis.

‡Values exclude twins and second pregnancies of mothers with previous live-born infants in the study.

§Values were adjusted for multiparity; previous spontaneous abortion; preeclampsia, eclampsia, and hypertension; smoking status; maternal age; socioeconomic status; race; average dosage of fluoxetine; gestational diabetes; use of other psychotherapeutic drugs; alcohol use; and evidence of maternal or neonatal infection near delivery.

‖Values were adjusted for prematurity; preeclampsia, eclampsia, and hypertension; smoking status; maternal age; socioeconomic status; race; average dosage of fluoxetine; gestational diabetes; mode of delivery; alcohol use; evidence of maternal or neonatal infection near delivery; and therapy with other psychotherapeutic drugs near delivery.

¶This analysis was restricted to patients for whom medical records were available.

**Values were adjusted for prematurity; use of preterm-labor medications; preeclampsia, eclampsia, and hypertension; smoking status; maternal age; socioeconomic status; race; average dosage of fluoxetine; gestational diabetes; alcohol use; evidence of maternal or neonatal infection near delivery; and therapy with other psychotherapeutic drugs near delivery.

(Courtesy of Chambers CD, Johnson KA, Dick LM, et al: Birth outcomes in pregnant women taking fluoxetine. *N Engl J Med* 335:1010–1015,)

Results.—There were no significant differences between women receiving fluoxetine and control subjects in spontaneous pregnancy loss or rate of major structural anomalies. There were 97 infants exposed to fluoxetine who were evaluated for minor anomalies. The frequency of 3 or more minor anomalies was significantly higher in the fluoxetine group, compared with 153 control infants who were evaluated similarly. A comparison between the 101 infants exposed to fluoxetine in the first and second trimesters only and the 73 infants exposed in the third trimester indicated that infants in the latter group had higher rates of premature delivery, more admissions to special-care nurseries, poor neonatal adaptation (including respiratory difficulty, cyanosis on feeding, and jitteriness), lower birth weight, and shorter birth length (Table 4).

Conclusions.—Women who took fluoxetine during pregnancy did not have an increased risk of spontaneous pregnancy loss or major fetal anomalies. Infants of fluoxetine-treated mothers had an increased incidence of 3 or more minor anomalies compared with control subjects. The combination of any 3 minor anomalies is considered rare. Perinatal complications are more frequent in women who take fluoxetine in the third trimester of pregnancy.

▶ There have been times when, confronted with a huge pile of articles requiring comments or selections for the YEAR BOOK, I have been tempted to reach for the fluoxetine. To date, I have been able to overcome that temptation. Unless there are dramatic anomalies, such as those attributable to thalidomide, it is difficult to establish a cause-and-effect relation between drugs (prescription or otherwise) taken by the mother and fetal anomalies. There has been a trend toward therapeutic nihilism during pregnancy and careful observation for defects when drug treatment is necessary for the mother. Hence, Chambers and her vigilant colleagues, through the auspices of the California Teratogen Information Service and Clinical Research Program, were able to gather information on 228 pregnant women taking fluoxetine and compare the outcomes of their pregnancies with those of 254 women not taking fluoxetine. The authors decided that "finding no increase in major anomalies in the infants of women taking fluoxetine in the first trimester is reassuring." Maybe so, but overall the outcome data were far from reassuring. The affected infants were lighter, shorter, and had more transitional problems. There were more premature infants and the incidence of 3 or more minor malformations was significantly higher than in the control subjects. None of these are cause for a 4-alarm–fire response, but they are likely to add significant stress to a fragile mother, already receiving antidepressant medication, who is anticipating a perfect outcome of her pregnancy.

The observation that there are 3 or more minor anomalies in 15.5% of women exposed to fluoxetine in the first trimester cannot be taken lightly. These minor anomalies may be associated with a major anomaly, such as aberrant brain development, that is not apparent at birth.

Close follow-up of this cohort will be important, but because the cases were gathered from a large number of centers, this may not happen. Further, if the children are not exactly up to par, how much can be attributed to the fluoxetine exposure during pregnancy, and what proportion will be the result of poor nurturing by a psychotropic-dependent mother?

In 1965, as many as 10% of pregnant women were taking psychotropic drugs during pregnancy. Publicity aimed at averting unnecessary medication use during pregnancy since then has been effective, and Larivaara and associates reported that the rate of psychotropic drug use during pregnancy is now 1.5%, with morbidity similar to that observed by Chambers' group.[1] The former authors concluded that "the use of psychotropic drugs during pregnancy may harm both the mother and infant and, therefore, the continuous decreasing trend in the usage is favorable." We concur. It is depressing to realize that if 1.5% of women in the United States need and/or use psychotropic drugs, then in excess of 40,000 fetuses are being exposed to these agents. Pass the Prozac.

A.A. Fanaroff, M.B.B.Ch.

Reference

1. Larivaara P, Hartikainen A-L, Rantakallio P: Use of psychotropic drugs and pregnancy outcome. *J Clin Epidemiol* 49:1309–1313, 1996.

Outcome of Children Born to Epileptic Mothers Treated With Carbamazepine During Pregnancy

Ornoy A, Cohen E (Hebrew Univ, Jerusalem)
Arch Dis Child 75:517–520, 1996 2–2

Objective.—Whether in utero exposure to carbamazepine increases the incidence of congenital and development abnormalities was investigated.

Methods.—From telephone calls by patients to a teratogen information service, 37 epileptic women were identified who had received carbamazepine monotherapy during pregnancy. They had a total of 49 children aged

TABLE 1.—Parental Socioeconomic Status, Gestational Age, Birth Weight, Age, Weight, and Head Circumference at Examination in 47 Research and 47 Control Children

	Children of epileptic mothers	*Controls*
Parental socioeconomic status	2.31 (0.8) [33]	2.14 (0.8) [43]
Gestational age (weeks)	39.3 (1.8) [47]	39.8 (1.6) [47]
Birth weight (g)	3187 (530) [47]	3162 (680) [47]
Age at examination (months)	31 (15) [45]	24 (16) [47]
Weight (centile)	43 (25) [37]	32 (22) [38]
Head circumference (centile)	24 (23) [43]	29 (21) [44]
Facial dysmorphism (carbamazepine syndrome)	6*	0

Note: Values are mean (SD). Figures in brackets are number of children.
*Significantly higher than controls, χ^2, $P < 0.05$.
(Courtesy of Ornoy A, Cohen E: Outcome of children born to epileptic mothers treated with carbamazepine during pregnancy. *Arch Dis Child* 75:517–520, 1996.)

TABLE 2.—Mental and Motor Scores of Control and Research Children in Bayley and McCarthy Tests

	Children of epileptic mothers	Controls
Bayley MDI	101.1 (14.8) [22]*	112.0 (10.0) [35]
Bayley PDI	97.5 (18.0) [20]	101.0 (11.6) [34]
McCarthy GCI	99.4 (21.1) [19]*	113.0 (15.0) [12]
McCarthy	52.4 (10.5) [13]	49.5 (7.0) [11]

Note: Values are mean (SD). Figures in brackets are number of children.
*Significantly lower than appropriate controls, $P < 0.05$.
Abbreviations: MDI, mental developmental index; *PDI*, psychomotor developmental index; *GCI*, general cognitive index.
(Courtesy of Ornoy A, Cohen E: Outcome of children born to epileptic mothers treated with carbamazepine during pregnancy. *Arch Dis Child* 75:517–520, 1996.)

6 months to 6 years. Two children were excluded because of prematurity. The remaining 47 children received physical and neurologic examinations, along with psychological examinations, using Bayley or McCarthy developmental scales for those 1 year of age or older. They were matched to 47 control children by birth weight, gestational age, and parental socioeconomic status as determined by profession and education.

Results.—The characteristics of the 2 groups are compared in Table 1. The significant difference was that in the research group, 6 children had facial dysmorphism (upslanting palpebral fissure, epicanthic folds, micrognathia, broad nasal bridge, high arched palate, and/or cleft palate). No children in the control group had these features. As shown in Table 2, the average mental and cognitive scores were lower in the research group. All 6 children with facial dysmorphism had a development quotient or intelligence quotient below 90. Neither facial dysmorphism nor low cognitive scores were associated with the incidence of maternal seizures during pregnancy or with the daily dose of carbamazepine.

Conclusions.—Children of women who receive carbamazepine during pregnancy may have "carbamazepine syndrome," which is characterized by facial dysmorphism and mild mental retardation. Neither the dose of carbamazepine nor the incidence of maternal seizures during pregnancy seems to affect the prevalence of this syndrome.

▶ The "carbamazepine syndrome" has been disputed as a pure entity. However, Jones et al. reported the following dysmorphic features: a short nose; long philtrum; upslanting, palpebral fissures; hypertelorism; epicanthal folds; and nail hypoplasia, together with developmental delay in women exposed to carbamazepine during pregnancy.[1] Ornoy has used the Israeli Teratogen Information Service to reexamine the question of whether carbamazepine exposure renders the fetus vulnerable to a specific syndrome. Through a case-matched control system, Ornoy and Cohen support Jones by noting specific facial features and lower average cognitive scores in the children born to epileptic mothers receiving carbamazepine monotherapy. No dose relationship was established and, like the phenytoin embryopathy, a genetic predisposition is queried. The epoxide hydrolase enzyme implicated in the phenytoin embryopathy or other enzymes may be involved; further analyses are planned.[2]

A.A. Fanaroff, M.B.B.Ch.

References

1. Jones KL, Lacro RV, Johnson KA, et al: Pattern of malformations in children of women treated with carbamazepine during pregnancy. *N Engl J Med* 320:1661–1666, 1989.
2. Buehler BA, Bick K, Delmont D: Prenatal prediction of risk of fetal hydantoin syndrome. *N Engl J Med* 329:1660–1661, 1993.

Periconceptional Multivitamin Use and the Occurrence of Conotruncal Heart Defects: Results From a Population-based, Case-Control Study

Botto LD, Khoury MJ, Mulinare J, et al (Ctrs for Disease Control and Prevention, Atlanta, Ga)

Pediatrics 98:911–917, 1996 2–3

Background.—Conotruncal heart defects are malformations of the cardiac outflow tract and a major cause of infant morbidity and mortality. There have been recent advances in medical and surgical treatment of these defects, but not all infants can be treated surgically. Also, the treatment itself is associated with substantial personal and economic costs and un-

TABLE 5.—Estimated Relative Risk for Periconceptional Multivitamin Use and Conotruncal Defects by Type of Conotruncal Defect and Overall Clinical Diagnosis, Using Infants With Other Congenital Anomalies as Control Infants, Atlanta Birth Defects Case-Control Study, 1968 Through 1980

Group	Use	No Use	Odds Ratio (95% Confidence Interval)
Control	561	1732	Reference
Conotruncal defects	15	72	0.64 (0.37–1.13)
Isolated	8	54	0.46 (0.22–0.95)
Multiple	5	15	1.03 (0.37–2.85)
Syndromic	2	3	2.06 (0.36–11.89)
Transposition of the great arteries	5	38	0.41 (0.16–1.01)
Isolated	4	32	0.39 (0.14–1.06)
Multiple	1	6	0.52 (0.06–4.12)
Syndromic	0	0	—
Tetralogy of Fallot	4	23	0.54 (0.19–1.53)
Isolated	2	16	0.39 (0.09–1.60)
Multiple	1	5	0.62 (0.07–5.19)
Syndromic	1	2	1.54 (0.14–16.75)
Truncus arteriosus	4	9	1.37 (0.42–4.45)
Isolated	1	4	0.78 (0.09–6.89)
Multiple	3	4	2.32 (0.54–9.95)
Syndromic	0	1	0.00

Note: Infants with neural tube defects were not included in control infant group.

(From Botto LD, Khoury MJ, Mulinare J, et al: Periconceptional multivitamin use and the occurrence of conotruncal heart defects: Results from a population-based, case-control study. *Pediatrics* 98:911–917, 1996. Reproduced by permission of *Pediatrics*, Copyright 1996.)

certain outcome. Studies have indicated that the use of multivitamins or folic acid alone around the time of conception can prevent neural tube defects and possibly some types of heart and other birth defects. The effect of periconceptional multivitamin use on the incidence of conotruncal defects was examined.

Methods.—A subset of the Atlanta Birth Defects Case-Control Study population was analyzed. A total of 158 infants with conotruncal defects and 3,026 unaffected, control infants were identified. The use of multivitamins from 3 months before pregnancy through the first 3 months of pregnancy was determined from telephone interviews. The relative risk of conotruncal defects associated with use of multivitamins was calculated.

Results.—The infants of mothers who reported taking multivitamins around the time of conception had a 43% lower risk of conotruncal defects than did infants whose mothers did not take multivitamins. Of the relative risks for isolated conotruncal defects and defects associated with noncardiac defects or a recognized syndrome, the relative risk for isolated conotruncal defects was the lowest (Table 5). The risk of anatomical subgroups of defects was also analyzed. The greatest reduction in risk was for transposition of the great arteries.

Discussion.—In these subjects, the use of multivitamins around the time of conception was associated with a lower risk of infant conotruncal defects. The protective effect was strongest for transposition of the great arteries and was somewhat weaker for tetralogy of Fallot. A lower risk of conotruncal defects was seen in mothers who used multivitamins around the time of conception but not in those who began taking multivitamins at or after the second month of pregnancy. Increasing the use of multivitamins during this critical time in pregnancy may prevent conotruncal defects and significantly lower infant morbidity and mortality. Large doses of vitamin A during pregnancy may be associated with birth defects and should be avoided.

► The beneficial effects of periconceptional multivitamin use, and folic acid in particular, are so profound that it must be a top priority to disseminate this knowledge. But as George Will, the noted columnist observed, "This is an age in which one cannot find common sense without a search warrant." The administrative wheels to implement universal supplementation turn so slowly that simple obstacles are converted into impossible hurdles. Botto and colleagues provide additional ammunition to an already loaded arsenal of benefits by documenting a reduced risk for conotruncal defects. The timing of the multivitamin use is critical, with protection evident only among mothers who reported periconceptional use, not later. There was better protection against transposition than against tetralogy of Fallot and stronger protection against isolated, rather than nonisolated, defects. Tetralogy might be part of CATCH 22 (characterized by cardiac defects, abnormal facies, thymic aplasia/hypoplasia, cleft palate, hypoparathyroidism, and microdeletion of 22q11), which would not be prevented by periconceptional vitamin use.

We must be able to take advantage of the ability to avoid such devastating malformations as neural tube defects and major heart lesions with something so safe and inexpensive. (Also see Abstract 2–5.)

In a cute commentary, Wald[1] has suggested that folic acid should be classified as B4—the B4 you conceive pill. However, in The Netherlands, folic acid is classified as B_{11}, whereas in France it is called B_9. No consensus yet, although logic would tend to place it as a B_{11}.

A.A. Fanaroff, M.B.B.Ch.

Reference

1. Wald N: The B4 you conceive pill. *Lancet* 348:1460, 1996.

Folate Levels and Neural Tube Defects: Implications for Prevention

Daly LE, Kirke PN, Molloy A, et al (Univ College Dublin; Trinity College Dublin)

JAMA 274:1698–1702, 1995 2–4

Background.—Research has shown conclusively that the use of folic acid during pregnancy substantially reduces the risk of neural tube defects (NTDs). Findings from a previous study were used to quantify the effect of various intervention strategies on the risk of NTD.

Methods and Findings.—Data from a recent case-control study demonstrated that NTD is associated with early pregnancy red blood cell folate levels in a continuous dose-response relationship. Through the use of these data, the reduction in NTD cases that could be expected to result from 2 different strategies to increase folate levels was calculated. Although targeting high-risk women had a small effect on population prevalence, this strategy markedly changed an individual's risk. When the population was targeted, individual risk changed minimally, but the population prevalence was greatly affected. The most efficient way to implement the high-risk strategy would be to provide folic acid supplementation for women at high risk. Food fortification would be preferable for the population approach. Current guidelines for preventing NTD—to increase folic acid intake by 0.4 mg per day—would reduce NTD cases by 48%.

Conclusions.—The high-risk strategy by itself is likely to be less effective than the population approach, but these 2 strategies may be viewed as complementary. The identification and supplementation of women with red blood cell folate levels of less than 340 nmol/L would reduce their risk of NTD by more than 85%.

► Commenting on this article is Louis P. Halamek, M.D., Professor of Pediatrics, Division of Neonatal and Developmental Medicine, Stanford University Medical Center, Palo Alto, California:

► The fact that low maternal serum folate levels are associated with an increased incidence of neural tube defects has been confirmed by numerous studies. The finding of a continuous dose-response relationship between red blood cell folate and the risk of neural tube defects has the potential to allow obstetricians and perinatologists to first identify and then selectively target women at high risk and optimize their folate intake and levels. This would represent an important preventive step beyond maternal serum α-fetoprotein and prenatal ultrasound.

L.P. Halamek, M.D.

Prepregnant Weight in Relation to Risk of Neural Tube Defects
Werler MM, Louik C, Shapiro S, et al (Boston Univ, Brookline, Mass)
JAMA 275:1089–1092, 1996 2–5

Objective.—It has been suggested that obesity may increase the risk of having a pregnancy affected by a neural tube defect (NTD). This is an important public health question, because obesity is common and NTDs are among the most frequent and severe congenital malformations. The role played by folate intake also is important to determine. The effect of maternal obesity on the risk of NTDs was evaluated in 2 case-control studies, one conducted as part of a birth defect surveillance program and the other as part of a population-based study.

Surveillance Study.—This study included 604 fetuses or infants with an NTD diagnosed within 6 months of birth, 1,658 control fetuses or infants with other major malformations, and 93 control subjects without major malformations. Women with body weights of 50–59 kg were used as the reference group. The relative risk of NTDs for women weighing 80–89 kg was 1.9 (95% confidence interval, 1.2–2.9). For women weighing 110 kg or more, the relative risk was 4 (95% confidence interval, 1.6–9.9). The risk of NTDs related to body weight applied to women who did and did not receive the recommended level of 400 μg of folate. For women with body weights of less than 70 kg who took 400 μg of folate or more, the risk of NTDs decreased by 40%. For women weighing more than 70 kg, taking the recommended folate level did not reduce the risk of NTDs.

Population-based Study.—This study included 538 fetuses and infants with NTDs and 539 control subjects without malformations. The mothers were interviewed within an average of 5 months after their term delivery date. The risk of NTDs was about doubled for obese women, compared with those with a body mass index of 29 kg/m^2 or less. The odds ratio was 1.9, with a 95% confidence interval of 1.3–2.9. The obesity-associated increase in risk was unrelated to use of vitamins containing folic acid, diabetes, use of diet pills, dietary folic acid intake, or a previous NTD pregnancy. The odds ratio was unaffected by adjustment for maternal age, education, gravidity, vitamin use, or alcohol use. The link between maternal obesity and NTDs was greater for spina bifida and other less common NTDs than for anencephaly.

Conclusions.—Mothers with heavier prepregnancy body weights are at increased risk for pregnancies affected by NTDs. The risk of NTDs appears to be doubled for obese women, independent of the effects of folate intake. This modest effect probably makes a significant contribution to the number of NTDs in the population, given that perhaps 10% of women are obese when they become pregnant.

► It has been almost a decade since Yates and colleagues[1] postulated that a disorder of folate metabolism might be the basis for the genetic predisposition to NTDs. The relation between periconceptional folate consumption and the prevention of NTDs emerged slowly. The MRC study group[2] documented a 71% reduction and, using samples obtained during that multinational trial, the authors attempted to correlate blood folate and vitamin B_{12} status with NTDs[3] (see Abstract 2–4). The data are consistent with other evidence that folic acid and vitamin B_{12} levels are lower in women with NTD pregnancies and consistent with evidence from randomized trials showing that folic acid is protective. As might be anticipated, the differences between affected and unaffected pregnancies were not pronounced in the first trimester of pregnancy. The risk of a woman having had 2 or 3 NTD pregnancies, compared with having had just 1, was significantly higher if her whole blood folic acid level was low. According to multiple regression analyses, there was no evidence of an independent association between low serum B_{12} levels and NTDs.[4]

Werler and associates now confound an already complex situation by demonstrating a relation between prepregnant weight and risk of NTDs. Simply stated, NTDs can be added to the already extensive reproductive risks for obese women. Their folate intake was adequate and there is no plausible explanation for the failure of folate supplementation to confer protection to the fetuses of obese women. We are forced, but lamely, to speculate that in this population, a genetic predisposition complemented by relative or absolute folate deficiency at a critical time in embryogenesis generates an NTD. Daily folate supplementation in the periconceptional period is essential to minimize these devastating defects.[5]

A.A. Fanaroff, M.B.B.Ch.

References

1. Yates JRW, Ferguson-Smith MA, Shenkin A, et al: Is disordered folate metabolism the basis for genetic predisposition to neural tube defects? *Clin Genet* 31:279–287, 1987.
2. MRC Vitamin Study Research Group: Prevention of neural tube defects: Results of the MRC vitamin study. *Lancet* 338:132–137, 1991.
3. Daly LE, Kirke PN, Molloy A, et al: Folate levels and neural tube defects: Implications for prevention. *JAMA* 274:1968–1702, 1995.
4. Kirke PN, Molloy AM, Daly LE, et al: Maternal plasma folate and vitamin B_{12} are independent risk factors for neural tube defects. *Q J Med* 86:703–708, 1993.
5. Wald N: Folic acid and neural tube defects: The current evidence and implications for prevention, in *Neural Tube Defects*. CIBA Foundation Symposium 181.

Risk of Neural Tube Defect–Affected Pregnancies Among Obese Women
Shaw GM, Velie EM, Schaffer D (March of Dimes Birth Defects Found, Emeryville, Calif; Kaiser Permanente, Oakland, Calif)
JAMA 275:1093–1096, 1996 2–6

Background.—Nutritional factors, particularly maternal folic acid intake, have been identified as important etiologic factors for neural tube defects. It has been hypothesized that overweight or underweight mothers may have suboptimal nutritional patterns, increasing their risk of having an infant with a congenital anomaly. This hypothesis was investigated in a population-based case-control study.

Methods.—The mothers of 538 case infants, defined as singleton infants or fetuses with a diagnosis of a neural tube defect, and of 539 randomly selected controls without congenital anomalies were interviewed. The interviews elicited information on medical, reproductive, and family history; vitamin intake; nutrient intake from diet; and body mass index (BMI).

Results.—Neural tube defects were linked to the following maternal factors: Hispanic race, age younger than 25 years, no college graduation, and alcohol consumption during the first trimester. Compared with women with a BMI no greater than 29 kg/m^2, women with a higher BMI had twice the risk of having an infant or fetus with a neural tube defect. This risk was not affected by simultaneous adjustment for maternal age, education, gravidity, vitamin use, and alcohol use. In analysis of specific diagnoses, the risk for anencephaly was not increased, but the risk for spina bifida and other neural tube defects was significantly increased in women with a BMI exceeding 29 kg/m^2. In particular, the use of vitamins including folic acid did not impact the association between BMI and neural tube defects.

Conclusions.—Prepregnancy maternal obesity is associated with an increased risk of neural tube defects in the infant or fetus. An explanatory covariable could not be identified.

▶ The prevalence of obesity in the United States exceeds that of other industrialized countries, and our tendency to obesity is increasing.[1] As many as 10% of women in the United States are obese at the time they become pregnant. In addition to the other complications associated with obesity, these investigators show a twofold increase in the risk of neural tube defects in such mothers. These women are, therefore, candidates for intense scrutiny during the early weeks of pregnancy.

Obesity is measured by the body mass index (weight in kilograms divided by the square of height in meters), and if your BMI is greater than 29 kg/m^2, the Institute of Medicine defines you as being obese. When the subject was raised, one of my mentors, who could be considered more than a little chubby, would quip "I am just short for my weight." I guess it depends on your point of view.

M.J. Maisels, M.B., B.Ch.

Reference

1. Kuczmarski RJ, Flegal KM, Campbell SM, et al: Increasing prevalence of overweight among US adults: The National Health and Nutrition Examination Surveys, 1960 to 1991. *JAMA* 272:205–211, 1994.

Chromosome 22q11 Microdeletions in Tetralogy of Fallot

Trainer AH, Morrison N, Dunlop A, et al (Duncan Guthrie Inst of Med Genetics, Glasgow, Scotland)

Arch Dis Child 74:62–63, 1996 2–7

Objective.—Although chromosome 22q11 microdeletions have been found in patients with tetralogy of Fallot, the most common cause of cyanotic congenital cardiac defects, the prevalence of these deletions is unknown. The prevalence of sporadic and familial 22q11 microdeletions was determined in patients with tetralogy of Fallot using the 22q11 fluorescence in situ hybridization (FISH) technique.

Methods.—Familial chromosome banding studies and clinical evaluations were performed and a 3-generation family tree was drawn for 33 patients, (15 females) on 33 children.

Results.—Microdeletions at 22q11 were detected in 7 patients by FISH. In addition to tetralogy of Fallot, 3 patients had velocardiofacial and 1 had partial DiGeorge syndrome. In the remaining 3 (11%), the deletions were not familial and only tetralogy of Fallot was present.

Conclusion.—Three patients had tetralogy of Fallot only, which had recently been associated with cardiac defects, abnormal facies, thymic aplasia/hypoplasia, cleft palate, hypoparathyroidism, and microdeletion of 22q11 (CATCH 22). Dysmorphic features were detected with difficulty and then only in some patients. Routine FISH studies in children with tetralogy of Fallot only would be useful in identifying this abnormality and can be an important aspect of total care.

► Fluorescence in situ hybridization studies have added a new dimension and changed the perspective for both the geneticist and the humble clinician. Syndromes and other constellations of anomalies that appeared to be randomly associated are, with seemingly great frequency, identified as specific problems. A prime example has been the 22q11 microdeletion and the newly recognized chromosome 22 deletion syndrome (CATCH 22) with due apologies to Kurt Vonnegut, whose classic book has been besmirched by a bad karyotype. The CATCH 22 is characterized by *c*ardiac defects, *a*bnormal facies, *t*hymic aplasia/hypoplasia, *c*left palate, *h*ypoparathyroidism, and microdeletion of 22q11. The infants may have learning disorders later. DiGeorge syndrome, tetralogy of Fallot, and the velocardiofacial syndrome may occur with or without a deletion and, in the clinical features, may be subtle enough that they are apparent only after the karyotype has been reported. The message to do a karyotype on infants with an isolated tetralogy is appropriate. The results help provide meaningful counseling with regard to future risk and long-term outcome. The use of FISH has helped demystify other enigmatic clinical entities, such as Williams syndrome, in which an elastin gene deletion has been identified (7q11,23 on chromosome 7).[1]

"One of the secrets of life is to make stepping stones out of stumbling blocks."—Jack Penn

A.A. Fanaroff, M.B.B.Ch.

Reference

1. Lowery MC, Morris CA, Ewart A, et al: Strong correlation of elastin deletions, detected by FISH, with Williams syndrome: Evaluation of 235 patients. *Am J Hum Genet* 57:49–53, 1995.

Intellectual Impairment in Children Exposed to Polychlorinated Biphenyls In Utero

Jacobson JL, Jacobson SW (Wayne State Univ, Detroit)

N Engl J Med 335:783–789, 1996 2–8

Background.—Polychlorinated biphenyls have been banned in the United States and most Western nations for more than 2 decades, but their residues persist in human tissues. A major source of exposure is the consumption of fatty sport fish. Two prospective studies, one conducted in Michigan and the other in North Carolina, link in utero exposure to polychlorinated biphenyls to adverse effects on neurologic and intellectual function. A study of children whose mothers had eaten Lake Michigan fish examined the persistence of these effects through school age.

Methods.—The 212 children examined represented 68% of newborns studied in 1980–1981. Mothers of 167 of these children had eaten at least 11.8 kg of Lake Michigan salmon or lake trout during the 6-year period preceding their child's birth. At age 11 years, the children were evaluated with a battery of intelligence quotient (IQ) and achievement tests. Concentrations of polychlorinated biphenyls in umbilical cord serum and maternal serum and milk provided a composite measure of prenatal exposure. At the time of delivery, these concentrations were slightly higher than in the general population. Twenty-four control variables, including other exposures and prenatal influences, also were evaluated.

Results.—Children who were breast-fed for extended periods accumulated substantial body burdens of the compounds, but serum concentrations had declined substantially by the age of 11 years. After controlling for potential confounding variables, prenatal exposure to polychlorinated biphenyls was associated with lower full-scale and verbal IQ scores (Fig 1), with the strongest effects related to memory and attention. Children with the highest exposure levels were 3 times as likely to have low average IQ scores and twice as likely to be at least 2 years behind in reading comprehension.

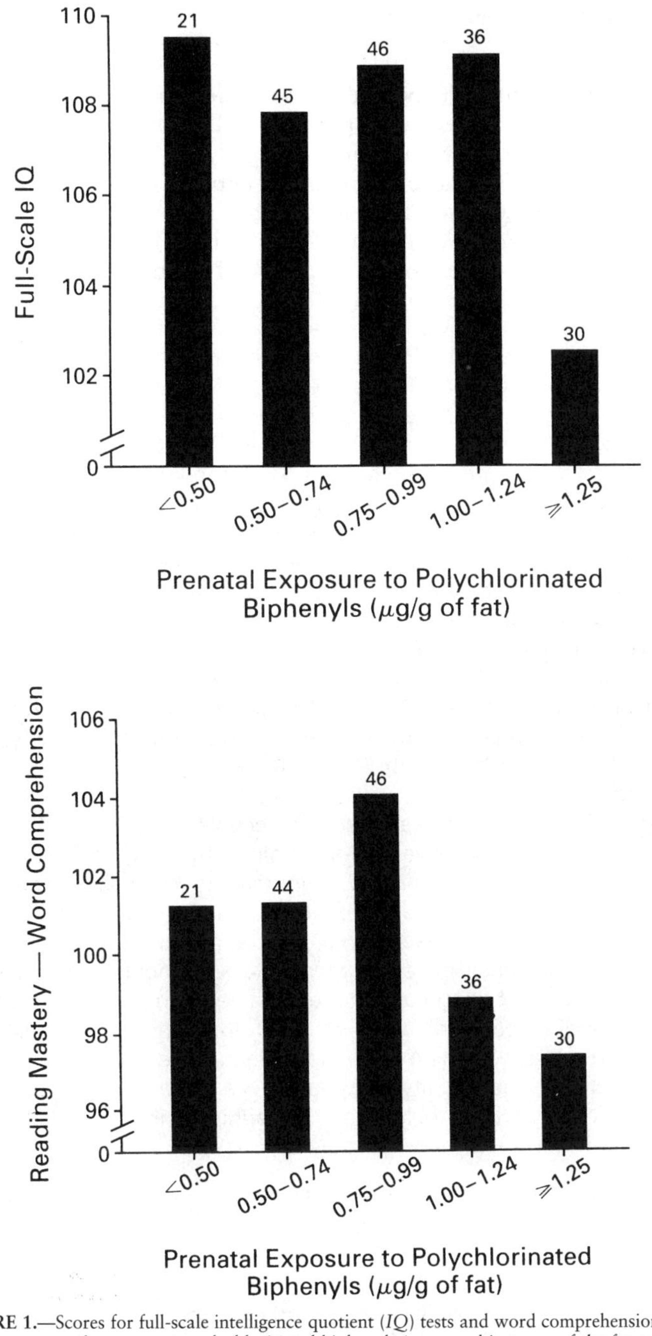

FIGURE 1.—Scores for full-scale intelligence quotient (*IQ*) tests and word comprehension in reading according to prenatal exposure to polychlorinated biphenyls (expressed in terms of the fat concentration of maternal milk). Scores were adjusted for the potential confounding variables listed in the footnotes to Table 3. The number of children in each group is given above the *bars*. One child was not tested for reading mastery. (Courtesy of Jacobson JL, Jacobson SW: Intellectual impairment in children exposed to polychlorinated biphenyls in utero. *N Engl J Med* 335:783–789, 1996. Copyright 1996, Massachusetts Medical Society. All rights reserved.)

Discussion.—In utero exposure to polychlorinated biphenyls and related contaminants was related to poorer intellectual function at the age of 11 years. The school-age children evaluated had deficits in short-term memory and in focused and sustained attention. These effects occurred even with levels of contaminants only slightly higher than those found in the general population. Women may accumulate these compounds from other food sources, and exposure is unrelated to socioeconomic status.

▶ Polychlorinated biphenyls, more familiarly known by the abbreviation PCBs, previously were the major insulating materials used in electrical transformers and capacitors. They have been banned since the 1970s in the United States and most of the Western world but persist as environmental contaminants. There is substantial evidence linking PCB exposure in utero to adverse neural development in children. The present study was an ongoing evaluation, at school age, of a cohort in whom deficits in fetal and postnatal growth and poor short-term memory at the age of 4 years had been noted.[1] The main objective was to determine whether the deficits had persisted and, if they had, how it had affected the acquisition of reading and arithmetic skills. Las Vegas odds-makers would have had no difficulty in setting heavy odds against these children learning normally and, as usual, they would have been correct. Ultimately, exposure in utero emerges as the culprit, and although larger quantities of PCBs are transferred postnatally through lactation than in utero, intellectual impairment occurred only in relation to in utero exposure. This is, no doubt, music to the ears of the La Leche League promoters.

The article is not a quick read. Table 1 occupies a full journal page, with more notations, such as 19 variables indicated by daggers, than a page of stock quotations in the *Wall Street Journal.* In correlating the prenatal exposure to PCBs, the calculated level per gram of fat is predictive of IQ score. With prenatal levels exceeding 1.25 mg per gram of fat, the intellectual impairment is small in terms of absolute IQ points, but functionally qualitative evidence of poor math and reading performance is evident so that the children are 2 years behind in word comprehension. The PCBs strike critical areas so that there is a general intellectual deficit, poorer short- and long-term memory, and inability to sustain focus and attention. There are still huge quantities of PCBs in older electrical equipment and landfills, and the environmental lobby will need to stay strong and vigilant to protect the unborn.

A.A. Fanaroff, M.B.B.Ch.

Reference

1. Jacobson JL, Jacobson SW, Humphrey HEB: Effects of in utero exposure to polychlorinated biphenyls and related contaminants on cognitive functioning in young children. *J Pediatr* 116:38–45, 1990.

▶ Our representatives should be aware of these sobering data as they debate regulations designed to protect us from this type of environmental contamination. The message is clear—once the contaminant is in the environment, it is extremely difficult to avoid it. As the authors point out, even women who do not eat fish from Lake Michigan accumulate these compounds from other food sources such as cheese, butter, beef, and pork. Furthermore, prenatal exposure to PCBs, unlike lead or illicit drugs, is completely unrelated to socioeconomic status. A recent Swedish study points out that there is a correlation between total and inorganic mercury levels in blood, the intake of fish, and the number of amalgam fillings in women who live in the north of Sweden.[1] There was also an association between levels of total mercury in blood and in the mothers' milk. Inorganic mercury is efficiently transferred from blood to milk and could form another environmental hazard to the developing brain.

M.J. Maisels, M.B., B.Ch.

Reference

1. Oskarsson A, SchÂultz A, Skerfving S, et al: Total and inorganic mercury in breast milk and blood in relation to fish consumption and amalgam fillings in lactating women. *Arch Environ Health* 51:234–241, 1996.

Synchronization of the Factors Critical for Diabetic Teratogenesis: An In Vitro Model

Reece EA, Wiznitzer A, Homko CJ, et al (Temple Univ, Philadelphia)
Am J Obstet Gynecol 174:1284–1288, 1996 2–9

Background.—An estimated 6% to 10% of infants of diabetic mothers reportedly have major congenital anomalies. This is twofold to fivefold higher than in the nondiabetic population. Research suggests that changed metabolic control associated with hyperglycemia during organogenesis is a teratogen. The relationship between critical factors and conditions such as gestational age and exposure time to increased glucose levels in diabetic embryopathy was investigated.

Methods.—The effect of various factors on embryonic development was studied in a model of postimplantation rat embryo culture. Experiments were performed with glucose concentrations increasing from 150 to 905 mg/dL, at gestational ages of 10–12 days, and for exposures of 30–180 minutes. The gross morphologic features of the yolk sac and embryo were studied.

Findings.—The malformations induced were dose related (Fig 1). Exposure to 950 mg/dL D-glucose significantly reduced the conceptus size. Embryos had gross anomalies, including open neural tube defects, microcephaly, dorsal tail flexion, heart defects, and pericardial effusion. At least 2 hours of exposure to hyperglycemia was needed to induce malformations. When exposure to the 100% teratogenic dose of hyperglycemia was begun on day 10, the malformations were primarily neural tube defects. When begun on day 11, they were primarily cardiac defects. When exposure was begun after day 11.5, no defects occurred (Fig 4).

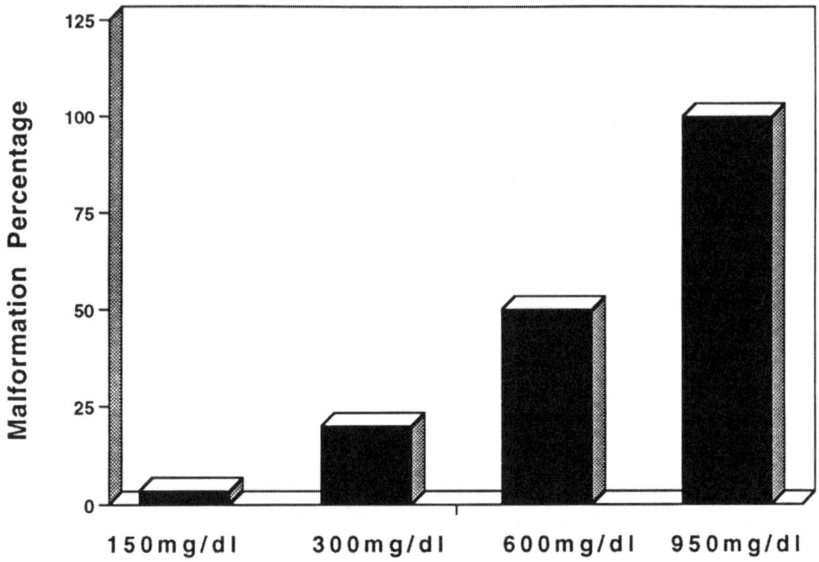

FIGURE 1.—Postimplantation rat embryo culture exposed to increasing concentrations of D-glucose. Glucose concentration of 150 mg/dL served as control. (Courtesy of Reece EA, Wiznitzer A, Homko CJ, et al: Synchronization of the factors critical for diabetic teratogenesis: An in vitro model. *Am J Obstet Gynecol* 174:1284–1288, 1996.)

Conclusion.—Diabetic teratogenesis occurs in a dose-related manner. A minimum exposure time and critical gestational age are needed. Embryonic malformation only occurs when these critical conditions occur together. Nonsynchronized aberrant conditions may result in an embryonic development that appears normal.

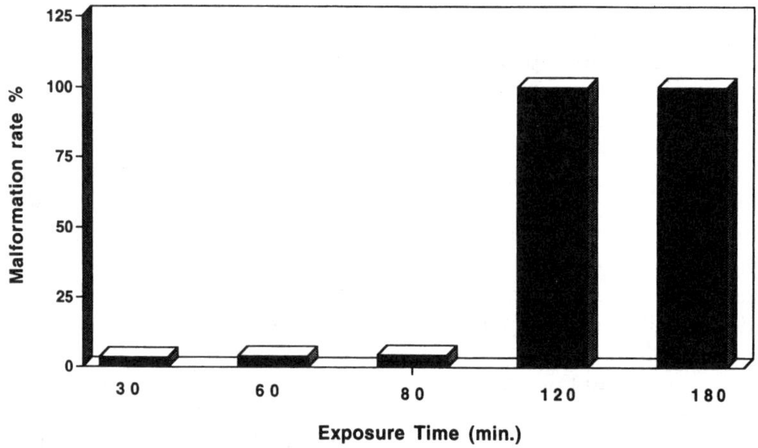

FIGURE 4.—Postimplantation rat embryo culture exposed to 100% teratogenic dose of glucose to produce hyperglycemia (950 mg/dL) for varying exposure times. A minimum exposure time of 2 hours was needed to induce malformations. (Courtesy of Reece EA, Wiznitzer A, Homko CJ, et al: Synchronization of the factors critical for diabetic teratogenesis: An in vitro model. *Am J Obstet Gynecol* 174:1284–1288, 1996.)

► The results of this elegant study in a rat embryo culture model cannot be extrapolated directly to the human fetus, but the message is both clear and consistent with what we know about the risk of diabetic pregnancies and congenital anomalies in the human infant. Reece et al. show a remarkable dose-response relationship between the degree of hypoglycemia and the risk of embryopathy. They also show that the insult must occur during a critical window of development (equivalent to the first 5–6 weeks of human pregnancy) and that a certain length of exposure is necessary before malformations will occur. Because the sensitive period in human development appears to be the first 5–6 weeks of pregnancy, it is important for women with diabetes to understand that compulsive control of their blood sugar levels is necessary in the earliest weeks of their pregnancy.

M.J. Maisels, M.B., B.Ch.

Patient Selection May Affect Gene Therapy Success: Dominant Negative Effects Observed for Ornithine Transcarbamylase in Mouse and Human Hepatocytes

Morsy MA, Zhao JZ, Ngo TT, et al (Baylor College of Medicine, Houston; McMaster Univ, Ont, Canada)

J Clin Invest 97:826–832, 1996 2–10

Background.—Ornithine transcarbamylase (OTC) deficiency is inherited as an X-linked recessive. It is the most common and serious of the urea cycle disorders. Frequent new mutations occur, ranging from deletions of the gene to point mutations affecting the activity and stability of the protein. Ornithine transcarbamylase deficiency is associated with citrulline and arginine depletion, orotic aciduria, hyperammonemia, and coma. If the hyperammonemia is not treated within 24–48 hours, patients deteriorate quickly. Dietary and pharmacologic treatments are inadequate, often resulting in death or mental retardation. Liver transplantation is possible in some cases, but it carries high morbidity and mortality rates. A gene transfer method of therapy for OTC deficiency was developed, and findings after in vivo gene transfer in a mouse model were reported.

Mouse Model.—The sparse fur–abnormal skin and hair mutant mouse model was used; this is 1 of 2 mouse models for OTC deficiency. Orotic aciduria is one of the characteristics of OTC deficiency in mice and humans and is the most sensitive marker for this deficiency in these mice.

Results.—Within 24 hours of treatment, significant reduction in orotic aciduria occurred. Metabolic correction was associated with later phenotypic correction and increase in enzymatic activity. In identifying the level of gene expression needed to achieve wild-type levels of enzyme activity, a dominant negative effect of the endogenous mutant protein on the activity of the delivered recombinant wild-type protein was discovered. This has implications for homomultimeric protein defects such as OTC deficiency, a difficult class of disorders for gene therapy.

Conclusions.—Adenoviral-mediated gene transfer may be effective short-term therapy for OTC deficiency in humans and may be effective during catabolic crisis. Careful patient selection based on mutation class may be critical for initial gene therapy trials of OTC deficiency as well as other homomultimeric enzyme deficiencies.

► A rapid publication in the *Journal of Clinical Investigation* represents ecstasy for these investigators. They have truly made a new observation worthy of immediate publication in the journal most highly regarded by their peers. Morsy and colleagues have published the maiden report demonstrating the "potential dominant negative effects as a consequence of a gene therapy attempt for homomultimeric protein defects." As the genes responsible for many complex disorders are identified, the hopes and dreams of the mutant/missing gene carriers rest on gene therapy. Ornithine transcarbamylase is the most severe of the urea cycle disorders and is inherited as an X-linked recessive with frequent new mutation occurrences. The deficiency is associated with citrulline and arginine depletion, orotic aciduria, hyperammonemia, and profound coma.

Metabolic correction can be achieved temporarily in a mouse model with OTC deficiency through adenoviral-mediated gene transfer of the human OTC complementary DNA. This suggests that gene therapy for humans with OTC deficiency may be just around the corner. But, as Morsy and colleagues indicate, many variables, including the mutation class, must be taken into consideration. Ornithine transcarbamylase complementary DNA mutations are frequently de novo, are heterogeneous, and result in differing OTC enzyme/protein levels, so phenotypically, patients range from asymptomatic or mild to severely affected. "The selection of patients may be critical to the evaluation of a gene transfer method when multimeric subunits constitute the active gene product."

Who gets cloned and who gets left behind, reduced to a mere solitary soul for all time?—Craig Wilson, USA Today

A.A. Fanaroff, M.B.B.Ch.

The Hazards of Reproduction in Space

Sullivan R (Univ College London)

Acta Obstet Gynecol Scand 75:372–377, 1996 2–11

Introduction.—Although the medical effects of space travel are well documented, there is little information on human reproduction in microgravity. Most space missions have been of short duration, and few female astronauts have participated. As missions are extended, manned space outposts are planned, and more women take part, successful space travel for long periods will require control of reproductive function and a thorough understanding of the effects of space environmental factors on reproduction. Space motion sickness, microgravity, closed life-support systems, and radiation affect all species, and research done in nonhuman species has provided valuable information about the hazards of space travel to human reproduction.

Space Motion Sickness.—The incidence of space motion sickness in astronauts is 40% to 50% in spite of intense desensitization programs. The pathophysiology of space motion sickness is not well understood, but it involves various neuroendocrinologic factors that interact with vestibular, ocular, proprioceptive, and cortical factors. Pregnancy-induced sickness involves endocrine, gastric stasis, immune, psychological, and other factors. The combined effects of space motion sickness and pregnancy-induced sickness are unknown. At best, there would be no increase in pregnancy-induced sickness, but at worst, space motion sickness may have a synergistic effect resulting in prolonged and more severe pregnancy-induced sickness. The latter would result in hyperemesis gravidarum and risk of dehydration, liver damage, multiple neuropathies, and Wernicke encephalopathy.

Electromagnetic Radiation.—The average person receives 125 mrem per year of radiation exposure, 40 mrem from cosmic radiation and the rest from medical and earth sources. Astronauts are exposed to substantially higher levels, which may cause reproductive dysfunction in both men and women. The cumulative teratogenic effects of radiation exposure on DNA must not be underestimated. Acute radiation exposure to a fetus between 8 and 25 weeks' gestation can result in microcephaly and mental retardation. Doses as low as 10 rad can have damaging effects. In children exposed to radiation in utero, there is a dose-dependent decrease in intelligence quotient. Radiation exposure also affects male fertility, and doses that cause azoospermia also can be fatal. However, recovery from damage in men does occur, unlike the irreversible damage to ovaries.

Discussion.—If manned space stations and interplanetary colonization are to become reality, they will have to proceed cautiously and gradually because of the unprecedented and potentially unforeseen hazards to reproduction. Research in space medicine is under way, although it is underfunded. The effects of microgravity and closed life-support systems also are important considerations.

► According to Sharon Begley, in *Newsweek,* January 27, 1997, "In science, it doesn't really count if you see it coming. The genuinely novel discovery is the one that takes researchers by surprise." At this time, it is difficult to envision human reproduction in space, but stranger things have happened. This discussion of some of the known potential hazards shows that human reproduction in space will be more than a daunting challenge. It makes for an interesting "what if" type of discussion. Will women ovulate in prolonged microgravity, and will men remain fertile? Will the radiation exposure in space create a hazard for the developing fetus? How real are the risks of rapid decompression, and will both mother and fetus get the bends? What sort of birthing suite will be required? Will microgravity protect against pregnancy-induced hypertension and edema? Nobody has the answers or wishes to address these questions hastily, but as the space program expands and journeys into space are extended, it is not too early to start the theoretical discussions. We can build on the knowledge gained from all the prior missions. Given that many astronauts still experience considerable nausea in space, the prospects for hyperemesis gravidarum loom large.

A.A. Fanaroff, M.B.B.Ch.

Reproductive Effects of Paternal Exposure to Chlorophenate Wood Preservatives in the Sawmill Industry

Dimich-Ward H, Hertzman C, Teschke K, et al (Univ of British Columbia, Canada)

Scand J Work Environ Health 22:267–273, 1996 2–12

Background.—Until 1989, dioxin-contaminated substances called chlorophenates were used as wood preservatives in the sawmill industry. Some previous studies have suggested that paternal exposure to dioxin-like substances can lead to malformations in offspring, although others have found no such link. A recent report suggested that offspring of sawmill workers were more likely to have heart defects, congenital hip dislocation, cleft lip, or obstructive renal defects. A cohort of sawmill workers was studied to determine whether paternal exposure to chlorophenates is related to adverse reproductive outcomes.

Methods.—The study cohort consisted of 9,512 fathers who had worked at least 1 year in sawmills at which chlorophenates were used. These men fathered 19,675 children from 1952 to 1988. The effects of chlorophenate exposure were assessed by comparing the sawmill workers' offspring to 5 referents matched for sex and year of birth. A panel of experienced workers estimated the men's chlorophenate exposure at intervals before and during pregnancy.

Results.—The prevalence of birth defects in the sawmill workers' offspring was nearly 5%, with many of the infants having multiple abnormalities. There was a significantly increased risk of eye anomalies, especially congenital cataracts. Depending on the exposure interval, the risk of anencephaly, spina bifida, or anomalies of the genitals also was increased. The offspring of sawmill workers were no more likely to have low birth weight, prematurity, stillbirth, or neonatal death.

Conclusions.—Male sawmill workers exposed to chlorophenates are more likely to have offspring with certain congenital anomalies. In particular, the risk of congenital anomalies of the eye increases along with estimated cumulative hours of chlorophenate exposure. The results strengthen the hypothesis that fetal developmental toxicity can be mediated through paternal occupational exposures.

▶ Epidemiologic studies usually do not get the fight-or-flight hormones flowing. They invariably conclude that further studies are warranted "in order to elucidate the mechanism" of whatever has been observed. This report is no exception in that regard; however, it has several redeeming features. First, the British Columbia malformation registry has "nearly 100%

reporting through multiple sources and emphasizes the quality control of diagnoses." This eliminates the possibility of selection bias on adverse reproductive outcomes, the primary objective of the survey. Second, the cohort size, ultimately 19,675 newborns fathered by 9,512 cohort members with validation of the potential exposure to chlorophenates, adds power to the conclusions. Third, it is important to establish that paternal health is a significant factor before conception and early in gestation, and that "male-mediated developmental toxicity" is a real entity.

Prior studies have yielded conflicting data on the role of potential exposure to dioxin-containing herbicides. Olshan and associates[1] used the same British Columbia population-based registry to identify paternal occupations that were associated with congenital anomalies in offspring. Sawmill work emerged as an occupation with an elevated odds ratio (greater than 1.5) of heart and renal defects, precipitating the present study, which addressed a more specific question: Are potential paternal occupational exposures to chlorophenate wood preservatives associated with an increased risk of congenital anomalies, stillbirth, prematurity, low birth weight, or perinatal mortality among offspring? There were 942 birth defects, a prevalence rate of 4.8%, among the progeny of the cohort of sawmill workers, with a strong association between high paternal exposure to chlorophenates before conception and during pregnancy, and offspring with congenital cataracts. Neural tube defects and genitourinary malformations also were increased in the children of heavily exposed workers.

There are many potentially toxic exposures at the sawmill, and maternal factors were not considered in this cohort. Nonetheless, there is strong circumstantial evidence that paternal exposure to toxins at critical times can be teratogenic.

The pessimist looks at opportunities and sees difficulties; the optimist looks at difficulties and sees opportunities.—Anonymous

A.A. Fanaroff, M.B.B.Ch.

Reference

1. Olshan AF, Teschke K, Baird PA: Paternal occupation and congenital anomalies in offspring. *Am J Ind Med* 20:457–475, 1991.

The Presence of Multinucleated Blastomeres in Human Embryos Is Correlated With Chromosomal Abnormalities

Kligman I, Benadiva C, Alikani M, et al (New York Hosp–Cornell Med Ctr)
Hum Reprod 11:1492–1498, 1996 2–13

Background.—Certain types of morphologic abnormalities have been invariably associated with chromosomal abnormalities. Multinucleated embryos have been found to contain a chromosomal abnormality, although whether the chromosomal aberration is limited to the multinucleated cell or is shared by the rest of the cells is unknown. Multinucleated blastomeres (MNBs) are arrested developmentally; thus, embryos with 1 or 2 of these may still develop normally, whereas those with many MNBs will not. Although MNBs have been the focus of some research, no one has investigated embryos in which multinucleation was observed at the first embryonic division. Whether the presence of 1 or more MNBs during early embryonic development is related to chromosomal abnormalities in sibling blastomeres of that embryo was investigated.

Methods.—Forty-seven embryos with multinucleated cells found on day 2 or 3 of development were compared with dividing embryos without multinucleation. Fluorescence in situ hybridization (FISH) with X, Y, 18, and 13/21 chromosome-specific probes was used to detect chromosome abnormalities.

Findings.—Chromosomal abnormalities were found in 76.6% of the embryos with multinucleated cells and in 50.9% of the control group. When aneuploidy was excluded, differences were even greater, with 74.5% of multinucleated embryos and 32.3% of the control group being chromosomally abnormal. The rate of chromosomal abnormalities in embryos with multinucleated cells was unaffected by day of the appearance of multinucleation, number of nuclei per cell, number of multinucleated cells per embryo, developmental quality of the embryos, or type of fertilization.

Conclusion.—Multinucleated embryos detected on day 2 or 3 of development have a much higher incidence of chromosomal abnormalities than embryos without multinucleation. Thus, embryos with MNBs observed on day 2 or 3 should not be replaced unless no other embryos are available.

▶ In this study using FISH, the authors investigated the presence of multinucleated blastomeres in human embryos as a screening tool for guiding the use of such embryos in in vitro fertilization cycles. Biopsies of the embryos were done on day 4 of development, and blastomeres were removed from each embryo by micromanipulation and subjected to FISH. The results were compared with those obtained from nonarrested embryos without multinucleation. The total number of chromosomal abnormalities in multinucleated embryos was significantly higher than in nonmultinucleated embryos, indicating that multinucleated embryos have a much higher incident of chromosomal abnormalities and that perhaps these should not be used for implantation in in vitro fertilization unless no other embryos are available.

Techniques such as this could permit earlier detection of chromosomal abnormalities in prospective embryos and would help decrease the morally difficult decisions that occur when fetal reduction procedures are indicated for chromosomal abnormalities. With this technique, the embryo would be prescreened and would be rejected for implantation.

D.K. Stevenson, M.D.

Enrichment of Fetal Trophoblast Cells From the Maternal Peripheral Blood Followed by Detection of Fetal Deoxyribonucleic Acid With a Nested X/Y Polymerase Chain Reaction

van Wijk IJ, van Vugt JMG, Mulders MAM, et al (Free Univ Hosp, Amsterdam)

Am J Obstet Gynecol 174:871–876, 1996 2–14

Background.—Early in pregnancy, fetal cells circulate in maternal blood. However, these cells are rare, and enrichment procedures are needed before noninvasive prenatal diagnosis can be done. A 2-step enrichment procedure for isolating trophoblast cells from 20 mL of peripheral blood was developed.

Methods and Findings.—Blood samples were obtained from 36 pregnant women at between 6 and 15 weeks' gestation. The success of isolating fetal cells was determined after enrichment by amplifying Y chromosome sequences. A highly specific X/Y polymerase chain reaction (PCR) was established. This PCR was sensitive enough to detect X and Y chromosome-specific sequences in 1 cell and in 1 male cell among 100,000 female cells. Compared with results from conventional karyotyping, sex determination by PCR had a 91.7% success rate.

Conclusions.—This technique demonstrates the feasibility of performing a rapid, reliable enrichment of mononuclear cytotrophoblast cells without specific antibodies to these fetal cells. Furthermore, because they occur in maternal blood early in pregnancy but not in normal adult blood and enable cell culturing after isolation from maternal blood, trophoblast cells are attractive target cells. The current approach for enriching fetal trophoblast cells may contribute to noninvasive prenatal diagnosis very early in gestation.

▶ This comment has been provided by Phyllis A. Dennery, M.D., Assistant Professor of Pediatrics, Stanford University School of Medicine; Lucille Salter Packard Children's Hospital at Stanford, Palo Alto, California:

▶ Early prenatal diagnosis of genetic disorders would be greatly enhanced by the ability to detect fetal cells from the maternal peripheral circulation. Presently, detection of fetal or paternally inherited gene polymorphisms (or mutations) is possible only because the mother lacks these genes and maternal cell contamination does not hinder the diagnosis. As Dr. Bianchi[1] and colleagues have pointed out, fetal progenitor cells may persist in maternal circulation for decades post partum, thereby hindering the ability to confirm that the condition detected is that of the fetus rather than reflecting a previous pregnancy.

In this article, van Wijk et al. describe the use of fetal trophoblast cells from the maternal peripheral blood as a means of approaching prenatal diagnosis. The circulating trophoblasts are unlikely to persist after delivery, including subsequent pregnancies, and have a short replication time, which makes these cells ideal for karyotyping. However, the correlation between the sex determination using enriched trophoblasts subjected to PCR reaction vs. detection with conventional karyotyping by chorionic villus sampling or amniocentesis was not perfect. The authors suggest that future use of in situ hybridization protocols might allow for better correlation. Other investigators have looked at the fetal erythrocyte as a cell source for prenatal diagnosis, and a recent report on prenatal diagnosis of Duchenne's muscular dystrophy using a single nucleated erythrocyte shows promise as well.[2] The definite advantage of techniques using maternal peripheral blood is that they could be used as early as the first trimester of pregnancy, much earlier than conventional amniocentesis and obviously less invasive than other procedures such as chorionic villus sampling.

P.A. Dennery, M.D.

References

1. Bianchi DW, Zickwolf GK, Weil GJ, et al: Male fetal progenitor cells persist in maternal blood for as long as 27 years post partum. *Proc Natl Acad Sci U S A* 93:705–708, 1996.
2. Sekizawa A, Kimura T, Sasamk M, et al: Prenatal diagnosis of Duchenne muscular dystrophy using a single fetal nucleated erythrocyte in maternal blood. *Neurology* 46:1350–1353, 1996.

Down's Syndrome-like Skeletal Abnormalities in *Ets2* Transgenic Mice

Sumarsono SH, Wilson TJ, Tymms MJ, et al (Monash Univ, Clayton, Australia; Peter MacCallum Cancer Inst, East Melbourne, Australia; Med Univ of South Carolina, Charleston; et al)

Nature 379:534–536, 1996 2–15

Background.—Ets2 is a proto-oncogene and transcription factor that is expressed in a variety of cell types. During murine development, *Ets2* expression is high in newly forming cartilage, such as in skull precursor cells and vertebral primordia. Located on human chromosome 21, *Ets2* is overexpressed in Down's syndrome.

Methods and Findings.—Transgenic mice were produced to determine the consequences of *Ets2* overexpression. Mice with less than twofold *Ets2* overexpression in certain organs were found to have neurocranial, viscerocranial, and cervical skeletal abnormalities. These abnormalities were similar to the skeletal anomalies found in trisomy-16 mice and human beings with Down's syndrome, in whom there is an increase in the gene dosage of *Ets2*.

Conclusions.—Ets2 appears to play a role in skeletal development. Furthermore, the overexpression of *Ets2* seems to be involved in the genesis of some skeletal abnormalities occurring in patients with Down's syndrome.

► This comment has been provided by Phyllis A. Dennery, M.D., Assistant Professor of Pediatrics, Stanford University School of Medicine; Lucille Salter Packard Children's Hospital at Stanford, Palo Alto, California:

▶ In this study, transgenic mice overexpressing *Ets2*, a proto-oncogene and transcription factor, were evaluated for similarities with human beings with Down's syndrome because the *Ets2* gene is expressed on chromosome 21 in human beings. The important point made in this study is that although *Ets2* is important in forming new cartilage and vertebral primordia, overexpression of this factor results in deleterious effects, such as abnormal skeletal development. This is another example of "too much of a good thing" in Down's syndrome. Infants with Down's syndrome additionally have an extra copy of the superoxide dismutase gene, which is seen to cause abnormal thymic development (i.e., early thymic involution).[1] Additionally, there are excesses in human carbonyl reductase in Down's syndrome.[2] This enzyme modulates oxygen-free radicals in cells and may contribute to the pathologic changes in Down's syndrome. It may be a monumental task to examine all of the factors that are overexpressed in Down's syndrome, but each new finding gives us insight into embryogenesis and its regulation.

P.A. Dennery, M.D.

References

1. Nabarra B, Cassanova M, Paris D, et al: Transgenic mice overexpressing the human Cu/Zn-SOD gene: Ultrastructural studies of a premature thymic involution model of Down's syndrome (trisomy 21). *Lab Invest* 74:617–626, 1996.
2. Limieux N, Malfory B, Forrest GL: Human carbonyl reductase (CBR) localized to band 21q22.1 by high–resolution fluorescence in situ hybridization displays gene dosage effects in trisome 21 cells. *Genetics* 15:169–172, 1993.

Morphologic Changes in Offspring of Female Mice Exposed to Ethanol Before Conception

Soltes BA, Anderson R, Radwanska E (Rush Presbyterian–St Luke's Med Ctr, Chicago)

Am J Obstet Gynecol 175:1158–1162, 1996 2–16

Introduction.—Some investigations have suggested that ethanol consumption causes mutagenic fetal effects. The mutagenic effects of long-term ethanol exposure before conception were evaluated using a mouse model.

Methods.—Fifty-three adult female CF-1 mice were randomly assigned to 1 of 5 groups: (1) a negative control group (10 mice maintained on a liquid diet containing sucrose), (2) a mutagenic positive control group (10 mice maintained on a liquid diet with sucrose and Trenimon, a known mutagen administered before mating), (3) a teratogenic positive control group (11 mice maintained on a liquid diet with sucrose before mating, then maintained on a liquid diet with 5% ethanol after mating), (4) a mutagenic ethanol treatment group (11 mice given a liquid diet with 5% ethanol before mating, then maintained on a liquid diet with sucrose during gestation), and (5) a mutagenic-teratogenic ethanol treatment group (11 mice maintained continuously on a liquid diet with 5% ethanol before and after mating). Mice were on special diets for 28 days, then were superovulated and mated. Mice were killed on day 14 of gestation and fetuses were removed and examined for abnormalities.

Results.—Compared with other groups, the teratogenic group (group 3) had significant differences in litter size, offspring birth weights, and crown–rump length. Mice in the continuous ethanol–treated group (group 5) had a lower pregnancy rate than other treatment groups. The highest mutation indices were detected in the teratogenic group (group 3) (56%) and continuous ethanol–treated group (group 5) (64%). At dissection, every mouse in the teratogenic group (group 3) had at least 1 anomaly. The percentages of anatomical anomalies for group 1 was 28%; for group 2, it was 67%; for group 3, it was 100%; for group 4, it was 50%; and for group 5, it was 50%. The most common anatomical characteristics of fetal alcohol syndrome were abdominal wall defects.

Conclusion.—This investigation was the first of its kind to compare the possible mutagenic effects with regard to morphological abnormalities on surviving offspring of female mice treated with ethanol before mating, during gestation, and both before and after conception. Findings suggest that chronic ethanol exposure in female mice before conception produces anatomical abnormalities in the offspring. Offspring are at increased risk when ethanol is consumed before or after conception in CF-1 mice.

▶ There is general professional and public awareness about fetal alcohol syndrome, which represents a spectrum of manifestations of specific anatomical, behavioral, and developmental anomalies in offspring born to mothers with alcoholism. Thus, there is also little dispute about the teratogenic effects on the fetuses of animals and humans exposed to ethanol after conception. The implication that all the detrimental effects might be avoided by cessation of ethanol consumption during the pregnancy has influenced maternal behavior. However, this study in female mice suggests that there may be mutagenic effects of preconception ethanol exposure that result in lethal mutations or interfere with organogenesis. Regardless of whether the results using this mouse model can be extrapolated to human circumstances, the abuse of ethanol should be considered a potential risk before and after conception. However, that occasional social drinking would contribute to measurable effects of the sort described in this study seems unlikely from a practical perspective. Nonetheless, everything in nature is a poison depending on the dose, and some things are more likely to be poisons than others. Some poisons may, in fact, be remedies under some conditions, and alcohol probably is no exception in this regard. However, pregnancy is probably the least favorable time to test this hypothesis.

D.K. Stevenson, M.D.

3 Medical Complications of Pregnancy

Multicenter Randomized Clinical Trial of Home Uterine Activity Monitoring: Pregnancy Outcomes for All Women Randomized

Corwin MJ, Mou SM, Sunderji SG, et al (Univ of Missouri, Kansas City; State Univ of New York, Syracuse; Univ of Illinois Hosp, Chicago; et al)

Am J Obstet Gynecol 175:1281–1285, 1996 3–1

Introduction.—An earlier trial evaluating a subgroup of women with premature labor indicated that women undergoing home uterine activity monitoring were more likely to have a cervical dilatation of less than 2 cm at the time of diagnosis of preterm labor, longer gestations, higher birth weight infants, and infants who required less care in the neonatal ICU (NICU) than women whose uterine activity was not being monitored at home. Reported now are the outcomes of home uterine activity monitoring for the entire enrolled sample.

Methods.—A total of 339 women with singleton gestations from 3 centers who were at high risk for preterm labor were randomly assigned to receive either high-risk prenatal care alone (not monitored) or high-risk prenatal care with twice-daily home uterine activity monitoring (monitored).

Results.—Complete data were available for 174 women in the monitored group and 165 women in the group that was not monitored. Women in the monitored group were significantly more likely to remain undelivered through 37 weeks of gestation compared with women in the group that was not monitored. There was about a 40% reduction of preterm birth (before 37 weeks of gestation) in the monitored group compared with the group not monitored. The mean birth weight of infants in the monitored group was 3,158 g, and the mean birth weight of infants in the group not monitored was 2,942 g. Infants born to women who were monitored had a significantly lower risk for referral to an NICU. Overall days spent in an NICU for infants of mothers in the monitored group was 125, and those in the nonmonitored group spent a total of 594 days.

Conclusion.—The beneficial effects of home uterine activity monitoring remain even when analyses are not limited to the subsample of women who experienced preterm labor. Women at high risk for preterm labor who were in the monitored group had longer gestations, about a 40% reduction in risk for preterm birth, infants with higher birth weights, and fewer infants who required NICU care compared with women at high risk for preterm labor who were in the group that was not monitored.

▶ The home uterine activity monitoring debate goes on. Many women are eliminated in these trials for a variety of factors that often are associated with preterm labor and delivery, so extrapolation to real-world circumstances is difficult. Also, the mechanism by which home uterine activity monitoring affects pregnancy outcome remains fundamentally mysterious. It is difficult to tell from the article whether the monitoring itself effects a change or alerts physicians to events that lead to different clinical practices. The latter, of course, is implied but not proven by the study.

D.K. Stevenson, M.D.

The Preterm Prediction Study: Maternal Stress Is Associated With Spontaneous Preterm Birth at Less Than Thirty-five Weeks' Gestation

Copper RL, Goldenberg RL, Das A, et al (Natl Inst of Child Health and Human Development, Bethesda, Md)

Am J Obstet Gynecol 175:1286–1292, 1996 3–2

Introduction.—Some reports indicate that the risk of low birth weight (LBW) and complications of pregnancy are associated with maternal psychosocial characteristics, such as stress, depression, anxiety, self-esteem, and poor social support. Other reports do not confirm these findings. It has been shown that women with high rates of prematurity and LBW are more likely to participate in maladaptive health behaviors, such as smoking, substance abuse, and poor weight gain during pregnancy. These maladaptive behaviors are more widespread in women who are stressed compared with women who are not stressed. The association between psychosocial status and pregnancy outcome was evaluated at 25–29 weeks of gestation in 2,593 gravid women.

Methods.—Participants were recruited from 10 participating centers before 24 weeks of gestation. Participants completed a psychosocial status in pregnancy 28-item Likert scale that evaluated anxiety, stress, self-esteem, mastery, and depression. Poor psychosocial status was defined by scores in the lowest quartile. Outcome measures of spontaneous preterm birth, LBW, and intrauterine growth restriction (IUGR) were compared in women with high and low psychosocial scores.

Results.—The mean maternal age was 22.6 years and the mean educational level was 11.9 years. The rate of LBW was 5.1%, and the rate of IUGR was 11.1%. High stress scores were significantly associated with spontaneous preterm birth and LBW. There was a nonsignificant correlation between women with preterm, growth-restricted, or LBW infants. Poor overall psychosocial status was significantly correlated with education less than 13 years and tobacco and drug use during pregnancy. Spontaneous preterm birth was significantly associated with black race, low education, and high stress. Black race, tobacco use, and single head of household were significantly associated with IUGR. Stress was the only psychosocial characteristic significantly associated with LBW.

Conclusion.—Women who consider themselves stressed during pregnancy are at a higher risk for premature birth and LBW than women who do not consider themselves stressed. Black race was a significant predictor of spontaneous preterm birth, fetal growth restrictions, and LBW.

▶ It is easy for individuals to accept that biological factors can perturb biological systems, which can, in turn, lead to biological consequences. However, it is often more difficult for individuals to understand that factors categorized as psychological can also affect biological systems profoundly. This study serves to demonstrate that stress is significantly associated with spontaneous preterm birth and LBW. The data would suggest that it is all right to be anxious, have low self-esteem, and be out of control or depressed as long as you are not stressed. Thus, the motto must be that whatever nature throws at you, just sit back, relax, and enjoy what life has in store for you.

D.K. Stevenson, M.D.

Fetal Fibronectin in Cervicovaginal Secretions as a Predictor of Preterm Birth

Malak TM, Sizmur F, Bell SC, et al (Univ of Leicester, England)
Br J Obstet Gynaecol 103:648–653, 1996 3–3

Background.—Although only 7% to 11% of births are preterm, such births are the cause of about 85% of deaths of normally developed neonates. Current methods of clinically diagnosing preterm labor are inaccurate. The predictive value of fetal fibronectin detection in cervicovaginal secretions of patients with symptoms suggesting preterm labor was investigated.

TABLE 1.—Fetal Fibronectin in Cervicovaginal Secretions Sampled at 24–37 Weeks of Gestation as a Predictor of Preterm Birth

Fetal fibronectin test	Preterm birth cases (<37 weeks)	Term birth cases (≥37 weeks)	Total
Positive	17	5	22
Negative	10	109	119
Total	27	114	141

(Courtesy of Malak TM, Sizmur F, Bell SC, et al: Fetal fibronectin in cervicovaginal secretions as a predictor of preterm birth. *Br J Obstet Gynaecol* 103:648–653, 1996, publisher, Blackwell Science Ltd.)

TABLE 3.—Fetal Fibronectin in Cervicovaginal Secretions Sampled at 24–34 Weeks of Gestation as a Predictor of Birth Within 7, 14, or 21 Days of Sampling Irrespective of the Gestation at Delivery

	Birth within 7 days	Birth within 14 days	Birth within 21 days
True positive cases	8	9	12
True negative cases	92	92	92
False positive cases	10	9	6
False negative cases	2	2	2
Sensitivity (%)	80.0	81.3	85.7
Specificity (%)	90.2	91.1	93.9
Positive predictive value (%)	44.4	50.0	66.7
Negative predictive value (%)	97.9	97.9	97.9

(Courtesy of Malak TM, Sizmur F, Bell SC, et al: Fetal fibronectin in cervicovaginal secretions as a predictor of preterm birth. *Br J Obstet Gynaecol* 103:648–653, 1996, publisher, Blackwell Science Ltd.)

Methods.—One hundred forty-one women seen between 24 and 37 weeks' gestation with symptoms suggesting preterm labor were studied. All subjects had intact membranes and cervical dilatation of less than 2 cm. Specimens of cervicovaginal secretions were obtained from the ectocervix and posterior fornix. An enzyme-linked immunosorbent assay was used to measure fetal fibronectin levels. Samples were considered positive if the level of fetal fibronectin was 0.05 μg/mL or higher.

Findings.—Birth before 37 weeks' gestation occurred in 19.1% of neonates. Preterm birth was predicted by fetal fibronectin with a sensitivity of 63%; a specificity of 95.6%; and positive and negative predictive values of 77.3% and 91.6%, respectively. Findings were similar in women at less than 34 weeks' gestation. Negative test results excluded the chance of subsequent birth in the 3 weeks after sampling with an accuracy of 97.9% (Tables 1 and 3).

Conclusion.—Fetal fibronectin in the cervicovaginal secretions of women with symptoms suggesting preterm labor indicates a significant risk for subsequent preterm birth. The absence of fetal fibronectin strongly indicates that subsequent preterm birth is unlikely. When combined with clinical findings, fetal fibronectin testing can play an important role in the clinical management of women with symptoms suggesting preterm labor.

▶ Dr. David Schwartz, Associate Professor of Obstetrics and Gynecology, Wayne State University School of Medicine, Detroit, Michigan comments:

▶ Because we know that prematurity is the most important factor influencing perinatal outcome, our inability to prevent preterm labor is frustrating. Risk scoring systems; home uterine activity monitoring; bed rest; prophylactic cerclage; and a variety of medications, including alcohol, β-mimetics, prostaglandin synthetase inhibitors, and calcium channel blockers have had little impact on reducing spontaneous premature labor. Although intensive short-term tocolysis and prenatal corticosteroid therapy have contributed significantly to a reduction in neonatal morbidity and mortality, the clinical dilemma is when this therapy should be initiated. The emerging literature on fetal fibronectin testing as an adjunctive diagnostic test is encouraging.

Fibronectin is an extracellular matrix glycoprotein that is present in fetal membranes and is released when the choriodecidual interface is disrupted. This paper from the United Kingdom suggests that the presence of a fetal fibronectin level greater than 0.05 μg/mL has some ability to predict birth before 37 weeks (a positive predictive value of birth within 7, 14, or 21 days of 44.4%, 50.0%, and 66.7%, respectively). However, the negative predictive value for all of these intervals was 97.9%. These results are similar to those of Iams et al.,[1] who found that the absence of fetal fibronectin was 99% accurate in predicting that delivery would not occur within the next 7 days.

Unfortunately, the ability of this test to predict that preterm birth will occur is far more limited and, as we currently have no effective treatment for preterm labor, the cost of widespread testing is difficult to justify. On the other hand, because of their very high negative predictive value, negative test results, when combined with clinical assessment, should allow us to avoid the unnecessary costs of hospitalization and treatment for a large group of patients whom we currently, and incorrectly, assume will deliver preterm. As in most interventions, we need randomized trials to answer the question: will measuring fetal fibronectin reduce costs, conserve resources, and improve pregnancy outcome?

D. Schwartz, M.D.

Reference

1. Iams JD, Casal D, McGregor JA, et al: Fetal fibronectin improves the accuracy of diagnosis of preterm labor. *Am J Obstet Gynecol* 173:141–145, 1995.

Fetal Fibronectin in Vaginal Specimens Predicts Preterm Delivery and Very-low-birth-weight Infants

Bartnicki J, Casal D, Kreaden US, et al (Adeza Biomedical, Berlin-Neukölln, Germany; Women's Hosp, Sunnyvale, Calif)

Am J Obstet Gynecol 174:971–974, 1996 3–4

Background.—Very low birth weight is highly correlated with preterm delivery, and both are strongly associated with perinatal morbidity and mortality. Diagnostic methods that can predict accurately the risk of premature delivery or low birth weight are needed. Recent studies have suggested that cervicovaginal expression of fetal fibronectin may be a sensitive indicator of preterm delivery. The accuracy of cervicovaginal fetal fibronectin expression as a predictive factor for preterm delivery and delivery of very low birth weight infants was evaluated in women seeking emergency obstetric care for symptoms of preterm labor.

Methods.—Vaginal specimens were obtained from the posterior fornix of 112 pregnant women with symptoms of preterm labor during their

22nd to 35th gestational week who had intact amniotic membranes and cervical dilatation not exceeding 2 cm. The vaginal specimens were analyzed with an immunoassay to determine fetal fibronectin concentrations; concentrations of at least 0.05 μg/mL were considered to be positive. Associations between subsequent preterm delivery and fetal fibronectin concentrations were analyzed.

Results.—There were premature deliveries in 40 (35.7%) of the patients and positive fetal fibronectin concentrations in 34 (30.4%). In the prediction of preterm delivery, fetal fibronectin had a sensitivity of 67.5%, a specificity of 90.3%, a positive predictive value of 79.4%, and a negative predictive value of 83.3%. Although cervical dilatation, uterine activity, and vaginal pH also were significantly associated with preterm delivery in univariate analysis, fetal fibronectin was the only significant independent predictor in multivariate analysis. In particular, a positive fetal fibronectin test result strongly predicted preterm delivery within 14 days of sampling. A positive fetal fibronectin test also increased the probability of delivery of a very low birth weight infant (less than 1,500 g) by 13-fold. In the prediction of very low birth weight, fetal fibronectin had a sensitivity of 85.7%, a specificity of 75.9%, a positive predictive value of 32.4%, and a negative predictive value of 97.5%.

Conclusions.—Cervicovaginal fetal fibronectin expression is an independent risk factor for preterm delivery and delivery of very low birth weight infants. This association has biological plausibility, because of its presence in the extracellular matrix of the choriodecidual interface, and has temporal significance, predicting delivery within 7–14 days.

The Preterm Prediction Study: Fetal Fibronectin Testing and Spontaneous Preterm Birth

Goldenberg RL, for the NICHD Maternal Fetal Medicine Units Network (Univ of Alabama, Birmingham; et al)

Obstet Gynecol 87:643–648, 1996 3–5

Background.—Previous studies have suggested that, among women in preterm labor, the finding of cervical or vaginal fetal fibronectin identifies a group at increased risk for preterm delivery. One study used fetal fibronectin testing to screen for risk of subsequent preterm labor and delivery in women with high-risk pregnancies. Although fetal fibronectin was significantly related to preterm labor, the test was not sensitive. The ability of fetal fibronectin testing as a screening test to predict spontaneous preterm birth in a relatively low-risk population was studied.

Methods.—The study included 2,929 pregnant women at 10 study centers. Beginning at 22–24 weeks' gestation and continuing through 30 weeks, the women underwent biweekly screening for cervical and vaginal fetal fibronectin. The data were analyzed to determine the link between a positive test result at various gestational ages and the risk of spontaneous preterm birth at various intervals after each test.

Results.—At each testing interval, 3% to 4% of fetal fibronectin test results were positive. There was about a 0.7 correlation between cervical and vaginal fetal fibronectin at each visit, and a 0.17–0.25 correlation between cervical or vaginal fetal fibronectin at successive visits. A positive fetal fibronectin test result at 22–24 weeks' gestation was 63% sensitive in predicting spontaneous birth at less than 28 weeks' gestation, with a relative risk of 59 for a positive vs. negative test result. Specificity was in the range of 96% to 98% as the definition of preterm birth was increased from before 28 to before 37 weeks. However, positive predictive value increased from 13% to 36% as this definition changed. The testing period considered and the definition of preterm birth used had a significant effect on the relative risk for spontaneous preterm birth after a positive vs. a negative fetal fibronectin test result. However, the relative risk was always significant at more than 4.

Conclusions.—Most spontaneous births occurring before 28 weeks' gestation are predictable by a positive cervical or vaginal fetal fibronectin test result at 22–24 weeks' gestation. The association remains significant, although not as strong, as the outer gestational limit of spontaneous preterm birth is extended and the fetal fibronectin test is performed at later gestational ages. Thus, cervical or vaginal fetal fibronectin is very effective in predicting spontaneous preterm birth. Further research will be needed to find an intervention that can actually reduce the rate of these births, however.

► Despite many interventions and prevention strategies, the rate of prematurity in the United States has remained constant. More recently, a chemical marker, fetal fibronectin (fFN), has been identified in the vaginal secretions of women who are about to experience premature labor.[1] Lockwood and colleagues reported that of 117 patients who presented to the hospital with possible premature labor and intact membranes, 60 subsequently delivered prematurely. Forty-nine of the 60 had elevated fFN from the cervix or vagina, whereas fFN was not present in 47 of 57 patients who went on to deliver at term. The fFN appears in the vagina, at most, 2–3 weeks before delivery, so current studies are using delivery within 1 week of evaluation as a more realistic end point.[2, 3] Iams and associates found that fFN was highly predictive of premature delivery within a week in symptomatic patients with cervical dilation of about 2 cm. The negative predictive value was 99.5%, but only after manipulation of the cohort. Fibronectin is a ubiquitous protein that has been referred to as the "handyman of the body." Fetal fibronectin appears to play a role in the extracellular interface between the mother and fetus, and may be of some importance in placental cleavage after delivery.

The report from Goldenberg and colleagues of the National Institutes of Health multicenter trial (Abstract 3–5) indicates that they could identify almost two thirds of the very early preterm births with a single positive fFN test result. The odds of delivery before 28 weeks with a single positive test result were increased by 59-fold. Morrison and associates[3] combined uterine contraction monitoring with determinations of fFN. They found that if there were more than 2 contractions per hour and the fFN test result was positive, the risk of preterm labor (before 34 weeks) increased exponentially as compared with the individual tests. The absence of contractions and a negative fFN test result had a 96% negative predictive value for premature labor.

In reviewing the various trials, my bias has been that fFN is a useful tool to predict premature labor. Thomas Kirschbaum, the editor responsible for the obstetric component of the YEAR BOOK OF OBSTETRICS, GYNECOLOGY, AND WOMEN'S HEALTH, is much more skeptical and has kindly permitted inclusion of his analyses of these same manuscripts.

A.A. Fanaroff, M.B.B.Ch.

References

1. Lockwood CJ, Wein R, Lapinski R et al: The presence of cervical and vaginal fetal fibronectin predicts preterm delivery in an inner city obstetric population. *Am J Obstet Gynecol* 169:798–804, 1993.
2. Iams J, Casal D, McGregor J, et al: Fetal fibronectin improves the accuracy of diagnosis of preterm labor. *Am J Obstet Gynecol* 173:141–145, 1995.
3. Morrison JC, Naef RW, Botti JJ, et al: Prediction of spontaneous preterm birth by fetal fibronectin and uterine activity. *Obstet Gynecol* 87:649–655, 1996.

▶ Thomas H. Kirschbaum, M.D., Professor, Department of Obstetrics and Gynecology, Albert Einstein College of Medicine, The Bronx, New York, commented on the Goldenberg article in the 1997 YEAR BOOK OF OBSTETRICS, GYNECOLOGY, AND WOMEN'S HEALTH:

▶ Although the predictability of vaginal-cervical fFN has been discussed previously in the YEAR BOOK,[1-3] this study by the Maternal Fetal Medicine Units Network of the National Institute of Child Health and Human Development is noteworthy for the nearly 3,000 patients enrolled in a well-designed and evaluated prospective trial. Women with single pregnancies without placenta previa, fetal anomaly, or cerclage were enrolled with US confirmation of gestational age before the 24th week. They were evaluated for the incidence of spontaneous premature delivery before 34 weeks, as a function of fFN test results at 2-week intervals. Two thirds of the enrolled women were black. In a group with a 10.3% prematurity rate, the incidence of either a positive cervical or vaginal test result for fFN was 4%. The issue here was not whether there was a correlative relation between fFN presence in the lower reproductive tract and preterm delivery (because there certainly was), but whether the relation was strong enough to be useful in screening asymptomatic women. The authors conclude that screening was not warranted for want of effective therapy for those screened, but this begs the issue of the strength of the predictive relation here. Sensitivity was low for each of the 4 aggregates studied (20% to 29%), and the incidence of false-positive test results ranged between 75% and 82%. In Table 3 in the original article, extended follow-up to 36 weeks is depicted, with an overall sensitivity of 10% and greater sensitivity in the 3 weeks after entry, a subset comprised of only 6% of cases of preterm delivery. Because false positive rates are not provided, the predictive value of a positive test cannot be calculated. In a companion paper, the role of the simultaneous presence of bacterial vaginosis cannot be shown to increase predictability to acceptable levels, with false positive values, even when both test results are positive, ranging from 95% to 100%.[4] No matter how regrettably, it seems that the large number of false positive results robs fFN assays of most of their clinical usefulness.

T.H. Kirschbaum, M.D.

References

1. Lockwood CJ, Wein R, Lapinski R, et al: The presence of cervical and vaginal fetal fibronectin predicts preterm delivery in an inner-city obstetric population. *Am J Obstet Gynecol* 169:798–804, 1993.
2. Nageotte MP, Casal D, Senyei AE: Fetal fibronectin in patients at increased risk for premature birth. *Am J Obstet Gynecol* 170:20–25, 1994.
3. Inglis SR, Jeremias J, Kuno K, et al: Detection of tumor necrosis factor-α, interleukin-6, and fetal fibronectin in the lower genital tract during pregnancy: Relation to outcome. *Am J Obstet Gynecol* 171:5–10, 1994.
4. Goldenberg RL, Thom E, Moawad AH, et al: The preterm prediction study: Fetal fibronectin, bacterial vaginosis, and peripartum infection. NICHD Maternal Fetal Medicine Units Network. *Obstet Gynecol* 87:656–660, 1996.

The Value of Fetal Fibronectin in Cervical and Vaginal Secretions and of Ultrasonographic Examination of the Uterine Cervix in Predicting Premature Delivery for Patients With Preterm Labor and Intact Membranes

Rizzo G, Capponi A, Arduini D, et al (Universita' di Roma "Tor Vergata")

Am J Obstet Gynecol 175:1146–1151, 1996 3–6

Background.—Increasing evidence suggests that the different mechanisms thought to promote preterm delivery share a common pathway characterized by changes in extracellular matrix that result in cervical modifications and the disruption of the chorionic-decidual interface. An increased risk of preterm labor has been associated with both fetal fibronectin and the US detection of a short uterine cervix or dilation of the internal os. The diagnostic performances of fetal fibronectin assay of cervical and vaginal secretions and of transvaginal US assessment of the uterine cervix in predicting preterm delivery of patients with preterm labor and intact membranes were compared.

Methods and Findings.—One hundred eight women were studied. Forty-seven gave birth before term. In a receiver characteristic curve analysis, fetal fibronectin levels of 60 ng/mL or greater in cervical secretions best predicted preterm delivery. In a multiple stepwise logistic regression analysis, the cervical index significantly improved the prediction of preterm delivery achieved by the fetal fibronectin assay. In patients with fibronectin levels in cervical secretion of 60 ng/mL or greater, survival analysis indicated a shorter admission-to-delivery interval in the presence of an abnormal cervical index.

Conclusion.—Assaying fetal fibronectin in cervical secretions is a better predictor of preterm delivery than US assessment of the uterine cervix. Diagnostic efficiency is improved by the combined use of the fetal fibronectin assay and the cervical index. The use of both techniques allows prediction of the admission-to-delivery interval and identification of a patient subgroup who may need aggressive therapy.

▶ Commenting on this article is Robert P. Lorenz, M.D., Director, Maternal Fetal Medicine, William Beaumont Hospital, Royal Oak, Michigan:

▶ A reduction in the rate of preterm birth remains the most important and resistant challenge in maternal and child health. Progress has been made in understanding the pathophysiology of preterm birth and the detection of patients destined to deliver early. Unfortunately, no significant advances have been made in the area of intervention.

Cervical fetal fibronectin measurement performed at 20–24 weeks of gestation has emerged as the single strongest predictor of preterm delivery. It is a better predictor than historical risk factors, other laboratory assays, or US. In this study, fetal fibronectin combined with cervical US was a better predictor than either alone.

What is the clinical application of the test today? Currently, it is as if we have invented gasoline but are awaiting the invention of the internal combustion engine. The test, as commercially available, has no obvious clinical application. The potential future uses await a proven intervention to reduce the risk of preterm birth or a fetal fibronectin test that can be completed within a few hours. The former is a considerable time in the future; the latter may be available in the next few years. The applications may be as follows:

1. screening asymptomatic outpatients; either pregnant women or patients who have risk factors based on history or pregnancy risks will be candidates for this test when we have a proven intervention that is clinically effective.
2. evaluation of a patient in preterm labor; because of the high cost of the test, it is currently only commercially available on a 24–48–hour turnaround time. If it could be done within a few hours, then many patients currently given a diagnosis of "preterm labor" could be identified by a negative fetal fibronectin test as low risk. This would potentially lower the number of mothers and fetuses exposed to tocolytics, steroids, and hospitalization. It would not impact on the preterm birth rate, however. Development of a rapid test is under way.

In summary, fetal fibronectin testing is an important research advance that, when coupled with proven interventions, may in the future help us to reduce the frequency of preterm birth.

R.P. Lorenz, M.D.

Plasma Ferritin and Pregnancy Outcome

Goldenberg RL, Tamura T, DuBard M, et al (Univ of Alabama, Birmingham; Univ of Alabama, Tuscaloosa)

Am J Obstet Gynecol 175:1356–1359, 1996 3–7

Introduction.—Iron deficiency is best measured by evaluation of plasma ferritin levels. Placental isoferritin has been correlated with pregnancy outcomes in several populations. Plasma ferritin and hematocrit values were obtained at 19, 26, and 36 weeks of gestation and were correlated with birth weight and preterm delivery.

Methods.—The mean age of the 580 indigent black women evaluated was 23.4 years. Patients were divided by quartiles of plasma ferritin levels. Birth weight gestational age, and preterm delivery were recorded.

Results.—There was no correlation between mean birth weight, mean gestational age, percent of preterm deliveries (32–37 weeks or less), and percent of infants weighing 1,500–2,500 g or less and hematocrit levels. There was no significant correlation between ferritin levels in the lowest or 3 higher quartiles and any outcome measures. Ferritin levels in the highest quartile were significantly correlated with lower mean birth weight than the 3 lower quartiles at every time point measured (19, 26, and 36 weeks). At 26 weeks, high plasma ferritin levels were strongly correlated with low birth weight and premature delivery.

Conclusion.—High plasma ferritin levels were associated with low birth weight at 19, 26, and 36 weeks of gestation. At 26 weeks, high plasma levels were also correlated with preterm delivery. It has yet to be determined whether plasma ferritin levels can be used clinically to predict preterm delivery or poor fetal growth and whether test results can be used to improve pregnancy outcome.

► In a never-ending search for predictors of preterm labor, investigators have found that ferritin appears to be another nonspecific indicator of inflammatory events and is probably associated with infection. Thus, high plasma ferritin levels are associated with subsequent preterm delivery and low birth weight. As there seem to be an almost unlimited number of acute phase reactants, I am sure that the list of associations will grow. Whether this will help physicians predict any better the onset of preterm labor and delivery or help serve as a sign that can be addressed by a specific intervention to prevent preterm labor and delivery remains a big question.

D.K. Stevenson, M.D.

Reduced Incidence of Preterm Delivery With Metronidazole and Erythromycin in Women With Bacterial Vaginosis

Hauth JC, Goldenberg RL, Andrews WW, et al (Univ of Alabama, Birmingham)

N Engl J Med 333:1732–1736, 1995 3–8

Background.—Bacterial vaginosis about doubles the risk of spontaneous preterm delivery. The possibility that treatment with antimicrobials during the second trimester would lower the incidence of preterm delivery in women at increased risk for preterm delivery was investigated in a prospective trial.

Methods.—The study group included 624 otherwise healthy women who were at risk for preterm delivery (based on a prior spontaneous preterm delivery or a weight of less than 50 kg before pregnancy). Vaginal and cervical cultures and other tests for bacterial vaginosis were done at a mean of 23 weeks' gestation. A 2:1 double-blind randomization was used: 433 women (the treatment group) received metronidazole for 1 week and erythromycin for 2 weeks, and 191 women received a placebo. Two to 4 weeks later, the tests were repeated. Women with vaginosis then received a second course of metronidazole and erythromycin.

Results.—Significantly fewer of the women in the treatment group (26%) were delivered of their infants prematurely compared with the women in the placebo group (36%). However, the lower rates of prematurity associated with antimicrobial treatment were present only in the 258 women with bacterial vaginosis (31% were delivered of their infants prematurely with treatment vs. 49% with placebo; $P = 0.006$). The premature delivery rate was similar in the 358 women without bacterial vaginosis (treatment group, 22%; placebo group, 25%).

Conclusions.—Women with risk factors for premature delivery and bacterial vaginosis are likely to deliver prematurely. Treatment with metronidazole and erythromycin in the second trimester reduces their risk for premature delivery.

▶ A ray of sunshine in the otherwise gloomy news about prematurity emerges from this article. Antimicrobial therapy administered to women with bacterial vaginosis reduces the rate of prematurity. However, the treatment was effective only when bacterial vaginosis was present. The administration of metronidazole and erythromycin to high-risk women without bacterial vaginosis did not reduce the prematurity rate, which was in excess of 20%. Low maternal weight at the time of conception and history of preterm delivery were identified risks for prematurity. There is a complex relation between infection and prematurity. Infection may precipate premature labor and also has been implicated in periventricular leukomalacia. Antimicrobial therapy is indicated for a select subgroup at risk for prematurity. As better markers of prematurity, such as fetal fibronectin, are established, a combination of treatments to forestall premature labor will emerge (see Abstract 3–4). We then can look forward to substantially reducing prematurity, with all its comorbidity. (See also Abstract 6–4.)

A.A. Fanaroff, M.B.B.Ch.

Antibiotic Treatment in Preterm Premature Rupture of Membranes and Neonatal Morbidity: A Metaanalysis

Egarter C, Leitich H, Karas H, et al (Univ of Vienna)

Am J Obstet Gynecol 174:589–597, 1996 3–9

Background.—Preterm premature rupture of fetal membranes occurs in a substantial portion of preterm births. Although there is some evidence that infection plays a role in preterm premature rupture of membranes, studies with significant statistical power to demonstrate an effect of antibody treatment are not available. This meta-analysis was performed to determine the effects of prophylactic antibiotics on neonatal morbidity. To evaluate the effects of antibiotics alone, studies including tocolytics or corticosteroids were excluded.

Methods.—In January 1995, 18 medical data bases were searched for literature on preterm premature rupture of fetal membranes and antibiotics. Investigations involving tocolytics and corticoteroids were not included.

Findings.—Seven clinical trials, published between 1989 and 1994, were found that met the inclusion criteria. These trials included 657 patients. Meta-analysis showed that prophylactic antibiotic therapy significantly reduced the risk of neonatal sepsis and of intraventricular hemorrhage. There was no significant effect of antibiotic therapy on respiratory distress syndrome, necrotizing enterocolitis, or overall mortality.

Conclusion.—This meta-analysis provides evidence from 7 clinical trials that prophylactic antibiotic therapy after preterm premature rupture of membranes significantly reduced the risk of sepsis and intraventricular hemorrhage among newborns. This suggests that antibiotics are useful in the treatment of this condition.

► Commenting on this article is William E. Benitz, M.D., Associate Professor of Pediatrics, Clinical Director of Intensive Care Nursery, Division of Neonatal and Developmental Medicine, Stanford University School of Medicine, Palo Alto, California:

► These authors present a technically fastidious meta-analysis of the effects of intrapartum antibiotic therapy on neonatal outcomes, concluding that the risk of neonatal sepsis is reduced by 68% in women who are so treated. Unfortunately, sepsis was defined as "clinical sepsis with fever, leukocytosis, and C-reactive protein elevation; positive blood cultures alone were considered insufficient." Because the studies analyzed did not report all of these variables, 1 did not report blood culture results, and fever, leukocytosis, and elevated C-reactive protein levels are nonspecific and insensitive indicators of neonatal infection, one is left to wonder exactly what this end point might represent. In addition, studies in which tocolytic therapy or corticosteroids were used were excluded from the analysis, even though it has not been shown that either of these influences the incidence of neonatal sepsis.

Given the current wide application of these therapies in women with preterm rupture of membranes, the relevance of this meta-analysis to current practice is doubtful. In spite of these shortcomings, the authors' conclusion that intrapartum treatment of women with preterm premature rupture of membranes substantially reduces the incidence of sepsis in their infants is correct (Benitz WE, unpublished meta-analysis). Because the sepsis rate in these infants is very high (approaching 50% in those whose mothers are colonized with group B streptococci in particular), I also recommend intrapartum antimicrobial therapy for women with preterm premature rupture of membranes.

W.E. Benitz, M.D.

The Accuracy of Late Antenatal Screening Cultures in Predicting Genital Group B Streptococcal Colonization

Yancey MK, Schuchat A, Brown LK, et al (Tripler Army Med Ctr, Honolulu, Hawaii; Ctrs for Disease Control and Prevention, Atlanta, Ga; et al)

Obstet Gynecol 88:811–815, 1996 3–10

Objective.—Because of concerns about the accuracy of prenatal cultures, screening strategies to prevent early-onset neonatal group B streptococcal sepsis have not gained wide acceptance. Collecting cultures later in gestation, i.e., at 35–37 weeks rather than at 26–28 weeks, might improve the accuracy of prenatal cultures. However, there is little information on the test performance of these cultures. The accuracy of late antenatal

TABLE 2.—The Effect of the Interval Between Antenatal and Intrapartum Cultures on Test Performance

Interval (wk)	Antenatal screen positive: Positive at delivery	Negative at delivery	PPV	Antenatal screen negative: Positive at delivery	Negative at delivery	NPV
1	10	0	100%	1	39	98%
2	60	3	91%	4	99	96%
3	30	4	88%	5	165	97%
4	66	10	87%	6	183	97%
5	29	4	88%	5	101	95%
≥6	3	4	43%	5	20	80%
Total	168	25	87%	26	607	96%

Abbreviations: PPV, positive predictive value; *NPV*, negative predictive value.

(Reproduced with permission from American College of Obstetricians and Gynecologists, from Yancey MK, Schuchat A, Brown LK, et al: The accuracy of late antenatal screening cultures in predicting genital group B streptococcal colonization. *Obstet Gynecol* 88:811–815, 1996.)

TABLE 3.—Estimated Predictive Values for Antenatal Group B Streptococcal Cultures for Populations With a Range of Colonization Rates

Prevalence of GBS colonization	Positive predictive value	Negative predictive value
10%	71%	99%
15%	79%	98%
20%	85%	97%
26.5% (current study)	87%	96%
30%	90%	95%
35%	92%	93%

Note: Estimates were based on assumption of test sensitivity of 87% and specificity of 96%.
Abbreviation: GBS, group B streptococcus.
(Reproduced with permission from American College of Obstetricians and Gynecologists, from Yancey MK, Schuchat A, Brown LK, et al: The accuracy of late antenatal screening cultures in predicting genital group B streptococcal colonization. *Obstet Gynecol* 88:811–815, 1996.)

cultures in predicting intrapartum colonization with group B streptococci was assessed.

Methods.—Vaginal and rectal swabs were obtained from 826 pregnant women making routine prenatal visits at 35–36 weeks' gestation. The swabs were cultured in broth media to detect the presence of group B streptococci. The cultures were repeated when the women were admitted to the hospital for delivery. The ability of the antenatal cultures to predict the results of the delivery cultures was assessed. The sensitivity and specificity of the antenatal cultures were analyzed, and their predictive value across a range of group B streptococcal carriage rates was estimated.

Results.—The overall rate of group B streptococcal colonization was 26.5%. Late antenatal cultures were 87% sensitive in predicting the women's colonization status at delivery, with a specificity of 96%, positive predictive value of 87%, and negative predictive value of 96%. The predictive ability of the test was about the same when performed anywhere from 1 to 5 weeks before delivery. However, test performance declined when the antenatal culture was made more than 6 weeks before delivery, to a sensitivity of only 43% (Table 2). Predictive values differed by colonization rate (Table 3). Estimated positive predictive value was 50% and negative predictive value 81% at a colonization rate of 20%. At a colonization rate of 15%, these values improved to 79% and 98%, respectively.

Conclusions.—Culture of anogenital swabs taken at 35–36 weeks' gestation can accurately predict group B streptococcal colonization at delivery in pregnant women. The predictive ability of these late antenatal cultures is significantly better than for earlier cultures. Late cultures may result in less pressure to prescribe antenatal antibiotics and may facilitate an informed discussion of the risks and benefits of intrapartum prophylaxis against group B streptococci.

▶ This series of cultures, or cultured series, whatever your preference, provides perspective on the limitations of screening protocols for group B streptococci (GBS). Even under ideal circumstances, i.e., the correct timing (35–37 weeks), cultures taken from appropriate sites (distal vagina and rectum), and use of the selective broth medium, a number of women (15% or more depending on rates of colonization with GBS) colonized when delivery takes place, will not be identified as GBS carriers. Various explanations, including intermittent seeding from chronic carriage in the gastrointestinal tract, are offered to account for the missing carriers. The study does provide support for cultures to be performed late in the third trimester as opposed to at 26–28 weeks' gestation when there are even more false negative results. The implications for intrapartum management, which is driven by GBS status, will have to be measured. Cost considerations and lack of availability of a reliable quick screen preclude universal screening during labor. In the meantime the Centers for Disease Control and Prevention guidelines[1] designed to eradicate GBS disease from neonates[2] have been broadly accepted and instituted. The screening has posed a number of ethical issues,[3] but equal weight is given to algorithm-driven risk identification or screening cultures. Close monitoring for GBS is in progress and the results will speak for themselves. See also Abstracts 5–13 and 14–2.

Something attempted, something done, has earned a night's repose.— Henry Wadsworth Longfellow

A.A. Fanaroff, M.B.B.Ch.

References

1. Schuchat A, Whitney C, Zangwill K: Prevention of perinatal group B streptococcal disease: A public perspective. *MMWR Morb Mortal Wkly Rep* 45:1–24, 1996.
2. Regan JA, Klebanoff MA, Nugent RP, et al: Colonization with group B streptococci in pregnancy and adverse outcome. *Am J Obstet Gynecol* 174:1354–1360, 1996.
3. Yancey MK, Schuchat A, Duff P: Ethical issues associated with routine screening and prophylaxis for group B streptococci in pregnancy. *Infect Dis Obstet Gynecol* 4:36–42, 1996.

Varicella During Pregnancy: Maternal and Fetal Effects

Katz VL, Kuller JA, McMahon MJ, et al (Univ of North Carolina, Chapel Hill)

West J Med 163:446–450, 1995 3–11

Background.—Varicella infection in pregnancy, estimated to occur in 1 to 5 per 10,000 pregnancies, can have devastating consequences. The spectrum of fetal manifestations, the incidence and severity of varicella pneumonia, and the use of antiviral agents in affected patients are debated. One series was reviewed.

Methods.—Obstetric admissions during a 5.5-year period were reviewed to identify cases of varicella infections during pregnancy. There were 31 affected pregnancies among 11,753 deliveries.

Findings.—The mean age of affected women was 19.6 years, significantly different from the mean of the overall population, which was 25.3

years. The racial composition among affected patients was also different, with more Hispanics and fewer whites and blacks. The mean gestational age at vesicle eruption was 25 weeks. Seven of the 31 affected women entered labor preterm within a week of infection, and 3 delivered prematurely. Three infants weighed less than 2,700 g at birth. Respiratory symptoms developed in 6 women. Pneumonia developed in 4 women, 2 of whom needed ventilatory support. None of the 8 women given acyclovir had sequelae. Overall, 6 infants had lesions and anomalies at birth, which may have been associated with varicella in 5.

Conclusion.—Varicella infection increases maternal and fetal morbidity. Fetal disease may result from maternal infection at any gestational age. Maternal consequences appear to be worse when infection occurs in the latter half of pregnancy. Varying incidences of varicella infections in different populations is probably the result of differences in vaccination programs.

▶ This comment has been co-authored by Daniel S. Seidman, M.D., of The Sheba Medical Center, Tel-Hashomor, Israel:

▶ The introduction of child vaccination programs for chickenpox is likely to change the epidemiology of varicella infection during the next few years. However, the availability of a safe and effective varicella vaccine has raised the question as to whether serologic screening and immunization for varicella should now be offered to all women of childbearing age, similar to routine programs performed for rubella. Although the teratogenicity of varicella is much lower than that associated with rubella, prenatal diagnosis of varicella infection during pregnancy is not available, and chickenpox may be associated with severe maternal complications. The cost-effectiveness of screening programs for varicella immunity in the United States is doubtful, because well over 95% of the adult population is seropositive. However, as is demonstrated in the above study, it must be remembered that in some minority and immigrant groups, such as Hispanics and or Pacific Islanders, adult immunity is much lower, and, thus, those pregnant women are at higher risk of infection.

D. Seidman, M.D.
D.K. Stevenson, M.D.

Low Dose Aspirin for the Treatment of Fetal Growth Restriction: A Randomized Controlled Trial

Newnham JP, Godfrey M, Walters BJN, et al (King Edward Mem Hosp for Women, Perth, Western Australia)

Aust N Z J Obstet Gynaecol 35:370–374, 1995 3–12

Background.—Fetal growth restriction is associated with higher perinatal morbidity and mortality and may predispose the fetus to health risks later in life. Therapy for fetal growth restriction secondary to placental insufficiency needs to be established. These conditions can now be identified by US and Doppler flow studies. They may be related to abnormal vasoactive prostaglandin metabolism and dominant thromboxane activity. In animal models, the administration of a thromboxane analogue has produced abnormal umbilical artery waveforms. Low-dose aspirin therapy inhibits platelet thromboxane production. In 1 study, birth weight significantly improved in women with abnormal umbilical artery flow velocity waveforms who were given aspirin compared with women who were given placebo. The effect of daily aspirin therapy on birth weight in women with fetal growth restriction and umbilical-placental insufficiency was studied in a double-blind, placebo-controlled, randomized trial.

Methods.—Aspirin, 100 mg/day, or placebo was given to 51 women at 28–36 weeks of gestation who had a diagnosis of restricted fetal growth and umbilical-placental insufficiency. Compliance was evaluated by assaying maternal serum thromboxane B_2 levels. Ultrasonographic examinations were conducted every 7 days for the remainder of the pregnancy. Birth weight and other measures of neonatal size were recorded for each infant.

Results.—The following measures were similar for both groups at birth: gestational age; birth weight and birth weight ratio; head, chest, and abdomen circumference; skinfold thickness; and neonatal morbidity. Doppler systolic-to-diastolic ratios were not changed by aspirin therapy. Mean thromboxane B_2 levels fell more than 80% after 14 days of therapy. The ingestion of aspirin was not verified biochemically in 10.5% of women, despite their reports of compliance.

Conclusions.—In the women studied, low-dose aspirin therapy for 3.5 weeks did not improve fetal birth weight. Doppler systolic-to-diastolic ratios were not improved by aspirin therapy. Although 100% compliance was expected, 10% of women did not have biochemical evidence of aspirin. This may be related to the general belief that aspirin is contraindicated during pregnancy and to the reluctance in most women to take medication while pregnant. Biochemical confirmation of aspirin ingestion is recommended in similar trials.

▶ The Italian Study of Aspirin in Pregnancy demonstrated no differences in the frequency of spontaneous abortion, therapeutic abortion, stillbirth, premature birth, perinatal mortality, or low birth weight, or in the frequency of pregnancy-induced hypertension (PIH).[1] The authors concluded that prophylactic low-dose aspirin "does not appear to provide any benefit to women at moderate risk of PIH or IUGR [intrauterine growth retardation]." It is true that the study had its share of flaws, including the fact that the control group was unblinded. Hence, Newnham and colleagues can justify their attempt to reverse fetal growth restriction and alter Doppler systolic-to-diastolic ratios with the daily administration of 100 mg of aspirin to the mother. Unfortunately, they, too, were forced to conclude that low-dose aspirin "is not of benefit in the treatment of pregnancies complicated by fetal growth restriction and umbilical placental insufficiency between 28 and 36 weeks' gestation." In 10% of the women who claimed to be fully compliant, there was no change in the thromboxane B_2 levels, suggesting that they had failed to ingest the aspirin. What, if any, is the role of aspirin in complicated pregnancies? The evidence appears to be mounting against its use other than in highly selected pregnancies, such as those complicated by collagen vascular disease. Furthermore, if compliance is not 100% in women who have been shown that their infants are undergrown, what sort of compliance can be expected from a lower-risk population? Also see reference 2.

A.A. Fanaroff, M.B.B.Ch.

References

1. Italian Study of Aspirin in Pregnancy: Low dose aspirin in prevention and treatment of intrauterine growth retardation and pregnancy induced hypertension. *Lancet* 341:396–400, 1993.
2. 1995 YEARBOOK OF NEONATAL AND PERINATAL MEDICINE, p 51.

Twin Births to Mothers Who Are Twins: A Registry Based Study

Lichtenstein P, Olausson PO, Källén AJB (Karolinska Inst, Stockholm; Natl Board of Health and Welfare, Stockholm; Univ of Lund, Sweden)

BMJ 312:879–881, 1996 3–13

Background.—Although genetic factors are generally thought to be important for dizygotic but not monozygotic twinning, this issue has not been studied thoroughly. The risk of having twins among mothers who are twins was investigated.

Methods.—Data were obtained from 2 national Swedish registries. Multiple births occurring among 31,586 deliveries between 1973 and 1991 to women who were twins were noted.

Findings.—Women who were dizygotic twins had a moderately increased risk of giving birth to twins, with a relative risk of 1.3. This increase in risk appeared to be completely the result of dizygotic twinning. Mothers who were monozygotic twins had a significantly increased risk of giving birth to twins of the same sex, with a relative risk of 1.47. This was the result of an excess of monozygotic twins.

Conclusion.—The risk of giving birth to twins is increased among women who are twins. The genetic components of monozygotic and dizygotic twinning appear to operate independently.

▶ David J. Aughton, MD, Chief, Division of Genetics, Department of Pediatrics, William Beaumont Hospital, Royal Oak, Michigan, comments:

▶ During the past few decades, geneticists have become accustomed to the idea that what is unassailable fact today may be quaint archaism tomorrow. Phenomena such as uniparental disomy, gonadal mosaicism, genomic imprinting, submicroscopic chromosomal deletion, and triplet repeat expansion have each successfully challenged some element of genetic dogma and, in the process, have each taught medicine something new about the manner in which DNA goes about doing its work. Hence, a paper that challenges still another cherished bit of conventional genetic wisdom, namely, that genetic factors are rarely, if ever, important in the occurrence of monozygotic twinning, may be received with considerably less skepticism than was the case only a few years ago.

In this retrospective study, the authors confirmed earlier observations that women who are themselves dizygotic twins have a moderately increased risk of giving birth to twins, noting that the increased risk appears to be the result exclusively of dizygotic twinning. More surprisingly, the authors also found that women who are themselves monozygotic twins have an increased risk of having same-sex twins (although their overall risk of having twins is not increased) and that this increased risk is the result of an excess of monozygotic twins. The authors' findings hence suggest that genetic factors are important to the occurrence of monozygotic, as well as dizygotic, twinning.

In my view, however, the study is much weakened by the methods used to determine zygosity. The article describes the methods used for zygosity determination only briefly, and the references it cites regarding zygosity determination were all published in the 1960s and 1970s, well before newer and more reliable molecular methods for zygosity determination were developed. Although the authors' findings are exciting and most certainly worthy of further investigation, I consider it premature to counsel a woman who is a monozygotic twin that she is at increased risk of having monozygotic twins—at least until as confirmatory follow-up studies, using the most accurate methods for zygosity determination available, can be designed and conducted.

D.J. Aughton, M.D.

The Maternal and Neonatal Outcome of Triplet Gestations

Albrecht JL, Tomich PG (Loyola Univ, Maywood, Ill)

Am J Obstet Gynecol 174:1551–1556, 1996 3–14

Background.—The number of triplet gestations is increasing. Up-to-date information is needed on maternal risks and neonatal outcomes for management and counseling purposes. One experience with triplet gestations was reviewed.

Methods and Findings.—Fifty-seven triplet deliveries between April 1, 1989, and July 31, 1994, were retrospectively reviewed. The mean gestational age at birth was 33 weeks. The mean weight at birth was 1,820 g. Preterm labor occurred in 86% of the mothers; anemia in 58.1%, preeclampsia in 33.3%; preterm premature rupture of the membranes in 17.5%, postpartum bleeding in 12.3%; and hemolysis, increased liver enzymes, and low platelets syndrome in 10.5%. Neonatal complications included hyaline membrane disease in 29.6% of the infants, transient tachypnea of the newborn in 20.1%, intraventricular hemorrhage in 7.7%, and major congenital anomalies in 7.1%. Birth order did not significantly affect the incidence of neonatal complications. The perinatal death rate was 41 in 1,000 infants.

Conclusion.—Maternal and neonatal risks should be explained to patients being counseled about triplet gestations. Maternal morbidity continues to be extensive, and although perinatal mortality has declined markedly in triplet gestations, it is still higher than the mortality among singletons.

▶ Commenting on this article is Louis P. Halamek, M.D., Professor of Pediatrics, Division of Neonatal and Developmental Medicine, Stanford University Medical Center, Palo Alto, California:

▶ Although the lay public may think of multiple births as "blessed events," perinatologists and neonatologists usually do not speak of them in quite the same terms. Although it is intuitive that the maternal and fetal/neonatal risks increase with an increasing number of fetuses, few contemporary studies have assigned numerical values to these risks. Reproductive technologies have provided, and will continue to provide, many opportunities to quantify the risks of the multiple-gestation pregnancy.

L.P. Halamek, M.D.

Exercise During Pregnancy and Pregnancy Outcome

Sternfeld B, Quesenberry CP Jr, Eskenazi B, et al (Kaiser Permanente Med Care Program, Oakland, Calif; Univ of California, Berkeley)

Med Sci Sports Exerc 27:634–640, 1995 3–15

Background.—Studies have shown that healthy pregnant women can safely tolerate the physiologic demands of exercise. However, the effects of maternal exercise on pregnancy outcome are more controversial. The relations between maternal aerobic exercise and pregnancy outcomes, including birth weight and pregnancy symptoms, were investigated.

Methods.—A quantitative exercise history was obtained from 388 healthy women with singleton pregnancies at 3 different time points, beginning at 16.5 weeks' gestation. Retrospective information about exercise patterns before pregnancy and during the first trimester of pregnancy was obtained at the initial interview. Data on the frequency, duration, and mode of exercise were evaluated to classify the exercise level as follows: level I was defined as aerobic training exercise excluding vigorous walking at least 3 times a week for at least 20 minutes; level II exercise included vigorous walking at the same frequency and duration as in level I; level III was defined as aerobic exercise including walking at least once a week; level IV was defined as aerobic exercise less than once a week. Outcome variables included symptoms of pregnancy, birth weight, gestational weight gain, complications of pregnancy, and perinatal complications. Multivariate analysis included potential confounders, such as race, education, parity, and history of adverse pregnancy outcome.

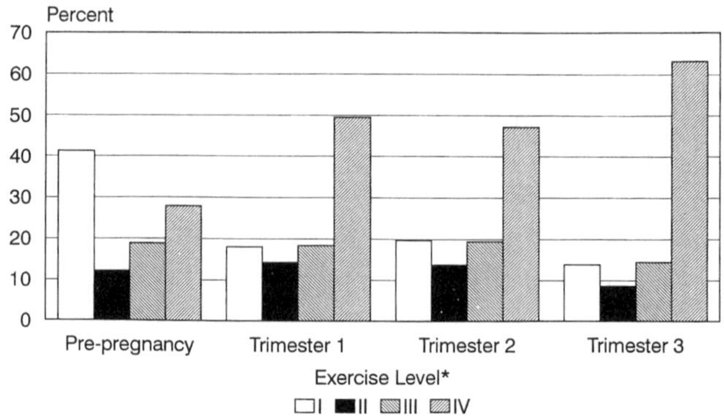

FIGURE 1.—Level of aerobic exercise before pregnancy and in trimesters 1, 2, and 3. Level I included aerobic exercise other than vigorous walking at least 3 times a week for 20 minutes at a time; level II included aerobic exercise at least 3 times a week for 20 minutes at a time only if walking was included; level III included aerobic exercise at least once a week but less than level I or II; and level IV included aerobic exercise less than once a week. (Courtesy of Sternfeld B, Quesenberry CP Jr, Eskenazi B, et al: Exercise during pregnancy and pregnancy outcome. *Med Sci Sports Exerc* 27(5):634–640, 1995.)

Results.—Overall, the women tended to exercise less during pregnancy than they had before pregnancy (Fig 1). Birth weight did not differ significantly in relation to levels of exercise before or during pregnancy in either univariate or multivariate analysis. Similarly, other pregnancy outcomes, including gestational age, gestational weight gain, percentage of cesarean sections, and perinatal or infant complications, were not associated with the level of aerobic exercise. However, the women who were getting level I or II exercise during the first trimester and/or third trimester experienced fewer symptoms of pregnancy than the women who were getting level III or IV exercise during the same period. Second-trimester exercise level was not associated with variations in symptoms of pregnancy. Higher levels of exercise during the first trimester also were associated with reduced symptoms in later pregnancy.

Discussion.—Aerobic exercise at a level sufficient for a physiologic training effect can reduce the symptoms of pregnancy without compromising birth weight or other pregnancy outcomes. Decreased activity levels tended to precede changes in pregnancy symptoms, suggesting that exercise had a direct causal effect on well-being.

▶ Exercise has become a multibillion-dollar industry. There is a constant barrage of glamorized commercials advertising athletic equipment and infomercials extolling the advantages of the latest exercise bike, treadmill, or stair-climbing equipment. In addition, you may purchase the latest gadget to give you thighs of steel, if that is what you desire, or an abdomen like a washboard. Not to mention the clothing. Well, what should the expectant mother do? Is exercise good for her and her unborn child?

Sternfeld and colleagues publish data to support the safety of exercise during pregnancy, with no adverse effects on fetal growth and enough endorphins generated to diminish the usual pregnancy-associated symptoms. McMurray and associates demonstrated that pregnant women between 21 and 28 weeks' gestation could perform 40 minutes of either aerobic dance or walking with fairly high intensity.[1] The walking seemed to be better for the fetus because there was less of an increase in fetal heart rate than occurred in response to aerobic dance. The fetal heart rates averaged 172 beats/min during aerobic dance vs.149 beats/min with walking. When the mom is exercising vigorously, the fetus is getting a stress test, too.

Hence, the answer to the question of whether exercise is good for the fetus is a resounding maybe. Pregnancy is not the time to become a couch potato, nor is it the time to start training for a marathon. Women who are used to daily vigorous exercise will go stir-crazy if they are totally restricted. Exercise should be done in moderation so that the mother is not overheating or overstressing the fetus.

A.A. Fanaroff, M.B.B.Ch.

Reference

1. McMurray RG, Katz VL, Poe MP: Maternal and fetal responses to low impact aerobic dance. *Am J Perinatol* 12:282–285, 1995.

Cigarette Smoking During Pregnancy

Stewart DE, Streiner DL (Univ of Toronto; McMaster Univ, Hamilton, Ont, Canada)
Can J Psychiatry 40:603–607, 1995 3–16

Background.—Although the deleterious effects of smoking on pregnancy have long been well documented, many pregnant women still smoke. A sample of women in prenatal care were studied to determine the

TABLE 1.—Relative Risks of Prenatal Smokers (n = 89) vs. Nonsmokers (n = 456)

VARIABLE (NUMBER)	RELATIVE RISK	95% CI
Age under 21 years (531)	6.08	3.55 – 10.41
Born in Canada (531)	1.38	1.17 – 1.61
Elementary school education or less (521)	4.55	2.96 – 6.98
Unemployed (532)	1.74	1.33 – 2.29
Unmarried (539)	4.00	2.84 – 5.63
Unplanned pregnancy (539)	2.25	1.81 – 2.79
Previous emotional problem (536)	7.29	4.09 – 12.98
Previous physical problem (537)	1.95	1.21 – 3.15
Unhealthy diet (535)	2.41	1.30 – 4.49
Alcohol drinking (465)	2.84	2.08 – 3.88
Nonprescription drug use (538)	1.85	1.36 – 2.52
Illicit drug use (539)	28.97	10.24 – 81.97
Physical abuse before pregnancy (492)	5.95	3.63 – 9.77
Physical abuse during pregnancy (542)	13.23	6.62 – 26.46
GHQ case status (524)	1.61	1.37 – 1.91

Abbreviations: CI, confidence interval; *GHQ*, General Health Questionnaire.
(Courtesy of Stewart DE, Streiner DL: Cigarette smoking during pregnancy. *Can J Psychiatry* 40:603–607, 1995.)

prevalence of smoking during the latter half of pregnancy, the psychosocial and demographic characteristics differentiating smoking and heavy-smoking patients, and the psychiatric morbidities and psychological attitudes of these smokers.

Methods.—A total of 545 women during the latter half of pregnancy completed a survey containing 3 questionnaires. The study questionnaire addressed sociodemographic features, past and present health, current pregnancy history, domestic violence, and health habits (including smoking) during pregnancy. The General Health Questionnaire measured mental distress and identified probable psychiatric cases. The Fetal Health Locus of Control measured the extent to which the woman believed the health of her fetus was controlled by internal control, powerful others, or chance. The responses of smokers and nonsmokers were compared.

Results.—Of the 545 women, 89 (16.33%) smoked during the second half of pregnancy. Compared with nonsmokers, the smokers were younger, had less education, and were more likely to be unemployed and unmarried, have poor nutritional habits, drink alcohol, use illicit drugs, have unplanned pregnancies, have histories of emotional and physical problems, and have histories of physical abuse (Table 1). Smokers also were more likely to have General Health Questionnaire scores indicating probable case status and to consider chance to be more important than internal control or powerful others to the health of their fetuses. These features were even more characteristic of heavy smokers, compared with smokers who smoked 10 or fewer cigarettes per day.

Conclusions.—Women who smoke during pregnancy tend to have several other health risk factors, making them a high-risk population requiring multidimensional intervention. Psychiatrists working with obstetric and gynecologic services can provide primary preventive measures (including education about the effects of smoking and more adaptive ways of coping) and secondary preventive measures (including identifying and treating psychiatric disorders).

► Facts should speak for themselves. The facts are that smoking may result in abortion, fetal death, abruptio placentae, fetal growth retardation, and perinatal death. The offspring have an increased risk of asthma, upper respiratory tract infections, and sudden infant death. Why, then, would anyone with reasonable intelligence continue this noxious habit when pregnant? The psychiatric approach to the problem reveals that the answer to this question is exponentially more complicated than one would have imagined. Smokers were more likely to drink alcohol, use nonprescription and illicit drugs, have unplanned pregnancies, have histories of emotional and physical problems, and have suffered physical abuse before and during pregnancy. Because one of the objectives of the study was to determine psychiatric morbidities with psychological attitudes associated with smoking and pregnancy, Pandora's box has been opened. Psychiatrists can have a field day addressing the public health problem posed by smoking. Education about the harmful effects of smoking is a good starting point. A more formidable task is to change perceptions about the social acceptability of smoking and to improve the self-esteem of these downtrodden women.

Pregnancy provides a unique opportunity to educate women, because it is one of the rare occasions when they receive regular contact with health care providers. More young women than ever are smoking, and we must persist in delivering the simple message that it is not only harmful for them, but also for their unborn children.

Values are not trendy items that are casually traded in.—Ellen Goodman

A.A. Fanaroff, M.B.B.Ch.

Validity of Self-reported Smoking Habits in Pregnancy: A Saliva Cotinine Analysis

Parazzini F, Davoli E, Rabaiotti M, et al (Istitute di Ricerche Farmacologiche 'Mario Negri,' Milano, Italy; Università di Milano, Italy)
Acta Obstet Gynecol Scand 75:352–354, 1996 3–17

Objective.—Although half of women smokers in Italy report that they stop smoking during pregnancy, the validity of those reports is questionable. The validity of self-reported cigarette smoking during the third trimester of pregnancy was examined using saliva cotinine as a marker of exposure.

Methods.—Interviews were conducted with 109 pregnant women aged 18–40 years and saliva samples were collected from current and self-reported former smokers. Saliva cotinine concentrations were determined.

Results.—There were 25 self-reported former smokers and 27 current smokers. Cotinine levels were less than 10 ng/mL in 20 of 25 self-reported former smokers. The 5 self-reported former smokers said their husbands smoked more than 10 cigarettes per day. Six of 26 current smokers had cotinine levels less than 10 ng/mL, 20 had levels of 10 ng/mL or greater. Mean levels were 20.4 ng/mL in smokers of less than 5 cigarettes per day and 50.8 ng/mL in smokers of more than 5 cigarettes per day.

Conclusion.—Measurement of saliva cotinine levels validates self-reported smoking habits of pregnant women.

▶ This comment was co-authored by Daniel S. Seidman, M.D., of The Sheba Medical Center, Tel-Hashomor, Israel:

▶ Smoking is currently recognized as the most important adverse environmental factor during pregnancy. A large volume of data collected during the past 3 decades has consistently revealed a quantitative effect of smoking on fetal growth in populations spanning the entire globe. The need to validate the number of cigarettes that the mother actually smoked during pregnancy is important to support associations revealed in epidemiologic studies. The well-recognized phenomena of maternal underreporting of smoking habits during pregnancy may actually reflect a more fundamental phenomenon of self-denial by the mothers. Thus, presenting results of objective measures of exposure to smoke to the mother may play an important role in patient education, especially for teenage mothers. Analysis of saliva cotinine, suggested in the present study to be highly accurate, has the advantage of being less invasive than measurements of serum thiocynate.

Another method of precisely assessing exposure to tobacco smoke without obtaining blood or urine samples is the assessment of carbon monoxide (CO) levels in the breath of the mother or newborn. A recently introduced portable machine used for detection of neonatal hemolysis (Baby's Breath, Natus, San Carlos) has been shown to allow rapid determination of CO levels in the mother's or newborn's breath. This instrument may be especially useful for educational purposes, as it provides the results of the measurements "on the spot." The need for accurate determination of smoke exposure is most apparent for assessment of passive smoking, because even responsible self-reporting may not provide a true estimate of the magnitude of environmental exposure.

D. Seidman, M.D.
D.K. Stevenson, M.D.

Drugs, Poverty, Pregnancy, and Foster Care in Los Angeles, California, 1989 to 1991

Lewis MA, Leake B, Giovannoni J, et al (Univ of California, Los Angeles)
West J Med 163:435–440, 1995 3–18

Background.—In previous research conducted by the Los Angeles Department of Children and Family Services, it was discovered that the vast majority of infants removed from their mothers at birth for referral to the juvenile court had been born to drug users who had several other children already under the court's jurisdiction. The characteristics and childbearing histories of women with infants entering foster care in Los Angeles County were reported.

Methods and Findings.—Data were obtained on 1,155 drug users whose infants were removed from them at birth by court order and 236 non–drug users whose infants were removed at birth. All were indigent. Fewer than half had graduated from high school. More than one fourth of the drug users were homeless. Criminal records were more common among drug users than non–drug users. Many of the women in the comparison group had mental health problems. Seventeen percent were teenagers under court custody. Eighty percent of all children born to both groups of women were under court jurisdiction. Twenty-two percent of a subgroup of 926 drug users had borne another infant placed in foster care. Half of these infants had had a positive drug immunoassay. Of 185 non–drug users, 7.6% had had another infant in foster care.

Conclusion.—The foster care population is increasingly one of drug users and adolescents and their children. Preventive programs for this population need to include family planning, mental health services, and drug prevention or rehabilitation services. Previous findings have shown that as many as 80% of infants exposed to drugs prenatally will be placed in foster care in the first year of life.

► Commenting on this article is William E. Benitz, M.D., Associate Professor of Pediatrics, Clinical Director of Intensive Care Nursery, Division of Neonatal and Developmental Care Medicine, Stanford University School of Medicine, Palo Alto, California:

► Here is another demonstration that social services and policies remain inadequate. Efforts to improve the prospects of high-risk newborn infants clearly must include activities in the political arena for addressing these issues. The scope of neonatal-perinatal medicine extends beyond the walls of the hospital!

W.E. Benitz, M.D.

The Safety of Calcium Channel Blockers in Human Pregnancy: A Prospective, Multicenter Cohort Study

Magee LA, Schick B, Donnenfeld AE, et al (Hosp for Sick Children, Toronto; Pennsylvania Hosp, Philadelphia; Univ of South Florida, Tampa; et al)

Am J Obstet Gynecol 174:823–828, 1996 3–19

Introduction.—Many unplanned pregnancies are terminated because of the fear that inadvertent drug exposure may have harmed the fetus. In the case of calcium channel blockers, there have been 55 reports of presumed or confirmed first-trimester exposure and 4 malformations. The potential teratogenicity of first-trimester exposure to these commonly prescribed drugs was assessed in a prospective, multicenter, cohort study.

Methods.—Patients were enrolled when they contacted teratogen information services about first-trimester exposure to any calcium channel blockers. The outcome of these pregnancies was compared with that of a group of control patients matched to case patients by maternal age and smoking habits. Control patients had been counseled about drugs or exposures not known or suspected of being teratogenic or fetotoxic.

Results.—Seventy-eight women were enrolled and followed up for pregnancy outcome. The most commonly ingested agents were nifedipine (44%) and verapamil (41%), and hypertension was the most common (57%) indication for treatment. There was a trend toward fewer live births in the group exposed to calcium channel blockers (79%) compared with the nonteratogenic control group (89%). Two women treated for hypertension with calcium channel blockers had stillborn infants. The incidence of major malformations did not differ significantly between control patients (0%) and patients with first-trimester exposure to calcium channel blockers (3%). Malformed infants were born to 2 women, both of whom had been treated with calcium channel blockers throughout pregnancy.

One woman had insulin-dependent diabetes and the other had systemic lupus erythematosus. Treatment with calcium channel blockers was associated with a decrease in gestational age, an increase in preterm delivery, and a trend toward lower birth weight.

Conclusions.—First-trimester exposure to calcium channel blockers, principally nifedipine or verapamil, did not lead to an increase in major malformations or excess neonatal health problems. A significant decrease in gestational age in the calcium channel blockers–treated group was attributed to maternal illness rather than to the therapy itself.

▶ The words "multicenter, prospective, cohort study" surely must be music to the toxicologist/geneticist/environmentalist's ears. It is difficult to conceive, but evidently true, that before 1960, birth defects were regarded as genetic in origin. The sanctuary of the womb was believed to protect the fetus from the toxic effects of environmental agents to which the mother was exposed. Since then, it has been established that the fetus may be injured by many chemicals, drugs, or other agents taken by the mother. Perhaps thalidomide has been the most dramatic example, but, unfortunately, the list of harmful products continues to expand. Awareness of the possible harm presented to the fetus by prescription or "street" drugs has led to an increased number of well-controlled scientific studies that supplement the extensive anecdotal literature. To this collection we can add this nice little piece of evidence from Magee and associates. They conclude that first-trimester exposure to calcium channel blockers (especially nifedipine and verapamil) does not represent a major teratogenic risk. The study, which included 66 women exposed to calcium channel blockers from the first trimester, ruled out a 5-fold increase in malformations (baseline 2%, $a = 0.05$, $B = 0.2$). There was an increase in low–birth weight infants that could be attributed to maternal disease for which the calcium channel blockers were prescribed.

Premarketing animal toxicology studies, in several species, consistently demonstrated digital or other limb defects, proving once again the limited predictive value of animal studies for human teratogenicity. The fallibility of postmarketing surveillance is discussed—the outcome of the exposure is known, but the relative risk cannot be assessed because the total number of drug-exposed, pregnant women is not known.

Women exposed to calcium channel blockers perceived their teratogenic risk to be significantly higher than that of control patients, but after counseling, the groups were indistinguishable in their teratogenic risk perception. The book has not been closed on calcium channel blockers and their risk to the fetus; however, the first chapter concludes in a satisfactory manner.

*Forget about transplants. In the not too distant future, people with failing tissues or organs may have new ones fabricated in the laboratory. The tools are already in hand.—Geoffrey Cowley (*Newsweek, *January 27, 1997)*

A.A. Fanaroff, M.B.B.Ch.

Antenatal Care in Pregnancies at Risk of Alloimmune Thrombocytopenia: Report of 19 Cases in 16 Families

Kanhai HHH, Porcelijn L, van Zoeren D, et al (Univ Hosp, Leiden, The Netherlands; Central Lab Bloodtransfusion, Amsterdam)

Eur J Obstet Gynecol Reprod Biol 68:67–73, 1996 3–20

Background.—Fetal/neonatal alloiummune thrombocytopenia (NAITP), a rare disease caused by alloimmunization of the mother against a platelet-specific antigen, is associated with a 2% to 20% chance of intracranial hemorrhage in the fetus. In the first pregnancy, immunization occurs in 10% to 50% of cases. Optimal antenatal care for these patients has not been established because of the lack of information on some crucial pathophysiologic aspects of NAITP. A protocol for the assessment and treatment of fetal thrombocytopenia was reported.

Methods.—Nineteen fetuses at risk for thrombocytopenia were identified and cordocentesis was done. When the fetal platelet count was less than 100 × 10^9/L, high-dose IV gamma globulin was administered to the mother.

Findings.—Platelet antagonisms were HPA-la in 15 patients. HPA-4a in 2, and HPA-3a in 1. Another woman had antibodies against a private antigen. All 18 multigravidas had previously given birth to an infant with NAITP, 2 of whom had severe bleeding. Findings for the offending antigen were negative in 2 fetuses. At first cordocentesis, the median and mean platelet counts were 26 and 75 × 10^9/L, respectively. Thirty-seven of the 46 cordocenteses were followed by platelet transfusions. There were no bleeding complications. Eight mothers received IV gamma globulin and 2 fetuses responded. Nine infants were delivered by cesarean section and 10 vaginally at 34–41 weeks' gestation (mean, 37 weeks). At birth, median and mean platelet counts were 141.5 and 140 × 10^9/L, respectively. Antenatal and postnatal ultrasound assessment showed no intracranial bleeding. One neonate died of procedure-related causes. Another had convulsions in the neonatal period, caused by a sinus thrombosis, possibly related to the platelet transfusions.

Conclusion.—Cordocentesis in NAITP can be postponed when obstetric history is considered. By following safety recommendations, cordocentesis can be performed without bleeding complications. However, the current findings do not support routine cordocentesis in patients with a history of NAITP. Clinicians must consider the risks of this procedure and the lack of prospective data on the magnitude of the risk of intrauterine or peripartal bleeding.

▶ Commenting on this article is Louis P. Halamek, M.D., Professor of Pediatrics, Division of Neonatal and Developmental Medicine, Stanford University Medical Center, Palo Alto, California:

▶ Alloimmune thrombocytopenia remains a difficult problem for the perinatologist. Up to 20% of affected fetuses have intracranial hemorrhage, half of which occur in utero before delivery. As in other areas of fetal therapy, including fetal surgery, how to select the subpopulation of fetuses at greatest risk for sequelae and how to limit invasive, risky interventions to this group are unkown. Progress is being made; genotyping of fetal platelet antigens with amniocytes is a technique that eliminates the need for cordocentesis in pregnancies found to be nonalloimmunized.[1] The findings in this report echo those of Paidas et al.,[2] indicating that obstetric history is a useful, noninvasive screening tool. While our perinatal colleagues wrestle with these issues, those of us on the other side of the umbilical cord—neonatologists and pediatricians—must continue to grapple with the questions of when to worry and what to do about "low" platelet counts in premature and full-term neonates.

L.P. Halamek, M.D.

References

1. Khouzami AN, Kickler TS, Bray PF, et al: Molecular genotyping of fetal platelet antigens with uncultured amniocytes. *Am J Obstet Gynecol* 173:1202–1206, 1995.
2. Paidas MJ, Berkowitz RL, Lynch L, et al: Alloimmune thrombocytopenia: Fetal and neonatal losses related to cordocentesis. *Am J Obstet Gynecol* 172:475–479, 1995.

Perinatal Consequences of Maternal Hypothyroidism in Early Pregnancy and Inadequate Replacement

Wasserstrum N, Anania CA (Baylor College of Medicine, Houston)
Clin Endocrinol (Oxf) 42:353–358, 1995 3–21

Objective.—Although hypothyroidism during pregnancy is rare, it frequently results in abortions, stillbirths, congenital malformations, maternal anemia, pregnancy-induced hypertension, and postpartum hemorrhage. Results of a retrospective study comparing the effect of hypothyroidism on maternal condition at the initial visit with near term perinatal outcome were assessed.

Methods.—Free thyroxine index (FTI), thyroid-stimulating hormone (TSH), and hematocrit were measured at the initial visit and several times during the 43 pregnancies of 42 women with hypothyroidism. Rate of cesarean section for fetal distress, neonatal weight and percentile at delivery, and gestational age were determined.

Results.—Five of 9 patients with severe hypothyroidism (FTI of 0.6 or less) at the initial visit, and 1 of 33 (34 pregnancies) patients with milder hypothyroidism at the initial visit, had a cesarean section. Severity of hypothyroidism at the initial visit was significantly associated with TSH level and an abnormally high TSH in late pregnancy but not with gestational age, neonatal weight percentile, or FTI in late pregnancy. Fetal distress was significantly associated with severity of hypothyroidism as measured by both low FTI and high TSH. Five of 6 women who had a cesarean section for fetal distress had FTI of 0.6 or less, whereas significantly fewer (4 of 36) women without fetal distress had severe hypothyroidism. Four of 6 women with fetal distress initially had TSH greater than 60, whereas significantly fewer (1 of 36) women without fetal distress had TSH greater than 60. Fetal distress was correlated with lower hematocrit during labor and delivery but not to near term FTI. There was 1 in utero fetal death and 1 preterm membrane rupture.

Conclusion.—Severe maternal hypothyroidism in early pregnancy frequently resulted in fetal distress during labor. Although near term FTI levels were normal in these women, TSH was elevated throughout pregnancy. Early treatment of hypothyroidism is important in this group of patients because early balances in maternal thyroxine level may have permanent and negative effects on the fetus.

▶ I had always been led to believe that severe hypothyroidism was characterized by anovulation, so pregnancy would be an uncommon association. However, Klein and associates[1] estimated the prevalence of thyroid deficiency in pregnant women was around 2.5%. Pregnancy complications attributable to hypothyroidism include abortions, stillbirths, maternal anemia, pregnancy-induced hypertension, postpartum hemorrhage, and congenital malformations. Man[2] reported ocular and neurologic defects in the progeny of hypothyroid women receiving "adequate replacement only later in gestation."

Wasserstrum and Anania present a strong correlation between very low FTI at initial antepartum presentation and fetal distress requiring surgical intervention. The total number of research subjects is small. Their initial presentation at around 19 weeks is surprisingly late for such a high-risk population, raising questions about the patients' understanding of their disease and compliance with medication. A number of possibilities are raised to explain the correlation. They were hypothetically sound, including anemia, diminished vascular reserve, and hypertension, but not very convincing.

It strikes me that our internal medicine colleagues or endocrinologists should be making a concerted effort to ensure better education of their hypothyroid patients and should ensure that they are euthyroid and well medicated before conception.

He who will not reason is a bigot; he who cannot is a fool; and he who dares not is a slave.—Sir William Drummond

A.A. Fanaroff, M.B.B.Ch.

References

1. Klein RZ, Haddow JE, Faix JD, et al: Prevalence of thyroid deficiency in pregnant women. *Clin Endocrinol* 35:41–46, 1991.
2. Man EB, Brown JF, Serunian, SA: Maternal hypothyroxinemia: Psychoneurological deficits of progeny. *Ann Clin Lab Science* 21:227–239, 1991.

4 Antepartum Fetal Surveillance

Improved Intrapartum Surveillance With PR Interval Analysis of the Fetal Electrocardiogram: A Randomized Trial Showing a Reduction in Fetal Blood Sampling

van Wijngaarden WJ, Sahota DS, James DK, et al (Univ of Nottingham, England; Ninewells Hosp, Dundee, Scotland; Prince of Wales Hosp, Hong Kong)

Am J Obstet Gynecol 174:1295–1299, 1996 4–1

Introduction.—Although the use of electronic fetal monitoring (EFM) has become a standard in assessing fetal health, no improvements in long-term neonatal outcome have been shown with its use. In addition, the introduction of fetal blood sampling has been associated with an increase in cesarean section rates. The limitations of these methods have shown a need for a better method of intrapartum surveillance to identify fetuses at risk for intrapartum hypoxia. In a prospective trial, the use of fetal ECG time-interval analysis in addition to conventional EFM was evaluated for its effect in reducing the need for fetal scalp blood sampling.

Methods.—Two hundred fourteen women with high-risk pregnancies were included in the trial. Patients were randomly assigned to undergo EFM alone (EFM group) or EFM with fetal ECG time-interval analysis (EFM with analysis). For patients receiving EFM alone, labor and interventions were managed by conventional practice. For patients undergoing monitoring and time-interval analysis, management was based on 3 criteria: EFM, conduction index, and ratio index. Interventions required (need for fetal blood sampling and operative delivery) and fetal outcomes were compared between the 2 groups.

Results.—Thirty of the 214 patients were excluded from the final analysis, primarily because of difficulties in obtaining fetal ECGs. Twenty-one patients in the EFM group underwent a total of 28 fetal blood samplings, whereas 5 patients in the EFM with analysis group underwent a total of 5 fetal blood samplings. These differences were statistically significant; the risk ratio for fetal blood sampling associated with EFM alone was 3.53. (Table 2). Fetal blood sampling was abnormal in only 1 sample in the EFM group, compared with 2 abnormal results in the EFM with analysis group;

TABLE 2.—Results

	Electronic fetal monitoring	*Electronic fetal monitoring and fetal electrocardiogram analysis*	*Risk ratio*	*95% Confidence interval*	*Significance*
Total recruited (No.)	102	112	—	—	—
Total included in analysis (No.)	100	84	—	—	—
Gestational age (No.)					
>37 wk	92	76	—	—	—
27–37 wk	8	8			
Patients undergoing fetal blood sampling (No.)	21 (21%)	5 (6%)	3.53	1.39–8.95	$p < 0.01$
Fetal blood sampling (No.)	28 (28%)	5 (6%)	—*	—*	—*
Fetal blood sampling with normal result (No.)	27 (96%)	3 (60%)	1.61	0.91–2.84	$p = 0.05$
Acidotic infants (No.)	14 (14%)	8 (9.5%)	1.47	—	NS
Missed acidosis (No.)	9 (9%)	4 (4.8%)	1.89	—	NS
Assisted deliveries (No.)	42 (42%)	36 (42.8%)	0.98	—	NS
Assisted deliveries for presumed fetal distress (No.)	16 (16%)	7 (8.3%)	1.96	—	NS

Abbreviation: NS, Not significant.

*These were not calculated, because the length of labor could distort comparisons.

(Courtesy of van Wijngaarden WJ, Sahota DS, James DK, et al: Improved intrapartum surveillance with PR interval analysis of the fetal electrocardiogram: A randomized trial showing a reduction in fetal blood sampling. *Am J Obstet Gynecol* 174:1295–1299, 1996.)

EFM alone was less likely to be associated with an abnormal fetal blood sampling result as compared with EFM with analysis, with a risk ratio of 0.62 for EFM alone. There were no significant differences in the number of acidotic infants, the number of assisted deliveries, or the number of assisted deliveries for presumed fetal distress. However, there was a trend for increased risk of these occurrences with EFM alone.

Conclusion.—In this study, the use of fetal ECG time-interval analysis in addition to conventional electronic fetal monitoring was associated with a significant decrease in the need for fetal scalp blood sampling. Electrocardiogram time-interval analysis also increased the effectiveness of fetal blood sampling, with more abnormal results as compared with conventional EFM. There were, however, no increases in adverse outcomes.

▶ The extensive use of EFM during the past 30 years has increased cesarean section rates dramatically without any measurable long-term benefit for the infant. In spite of this well-documented fact, obstetricians seem wedded to the use of EFM, and their enthusiasm for it is exceeded only by that of plaintiffs' attorneys. It has been possible for some time to analyze the fetal ECG, but only recently has its clinical usefulness been determined.[1] Normally, as one might expect, when the heart rate increases, the PR interval decreases. However, when fetal acidosis is present, the PR interval *increases* as the fetal heart rate increases. This is expressed as the conduction index, and a persistently positive index indicates an increased risk of fetal compromise. The relationship can be quantified by calculating the ratio index, which reflects the percentage of time that the conduction index is more than 2 standard deviations above the mean.

High-risk mothers were recruited and randomly assigned to a group that received conventional EFM alone or EFM plus fetal ECG time-interval analysis. Although the fetal ECG group had less need for fetal blood sampling and fewer abnormal fetal blood samples, it is disappointing that there was no difference in the number of "assisted deliveries" (forceps, ventouse, or cesarean section). However, only half as many patients in the fetal ECG monitoring group required assisted delivery for presumed fetal distress, although the numbers were too small to achieve statistical significance. The ultimate benefit of fetal ECG monitoring combined with EFM can be demonstrated only in a clinical trial that compares labors monitored in that manner with those monitored by standard intermittent auscultation. Failing this, a study of a larger sample size might demonstrate a significant reduction in cesarean sections for presumed fetal distress. The authors indicate that they are currently embarking on such a trial. Stay tuned.

M.J. Maisels, M.B.B.Ch.

Reference

1. Westgate J, Harris M, Curnow JSH, et al: Plymouth randomized trial of cardiotocography only versus ST waveform plus cardiotography for intrapartum monitoring in 2400 cases. *Am J Obstet Gynecol* 169:1151–1160, 1993.

The Potential Impact of PR Interval Analysis of the Fetal Electrocardiogram (FECG) on Intrapartum Fetal Monitoring

Reed NN, Mohajer MP, Sahota DS, et al (Univ Hosp, Nottingham, England)
Eur J Obstet Gynecol Reprod Biol 68:87–92, 1996 4–2

Introduction.—Although continuous electronic fetal heart rate monitoring (EFM) is considered an indicator of fetal well-being, its use alone is questioned. The potential value of PR interval analysis of the fetal ECG (FECG) was assessed and compared with conventional intrapartum assessment using EFM.

Methods.—The labors of 265 women were selected for intrapartum monitoring on the basis of high risk for fetal hypoxia. These outcome measures were recorded for each woman: fetal scalp blood sampling (FBS), the mode of delivery and whether delivery was expedited for EFM abnormality or low scalp pH, and the condition of the fetus at delivery (pH, base excess, partial pressure of carbon dioxide, and partial pressure of oxygen of umbilical cord blood). Arterial and venous cord blood was collected immediately after delivery. The PR interval and heart rate of the FECG waveform were recorded.

Results.—The FECG signals of 246 labors were suitable for analysis. Fetal blood sampling was obtained on 83 occasions in 61 patients (24.8% of labors) to evaluate abnormality of the fetal heart rate pattern. Twelve samples (14.5%) had a scalp pH of greater than 7.25. Of these, 7 (8.4%) had a pH of 7.20, prompting delivery, and 71 (85.6%) had normal scalp pH. With a normal fetal heart rate pattern, both FECG parameters would have to be abnormal to necessitate an FBS. There were 36 instances of cord arterial pH being 7.15 (14.6%) or greater at delivery. Of 53 (21.5%) instances of deliveries being expedited for either suspected fetal distress on EFM interpretation or an abnormal scalp pH, 38 (15.4%) had an arterial pH of less than 7.15 and 21 (8.5%) instances of acidosis were missed by EFM alone.

TABLE 4.—The Ability of Fetal ECG Parameters to Predict a Scalp pH of Less Than 7.20 Either Alone or When Used in Conjunction With Electronic Fetal Monitoring (EFM) Interpretation

Test	Sensitivity	Specificity	Positive predictive value	Negative predictive value	Accuracy
Single tests					
Abnormal EFM†	N/A*	N/A	8%	N/A	N/A
Abnormal ratio index‡	60%	77%	16%	96%	76%
Abnormal conduction index§	25%	60%	4%	94%	64%
Combined tests					
ABEFM + (ABRI or ABCI)	75%	62%	23%	98%	65%

**N/A* indicates not applicable because fetal scalp pH would be assessed only when EFM was abnormal.
†Abnormal EFM (*ABEFM*): pathologic trace diagnosed by labor suite staff.
‡Abnormal ratio index (*ABRI*): ratio index greater than 4%.
§Abnormal conduction index (*ABCI*): sustained conduction index for more than 20 minutes.
(Courtesy of Reed NN, Mohajer MP, Sahota DS, et al: The potential impact of PR interval analysis of the fetal electrocardiogram (FECG) on intrapartum fetal monitoring. *Eur J Obstet Gynecol Reprod Biol* 68:87–92, 1996.

Conclusions.—The addition of PR interval assessment possibly could reduce the number of normal FBSs being performed from 85.5% to 26.8% (Table 4) and the instances of missed acidosis at delivery from 8.5% to 4.5%. PR interval analysis of the FECG may improve the interpretation of intrapartum fetal monitoring.

▶ Electronic fetal monitoring, the mainstay of fetal evaluation, is unsatisfactory in its original format.[1] No ifs, ands, or buts. It needs to be upgraded either by considering it obsolete and moving on to the next generation of monitors, such as the near-infrared spectroscopy (see this year's Special Article and Abstract 5–5), or by complementing it with the FECG or parts thereof.[2–4] There is a significant body of evidence supporting such a move, and Reed and associates in this retrospective analysis confirm that the addition of PR interval analysis (measured from the peak of the P wave to the peak of the R wave) reduces the need for fetal blood gas sampling as well as the proportion of cases with "missed acidosis" at birth. The need for caution in the title and use of the word "potential" are necessary because this was a theoretical application of the findings. Time interval measurements of the FECG are robust and not subject to the problems of measuring changes in amplitude. The inevitable call for a prospective trial is muted by the final sentence of the manuscript informing the reader that a prospective multicenter trial has been launched. The power analysis for such a trial is presented, with 596 patients needed in each limb of the trial aimed at identifying fetal acidosis but reducing unnecessary blood gas measurements. We look forward to that publication.

Some people change their ways when they see the light; others when they feel the heat.—Caroline Schoeder

A.A. Fanaroff, M.B.B.Ch.

References

1. Neilson JP: Cardiotocography during labour (an unsatisfactory technique but nothing better yet). *BMJ* 306:347–348, 1993.
2. Westgate J, Harris M, Curnow JSH: Randomized trial of cardiotocography alone or with ST waveform analysis for intrapartum monitoring. *Lancet* 340:194–198, 1992.
3. Westgate J, Harris M, Curnow JSH, et al: Randomized trial of cardiotocography alone or versus ST waveform analysis plus cardiotogram for intrapartum monitoring in 2400 cases. *Am J Obstet Gynecol* 169:1151–1160, 1994.
4. Mohajer MP, Reed NN, Sahota DS, et al: Cumulative changes in the fetal electrocardiogram and biochemical indices of fetal hypoxia. *Eur J Obstet Gynecol Reprod Biol* 55:63–70, 1994.

Fetal Heart Rate Tracings: Observers Versus Computer Assessment

Todros T, Preve CU, Plazzotta C, et al (Discipline Ginecologiche e Ostetriche, Torino, Italy)

Eur J Obstet Gynecol Reprod Biol 68:83–86, 1996 4–3

Background.—Cardiotocography (CTG) is commonly used even though its reported sensitivity varies from 30% to 100% and its reported specificity varies from 60% to 100%. These variations result from differences in study populations and differences in the end points used to calculate the accuracy. Sensitivity and specificity also are affected by observer variation, which could be eliminated by computerized fetal heart rate analysis. The reproducibility of CTG readings by expert and nonexpert observers, and by a computerized system, was determined.

Methods.—Four clinicians, 2 experts and 2 nonexperts, and the 2CTG computerized system analyzed 63 randomly chosen fetal heart rate recordings from high- and low-risk pregnancies. The recordings were analyzed for baseline heart rate, long-term variability, number of large accelerations, and number and type of decelerations. Interobserver and intraobserver variability, and variability between observers and the computer system were analyzed.

Results.—The agreement among observers was fair to good. For the following values for agreement between observers and the computer system, less than 0.40 indicates poor agreement, 0.40–0.75 indicates fair to good agreement, and greater than 0.75 indicates excellent agreement. It is assumed that no method is a measure of truth. Agreement between each observer and the computer system was 0.18–0.48 for fetal heart rate baseline, 0.16–0.74 for variability, 0.37–0.64 for number of accelerations, and 0.41–0.54 for number of decelerations. Agreement on type of decelerations was 0.01–0.25.

Conclusions.—The poor agreement on type of decelerations has been reported in other studies. Experience in CTG readings does not affect reproducibility. There are some advantages to the computerized CTG system over traditional electronic fetal heart rate recordings, but it is unclear exactly how and to what degree it can improve electronic fetal monitoring.

▶ Cardiotocography, or fetal heart rate monitoring, is used extensively to monitor fetal condition before and during labor. Interpretation of CTG is imprecise and often inconsistent, with significant documented intraobserver and interobserver variation. Computer programs have been developed to reduce this inconsistency and make the decisions for intervention more rational. This manuscript compares the interpretation of a small number of fetal heart rate tracings by 2 experts (consultants/attending obstetricians), 2 nonexperts (obstetric residents with a year's experience), and the computer. As expected, there is considerable interobserver variability among both the experts and the nonexperts. Experience does not equate with reproducibility. The computer cannot help but be consistent. Before rushing to accept the computer as the gold standard, however, remember that the CTG does not have a rating system, and that artifacts can "heavily affect the computer reading." Somebody, expert or not, has to look at the tracing and decide that it is acceptable for analysis by the computer. This may prove to be cumbersome when accute life- or brain-threatening fetal distress develops requiring urgent operative intervention. In the meantime, the next generation of monitors is now being tested (see Abstract 5–1), and near-infrared spectroscopy (NIRS) may yield more consistent and reliable information concerning fetal jeopardy.

A.A. Fanaroff, M.B.B.Ch.

Efficacy of Fetal Echocardiography and Yield by Risk Category

Buskens E, Stewart PA, Hess J, et al (Erasmus Univ, Rotterdam, The Netherlands)

Obstet Gynecol 87:423–428, 1996 4–4

Background.—Advanced US equipment has made prenatal examinations possible, but full fetal examinations are often restricted to teaching hospitals because it is difficult to obtain both high-quality equipment and qualified personnel to perform the examinations. An extensive fetal examination may be indicated when risk factors for congenital heart disease are present. The outcome of fetal echocardiography may result in further tests and a change in obstetric management. The policy for prenatal examinations may need to be reevaluated as the cause of congenital heart disease becomes more clear. The effectiveness of fetal echocardiography in pregnant women who are at increased risk for congenital heart disease in their offspring was assessed.

Methods.—During a period of 2 years, 3,246 consecutive women underwent scanning for known risk factors for congenital heart disease in their offspring. Examinations were performed between 16 and 25 weeks' gestation in 83% of women. Maternal and gestational age, prenatal and postnatal diagnoses, and follow-up information was recorded. Sensitivity, specificity, and predictive values were calculated for fetal echocardiography. The relative yield was established for high-risk patients.

Results.—Follow-up information was available for 99% of cases. Of 47 cases of cardiac malformation, 20 were detected, which yielded a sensitivity of 43%. The sensitivity increased to 51% when cases that were undetected because of unfavorable scanning conditions were considered. Specificity and predictive values were more than 95%. The relative yield for high-risk patients was high in cases of parental congenital heart disease and maternal diabetes mellitus (Table 4). The relative yield equaled the prevalence of congenital heart disease in the general population in cases of a previous infant or other relatives affected, maternal antiepileptic drug use, maternal drug abuse, and other reasons for referral. No additional anomalies were detected in a separate validation study of 777 women.

TABLE 4.—Estimated Relative Risks of Making a Diagnosis of Congenital Heart Disease by Indication; Prenatal Diagnosis and Definite (Postnatal) Diagnosis (Adjusted for Gestational Age and Maternal Age)

	RR prenatal diagnosis		95% CI		RR definite diagnosis		95% CI	
Indication	Crude	Adjusted	Crude	Adjusted	Crude	Adjusted	Crude	Adjusted
Previous infant with CHD	0.088	0.084	0.012–0.66	0.011–0.64	0.51	0.55	0.25–1.03	0.27–1.13
Paternal CHD	4.24	4.45	1.40–12.8	1.46–13.6	3.33	3.31	1.46–7.61	1.44–7.59
Maternal CHD	3.37	3.38	1.28–8.83	1.27–8.99	1.52	1.40	0.67–3.44	0.61–3.12
Other relatives with CHD	*	*			0.43	0.42	0.058–3.12	0.057–3.09
Anti-epileptic drug use	*	*			0.30	0.30	0.072–1.24	0.73–1.27
Diabetes mellitus	3.90	3.79	1.54–9.84	1.50–9.59	2.82	2.77	1.44–5.55	1.41–5.46
Morphomimetic abuse	0.80	0.71	0.11–5.98	0.090–5.55	1.56	1.27	0.55–4.43	0.43–3.72
Miscellaneous	0.61	0.58	0.081–4.59	0.077–4.37	*	*		

*Number of cases affected too low for estimation of relative risk.

Abbreviations: CHD, congenital heart disease; *CI*, confidence interval; *RR*, relative risk.

(Reprinted with permission from American College of Obstetricians and Gynecologists, from Buskens E, Stewart PA, Hess J, et al: Efficacy of fetal echocardiography and yield by risk category. *Obstet Gynecol* 87:423–428, 1996.)

Conclusions.—When fetal echocardiography is performed because of known increased risk factors, it is moderately effective. There are differences in relative yield across various accepted risk categories.

► To separate the trees from the forest, it is desirable to read Stümpflen (Abstract 4–5) and Buskens, not necessarily in random order. Stümpflen and associates will leave you elated and with the impression that the technology are available. All that is required to detect all the cardiac lesions in the fetus are the time and resources to train sufficient sonographers. Resources become the rate-limiting step. Buskens and colleagues bring us back from space to terra firma with a stolid report indicating that even in a "more or less optimal clinical setting (i.e., expert staff) with state-of-the-art ultrasound equipment and sufficient scanning time per patient," only approximately half the cardiac lesions will be found. They are to be complimented on the consistency of their staff. The same sonographers dutifully remained at their stations for the duration of the 12-year study. They scanned a high-risk population based on family history, previous infant with congenital heart disease, maternal diseases (diabetes, collagen disease, rubella, phenylketonuria), genetic diseases, or maternal teratogen exposure. The overall detection rate of congenital heart disease was twice that expected, yet few complex heart lesions were encountered. Small lesions, unfavorable fetal position, and maternal obesity contributed to some of the "missed diagnoses." Ventricular septal defect was the most common undetected lesion. The psychological impact of the wrong diagnosis, missing the diagnosis, or overcalling a lesion all need to be measured. In summary, the technology is there, and we are very dependent on reliable technicians.

A.A. Fanaroff, M.B.B.Ch.

Effect of Detailed Fetal Echocardiography as Part of Routine Prenatal Ultrasonographic Screening on Detection of Congenital Heart Disease

Stümpflen I, Stümpflen A, Wimmer M, et al (Univ of Vienna, Austria)

Lancet 348:854–857, 1996 4–5

Introduction.—Because detailed fetal echocardiography is a time-consuming procedure requiring skilled investigators with special experience in fetal cardiology, it is reserved for cases known to be at high risk of congenital heart disease. Routine prenatal US examinations, however, can miss serious cardiac abnormalities. The prenatal detection rate of congenital heart disease when detailed fetal echocardiography was offered in routine screening was assessed in a prospective study.

Methods.—All women attending an antenatal-care unit from January 1993 through September 1994 were offered a detailed fetal echocardiography examination at 18–28 weeks' gestation. The procedure included the 4-chamber view, outflow-tract scans, and color-flow mapping. When appropriate, additional Doppler and M-mode investigations were performed. Of the 3,085 consecutive women who were screened, 2,181 had no known risk factor for congenital heart disease, 540 had maternal risk factors for congenital heart disease, and 364 had abnormalities detected at US.

Results.—Detailed echocardiography detected congenital heart disease in 46 fetuses (14.9% per 1,000). The group with no risk factors accounted for 15, or one third of all diagnosed cases. Only 3 heart defects were identified in the group with maternal risk factors. The highest rate of cardiac abnormalities (61%) occurred in the group examined because of known fetal abnormalities. Seventeen fetuses with cardiac defects (37%) had a concomitant chromosomal abnormality. Pregnancy was terminated in 22 of the 46 cases with prenatally detected cardiac malformations. Six cases of congenital heart disease were not detected before delivery, but all were minor abnormalities that did not require surgical intervention. The overall sensitivity of detailed fetal echocardiography was 88.5%; both specificity and positive predictive value were 100%.

Discussion.—Detailed fetal echocardiography is a costly procedure reserved for high-risk cases. In this series of patients, however, the incidence rate of congenital heart disease was greater in the group with no known risk factors than in the group with maternal risk factors. In 4 cases, the finding of an isolated cardiac malformation led to detection of an abnormal karyotype. The most important outcome of routine detailed fetal echocardiography is early diagnosis of critical cardiac defects.

▶ Technical advances and experience with fetal US and echocardiography have vastly improved the ability to recognize a multitude of fetal anomalies.[1, 2] However, the usefulness of fetal echocardiography as a screening tool has remained controversial. It is important to distinguish between what is feasible and practical. Hence, to reproduce the results reported by Stümpflen and colleagues (sensitivity of 88.5% and positive predictive value of 100%) would require approximately 400 additional fetal cardiac specialists in the United Kingdom alone. How many more would be required to screen the more than 4 million fetuses in the United States each year? These are unrealistic goals and expectations in the current medical economic climate.

More realistic objectives might be to add the evaluation of the great vessels to the standard 4-chamber view, which can be performed by the current army of obstetric ultrasonographers. However, even this may be beyond the scope of the average office ultrasonographer who is performing the bulk of routine antenatal scans. Furthermore, there are no data regarding the outcome if detailed echocardiography were possible in all pregnant women. The available reports on postnatal outcomes of infants with antenatally detected lesions reflect many variables including the presence of extracardiac lesions, pregnancy terminations, and the attitudes and skills of the team. The intriguing possibility of intrauterine cardiac interventions[3] adds a new perspective and a glimmer of optimism to the debate. As many lesions worsen, early correction, such as in the fetus, might significantly improve the outcome. Such therapy is still very experimental, and a long latent period can be anticipated until it becomes available for human fetuses.

A.A. Fanaroff, M.B.B.Ch.

References

1. Ott WJ: The accuracy of antenatal fetal echocardiography screening in high and low risk patients. *Am J Obstet Gynecol* 172:1741–1747, 1995.
2. Rustico MA, Benettonie A, D'Otavio G, et al: Fetal heart screening in low-risk pregnancies. *Ultrasound Obstet Gynecol* 6:313–319, 1995.
3. Hanley FL: Fetal cardiac surgery. *Adv Cardiac Surg* 5:47–74, 1994.

Common Iliac Artery Flow Velocity Waveforms in Fetuses With a Single Umbilical Artery: A Longitudinal Study

Sepulveda W, Nicolaidis P, Bower S, et al (Queen Charlotte's and Chelsea Hosp, London; Mitera Maternity Hosp, Athens, Greece)

Br J Obstet Gynaecol 103:660–663, 1996 4–6

Introduction.—Single umbilical artery (SUA) now can be diagnosed prenatally using US equipment, as can the fetal hemodynamic aspects of this condition. In normal conditions, the placenta is supplied with blood by both fetal common iliac arteries through the internal iliac arteries. However, in SUA, the entire blood flow to the placenta is supplied through the common and internal iliac arteries from the side of the single artery. In terms of fetal origins of adult disease, intrauterine circulatory alterations in fetuses with SUA may be relevant. The effect of gestational age on pelvic arterial blood flow in fetuses with SUA was investigated.

Methods.—Using high-resolution color Doppler US, common iliac artery flow velocity waveforms were studied longitudinally in 15 fetuses with SUA. They were studied at 3 gestational ages: 18–20 weeks, 28–30 weeks, and 35–37 weeks. In each common iliac artery, the pulsatility index was measured. To examine the effect of gestational age and side, a mixed-model analysis of variance was used.

Results.—The missing artery was on the right in 7 fetuses and on the left in 8 fetuses. At all gestational ages, there was a highly significant difference in pulsatility index between common iliac arteries. On the side that did not participate in the fetoplacental circulation, the values were always higher. On the SUA side, the pulsatility index fell significantly (mean decrease, 39%) for increasing gestation. In the non-SUA side, the pulsatility index remained high. At pediatric evaluation, all infants were normal after delivery, with the exception of 1 infant with hypospadias.

Conclusions.—As pregnancy progresses, asymmetry in the pelvic arterial blood flow in fetuses with SUA increases. This is consistent with increasing resistance in the lower extremities and decreasing vascular resistance in the placenta. Further research should be conducted on the vascular and structural development of the pelvic organs and lower extremities in infants with SUA.

► Funicular vascular anomaly is the pompous way of referring to SUA. Sepulveda and associates present an update and elaboration on their initial reports, which detailed the identification of SUA and discordant iliac and femoral artery flow velocity waveforms in fetuses. They validate their earlier observations and conclude that "the asymmetry in the pelvic arterial blood flow in fetuses with SUA increases as pregnancy progresses, consistent with decreasing vascular resistance in the placenta and increasing resistance in the lower extremities." These observations are of only theoretical interest unless they can be linked to subsequent morbidity. There is much speculation that aberrant prenatal hemodynamics influences long-term vascular development and disease. Meyer and Long's report of artherosclerotic lesions in children with SUA was provocative, but where is the validation?[1] Establishing a link between prenatal pathology and morbidity in adults is a daunting challenge for the epidemiologists. We await the fruits of their efforts and confirmation of concepts such as the one proposed by Law and associates that the initiation of hypertension is in utero and is amplified throughout life.[2] Barker and colleagues long have preached on the association between in utero and growth retardation and hypertension.[3]

A.A. Fanaroff, M.B.B.Ch.

References

1. Meyer WW, Long J: Iliac arteries in children with a single umbilical artery: Structure, calcifications, and early atherosclerotic lesions. *Arch Dis Child* 49:671–679, 1974.
2. Law CM, De Swiet M, Osmond C, et al: Initiation of hypertension in utero and its application throughout life. *BMJ* 306:24–27, 1993.
3. Barker DJP, Osmond C, Golding J, et al: Growth in utero, blood pressure in childhood and adult life, and mortality from cardiovascular disease. *BMJ* 298:564–567, 1989.

Uterine Doppler Wave Form and the Prediction of the Recurrence of Pre-eclampsia and Intra-uterine Growth Retardation in Patients Treated With Low-dose Aspirin

Haddad B, Uzan M, Bréart G, et al (Hôpital Cochin, Paris; Inserm U 149, Paris)

Eur J Obstet Gynecol Reprod Biol 62:179–183, 1995 4–7

Background.—Doppler US performed between 22 and 26 weeks of amenorrhea is useful for identifying women at high risk of preeclampsia and intrauterine growth retardation. The pathogenesis of these complications is associated with an imbalance of the thromboxane A_2/prostacyclin system. Low-dose aspirin appears to decrease these vascular complications in pregnant women with a high risk of vascular complications determined by poor outcomes in previous pregnancies or an early abnormal uterine Doppler US result. Whether midtrimester uterine Doppler US can predict recurrence of vascular complications in pregnant women given aspirin because of poor outcomes in previous pregnancies was determined.

Methods and Findings.—All 48 pregnant women seen between 1991 and 1992 and receiving 100 mg of aspirin daily were included. Uterine Doppler US assessment was performed at 23.8 weeks. Fifty-four percent of the patients had abnormal early uterine Doppler US results. Vascular complications occurred in 18.7%. Such complications occurred more frequently in women with an abnormal uterine Doppler US finding. Mean birth weight was reduced in the infants of women with a pathologic uterine Doppler US finding.

Conclusion.—Among pregnant women receiving early low-dose aspirin because of poor previous pregnancy outcomes, early uterine Doppler US was able to predict which patients had a high risk of recurrence of vascular complications. Consistent with previous findings, the current data showed a strong correlation between abnormal early uterine Doppler US results and the occurrence of serious vascular complications.

► This comment has been co-authored by Daniel S. Seidman, M.D., of The Sheba Medical Center, Tel-Hashomer, Israel:

► Low-dose aspirin was hailed only a few years ago as a major breakthrough in the prevention of preeclampsia, a leading cause of maternal and perinatal morbidity and mortality. However, large, randomized, prospective trials failed to demonstrate a beneficial effect of aspirin administration during pregnancy. The presumed effectiveness of aspirin treatment is based on the prevailing view of preeclampsia as an endothelial disease associated with an imbalance of thromboxane A_2 and prostacyclin. The search is ongoing to identify women "at risk," who are more likely to benefit from aspirin during pregnancy. The use of Doppler US examination of the uterine and umbilical arteries has been shown to detect at mid-pregnancy women in whom severe pregnancy-induced hypertension (PIH) is likely to develop.

This study shows that early treatment with low-dose aspirin does not preclude the usefulness of uterine artery Doppler US in predicting recurrence of preeclampsia and intrauterine growth retardation. It should be noted that the study was conducted in a high-risk population with poor previous pregnancy outcome. In a recent multicenter study, Doppler US was not found useful for screening a low-risk population in whom the prevalence of PIH was low.[1] Furthermore, a randomized trial of low-dose aspirin in patients with abnormal uterine artery Doppler studies failed to demonstrate a reduction in pregnancy complications in women with uteroplacental insufficiency.[2] Although the use of Doppler US as a predictor of PIH recurrence is limited to high-risk patients, its use in guiding clinical action in these patients has been shown in a meta-analysis of randomized trials to reduce the odds of perinatal death by 38% and to significantly reduce the number of antenatal admissions, inductions of labor, and cesarean sections for fetal distress.[3]

D. Seidman, M.D.
D.K. Stevenson, M.D.

References

1. Todros T, Ferrazzi E, Arduini D, et al. Performance of Doppler ultrasonography as a screening test in low risk pregnancies: Results of a multicentric study. *J Ultrasound Med* 14:343–348, 1995.
2. Morris JM, Fay RA, Ellwood DA, et al: A randomized controlled trial of aspirin in patients with abnormal uterine artery blood flow. *Obstet Gynecol* 87:74–78, 1996.
3. Alfirevic Z, Neilson JP: Doppler ultrasonography in high-risk pregnancies: Systematic review with meta-analysis. *Am J Obstet Gynecol* 172:1379–1387, 1995.

Prenatal Diagnosis of the Fetal RhD Blood Type Using a Single Fetal Nucleated Erythrocyte From Maternal Blood

Sekizawa A, Watanabe A, Kimura T, et al (Kohnodai Hosp, Chiba, Japan; Showa Univ, Tokyo)
Obstet Gynecol 87:501–505, 1996 4–8

Introduction.—Nucleated erythrocytes appear to be suitable for prenatal diagnosis because they are uncommon in the peripheral blood of normal adults and are abundant among these fetal cells in the maternal circulation. Until a technique was developed for retrieving nucleated erythrocytes from the maternal blood using a discontinuous density gradient method with Percoll and a micromanipulator under microscopic observation in 1995, there was no evidence that fetal cells could be retrieved selectively and individually at the single-cell level. A method that allows prenatal diagnosis of the fetal RhD blood type from maternal blood was developed.

Methods.—At 8–31 weeks' gestation, maternal blood was obtained from 10 pregnant women. Using a discontinuous density gradient method, nucleated erythrocytes were separated with Percoll and were collected individually under microscopic observation using micromanipulation. A nested polymerase chain reaction was used to amplify exon 7 of the RhD and RhCe, as well as the ZFX/ZFY loci, after whole genome amplification with primer extension preamplification.

Results.—In 9 of 10 maternal blood samples, nucleated erythrocytes were detected. In 13 of 21 nucleated erythrocytes, sex was determined. In 12 of 13 nucleated erythrocytes in which sex could be determined, RhD genotype was diagnosed. In nucleated erythrocytes obtained from maternal blood, the results of RhD blood type and sex were identical with those of the newborns. In 6 of 10 maternal blood samples, fetal RhD blood type could be determined.

Conclusions.—Using a single nucleated erythrocyte isolated from maternal blood, a new method for noninvasive prenatal diagnosis of the fetal RhD blood type was demonstrated. Extremely useful information for the management of Rh-negative pregnant women is provided by this diagnostic method. Other genetic disorders may be amenable to this method of prenatal diagnosis, which could become the preferred method of noninvasive prenatal diagnosis of DNA. The polymerase chain reaction can cause contamination of samples with an exogenous target DNA template, so appropriate measures must be taken to prevent this problem. To improve the sensitivity of this method, suitable micromanipulation techniques are needed.

► Writing in *Newsweek,* George Will said, "The pursuit of perfection often impedes improvement." If the ability to make a prenatal ascertainment of the RhD status of the fetus from a single cell does not represent perfection, then it surely comes pretty close. Identification of the Rh gene on chromosome 1 has enabled the application of recombinant DNA techniques to fetal cells isolated from maternal blood during pregnancy. A fluorescein tag is applied to fetal nucleated red blood cells found in maternal blood using a monoclonal antibody specific to fetal cell nuclei. Then a fluorescent activated sorter is used to collect an enriched sample of fetal cells. Thereafter, a polymerase chain reaction is applied to the D portion of the Rh gene or other genes of interest. I applaud these authors, who detected nucleated erythrocytes in 9 of 10 maternal blood samples and correctly determined sex in 13 of 21 nucleated erythrocytes. The RhD genotype could be diagnosed in 12 of the 13 nucleated erythrocytes in which sex could be accurately determined.

The ability to isolate fetal cells from circulating maternal blood allows "noninvasive" fetal genetic analysis. From as little as a single fetal cell, the genetic material can be amplified and aneuploidies or a host of inherited disorders identified. Obviously, the fetal cells need to be free of maternal contamination and without problems of contamination from prior pregnancies. There are still some wrinkles to be ironed out, and the issue of false negative results has to be resolved,[1] but the golden era of fetal diagnosis is dawning rapidly.

A.A. Fanaroff, M.B.B.Ch.

Reference

1. Geifman-Holtzman O, Bernstein IM, Berry SM: Fetal RhD genotyping in fetal cell flow sorted from maternal blood. *Am J Obstet Gynecol* 174:818–822, 1996.

Fetal RhD Genotyping in Fetal Cells Flow Sorted From Maternal Blood

Geifman-Holtzman O, Bernstein IM, Berry SM, et al (Med Ctr Hosp of Vermont, Burlington; Hutzel Hosp, Detroit; Massachusetts Gen Hosp, Boston, et al)

Am J Obstet Gynecol 174:818–822, 1996 4–9

Background.—Even with the availability of prophylactic Rh immunoglobulin, RhD hemolytic disease of the newborn still results in an incidence of 10.6 per 10,000 live births. If fetal RhD status could be determined from fetal cells circulating in the maternal blood, it would avoid multiple invasive procedures and exposure to Rh immune globulins. The accuracy of noninvasive fetal RhD typing in cells obtained by fluorescence-activated cell sorting from the maternal blood was evaluated.

Methods.—The study included fetal cells from 18 Rh-negative pregnant women referred for amniocentesis or cordocentesis. There was 1 twin pregnancy. Fetal cells were isolated from the maternal blood by fluorescence-activated cell sorting. The sorted cells then underwent polymerase chain reaction amplification of a 261–base pair fragment of the RhD gene. Fetal cells showing a positive RhD-amplification product were considered to predict an RhD-positive genotype in the fetus.

Results.—The noninvasive procedure correctly predicted the fetal genotype in 16 of 19 cases: 10 Rh-positive and 6 Rh-negative fetuses. The other 3 fetuses were RhD positive, but no amplification product was detected. The relation between the amplification product and the RhD-positive genotype was significant.

Conclusions.—Fetal RhD genotyping can be performed noninvasively using fetal cells obtained from the maternal blood by fluorescence-activated cell sorting. If no amplification product appears, the presence of fetal material in the specimen must be confirmed. The noninvasive test already has a positive predictive value of 100% and a negative predictive value of 67%, and its accuracy should improve further with advances in fetal cell purity and yield.

▶ As a consequence of the widespread use of prophylactic Rh immunoglobulin, only 1 in 1,000 live births is affected with RhD hemolytic disease of the newborn.[1] The Rh gene has been located on chromosome 1p34; it consists of 2 genes, 1 of which encodes the C/c and E/c polypeptides and the other of which encodes the D antigen. Determining the fetal RhD status before 1993 required an invasive procedure. Since then, fetal RhD genotyping has been established with increasing efficiency, from fetal cells flow sorted from maternal blood and subjected to polymerase chain reaction of a 261–base pair fragment of the RhD gene.

Noninvasive prenatal diagnosis of the fetal RhD genotype is feasible.[2] The trick is to avoid false negative results (3 of 19 in this series). Absence of amplification in the 3 false positive cases in this report reflected failure to capture fetal cells from the maternal circulation, the biological absence of fetal cells in the maternal sample, failure of DNA isolation from fetal cells, or problems with the polymerase chain reaction.

The implications of this study are that the analysis of fetal cells from maternal blood could be the initial step, with amniocentesis/cordocentesis reserved for situations in which the results are negative or inconclusive and for monitoring Rh-affected pregnancies.

A.A. Fanaroff, M.B.B.Ch.

References

1. Chavez GF, Mulinare J, Edmonds LD: Epidemiology of Rh hemolytic disease of the newborn in the United States. *JAMA* 265:3270–3274, 1991.

2. Low Y-MD, Bowell PJ, Selinger M, et al: Prenatal determination of fetal RhD status by analysis of peripheral blood of rhesus negative mothers. *Lancet* 341:1147–1148, 1993.

First-trimester Biochemical Screening for Down Syndrome With the Use of PAPP-A, AFP, and β-hCG

Casals E, Fortuny A, Grudzinskas JG, et al (Univ of Barcelona; London Hosp Med College; Odense Univ, Denmark)

Prenat Diagn 16:405–410, 1996 4–10

Background.—Prenatal screening for Down syndrome (DS) is effective in the second trimester of pregnancy, but its value in the first trimester is uncertain. In the second trimester, DS-affected pregnancies show changes in maternal serum α-fetoprotein (AFP) and human chorionic gonadotropin (hCG) levels. Recent studies indicate that first-trimester DS-affected pregnancies exhibit depressed maternal serum levels of pregnancy-associated plasma protein A (PAPP-A) and elevated maternal serum levels of free β-hCG (Fβ-hCG). Maternal serum samples collected from women referred for first-trimester chorionic villus sampling were evaluated for PAPP-A, AFP, and β-hCG.

Methods.—The 1,138 women had been referred largely for advanced (older than 35 years) maternal age. First-trimester serum samples were available for 19 women carrying a fetus with DS. The weekly medians of serum analyte levels in continuing chromosomally normal pregnancies were determined for weeks 10 through 13 of gestation and compared with results in DS pregnancies.

Results.—The mean of the multiples of the median in DS pregnancies was significantly lower for AFP and PAPP-A and significantly higher for β-hCG compared with normal pregnancies (Table 3). No significant correlations were found between the different analytes (AFP vs. β-hCG, AFP vs. PAPP-A, or β-hCG vs. PAPP-A). For a 5% false positive rate, the detection rates for DS were 18% for AFP, 9% for β-hCG, and 66% for PAPP-A. Assuming a 10% false positive rate, the detection rates were

TABLE 3.—Mean Values of Multiples of the Median for Maternal Serum Levels of Biochemical Markers in Down Syndrome Pregnancies in the First Trimester

Biochemical marker	Mean MOM in normal	Mean MOM in DS	Mann-Whitney (two-tailed probability)
AFP	1·03	0·90	<0·05
β-hCG	1·07	1·38	<0·001
PAPP-A	0·93	0·42	<0·001

Abbreviations: MOM, multiples of the median; *DS*, Down syndrome; *AFP*, α-fetoprotein; *β-hCG*, β-human chorionic gonadotropin; *PAPP-A*, pregnancy-associated plasma protein A.

(Courtesy of Casals E, Fortuny A, Grudzinskas JG, et al: First-trimester biochemical screening for Down syndrome with the use of PAPP-A, AFP, and β-hCG. *Prenat Diagn* 16:405–410, copyright 1996, reprinted by permission of John Wiley & Sons, Ltd.)

27%, 16%, and 73%, respectively. The best detection rate (85%) was obtained with a combination of PAPP-A and AFP and a 10% false positive rate.

Conclusion.—Early diagnosis of DS would be desirable, but women have had to wait until the second trimester to undergo biochemical screening. The findings of this study support the value of PAPP-A as a biochemical marker for DS and suggest that the combination of PAPP-A and AFP values offers the best detection rate.

► Screening for fetal abnormality is a growth industry, according to Steer.[1] The search for more sensitive and specific means of detecting the abnormal fetus is starting to narrow down. The yearning to detect the fetus with an abnormal karyotype, noninvasively during the first trimester, is the focus of this article. A relatively new player emerges, namely PAPP-A. This marker is detectable in maternal serum by the 30th day of gestation, its levels increase exponentially until term, then its levels decline until they are undetectable by the sixth postpartum week.

Levels of PAPP-A, like AFP, are depressed in pregnancies complicated by DS and probably are the single most effective biochemical marker in first-trimester screening for DS. The receiver operating curves generated in this study demonstrate that the combination of PAPP-A and AFP enhances the detection rate for DS to greater than 80%, with false positive rates between 5% and 10%. The detection rate with PAPP-A alone is 66%. α-Fetoprotein and β-hCG have established roles in the identification of pregnancies at risk for neural tube defects and other abnormalities; PAPP-A increases these detection capabilities. An advantage of identifying new biochemical markers is that many stored samples are available to verify the finding. The study draws our attention to PAPP-A as the most sensitive and specific marker for DS in the first trimester, which becomes less discriminatory as the pregnancy progresses. The next logical step, which is to examine the combination of US markers and these analytes, is being explored by the authors. Because nuchal skinfold thickness and serum markers are not correlated, their combination promises to provide increased sensitivity and specificity.[2] Time alone will tell. (See also Abstract 4–11.)

Not only is screening for fetal anomalies expensive and of unproved efficacy (there are no prospective randomized controlled trials), it is also contentious.—Philip Steer

A.A. Fanaroff, M.B.B.Ch.

References

1. Steer P: Obstetrics—recent advances. *BMJ* 311:1209–1212, 1995.
2. Brizot ML, Snijders RJM, Butler J, et al: Maternal serum hCG and fetal nuchal transparency thickness for the prediction of fetal trisomies in the first trimester of pregnancy. *Br J Obstet Gynaecol* 102:127–132, 1995.

Prenatal Screening for Down's Syndrome Using Inhibin-A as a Serum Marker

Wald NJ, Densem JW, George L, et al (St Bartholomew's Hosp, London; Univ of Reading, England)

Prenat Diagn 16:143–153, 1996 4–11

Purpose.—The 4-marker method of prenatal serum screening for Down syndrome provides good results, with an estimated detection rate of 65% and a false positive rate of 5%. Another potentially useful marker is inhibin-A (the $\alpha\beta_A$/dimeric form), which requires a much smaller volume of serum. Inhibin-A, alone and in combination with other serum markers, was investigated as a screening marker for Down syndrome.

Methods.—The study included stored serum samples obtained at 15–22 weeks' gestation from 77 singleton pregnancies with Down syndrome and 385 unaffected pregnancies. The 2 groups were matched for maternal age, gestational age, and length of serum storage. Supplementary data were obtained from 970 white women with unaffected pregnancies. Markers measured were the $\alpha\beta_A$/dimer of inhibin-A; human chorionic gonadotropin (hCG), both total hCG and the subunits free α-hCG and β-hCG; α-fetoprotein (AFP); and unconjugated estriol (uE_3).

Results.—The Down syndrome pregnancies had elevated serum inhibin-A levels, with a median of 1.79 multiples of the median (Fig 1). Using AFP, UE_3, total hCG, and inhibin-A together with maternal age correctly identified 70% of pregnancies affected with Down syndrome, with a 5% false positive rate. This compared favorably to a 59% detection rate with the conventional triple test (i.e., AFP, uE_3, and total hCG plus maternal age). Using a US-based estimation of gestational age would improve the detection rate of the 4-marker test to 77%, compared with 67% with the triple test or 79% if the marker values were adjusted for maternal weight. Using the 4-marker test with a detection rate of 70% and a US estimate of gestational age was associated with a false positive rate of only 6%, compared with 3% with the triple test. The use of free β-hCG vs. total hCG made little difference in the results.

Conclusions.—The 4-marker screening test for Down syndrome—including inhibin-A, AFP, uE_3, and total hCG—appears to be the most effective test for routine clinical use. The use of inhibin-A rather than free α-hCG would reduce the number of fetal losses to amniocentesis per case detected. This test would be cost-effective if the extra cost incurred were less than about £3 per patient.

► Down syndrome is the most common chromosomal abnormality in liveborn infants. Screening for Down syndrome, or trisomy 21, is undergoing constant refinement. Just when it appeared that the combination of the triple screen (AFP, uE_3, and hCG), together with maternal age, was settling in as the "standard," it became apparent that the 4 markers (AFP, uE_3, total hCG, and α-hCG) detected more abnormal fetuses. Screening performance may be enhanced further if inhibin-A is used as 1 of the serum markers. If

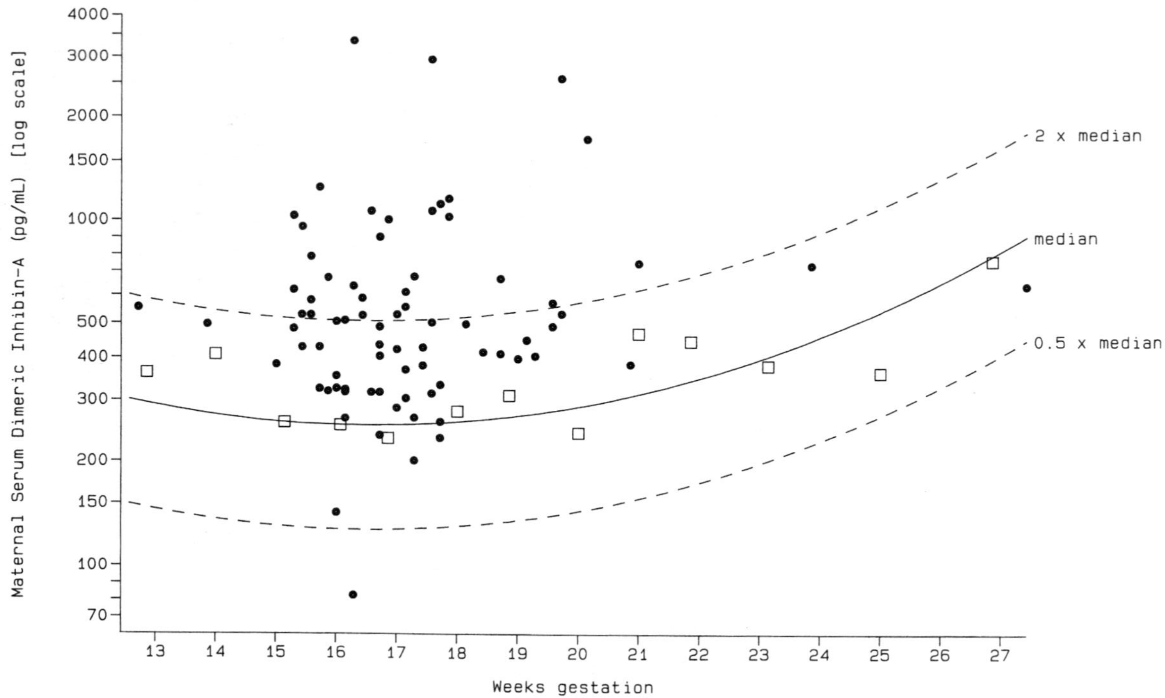

FIGURE 1.—Inhibin-A concentration in maternal serum at 13–27 weeks' gestation in 77 pregnancies with Down syndrome and regressed median for unaffected singleton pregnancies in relation to gestational age. The *squares* are the observed medians for unaffected pregnancies at each completed week of gestation. The *solid circles* are the values for each of the affected pregnancies. The *dashed lines* show twice and half the regressed median value. (Courtesy of Wald NJ, Densem JW, George L, et al: Prenatal screening for Down's syndrome using inhibin-A as a serum marker. *Prenat Diagn* 16:143–153, 1996. Reprinted by permission of John Wiley & Sons, Ltd.)

80% of mothers would undergo serum testing, it would result in a 61% detection rate in women younger than 35 years of age years and a 91% detection rate in women older than 35 years of age, for an overall detection rate of 70%.[1]

According to Wyllie and colleagues,[2] even if maternal screening and fetal echocardiography achieve their predicted potential, about half of all the pregnancies affected by Down syndrome will result in live-born babies. This prediction has major implications for the provision of resources for people with Down syndrome, whose life expectancy is increasing.

Every start upon an untrodden path is a venture which, only in unusual circumstances, looks sensible and likely to be successful.—Albert Schweitzer

A.A. Fanaroff, M.B.B.Ch.

References

1. Crossley JA, Aitken DA, Berry E, et al: Impact of a regional screening programme using maternal serum a feto-protein (AFP) and human chorionic gonadotrophin (hCG) on the birth incidence in the West of Scotland. *J Med Screen* 1:180–183, 1994.
2. Wyllie JP, Madar RJ, Wright M, et al: Strategies for antenatal detection of Down syndrome. *Arch Dis Child* 76:F26–F30, 1997.

Small or Absent Fetal Stomach: Prognostic Significance

McKenna KM, Goldstein RB, Stringer MD (Mills-Peninsula Hosps, San Mateo, Calif; Univ of California, San Francisco; Gen Infirmary at Leeds, England)

Radiology 197:729–733, 1995 4–12

Introduction.—The American Institute of Ultrasound in Medicine has recommended that a view of the fluid-filled stomach (Fig 1) be taken in every obstetric sonogram performed. A small or absent fetal stomach on sonogram is associated with abnormal outcomes, but the clinical significance of these findings has not been determined. Medical records were retrospectively reviewed to define the prognostic significance of a small or absent fetal stomach on sonographic examination.

Methods.—The medical records and sonograms of 87 fetuses with small or absent stomachs were reviewed for information regarding gestational age, amniotic fluid volume, stomach size, morphological defects, and karotypes. These data were correlated with clinical follow-up and autopsy findings.

Results.—The 87 fetuses with small or absent stomachs represented 1.4% of all fetuses who underwent sonographic examination in a time period of almost 4 years. Eight fetuses were eliminated because of diagnoses of ruptured membranes and oligohydramnios: thus, diminished fluid was available for swallowing. There were 52 fetuses with small stomachs (Fig 3) and 27 fetuses with absent stomachs (Fig 2). Of the 79 pregnancies

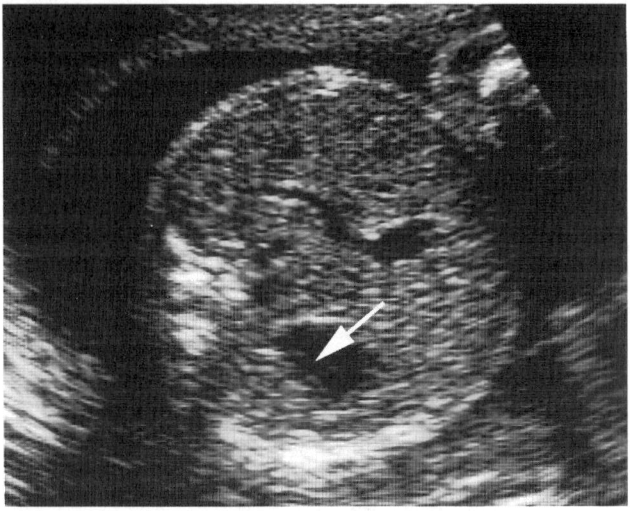

FIGURE 1.—Sonogram obtained at 20 weeks of gestation shows a normal fluid-filled stomach (*arrow*) that is easily visualized in the left upper abdomen of the fetus. (Courtesy of McKenna KM, Goldstein RB, Stinger MD: Small or absent fetal stomach: Prognostic significance. *Radiology* 197:729–733, 1995. Radiological Society of North America.)

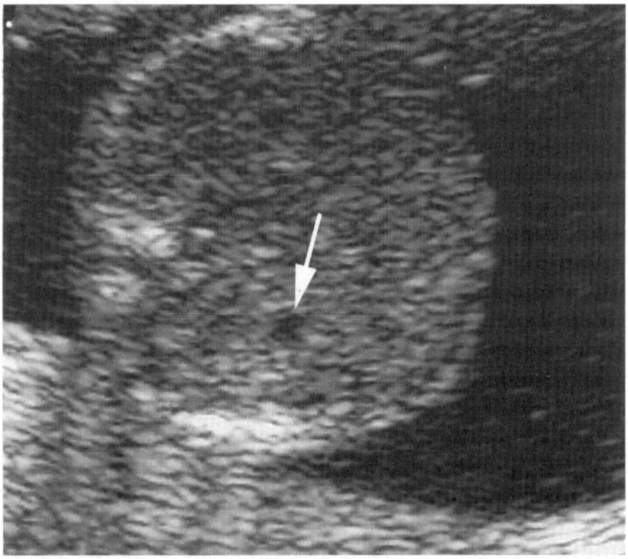

FIGURE 3.—Sonogram obtained at 19 weeks of gestation shows a persistently small fetal stomach (*straight arrow*) that could be identified only after a diligent search. A neck mass was also detected in the fetus. (Courtesy of McKenna KM, Goldstein RB, Stringer MD: Small or absent fetal stomach: Prognostic significance. *Radiology* 197:729–733, 1995. Radiological Society of North America.)

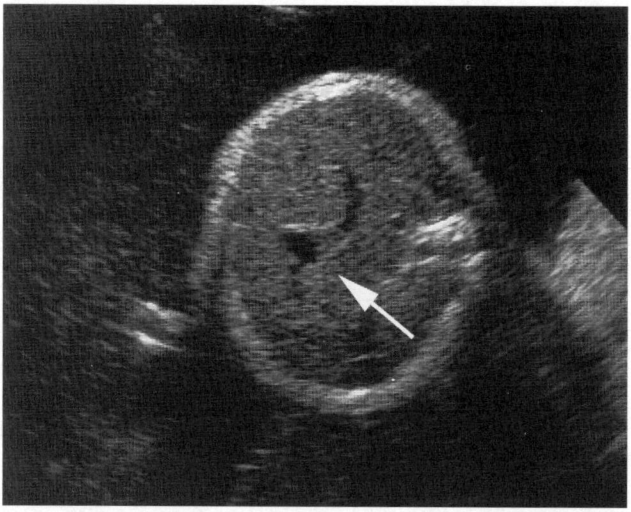

FIGURE 2.—Sonogram obtained at 34 weeks of gestation (different pregnancy) shows that an absent fetal stomach is a fairly straightforward sonographic observation when no fluid-filled structure can be identified in the expected location (*curved arrow*) of the stomach. The fetus had fetal akinesia syndrome with an absent stomach secondary to impaired neuromuscular function including swallowing. (Courtesy of McKenna KM, Goldstein RB, Stringer MD: Small or absent fetal stomach: Prognostic significance. *Radiology* 197:729–733, 1995. Radiological Society of North America.)

evaluated, 50 (63%) had abnormal outcomes; 23 (85%) of the fetuses with absent stomachs and 27 (52%) of the fetuses with small stomachs had abnormal outcomes (Table 1). Eight (38%) fetuses with absent stomachs and 2 (4%) fetuses with small stomachs had abnormal karotypes.

Conclusion.—The importance of finding small or absent stomachs in fetuses is evidenced by findings of abnormal outcomes that include structural abnormalities and intrauterine fetal or postnatal death in 85% of fetuses with absent stomachs and in 52% of fetuses with small stomachs.

▶ The bottom line is that an absent or small fetal stomach after 18 weeks of gestation is associated with a guarded prognosis. I could have guessed as

TABLE 1.—Outcomes of Fetuses With Small or Absent Stomachs

Outcome	Small (n = 52)	Absent (n = 27)	Total (n = 79)
Healthy term newborn	17 (33)	2 (7)	19 (24)
Premature newborn	11 (21)	2 (7)	13 (16)
Structural abnormalities with or without IUFD	24 (46)	23 (85)	47 (60)
Abnormal karyotype*	2/46 (4)	8/21 (38)	10/67 (15)
Survivors	36 (69)	9 (33)	45 (57)

Note: Numbers in parentheses are percentages.

*Data are presented as numbers of fetuses with an abnormal karotype/number tested plus those presumed normal by phenotype.

Abbreviation: IUFD, intrauterine fetal death.

(Courtesy of McKenna KM, Goldstein RB, Stringer MD: Small or absent fetal stomach: Prognostic significance. *Radiology* 197:729–733, 1995. Radiological Society of North America.)

much but would never have taken the time to wonder about all the other associations had someone not wondered for me. The article provides a good reference for an unusual problem.

D.K. Stevenson, M.D.

Acute and Chronic Fetal Hypoxia in Monochorionic and Dichorionic Twins

Maier RF, Bialobrzeski B, Gross A, et al (Humboldt Univ, Berlin, Germany)
Obstet Gynecol 86:973–977, 1995 4–13

Introduction.—From about 20 weeks of gestation, increased erythropoietin production is caused by a hypoxic stimulus. There are no stores for rapid erythropoietin release, so an increase in erythropoietin serum concentration in umbilical venous blood is indicative of prolonged fetal hypoxia of several hours to several days. Changes in umbilical arterial pH are more rapid, reflecting a more acute hypoxic episode. The risk for acute and chronic fetal hypoxia was assessed in monochorionic and dichorionic twin pregnancies using umbilical arterial pH and erythropoietin concentrations.

Methods.—Fifty of 156 sets of twins born in a 30-month period were admitted to the neonatal intensive care unit. The gestational age of the 50 sets of twins was 24–38 weeks, and birth weights ranged from 660 to 3,200 g. Of 100 infants, 76 were appropriate for gestational age (AGA), 20 were small for gestational age (SGA), and 4 were large for gestational age. Twenty-six AGA term singleton newborns acted as controls. Umbilical arterial pH was used to evaluate acute fetal hypoxia, and umbilical venous erythropoietin concentration was used to evaluate chronic fetal hypoxia.

Results.—There were 40 sets of diamniotic–dichorionic twins and 10 sets of diamniotic–monochorionic twins with transplacental vascular shunts. The umbilical arterial pH was significantly lower in second-born twins compared with first-born twins (7.29 vs. 7.31). The same trend was observed in infants with pH values below 7.20 (19% vs. 11%). Two second-born infants but no first-born infants had umbilical arterial pH values less than 7.05. The erythropoietin concentration was significantly more elevated in SGA twins compared with AGA twins. The erythropoietin concentration was similar in AGA twins and AGA singleton newborns. The erythropoietin concentration was higher in the smaller twin in 12 of 17 twin sets with weight difference greater than 15% and in all 5 sets of twins with weight difference greater than 25%. The incidence of increased erythropoietin concentration was significantly higher in monochorionic than dichorionic pregnancies. None of the singleton controls had elevated erythropoietin concentrations.

Conclusion.—There is an increased risk of acute birth asphyxia for the second-born twin. Fetal growth restriction in twin pregnancies was correlated with chronic fetal hypoxia. There was a higher risk of chronic fetal hypoxia in monochorionic twins compared with dichorionic twins.

► The diagnosis of twinning is often a joyous occasion, but individuals need to be reminded from time to time that twins represent a high-risk circumstance. Once again, monochorionic twinning is associated most often with evidence of chronic fetal hypoxia. Whenever such information is reviewed, it is impressive that twinning yields as much success as it does most of the time.

D.K. Stevenson, M.D.

The Prognostic Factors in the Prenatal Diagnosis of the Echogenic Fetal Lung

Barret J, Chitayat D, Sermer M, et al (Univ of Toronto, Canada)

Prenat Diagn 15:849–853, 1995 4–14

Background.—The use of high-resolution US for prenatal diagnosis has led to increased detection of echogenic fetal lung (EFL) in the early second trimester. This US finding usually is indicative of congenital cystic adenomatoid lung malformation, intrapulmonary lung sequestration, or major airway obstruction. As an aid to parental counseling in these cases, the outcomes of 11 recent cases and a series of cases derived from a literature review were discussed.

Study Group.—The study group consisted of 11 patients referred to the University of Toronto perinatal complex from 1992 to 1993. Repeated detailed fetal US was performed and associated structural abnormalities, lesion size, lung location laterality, mediastinal shift, and the presence of nonimmune hydrops fetalis (NIHF) were recorded for each case. The English literature was reviewed and patient series containing at least 5 prenatally diagnosed cases of EFL were extracted for purposes of comparison.

Findings.—The gestation at diagnosis for the 11 cases in the study group was 17–32 weeks. Five of the cases were solid and 6 had cystic components. Seven cases had a mediastinal shift, but only 1 case had hydrops associated with it. Three pregnancies were terminated. All the remaining 8 patients survived without the development of NIHF. In 3 cases, the lung lesions resolved by the third trimester. In 1 case, operation was required in the immediate postnatal period. In the remaining 4 cases, the patients are being treated conservatively and have had no complications during a follow-up period of 6 weeks to 6 months.

Literature Review.—From an English language literature review, 60 EFL cases in 3 series were selected. Of these 60 pregnancies, 10 were terminated. Of the remaining 50 cases, 32% survived past the immediate neonatal period. Among these, 5 had resolution of the lesion in utero and 14 did not require operation. Only 3 cases that did not have hydrops at diagnosis saw its development during the subsequent pregnancy.

Conclusions.—The results of a literature review and analysis of the outcome of a current series of 11 patients with a prenatal diagnosis of EFL indicate that, in the absence of fetal hydrops or other abnormalities, these fetuses have a good prognosis. If NIHF is absent at diagnosis, the chance that it will develop subsequently during the pregnancy is low. There is a significant chance that EFL will resolve before delivery. In cases of NIHF, the prognosis is poor.

▶ There is a remote chance that an EFL will resolve spontaneously. More than likely, the EFL indicates the presence of either a congenital cystic adenomatoid malformation of the lung or a pulmonary sequestration. In the absence of NIHF or other major malformations, the prognosis is very good and the families should be counseled accordingly. (See also Abstract 1–10 and reference 1.)

A.A. Fanaroff, M.B.B.Ch.

Reference

1. 1994 YEAR BOOK OF NEONATAL AND PERINATAL MEDICINE, p 11.

Antenatal Sonographic Diagnosis of Clubfoot: A Six-year Experience

Pagnotta G, Maggi E, Maffulli N, et al (Ospedale del Bambin Gesu, Rome; Univ of Aberdeen, Scotland; Univ 'La Sapienza,' Rome)

J Foot Ankle Surg 35:67–71, 1996 4–15

Introduction.—Many children with clubfoot have other anomalies. Although early prenatal detection of congenital talipes equinovarus, or clubfoot, does not significantly influence its treatment and prognosis, there is some thought that oligohydramnios or constriction rings may be important in idiopathic clubfoot. A 6-year experience with prenatal US diagnosis of clubfoot in a specialized, secondary referral center was reported.

Methods.—A total of 6,351 pregnant women were referred for suspected fetal anomalies or maternofetal problems. All women underwent abdominal and/or transvaginal US scanning at 12, 24, and 38 weeks of pregnancy. If a clubfoot was suspected, another US scan was performed in 2 hours to exclude a positional false positive diagnosis. When a clubfoot was detected, the foot was inverted and the metatarsal rays were visualized as being in the same plane of the tibia and fibula. Patients with US diagnosis of clubfoot underwent amniocentesis or fetal cord venous blood sampling for karyotyping.

Results.—Of 6,351 women evaluated, 235 had fetal malformations, such as hydrocephalus or cardiac or musculoskeletal malformations. Forty-one clubfeet were discovered in 27 pregnancies by the early part of the second trimester. Fourteen feet in 8 patients were isolated and classified as idiopathic. Clubfoot was found in association with neural tube defects in 6 patients, anomalies of the urinary and/or digestive system in 6 patients, cystic hygroma in 2 patients, and other musculoskeletal abnormalities in the remaining 6 patients. An abnormal karyotype was detected in 6 fetuses. Two patients had oligohydramnios and a fetal urinary tract malformation. Eighteen of the 27 women carrying fetuses with clubfoot had polyhydramnios. The remaining 7 had normal amounts of amniotic fluid. Polyhydramnios was found in 6 of 8 fetuses with idiopathic clubfoot.

Conclusions.—Clubfoot often is found in the presence of musculoskeletal and visceral anomalies. The finding of polyhydramnios in the presence of clubfoot cannot be considered an etiologic factor in its development. The detection of clubfoot on prenatal US should prompt amniocentesis.

▶ A plethora of data have been gathered by systematically recording the findings of women referred for US evaluation when fetal anomalies or maternal problems are suspected. Pagnotta and colleagues share with us their experience with 41 cases of congenital talipes equinovarus, or clubfoot, identified in 27 pregnancies in the early part of the second trimester during a 5-year period at a single referral center. If a clubfoot was detected, the scan was repeated 2 hours later to rule out a positional false positive diagnosis. The scans then were reviewed carefully by both a radiologist and an orthopedic surgeon before counseling of the family. Notable findings from this survey were that 22% of the patients had an abnormal karyotype; isolated or idiopathic clubfoot was a feature in 8 patients and oligohydramnios was present in only 2 patients, mitigating against external compression in utero playing an important role in the etiology.[1] Polyhydramnios was much more prevalent, perhaps reflecting other malformations. Talipes equinovarus may be diagnosed early in the second trimester. We concur that the fetus should be evaluated extensively, and if other anomalies are present, karyotyping is warranted.

A.A. Fanaroff, M.B.B.Ch.

Reference

1. Barlow IW, Clark NMP: Congenital talipes equinovarus. *Surgery* 27:211–215, 1994.

5 Labor and Delivery

Fetal Heart Rate Changes and Cerebral Oxygenation Measured by Near-infrared Spectroscopy During the First Stage of Labour

Aldrich CJ, D'Antona D, Spencer JAD, et al (Univ College London)
Eur J Obstet Gynecol Reprod Biol 64:189–195, 1996 5–1

Background.—It is uncertain whether the alterations in fetal heart rate (FHR) often detected by continuous electronic FHR monitoring during labor are associated with changes in cerebral oxygenation. Near-infrared spectroscopy monitoring was used to measure alterations in fetal cerebral oxygenation that occurred with changes in FHR during the first stage of labor.

Methods.—Thirty healthy women in uncomplicated labor, and with ruptured amniotic membranes, underwent application of an optical probe

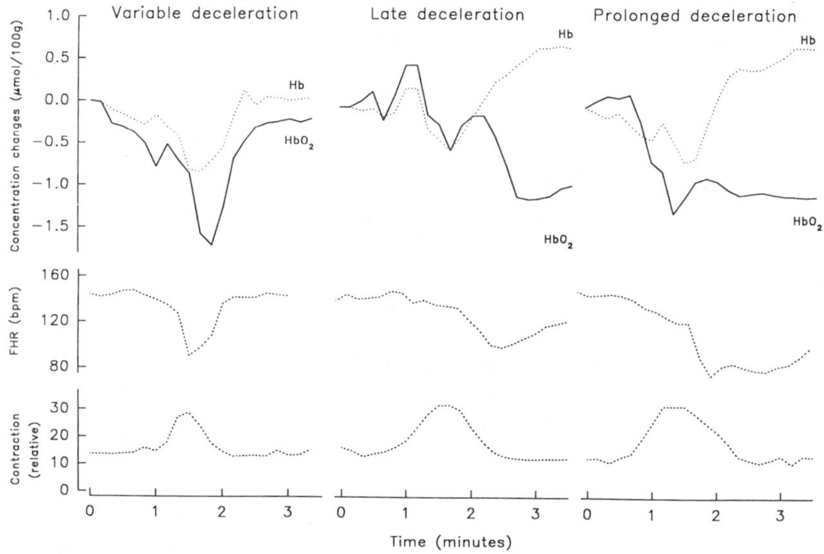

FIGURE 2.—Representative changes from baseline in cerebral oxyhemoglobin (HbO_2) and deoxyhemoglobin (*Hb*) from 3 fetuses demonstrating either a variable, late, or prolonged fetal heart rate (*FHR*) deceleration. (Courtesy of Aldrich CJ, D'Antona D, Spencer JAD, et al: Fetal heart rate changes and cerebral oxygenation measured by near-infrared spectroscopy during the first stage of labour. *Eur J Obstet Gynecol Reprod Biol* 64:189–195, copyright 1996. (With kind permission from Elsevier Science Ireland Ltd., Bay 15K, Shannon Industrial Estate, Co. Clare, Ireland.)

to the fetal scalp in addition to standard cardiotocographic monitoring. The probe measured changes in the attenuation of near-infrared light to monitor continuously concentrations of fetal cerebral oxyhemoglobin (HbO_2) and deoxyhemoglobin (Hb) before, during, and for 50 seconds after each contraction. Mean changes in the hemoglobin oxygenation index (Hb_{diff}) and the total cerebral hemoglobin concentration (Hb_{tot}) were calculated for the same periods.

Results.—For contractions associated with no change, acceleration, or early deceleration of FHR, HbO_2 and Hb both fell significantly, but there was no significant change in Hb_{tot} or Hb_{diff} and, therefore, no change in cerebral oxygenation. A significant drop in Hb_{diff} was seen during and after contractions with variable decelerations, and after contractions with late or prolonged decelerations, implying a significant decrease in fetal cerebral oxygenation (Fig 2). At delivery, no infant had severe umbilical artery acidemia ($pH < 7.05$).

Conclusion.—During the first stage of labor, variable, late, and prolonged changes in FHR are associated with a transient decrease in fetal cerebral oxygenation.

▶ Despite years of experience and a multitude of clinical trials, there is no concrete evidence that FHR monitoring has reduced perinatal hypoxic-ischemic brain injury. There are data indicating that difficulty in interpretation of the monitoring strips has led to more operative deliveries. The next generation of monitors, which incorporates near-infrared spectroscopy (NIRS), permits direct and continuous observation of cerebral oxygenation and perfusion during labor. This report from Aldrich and colleagues describes some initial observations with NIRS during the first stage of labor. The probe was well tolerated and 300 of 555 contractions were suitable for analysis; 48% of the others had poor-quality contractions, 24% had poor-quality NIRS, and 28% had such frequent uterine contractions that the baseline could not be identified between contractions. Variable patterns of NIRS were observed with contractions, such that if there were no alterations in the FHR, either accelerations or early decelerations, there was no evidence of a reduction in fetal cerebral oxygenation. Variable, late, or prolonged decelerations of the FHR were associated with significant but transient decreases in cerebral oxygenation. Thus, NIRS allows the physiologic effects of FHR changes in the brain to be monitored. Other factors, such as the frequency of uterine contractions, the duration and severity of the hypoxia, and the susceptibility of the brain, would determine whether any insult translates into brain injury.

The feasibility of NIRS monitoring during the first stage of labor has been established. More experience with complicated pregnancies and the mandatory randomized trial will determine the role and value of NIRS in labor.

Every start upon an untrodden path is a venture which only in unusual circumstances looks sensible and likely to be successful.—Albert Schweitzer.

A.A. Fanaroff, M.B.B.Ch.

Maternal Position During Labor: Effects on Fetal Oxygen Saturation Measured by Pulse Oximetry

Carbonne B, Benachi A, Lévèque M-L, et al (Université René Descartes, Paris; Nellcor France, Jouy-en-Josas, France)

Obstet Gynecol 88:797–800, 1996 5–2

Objective.—Previous reports have suggested that late decelerations of the fetal heartbeat occur when the mother lies in the supine position. These decelerations, which resolve when the mother shifts to the left lateral position, have been attributed to aortocaval compression. Pulse oximetry can detect changes in fetal oxygen saturation under varying conditions, such as maternal oxygen administration or uterine contractions. This tool was used to assess the effects of maternal position during labor on fetal oxygenation.

Methods.—The study included 15 women in uncomplicated labor. Fetal arterial oxygen saturation was measured by placing a sensor through the cervix and against the side of the fetus' head. Measurements of fetal oxygen saturation were made as the mothers were lying in the left lateral, supine, and right lateral positions for 10 minutes each, in random order. The results were analyzed by repeated measures for analysis of variance.

Results.—Successful readings were obtained during all 3 positions in 12 women. Fetal oxygen saturation was significantly lower when the mother was in the supine position than in the left lateral position. It was nonsig-

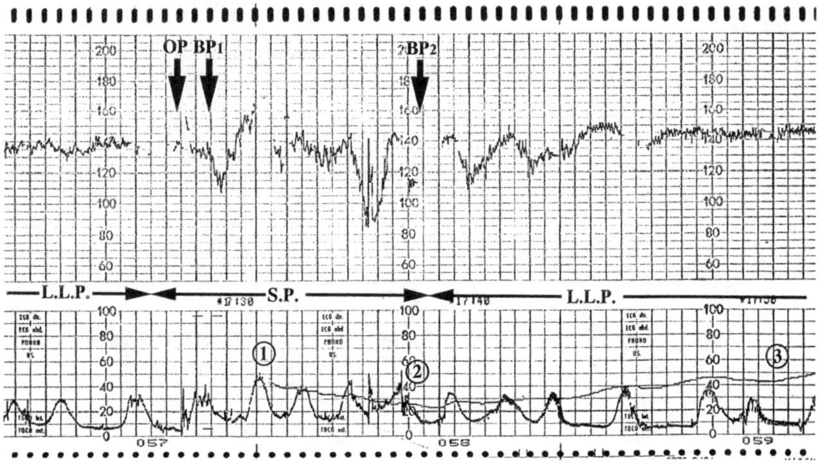

FIGURE 1.—Evolution of fetal heart rate, fetal oxygen saturation, and maternal blood pressure in 1 case of supine hypotension syndrome. Initially, the patient was in left lateral position (*L.L.P.*), then adopted the supine position (*S.P.*) for oximetry sensor placement. Fetal heart rate decelerations occurred in the supine position, with a drop in maternal blood pressure from 120/77 (BP_1) to 65/39 mm Hg (BP_2), and in fetal oxygen saturation from 42% (*1*) to 22% (*2*). When left lateral position was adopted again, the decelerations disappeared and oxygen saturation increased to 48% (*3*). *Abbreviation: OP,* oximetry sensor placement. (Reprinted with permission from American College of Obstetricians and Gynecologists from Carbonne B, Benachi A, Lévèque M-L, et al: Maternal position during labor: Effects on fetal oxygen saturation measured by pulse oximetry. *Obstet Gynecol* 88:797–800, 1996.)

nificantly lower in the right lateral position vs. the left lateral position. There was 1 case of supine hypotensive syndrome associated with fetal heart rate decelerations when the mother shifted from the left lateral to the supine position (Fig 1). In all other cases, fetal heart rate was normal in all maternal positions.

Conclusions.—Fetal oxygen saturation is lower when the mother lies in the supine position, compared to the left lateral position, during labor. As suggested by previous studies using fetal heart rate monitoring, lying in the left lateral position improves fetal oxygenation. Studies of the clinical value of pulse oximetry for fetal monitoring are under way.

▶ The assumption that late decelerations observed when the mother was in the supine position, which disappeared when the left lateral position was adopted, resulted from aortocaval compression has not been seriously challenged. Adaptation of the pulse oximeter to assist fetal oxygenation provides the opportunity to document the effects of maternal position during labor on fetal oxygenation. A low-risk group of women were recruited and randomly rotated into various positions with the sensor in position against the fetal temple or cheek. Adequate recordings were obtained on 12 of 15 subjects and verified that fetal oxygen saturation was lowest with the mother in the supine position. This finding was not dependent on maternal blood pressure. The fetal heart rate remained normal except in a single patient with the supine hypotensive syndrome. A dramatic decline (from 42% to 22%) in fetal saturation was noted in addition to variable decelerations in this subject.

This simple study supports the clinical practice of encouraging mothers to avoid the supine position and assume the left lateral position even in uncomplicated labor. The ability to better monitor oxygenation with the infrared spectroscopy may aid in the earlier detection of fetal compromise. See also Abstract 5–1.

It is better to ask the questions than to know all the answers.—James Thurber

A.A. Fanaroff, M.B.B.Ch.

Randomised, Controlled Trial of Efficacy of Midwife-managed Care

Turnbull D, Holmes A, Shields N, et al (Glasgow Royal Maternity Hosp, Scotland; Greater Glasgow Health Board, Scotland; Univ of Glasgow, Scotland)

Lancet 348:213–218, 1996 5–3

Background.—The efficacy of midwife-managed care programs, which are increasing in popularity, has not been studied sufficiently. The clinical efficacy of and patient satisfaction with midwife-managed care were compared with those of care divided among midwives, hospital physicians, and general practitioners.

TABLE 5.—Fetal and Neonatal Interventions and Outcomes

	Shared care (n=603)	Midwife care (n=613)	Difference (95% CI)
Readmissions	7 (1·2%)	12 (2·0%)	−0·8% (−2·3 to 0·6)
Birthweight centile for gestational age[19]			
<5th centile	29 (4·8%)	25 (4·1%)	0·7% (−1·6 to 3·0)
5th–9th centile	534 (88·6%)	540 (88·1%)	0·5% (−3·1 to 4·1)
-Apgar score			
8–10 at 1 min	449 (75·7%)	474 (78·2%)	−2·5% (−7·2 to 2·2)
8–10 at 5 min	565 (96·6%)	589 (97·8%)	−1·2% (−3·1 to 0·6)
Neonatal standby requested	302 (50·1%)	298 (48·6%)	1·5% (−4·1 to 7·1)
Preadmission observation in SCBU			
At birth	104 (17·2%)	119 (19·4%)	−2·2% (−6·5 to 2·2)
Postnatally	33 (5·5%)	34 (5·6%)	−0·1% (−2·6 to 2·5)
Admission to SCBU			
At birth	40 (6·6%)	33 (5·4%)	1·2% (−1·4 to 3·9)
Postnatally	18 (3·0%)	23 (3·8%)	−0·8% (−3·0 to 1·3)

Note: Denominators exclude missing data.
Abbreviation: SCBU, special-care baby unit.
(Courtesy of Turnbull D, Holmes A, Shields N, et al: Randomised, controlled trial of efficacy of midwife-managed care. *Lancet* 348:213–218. Copyright 1996 by The Lancet Ltd.)

Methods.—A total of 1,299 pregnant women were enrolled in the randomized, controlled study. At enrollment, none had any pregnancy complications. Six hundred forty-eight women were assigned to midwife-managed care and 651 to shared care. Data were collected by retrospectively reviewing medical records and self-report questionnaires.

TABLE 6.—Neonatal Complications and Fetal and Neonatal Loss

	Shared care (n=603)	Midwife care (n=613)	Difference (95% CI)
Neonatal complication*			
Birth asphyxia	5 (0·8%)	4 (0·6%)	0·2% (−0·8 to 1·1)
Bowel obstruction	1 (0·2%)	0	0·2% (−0·2 to 0·5)
Cardiac problems	4 (0·7%)	4 (0·6%)	0 (−0·9 to 0·9)
Fitting/seizures	1 (0·2%)	0	0·2% (−0·2 to 0·5)
Hypoxic encephalopathy	1 (0·2%)	0	0·2% (−0·2 to 0·5)
Jaundice requiring phototherapy	53 (8·8%)	59 (9·6%)	−0·8% (−4·1 to 2·4)
Meconium aspiration	0	1 (0·2%)	−0·2% (−0·5 to 0·2)
Pneumothorax	0	1 (0·2%)	−0·2% (−0·5 to 0·2)
Fetal loss before 24 weeks			
Spontaneous abortion	23 (3·8%)	19 (3·1%)	0·7% (−1·3 to 2·8)
Induced abortion	1 (0·2%)	1 (0·2%)	0 (−0·4 to 0·5)
Fetal loss after 24 weeks			
Stillbirth†	4 (0·7%)	1 (0·2%)	0·5% (−0·2 to 1·2)
Neonatal death‡	5 (0·8%)	3 (0·5%)	0·3% (−0·6 to 1·2)

*At birth and in the postnatal period, additional to those that resulted in fetal or neonatal loss, and defined as diagnosed by clinician at that time.
†Baby born dead after 24 completed weeks of pregnancy.
‡Death within 28 days of live birth.
(Courtesy of Turnbull D, Holmes A, Shields N, et al: Randomised, controlled trial of efficacy of midwife-managed care. *Lancet* 348:213–218. Copyright 1996 by The Lancet Ltd.)

TABLE 8.—Satisfaction With Choice, Information, Decision-making, and Individualized Care

Care period	Percentage response						p
	Shared care			Midwife care			
	Strongly agree/ agree	Not sure	Strongly disagree/ disagree	Strongly agree/ agree	Not sure	Strongly disagree/ disagree	
Antenatal*							
I'm offered little choice about my care (C)	25·5	22·5	52·0	8·0	8·2	83·8	<0·00001
I feel I get too little information (I)	20·9	14·0	65·1	4·9	5·1	90·0	<0·00001
I can be in control of decisions about my care when I want to (D)	62·8	27·8	9·4	87·3	11·2	1·5	<0·00001
I feel staff are interested in me and not just my pregnancy (IC)	56·2	18·8	25·0	80·2	6·5	13·3	<0·00001
Intrapartum†							
I felt I had little choice about what happened to me (C)	18·2	9·4	72·4	10·6	6·6	82·8	0·001
I was always asked what I thought about things (I)	66·0	14·6	19·4	80·3	10·4	9·3	0·00002
I felt little attention was paid to my wishes (D)	11·8	6·9	81·3	6·8	2·1	91·1	0·00008
I was treated like an individual (IC)	82·4	8·5	9·1	90·5	3·6	5·9	0·002
Hospital-based postnatal†							
I felt I was given choices about what I could do (C)	65·6	14·7	19·7	86·3	8·4	5·3	<0·00001
Staff took time to discuss any information I wanted (I)	73·2	12·2	14·6	92·5	2·7	4·8	<0·00001
Little attention was paid to my wishes (D)	13·6	7·2	79·2	4·3	1·8	93·9	<0·00001
There was little interest in me after my baby was born (IC)	15·4	6·1	78·5	5·2	0·9	93·9	<0·00001
Home-based postnatal†							
I felt I was given choices about what I could do (C)	79·6	11·2	9·2	89·4	6·0	4·6	0·0006
Staff took time to discuss any information I wanted (I)	91·6	3·2	5·2	95·8	2·1	2·1	0·03
Little attention was paid to my wishes (D)	4·6	4·8	90·6	1·8	2·1	96·1	0·007
There was little interest in me after my baby was born (IC)	4·3	3·5	92·2	2·8	0·9	96·3	0·02

**n* = 487 shared care, 534 midwife care.
†*n* = 380 shared care, 445 midwife care.
Abbreviations: C, choice; *I* information; *D*, decision-making; *IC*, individualized care.
(Courtesy of Turnbull D, Holmes A, Shields N, et al: Randomised, controlled trial of efficacy of midwife-managed care. *Lancet* 348:213–218. Copyright 1996 by The Lancet Ltd.)

Findings.—Twenty-four percent of the women receiving midwife care had induced labor, compared with 33.3% of those receiving shared care. Women in the midwife-managed group were also more likely to have an intact perineum and less likely to have an episiotomy than those in the shared-care group, with no significant between-group difference in perineal tears. Thirty-three percent of women receiving midwife care were transferred permanently to shared care—28.7% for clinical reasons and 3.7% for nonclinical reasons. Overall, women in both groups were satisfied with their care. However, those receiving midwife care were significantly more satisfied with their antenatal, intrapartum, hospital-based postnatal, and home-based postnatal care (Tables 5, 6 and 8).

Conclusion.—Compared with shared care, midwife-managed care resulted in similar or decreased rates of interventions, similar outcomes, comparable maternal and infant complications, and better satisfaction with care. There were no significant between-group differences in complications or outcomes. Thus, midwife-managed care for healthy pregnant women, integrated with existing services, is a clinically effective approach which increases patient satisfaction.

► The overwhelming majority of mothers in the United States are delivered by obstetricians, but in the United Kingdom, participation by midwives in antepartum, intrapartum, and postpartum care is the rule rather than the exception. The standard model in the United Kingdom is one of shared care— divided among midwives, obstetricians, and family practitioners. Virtually every study of care delivered by nurse practitioners and physician assistants in pediatrics and obstetrics has shown not only that these professionals deliver excellent care, but also that there is a high level of patient satisfaction.

The current, intense drive to contain the cost of medical care will probably lead to a greater role for nurse midwives in the United States. Turnbull, et al. did not compare midwives with physicians, but they compared care by midwives with "shared care" in which midwives, obstetricians, and family physicians all participated. Thus, the results are all the more remarkable. Certainly, it is not easy to conduct this type of randomized, controlled trial, and the authors are to be congratulated on having tested an important hypothesis in this carefully controlled manner. The results are not surprising and confirm, again, that given the appropriate environment and support services where needed, medical outcomes for mothers cared for by midwives are not only as good as the standard physician-directed model, but significantly better when patient perceptions regarding choice, information, decision-making, and individualized care are analyzed.

M.J. Maisels, M.B.B.Ch.

► The data generated by this trial will add weight to the argument for less primary care from the obstetric specialist. However, in the United States, it will be some time before the baton for routine obstetric care is handed over to midwives and family practitioners. There are insufficient such personnel and, until there is major tort reform, don't expect a rush of volunteers to do obstetrics.

The concept of primary low-risk obstetric care being provided by midwives and family practioners is not novel. The Dutch have, for many years, had such a system in place. Turnbull and colleagues needed to refer almost one-third of their patients for consultation and care by the obstetric specialists, very similar to the Dutch report.[1] In the Dutch experience, van Alten reported that 74.3% of patients were delivered by midwives, 17.7% required transfer to a physician during pregnancy, and 7.9% required transfer to the physician service during labor. Hundley and associates, from Aberdeen, Scotland, performed a randomized trial with low-risk pregnancies assigned either to the midwives' unit or the physician-run labor ward. A number of the midwife-assigned women required transfer to the labor ward because of complications before or during labor. There were significant differences in intrapartum management with less intervention by the midwives.[2] The outcomes for mothers and infants were similar. The conclusion was that patients could be safely delivered by midwives, but a number of apparently low-risk women will experience problems requiring transfer to a physician-led unit. Butler and colleagues reported fewer labor abnormalities, and the diagnosis of fetal distress was less common among patients who were cared for by nurse-midwives than among those in a physician's care. Nurse-midwife care was associated with a lower incidence of cesarean delivery.[3]

A.A. Fanaroff, M.B.B.Ch.

References

1. van Alten D, Eskes M, Treffers PE: Midwifery in the Netherlands: The Wormeveer study: Selection, mode of delivery, perinatal mortality and infant morbidity. *Br J Obstet Gynecol* 96:656–662, 1989.
2. Hundley VA, Cruickshank FM, Lang GD, et al: Midwife managed delivery unit: A randomized controlled comparison with consultant-led care. *BMJ* 309:1400–1404, 1994.
3. Butler J et al: Supportive nurse-midwife care is associated with a reduced incidence of cesarean section. *Am J Obstet Gynecol* 168:1407–1413, 1993.

Comparison of a Trial of Labor With an Elective Second Cesarean Section

McMahon MJ, Luther ER, Bowes WA Jr, et al (Univ of North Carolina, Chapel Hill; Dalhousie Univ, Halifax, NS, Canada)
N Engl J Med 335:689–695, 1996 5–4

Background.—About 50% of cesarean section deliveries in the United States and Canada are performed only to avoid labor after a previous cesarean section. Several conferences have concluded, however, that vaginal delivery can be safe for women who have had a previous low transverse cesarean section. A population-based, longitudinal study was conducted to determine how morbidity and mortality associated with a trial of labor compared with those related to an elective cesarean section.

Methods.—Study data were obtained from records of the Reproductive Care Program of Nova Scotia, Canada. From 1986 through 1992, 6,457 women who delivered a live singleton infant previously had undergone 1 cesarean section; 6,138 met eligibility requirements. Of these women, 3,249 attempted vaginal delivery after a previous low transverse cesarean section and 2,889 elected to undergo a second cesarean section. These 2 groups were compared for demographic and maternal characteristics and for the type and incidence of complications.

Results.—Women more likely to attempt a trial of labor were either 19 years of age or younger or 30 years of age or older, had had a previous vaginal delivery in addition to a cesarean section, and had attended prenatal classes. The perinatal mortality rate was 5 per 1,000 live births in the elective cesarean section group and 9 per 1,000 in the trial of labor group. There were no maternal deaths. Complications occurred in 8.1% of women and were major in 1.3%. The trial of labor group was 1.8 times as likely to have major complications but 20% less likely to have minor complications. The risk of puerperal fever was 25% higher in the elective cesarean section group. Of those who underwent a trial of labor, vaginal delivery was accomplished in 60.4%; women 35 years of age or older were less likely than younger women to have a successful trial of labor.

Discussion.—Major maternal complications are almost twice as likely among women who undergo a trial of labor after a previous cesarean section than among those who have a second cesarean section. Morbidity is greatest when the trial is unsuccessful and a second cesarean section is required. Apgar scores, admission to neonatal ICU, and perinatal mortality were similar among infants in the trial of labor and second cesarean section groups.

Trial of Labor in Patients With a Previous Lower Uterine Vertical Cesarean Section

Adair CD, Sanchez-Ramos L, Whitaker D, et al (Univ of Florida, Jacksonville)
Am J Obstet Gynecol 174:966–970, 1996 5–5

Background.—There are substantial data confirming the safety of a trial of labor after a previous low transverse cesarean section, and this strategy has been recommended by consensus bodies. However, there are no recommendations and scarce data regarding a trial of labor after a prior low vertical cesarean section. The efficacy and safety of a trial of labor in this population were evaluated, retrospectively.

Methods.—Medical records were searched to identify 77 patients with a history of low vertical uterine incision cesarean section who underwent a trial of labor, and the next 2 patients without a scarred uterus to deliver after each case patient. The delivery outcomes were reviewed in both groups.

Results.—During the 6-year study, there was an overall cesarean section rate of 8.6% and a repeated cesarean section rate of 17%. There were no significant differences between the 2 study groups in gravidity, parity, or maternal age. The course of labor was similar in the 2 groups, with a similar duration of the first and second stages of labor and similar total doses and maximal rates of oxytocin. Vaginal deliveries occurred in 85.7% of the cesarean section group and 90.9% of the comparative group. There were no differences in operative vaginal delivery rates. The 2 groups had no significant differences in maternal or perinatal morbidity. There was only 1 occurrence of uterine rupture in the cesarean section group.

Conclusions.—A trial of labor is generally as safe for patients with a history of prior low vertical cesarean section as for patients with an unscarred uterus, with an incidence of uterine rupture that is comparable. However, further study is needed before the routine use of a trial of labor can be recommended in patients with a previous low vertical uterine incision.

► It should be sobering to realize that cesarean section is the most common major surgical procedure in the United States. About 1 million infants each year are delivered in this manner, and if Craigin's dictum, "once a cesarean, always a cesarean," still held true, the number of operative deliveries would continue to escalate. This dictum, enunciated in 1916, dominated obstetric practice for nearly 70 years, and elective cesarean sections currently account for 38% of operative deliveries. It is now important to examine and take heed of the mounting evidence documenting the safety of vaginal birth after cesarean delivery and to heed the American College of Obstetricians and Gynecologists recommendations.[1-3] It is particularly gratifying to read the report by Adair and associates (Abstract 5–5) that even after a lower uterine vertical cesarean section, vaginal birth is not only possible, but safe.

It is safe for most women, unless there are specific contraindications, to undergo a trial of labor after a previous lower transverse cesarean section. After a previous cesarean section, about two-thirds of women will deliver vaginally, with a slight increase in uterine rupture (0.2%) as the major risk factor. The women subjected to repeated elective cesarean section (ERCS) may have increased risks for infection and hemorrhage. In the current climate in which cost savings head the priority list, it is noteworthy that cesarean section is substantially more expensive than vaginal delivery. The costs, however, may be greatest for a failed trial of labor necessitating a cesarean birth. Trial of labor was most successful when the initial indication for the cesarean section was breech presentation. We recently examined, in detail, the spectrum of neonatal morbidity after ERCS compared with a trial of labor. Sixty-nine percent of mothers (342) attempting a trial of labor (after previous cesarean birth) delivered vaginally, and 31% (157) required a repeated cesarean section. Infants delivered by ERCS had an increased risk of respiratory problems, but these were minor, whereas failed trial of labor infants had increased rates of suspected and proven sepsis. The overall morbidity was very low.[4]

More obstetric units should establish policies that women who have had a prior cesarean section, but not for cephalopelvic disproportion, are offered the opportunity and encouraged to undergo a trial of labor.

Statistics are like alienists—they will testify for either side.—F.H. La Guardia.
A.A. Fanaroff, M.B.B.Ch.

References

1. Rosen MG, Dickinson JC, Westhoff CL: Vaginal birth after cesarean: A meta-analysis of morbidity and mortality. *Obstet Gynecol* 77:465–470, 1991.
2. American College of Obstetricians and Gynecologists Committee on Obstetrics, Maternal and Fetal Medicine: *Fetal Maturity Assessment Prior to Elective Repeat Cesarean Delivery.* ACOG Committee Opinion No. 98. Washington, DC, American College of Obstetricians and Gynecologists, 1991.
3. Flamm BL, Goings JR, Liu Y, et al: Elective repeat cesarean delivery versus trial of labor: A prospective multi-center study. *Obstet Gynecol* 83:927–932, 1994.
4. Hook B, Kiwi R, Amini S, et al: Neonatal morbidity following elective repeat cesarean section and trial of labor. *Pediatrics* 1997, still in press.

Elective or Selective Caesarean Delivery of the Small Baby? A Systematic Review of the Controlled Trials

Grant A, Penn ZJ, Steer PJ (Univ of Aberdeen, Scotland; Chelsea and Westminster Hosp, London)
Br J Obstet Gynaecol 103:1197–1200, 1996 5–6

Introduction.—A systematic review of controlled trials was conducted to compare policies of elective cesarean delivery with those of selective cesarean delivery for women in spontaneous preterm labor.

Methods.—Reports were chosen for review if they compared elective cesarean delivery with selective cesarean delivery for infants at less than 37 weeks' gestation if the choice of policy was made by random assignment. Data from 122 women from 6 trials were analyzed. The main outcome measures were actual use of cesarean delivery, low Apgar score, neonatal intubation, intracranial pathologic findings, perinatal death, and major maternal complications.

Results.—Of those women allocated to elective cesarean delivery, 16% were delivered vaginally and 18% of women allocated to selective cesarean delivery were delivered by cesarean section, usually because of fetal distress. General anesthesia was used more often for patients who underwent elective cesarean delivery. The odds ratios for adverse neonatal outcome typically favored the elective group, but the confidence intervals were wide for all outcomes and did not exclude clinically important hazards of the policy.

Conclusion.—A policy of elective cesarean delivery was associated with increased maternal morbidity and may have occasionally led to the early delivery of a small infant in a pregnancy in which preterm labor would otherwise have stopped. It may be that a policy of elective cesarean delivery is associated with important benefits for some infants. The size of any beneficial effect is not known and it is not clear whether these benefits outweigh the maternal risks.

▶ Adrian Grant has helped make the review of controlled trials fashionable. The above review tackles the ticklish problem of elective or selective cesarean section delivery of the small baby. Are the deliveries ever truly elective for this population? The review was a concession because his group was unable to recruit sufficient patients for a prospective randomized trial. Indeed, all 6 trials of elective preterm cesarean delivery were terminated before reaching projected sample size, in 5 because of difficulty in recruitment. Grant and colleagues sought additional information from the investigators of all studies identified, all of whom were acknowledged for "generously giving access to unpublished data." With the large number of cesarean deliveries, it seems improbable that a randomized trial could not be successfully mounted.

Grant et al. performed a comprehensive analysis of the available data and concluded that the typical odds ratio tended to favor the elective group; but there were wide confidence intervals, and clinically important hazards could not be excluded. Nothing was statistically significant. In weighing the evidence, one must take into consideration the increased odds of serious maternal morbidity in the cesarean section group, which was statistically significant.

It is noteworthy that 2 women recruited to Penn's[1] trial who were allowed to labor delivered weeks later, so a policy of elective cesarean section delivery may occasionally result in iatrogenic prematurity. Also, a number of fetuses thought to be in the breech position were not. There remains an obvious need for properly controlled trials to determine whether an elective cesarean can help the small baby. I suspect we are dealing with a military type of situation, and no volunteers will step forward to tackle this task.

A.A. Fanaroff, M.B.B.Ch.

References

1. Penn Z, Steer P, Grant A: A multi-center randomized controlled trial to compare elective versus selective cesarean section for delivery of the preterm breech infant. *Br J Obstet Gynaecol* 103:684-689, 1996.

Reductions in Cost and Cesarean Rate by Routine Use of External Cephalic Version: A Decision Analysis

Gifford DS, Keeler E, Kahn KL (RAND, Santa Monica, Calif; Univ of California, Los Angeles)

Obstet Gynecol 85:930–936, 1995 5–7

Objective.—The percentage of breech births delivered by cesarean section has increased from 15% in 1970 to 84% in 1989. Other birth methods have been advocated as a means of lowering the cesarean section rate. A decision analysis based on a literature review of clinical trials estimates the changes that would occur in the mode of delivery and the cost after 4 methods of managing term breech births without contraindications to labor or external version.

Methods.—A MEDLINE and Health Planning and Administration search yielded 217 articles representing 4 management options including (1) external cephalic version followed by a trial of labor for those meeting criteria; (2) external cephalic version followed by scheduled cesarean delivery for infants who remain breech; (3) trial of labor for those meeting criteria and scheduled cesarean delivery for those who do not; and (4) scheduled, elective cesarean for all breech infants. Probabilities were calculated for delivery outcomes and costs based on the 4 management options.

Results.—Using the external cephalic version and trial of labor resulted in a cesarean rate of 25.4% and an expected cost of $8,071 per patient. With the external cephalic version and cesarean delivery, the cesarean rate was 31.9% with an expected cost of $8,276 per patient. Using trial of labor for those meeting criteria and scheduled cesarean for those who did not, the cesarean rate was 62.6% with an expected cost of $8,755. For patients with a scheduled, elective cesarean, the rate was 88.6% with an expected cost of $9,544.

Conclusion.—Use of the external cephalic version increases the number of vaginal deliveries and concurrently lowers the cost per patient. Routine cesarean deliveries unnecessarily increase costs and patient morbidity.

► This comment was co-authored by Daniel S. Seidman, M.D., of The Sheba Medical Center, Tel-Hashomer, Israel:

► Vaginal delivery of the breech infant is becoming a rare art in the United States. Most women with a breech pregnancy are thus destined to undergo a cesarean section and risk the associated morbidity. For these women, the only way to avoid an inevitable cesarean is a successful external cephalic version. The success rate reported for external cephalic version among the U.S. trials is approximately 65%, and once a version succeeds, almost all fetuses stay in the vertex position until birth.[1] External cephalic version, using tocolysis and cardiotocography, is a safe procedure with potential complications, such as placental abruption, rupture of the membranes, fetomaternal transfusion, and umbilical cord entanglement, only rarely being reported.[1] This study shows that even with the liberal use of vaginal delivery for term breech infants, the routine use of external version is likely to be translated to a significant decrease in the cesarean rate, with matching cost savings.

D. Seidman, M.D.
D.K. Stevenson, M.D.

References

1. Zhang J, Bowes WA, Fortney JA: Efficacy of external cephalic version. A review. *Obstet Gynecol* 82:306–312, 1993.

Breech at Term: Mode of Delivery? A Register-based Study

Krebs L, Langhoff-Roos J, Weber T (Univ of Copenhagen; Hvidovre Hosp, Denmark)

Acta Obstet Gynecol Scand 74:702–706, 1995 5–8

Background.—The best mode of delivery of term fetuses in the breech position is still debated. Neonatal mortality and morbidity in nonmalformed singleton term infants delivered in breech presentation were reported, and possible correlations between outcome and mode of delivery, parity, and birth weight were investigated.

Methods.—Data were obtained from a Danish cohort of 15,718 normal, singleton term infants presenting in the breech position and delivered between 1982 and 1990. All were alive at the onset of labor.

Findings.—Deliveries were vaginal for 3,247 infants (20.7%), elective cesarean in 7,106 (45.3%), and emergency cesarean in 5,356 (34.1%). Compared with those delivered by elective cesarean section, infants delivered vaginally and by emergency cesarean section had significantly greater rates of mortality—including intrapartum and early neonatal death—and morbidity, as evidenced by low Apgar scores. Parity was unassociated with outcome among vaginal deliveries. However, infants with birth weights of more than 4,000 g had significantly greater rates of low Apgar scores.

Conclusion.—Vaginal delivery of nonmalformed, term infants in breech presentation appears to be associated with increased mortality and morbidity. These findings need to be validated and more information must be obtained from the medical records before it is clear whether selection of parturients, structure of perinatal care, or professional skills need to be improved, or whether all singleton term infants in breech presentation should undergo cesarean delivery.

▶ This comment was co-authored by Daniel S. Seidman, M.D., of The Sheba Medical Center, Tel-Hashomer, Israel:

▶ Breech presentation accounts for approximately 4% of deliveries. In the United States, most hospitals report that 60% to 90% of their breech infants are delivered by cesarean section.[1] Furthermore, breech presentation is the third most important cause of the rise in cesarean section birth rate during the past 2 decades, accounting for 10% to 15% of cesareans. The decision to abandon the practice of allowing a trial of labor for breech infants has been based on the assumption that vaginal delivery is associated with increased mortality and morbidity. Unfortunately, the validity of the data supporting this view is questionable because of the retrospective nature of most studies, including this one from the Danish National Medical Birth Register.

All retrospective studies on this subject are fraught with a strong bias, as, over the years, obstetricians have been redefining the selection criteria of parturients for whom a vaginal delivery is planned. Vaginally delivered infants enrolled in such studies include undiagnosed breeches and very rapid deliveries for which an elective cesarean section may have been intended. It must also be remembered that the abnormal presentation itself may reflect some fetal abnormality, independent of the mode of delivery.

A long-awaited multinational, prospective study is under way, and it is hoped that, for the first time, it will achieve the sample size required to detect differences in low-incidence outcome variables, such as intrapartum and early neonatal death in nonmalformed fetuses. However, as few of the obstetricians currently trained in the United States receive adequate experience in vaginally delivering breech infants, it seems doubtful whether a study attesting to the safety or desirability of this approach will reverse the current practice of delivering breech infants by cesarean section.

D. Seidman, M.D.
D.K. Stevenson, M.D.

References

1. Zhang J, Bowes WA, Fortney JA: Efficacy of external cephalic version: A review. *Obstet Gynecol* 82:306–312, 1993.

Maternal and Neonatal Outcome of 846 Term Singleton Breech Deliveries: Seven-year Experience at a Single Center

Schiff E, Friedman SA, Mashiach S, et al (Tel-Aviv Univ, Israel; Univ of Tennessee, Memphis)

Am J Obstet Gynecol 175:18–23, 1996 5–9

Background.—Although breech presentations are not uncommon—occurring in about 3% of all term singleton pregnancies—their management is still debated. Some institutions have established policies for identifying women at low risk for complications to avoid a high rate of cesarean delivery, whereas other authorities argue that, even after careful selection, neonatal outcomes are better after abdominal delivery than after vaginal delivery. A retrospective study compared maternal and neonatal outcomes after term vaginal and abdominal deliveries of singleton breech infants at a center where uniform criteria for selecting delivery mode were in place.

Methods.—The records of all mothers delivering singleton breech infants between 1984 and 1990 were reviewed. The records of the neonates were also examined. Six hundred thirteen women (group 1) fulfilled the criteria for a trial of labor, and 233 (group 2) underwent scheduled cesarean section.

Findings.—Fifty-three percent of the women in group 1 were delivered vaginally. None of the mothers died. Febrile morbidity and length of hospital stay were significantly greater among those needing cesarean section in labor than in those delivered vaginally. None of the infants were stillborn. There were 8 neonatal deaths, 6 occurring in infants with major malformations incompatible with life. The other 2 deaths occurred in group 1. Overall, the group 1 infants had a higher trauma rate, with borderline significance. There were no significant differences in the rates of low Apgar scores, intubation, or ICU admission.

Conclusion.—These findings are not conclusive enough to support routine cesarean section for term breech presentation. Large randomized studies of short- and long-term outcomes are needed.

▶ Dr. Robert Lorenz, Director of Maternal Fetal Medicine, William Beaumont Hospital, Royal Oak, Michigan, comments:

▶ The appropriate mode of delivery for the term singleton breech is one of the major ongoing unresolved issues in modern obstetrics. Some things are certain:

1. In the absence of good data it is easy to speculate, but there are insufficient well-designed, randomized, controlled trials to permit an evidence-based clinical decision regarding the mode of delivery.
2. If you have a choice as a fetus, don't be breech. Regardless of mode of delivery, breech fetuses have higher rates of lethal and nonlethal anomalies and perinatal morbidity and mortality.
3. Mother Nature usually does a good job. A systematic approach to selective use of planned vaginal delivery will result in a good outcome in a majority of cases.
4. There are no zero-risk options (snake oil doesn't work for everyone). Significant birth trauma can occur with abdominal delivery of a breech.
5. How many drivers on the road can operate a manual transmission, and why? Despite efforts by teaching programs and the Residency Review Committee for Obstetrics and Gynecology, the overall level of experience, expertise, and comfort with vaginal breech deliveries among obstetricians has declined significantly over the past 20 years.
6. There is no free lunch. A policy of planned cesarean births for all singleton breech deliveries increases maternal minor and major morbidity and is one factor in the concern regarding the rate of cesarean birth in the United States.
7. This study is the largest retrospective investigation of vaginal breech delivery in term singletons to date. It shows that, with proper selection at an institution actively supporting this mode of delivery, many patients can be safely delivered vaginally. Even in such ideal circumstances, however, it appears that there is some increase in fetal/neonatal morbidity, and possibly mortality, that must be balanced against the higher maternal risks of routine abdominal delivery.
8. Although not addressed in this study, antepartum external version should be considered selectively as another tool for reducing the cesarean birth rate related to malpresentation. Unfortunately, in the absence of controlled trials, we must continue to rely on such large, descriptive studies as the next best resource for counseling patients regarding their options.

R. Lorenz, M.D.

Obstetric Brachial Plexus Palsy Associated With Breech Delivery: A Different Pattern of Injury

Geutjens G, Gilbert A, Helsen K (Institut Français de La Main, Paris)
J Bone Joint Surg Br 78B:303–306, 1996 5–10

Introduction.—Most cases of obstetric brachial plexus palsy occur in infants whose delivery is complicated by shoulder dystocia. The injury is rupture of the upper nerve roots, which responds well to early surgical exploration and grafting. The pattern of injury is different, and the prognosis is worse, for infants with obstetric brachial plexus palsy after breech delivery. Thirty-six such patients were reviewed.

Patients.—Of 379 infants treated for obstetric brachial plexus palsy from 1979 to 1993, 36 (9.5%) were born by breech delivery. Eight patients initially had bilateral injuries. The patients were 20 girls and 16 boys, with a mean birth weight of 2,912 g. The pattern of injury was analyzed at surgical exploration. Eighty-one percent of the cases had avulsion of the C5 and C6 nerve roots and sometimes also the C7 nerve root. Obvious avulsions were treated by immediate neurotization of the musculocutaneous nerve. In some cases with suspected in situ avulsion, neurotization was delayed in the hope of spontaneous recovery. Although this did occur in some cases, most patients had neurotization of the musculocutaneous nerve at a later operation. Most of the children for whom follow-up information was available required 2 or 3 additional procedures to improve shoulder function.

Conclusions.—Obstetric brachial plexus palsy occurring during breech delivery is different from that occurring during cephalic delivery. Avulsion of the upper nerve roots, which cannot be treated by microsurgical grafting, is common and carries a poor prognosis. Care should be taken to avoid these injuries in breech deliveries, particularly in premature infants.

► Fortunately, for the obstetrician, the patient, and the neonatologist (not necessarily in that order), most injuries to the brachial plexus recover without surgical intervention. If there has been no resolution or significant improvement after 3–4 months, surgical exploration may be warranted.[1, 2]

The most common pattern of injury found at surgical exploration is postganglionic rupture of the C5 and C6 nerve roots, sometimes including C7, which usually appears as neuroma in continuity. These are the simplest lesions to repair. This is not true of the pattern of injury associated with breech delivery, and notably in many premature infants. Eighty-one percent in this series had avulsion of the C5 and C6 roots, which carries a worse prognosis and requires multiple salvage surgical procedures.

The plea for caution when delivering a premature infant who is in the breech position already has been heeded. Similar care is necessary even when delivering a premature infant in the breech position by cesarean section.

A.A. Fanaroff, M.B.B.Ch.

References

1. Boome RS, Kaye JC: Obstetric traction injuries of the brachial plexus: Natural history, indications for surgical repair and results. *J Bone Joint Surg BR* 70B:571–576, 1988.
2. Gilbert A, Brockman R, Carlioz H: Surgical treatment of brachial plexus birth palsy. *Clin Orthop* 264:39–47, 1991.

Neonatal Complications in Newborns With an Umbilical Artery pH <7.00

van den Berg PP, Nelen WLDM, Jongsma HW, et al (Univ Hosp Nijmegen, The Netherlands)

Am J Obstet Gynecol 175:1152–1157, 1996 5–11

Introduction.—The fact that there is no consensus on the definition of neonatal acidosis makes it difficult to determine the relationship between umbilical artery pH as a measure of intrapartum asphyxia and newborn morbidity. Using an umbilical artery pH of less than 7.00 as a measure of severe intrapartum asphyxia, a retrospective matched cohort design was used to define the association between severe acidosis and neonatal morbidity and mortality.

Methods.—Between 1986 and 1993, arterial umbilical cord blood samples of 10,699 neonates were evaluated for pH. Eighty-four infants had umbilical artery pH values of less than 7.00. These neonates were individually matched with neonates with umbilical artery pH values greater than 7.24. Matching variables were birth date, sex, mother's

TABLE 2.—Umbilical Cord Acid-base Parameters

		Matched cases		
	Total population (N = 14,025)*	*Study group (n = 84)*	*Control group (n = 84)*	*Unmatched acidotic cases (n = 33)*
Arterial				
pH (mean ± SD)	7.24 ± 0.08 (N=14,025)	6.91 ± 0.09 (81)	7.29 ± 0.03 (84)	6.87 ± 0.13 (31)
P_{CO_2} (mm Hg) (mean ± SD)		12.0 ± 3.3 (80)	6.6 ± 1.2 (77)	
Base deficit (mmol/L) (mean ± SD)		18.2 ± 4.3 (81)	3.6 ± 2.4 (78)	
Venous				
pH (mean ± SD)		7.02 ± 0.12 (84)	7.35 ± 0.04 (84)	
P_{CO_2} (mm Hg) (mean ± SD)		9.5 ± 3.1 (81)	5.2 ± 0.9 (78)	
Base deficit (mmol/L) (mean ± SD)		15.5 ± 4.3 (82)	3.8 ± 2.0 (79)	

Values in parentheses indicate number.
*Total investigated population delivered in University Hospital Nijmegen between 1986 and 1993.
Abbreviation: P_{CO_2}, partial pressure of carbon dioxide.
(Courtesy of van den Berg PP, Nelen WLDM, Jongsma HW, et al: Neonatal complications in newborns with an umbilical artery pH < 7.00. *Am J Obstet Gynecol* 175:1152–1157, 1996.)

TABLE 3.—Neonatal Complications in Newborns With Umbilical Artery pH <7.00 Versus Umbilical Artery pH >7.24

Complication	*Study cohort (n = 84)*	*McNemar test (significance)*	*Control group (n = 84)*
Poor condition after delivery	63 (75)	p <0.001	10 (12)
Resuscitation	51	p <0.001	6
Intubation	24	p <0.001	2
Apgar score <7 at 1 min	56	p <0.001	8
Apgar score <7 at 5 min	26	p <0.001	2
Neurologic	19 (23)	p <0.01	6 (7)
Abnormal tone	12	p <0.02	2
Seizures	9	p <0.01	1
Intracranial hemorrhage	5	NS	2
Periventricular leukomalacia	2	NS	1
Abnormal EEG-cranial ultrasonography	12	p <0.05	3
Pulmonary	26 (31)	p <0.01	9 (11)
Recurrent apnea	4	NS	4
Aspiration	18	p <0.01	3
Pneumothorax	3	NS	1
Idiopathic RDS	8	p <0.02	3
Bronchopulmonal dysplasia	2	NS	1
Persistent pulmonary hypertension	1	NS	0
Cardiovascular	13 (15)	p <0.01	7 (8)
Treated open ductus arteriosus	2	NS	1
Bradycardia or tachycardia	7	NS	6
Hypotension	9	p <0.02	2
Renal	4 (5)	NS	1 (1)
Gastrointestinal	14 (17)	p <0.001	0
High liver enzyme values	14	p <0.001	0
Necrotizing enterocolitis	1	NS	0
Death	2 (2)	NS	1 (1)
NICU admission	27 (32)	p <0.001	7 (8)

Values in parentheses indicate percent.

Abbreviations: EEG, electroencephalogram; *NS,* not significant; *RDS,* respiratory distress syndrome; *NICU,* neonatal intensive care unit.

(Courtesy of van den Berg PP, Nelen WLDM, Jongsma HW: Neonatal complications in newborns with an umbilical artery pH < 7.00. *Am J Obstet Gynecol* 175:1152–1157, 1996.)

parity, gestational age, mode of delivery, fetal presentation, and birth weight. There were 33 unmatched neonates with acidosis. Between-group differences in neonatal complications were analyzed.

Results.—The pH value of the total population was 7.24, the pH value of the study group was 6.91, the pH value of the control group was 7.29, and the pH value of the unmatched neonates with acidosis was 6.87 (Table 2). The group with acidosis had significantly greater neonatal morbidity (poorer condition after delivery and neurologic, pulmonary, gastrointestinal, and cardiovascular complications), and neonatal intensive care admissions compared with the group without acidosis (Table 3). In the neonatal group with acidosis, 87.5% of infants had mixed acidosis, 2.5% had respiratory acidosis, and 10% had metabolic acidosis (Fig 1). There were no neurologic complications in neonates with metabolic acidosis. Fifteen of the 16 neurologic complications observed in neonates with mixed acidosis had a base deficit of 15 mmol/L or more. The proportion of neonates with neurologic complications increased with increasing hypercarbia or base deficit. Neurologic dysfunction was detected in all except 1

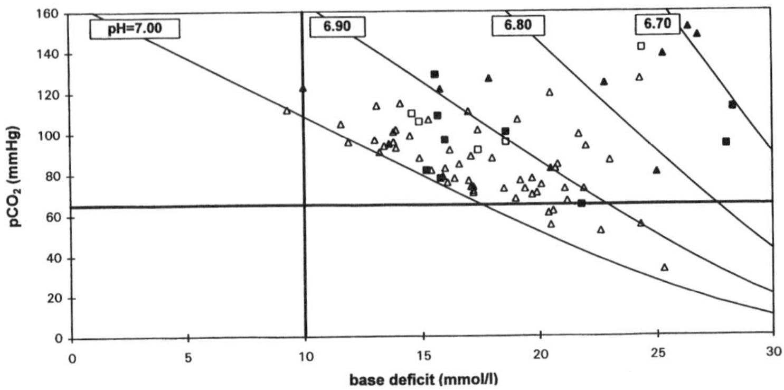

FIGURE 1.—Base deficit vs. partial pressure of carbon dioxide (PCO_2) in umbilical artery with subdivision for gestational age and neurologic dysfunction. Iso-pH lines were drawn at pH 7.00, 6.90, 6.80, and 6.70. *Solid square*, preterm infants with neurologic complications; *open square*, preterm infants without neurologic complications; *solid triangle*, term infants with neurologic complications; *open triangle*, term infants without neurologic complications. (Courtesy of van den Berg PP, Nelen WLDM, Jongsma HW, et al: Neonatal complications in newborns with an umbilical artery pH < 7.00. *Am J Obstet Gynecol* 175:1152–1157, 1996.)

neonate, and umbilical artery pH values ranged between 6.90 and 7.00. Of 24 neonates in the group with acidosis with a 1-minute Apgar score of 3 or less, 15 had neurologic complications (Fig 2). In 26 neonates with a 5-minute Apgar of less than 7, 13 had neurologic complications (Fig 3). All neonates with umbilical artery pH values less than 6.80 were born severely depressed. In neonates with an umbilical artery pH value greater than 6.80, there was no relationship between pH and 1- or 5-minute Apgar scores. In the group with acidosis, 25% of neonates were born in good condition. There were no 1-minute Apgar scores of 3 or less in the group without acidosis.

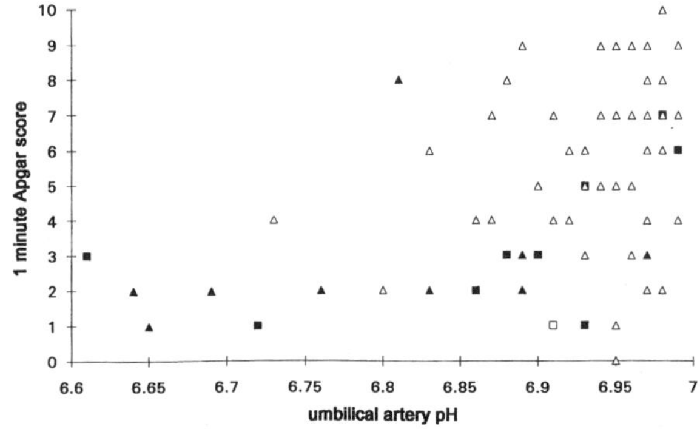

FIGURE 2.—Umbilical artery pH vs. 1-minute Apgar score with subdivision for gestational age and neurologic dysfunction. *Solid square*, preterm infants with neurologic complications; *open square*, preterm infants without neurologic complications; *solid triangle*, term infants with neurologic complications; *open triangle*, term infants without neurologic complications. (Courtesy of van den Berg PP, Nelen WLDM, Jongsma HW, et al: Neonatal complications in newborns with an umbilical artery pH < 7.00. *Am J Obstet Gynecol* 175:1152–1157, 1996.)

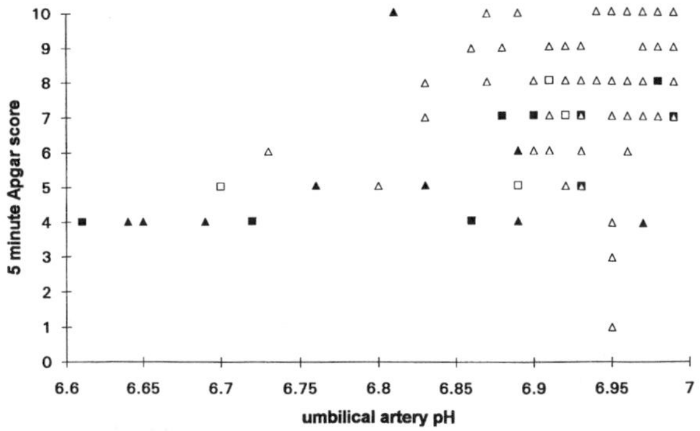

FIGURE 3.—Umbilical artery pH vs. 5-minute Apgar score with subdivision for gestational age and neurologic dysfunction. *Solid square*, preterm infants with neurologic complications; *open square*, preterm infants without neurologic complications; *solid triangle*, term infants with neurologic complications; *open triangle*, term infants without neurologic complications. (Courtesy of van den Berg PP, Nelen WLDM, Jongsma HW, et al: Neonatal complications in newborns with an umbilical artery pH < 7.00. *Am J Obstet Gynecol* 175:1152–1157, 1996.)

Conclusion.—Neonates with umbilical artery pH values of less than 7.00 had significantly more need for resuscitation and intubation and a significantly greater incidence of respiratory, gastrointestinal, cardiovascular, and neurologic complications compared with neonates with umbilical artery pH values of greater than 7.24. These findings are in concordance with other reports.

▶ This article is important for neonatologists and pediatricians because it further clarifies the importance of the umbilical artery pH as well as the nature of the acidosis as they relate to the immediate outcome of the newborn. One of the conclusions is that the determination of the umbilical artery pH should be performed in every newborn because using only Apgar scores would overestimate the role of acidemia as a causative factor for neonatal morbidity. The article points out that, of the newborns with acidosis, 87.5% had mixed acidosis, 2.5% had respiratory acidosis, and 10% had metabolic acidosis (see Fig 1). Interestingly, all of the neurologic complications were observed in the group with mixed acidosis, and none were observed in the acidosis group alone. All neonates whose umbilical artery pH was less than 6.80 were born severely depressed. However, 27% of the neonates born with a pH between 6.80 and 7.00 had no neonatal problems. The authors suggest that host factors may be important in determining whether a particular infant is compromised, which is just another way of saying that we cannot predict individual outcomes with any medical confidence. Our legal colleagues often require less confidence.

D.K. Stevenson, M.D

Epidural Analgesia for Labour and Delivery: Fentanyl or Sufentanil?
Cohen S, Amar D, Pantuck CB, et al (Mem Sloan-Kettering Cancer Ctr, New York)
Can J Anaesth 43:341–346, 1996 5–12

Objective.—Both epidurally infused fentanyl and sufentanil, combined with other drugs, provide satisfactory analgesia during labor and delivery, although patients experience lower-extremity sensory loss. Fentanyl and sufentanil were compared with regard to effectiveness of analgesia during labor and delivery, neonatal outcome, and opioid accumulation in the blood of the mother and the neonate.

Methods.—In a double-blind, randomized study, 100 women received either 2 µg/mL of fentanyl (n = 50, group I) or 2 µg/mL of sufentanil (n = 50, group II) in combination with bupivacaine 0.015% and epinephrine 2 µg/mL. Patients assessed pain intensity on a 0-to-10 (no pain to worst pain) scale, satisfaction on a 0-to-10 (no satisfaction to best satisfaction) scale, and side effects (pruritus, sedation, nausea, and vomiting) on a 1-to-3 (mild to severe) scale every hour. Infusion rates were adjusted as needed. Plasma opioid concentrations were obtained from selected patients in each group at the end of the infusions.

Results.—Patients in group I reported significantly higher pain scores in both the first and second stages of labor than did patients in group II. Additional bupivacaine was requested by significantly more patients in group I (42%) than in group II (6%). Group I required significantly more bupivacaine than did group II. There was no difference between groups with respect to lower sensory levels, time from discontinuation of infusion to delivery, durations of first and second stages of labor, or incidence of side effects. Maternal and umbilical vein plasma concentrations of fentanyl were 0.28 and 0.18 µg/mL and those of sufentanil were 0.11 and 0.09 µg/mL, respectively. Neonatal outcomes were uneventful.

Conclusions.—Patients receiving fentanyl reported less pain and required less bupivacaine rescue. There were no serious maternal or fetal side effects.

▶ The ability to relieve pain effectively during labor and delivery without harming the mother or the fetus continues to improve. Epidural anesthesia, in many institutions, has become the standard of care. Epidurals continue to be refined, and this manuscript reports the first double-blind study comparing the analgesic effects of epidural fentanyl and sufentanil combined with very low dose bupivacaine and epinephrine. Pain scores and patient satisfaction were greater with the sufentanil, with side effects including pruritus, sedation, and urinary retention noted in most patients and an overall cesarean delivery rate of 24%. It is somewhat surprising that patient satisfaction should be that great despite all these side effects. I would reiterate the plea of my now-retired colleague, Marshall Klaus, that patients should be informed that with epidural anesthesia, the length of labor is prolonged, there are more operative deliveries, and maternal temperature may be elevated.[1, 2]

However, apparently the ecstasy of pain relief outweighs the agony of these side effects.

There is nothing more vulnerable than entrenched success.—George Romney.

A.A. Fanaroff, M.B.B.Ch.

References

1. Klaus M: 1996 YEAR BOOK OF NEONATAL AND PERINATAL MEDICINE, pp 114–115.
2. 1995 YEAR BOOK OF NEONATAL AND PERINATAL MEDICINE, p 116.

Group B *Streptococcus* and Preterm Premature Rupture of Membranes: A Randomized, Double-blind Clinical Trial of Antepartum Ampicillin

Grable IA, Garcia PM, Perry D, et al (Northwestern Univ, Chicago; Northwestern Mem Hosp, Chicago)
Am J Obstet Gynecol 175:1036–1042, 1996 5–13

Introduction.—Several reports have shown that the use of antibiotics prolongs the latency period in patients with preterm premature rupture of membranes. It is not known whether patients colonized with group B streptococcus experience this benefit. The first prospective, double-blind, placebo-controlled investigation was undertaken to determine whether ampicillin prolongs the latency period after preterm premature rupture of membranes in patients colonized with group B Streptococcus.

Methods.—Sixty patients with preterm premature rupture of membranes at 35 or more weeks' gestation underwent cervical, vaginal, and perianal cultures for group B streptococcus. Participants were randomly assigned to receive either ampicillin or placebo intravenously for 24 hours, then oral ampicillin until hospital discharge or delivery. No patients received tocolytic medications.

Results.—Fifteen of 60 patients with preterm premature rupture of membranes had cultures positive for group B streptococcus (53% cervical, 73% vaginal, and 100% perianal). Of the 15 patients with positive cultures, 8 received ampicillin and 7 received placebo. Patients with positive cultures who received ampicillin were significantly more likely to remain undelivered 48 hours after membrane rupture than were patients who received placebo. There was a similar trend for patients with negative cultures who received ampicillin, compared with patients who received placebo, but the difference was nonsignificant. The treatment effect of ampicillin was lost after 7 days for patients with both positive and negative cultures. There was no difference between patients treated with ampicillin or placebo who had either positive or negative cultures in incidence of cesarean section, chorioamnionitis, postpartum endometritis, or neonatal infectious morbidity.

Conclusion.—The percentage of patients undelivered at 48 hours with group B streptococcus was significantly higher in patients treated with ampicillin than in patients who received placebo. It may be that antepartum antibiotic therapy offers a window of opportunity for maternal treatment with corticosteroids to reduce the risk of neonatal mortality among these preterm gestations.

► Contemporary obstetric practice is obsessed with a desire to totally eradicate group B streptococcal (GBS) disease.[1] As a vaccine, the ideal methodology, languishes on the drawing boards, and postpartum therapy is ineffective, intrapartum prophylaxis has almost by default become the strategy of choice. Benitz, in an invited contribution,[2] has summarized the various permutations to be considered in determining cost-effectiveness for reducing GBS infection, strategies, and what might be anticipated. The model addresses the key components, including the identification of infants at risk, the determination of relative risk and prevalence for each identified risk factor, the assessment of possible effectiveness of each intervention, the anticipation of costs, and the evaluation of how risk ascertainment and intervention strategies could be combined to optimize the benefits and costs of an integrated prevention program.

Grable and colleagues wished to determine whether ampicillin would prolong the latency period after preterm premature rupture of membranes in patients colonized with group B streptococcus. In a small series, they document that more GBS-positive women who receive ampicillin remain undelivered 48 hours after preterm rupture of membranes than the untreated controls. This enhances the window of opportunity for antepartum steroid administration to reduce neonatal mortality and morbidity.

The rationale for antibiotic therapy in preterm labor is sound. Infection generates prostaglandins, which, in turn, stimulate the release of cytokines such as tumor necrosis factor and interleukins 1 and 6, capable of inducing preterm labor. Cox[3] attempted to prevent preterm birth through the administration of antimicrobial therapy. The study was conducted in Dallas between 1989 and 1992, when women in preterm labor, between 24 and 34 weeks' gestation, received neither tocolytics nor antenatal steroids. The power analysis was based on the assumption that 30% of women treated with antimicrobials would deliver at term. Indeed, 40% of the placebo group achieved this goal. Amniocentesis, under US guidance, was done on the first 18 women to ascertain bacterial colonization of the amniotic fluid, but it was considered too invasive and high risk and was discontinued when a cesarean section for fetal distress was prompted by the amniocentesis. Cox concluded that antimicrobial therapy given to women in preterm labor was ineffective in the prevention of preterm birth. There is a relationship between infection and preterm labor; however, by the time labor starts, it is too late to start antibiotic therapy. To add insult to injury, 68% of the women randomized to antimicrobial therapy had symptomatic *Candida* vulvovaginitis. Hence, whereas antimicrobials effectively prolonged the latent period when membranes ruptured early in women colonized with GBS, they were ineffective once labor commenced. See also Abstract 14–2.

Play for more than you can afford to lose, and you will learn the game.—Winston Churchill.

A.A. Fanaroff, M.B.B.Ch.

References

1. Schuchat A, Whitney C, Zangwill K: Prevention of perinatal group B streptococcal disease: A public perspective. *MMWR Morb Mortal Wkly Rep* 45:1–24, 1996.
2. Benitz W, Druzin M, Gould J: Cost effective strategy for reducing neonatal GBS infection.
3. Cox SM, Bohman VR, Sherman ML, et al.: Randomized investigation of antimicrobials for the prevention of preterm birth. *Am J Obstet Gynecol* 174:206–210, 1996.

Amniotic Fluid Meconium: A Fetal Environmental Hazard

Ramin KD, Leveno KJ, Kelly MA, et al (Univ of Texas, Dallas)

Obstet Gynecol 87:181–184, 1996 5–14

Introduction.—Meconium passage was regarded as a sign of fetal death or impending death in obstetric texts from the 17th to 19th centuries. From early in this century, it has been linked to fetal hypoxia. In reality, most fetuses exposed to meconium are born in good condition. Umbilical artery blood gases were measured in 7,816 term pregnancies to determine

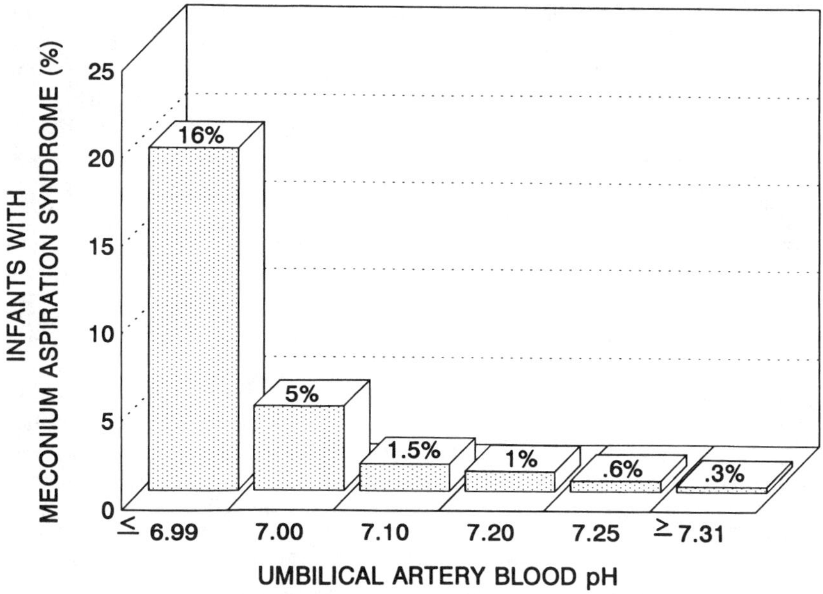

FIGURE 1.—Percentage of infants who aspirated meconium from their amniotic fluid in relation to their umbilical blood pH at birth. (Mantel-Haenszel χ^2 analysis, $P < 0.001$). (Reprinted with permission from American College of Obstetricians and Gynecologists, from Ramin KD, Leveno KJ, Kelly MA, et al: Amniotic fluid meconium: A fetal environmental hazard. *Obstet Gynecol* 87:181–184, 1996.)

TABLE 2.—Condition of Newborns at Delivery and Subsequent Neonatal Morbidity

Outcome	Infants with meconium in the AF and no MAS (*N* = 7747)	Infants with meconium in the AF and MAS (*N* = 69)	*P**
Apgar scores			
≤3 at 1 min	97 (1.3%)	12 (17%)	<.001
≤3 at 5 min	10 (0.1%)	3 (4%)	<.002
Ventilation at birth†	715 (9%)	29 (42%)	<.001
Seizure(s) first 24 h	11 (0.1%)	5 (7%)	<.001
Deaths	4 (0.05%)	4 (6%)	<.001

*χ^2 analysis and Fisher exact test (two-tailed), as indicated.
†Assisted with ambu bag.
Abbreviations: AF, amniotic fluid; *MAS*, meconium aspiration syndrome.
(Reprinted with permission from American College of Obstetricians and Gynecologists, from Ramin KD, Leveno KJ, Kelly MA: Amniotic fluid meconium: A fetal environmental hazard. *Obstet Gynecol* 87:181–184, 1996.)

whether meconium exposure was associated with superimposed fetal acute acidemia.

Methods.—Amniotomy was performed to assess the amniotic fluid (AF) for meconium when the fetal head was considered safely in the pelvis and the cervix was sufficiently dilated. Intrapartum and neonatal outcomes were correlated between infants with and without meconium aspiration syndrome.

Results.—Of 59,216 women delivered during the 4-year investigation, 8,136 (14%) had meconium-stained AF. Infants with pH values less than 7.20 were significantly more likely to have meconium aspiration syndrome than infants with pH values about 7.20 (Fig 1). Of 69 infants who had meconium aspiration syndrome, 31 (45%) were acidemic at birth. Analysis of fetal acidemia suggested that the fetal compromise associated with meconium aspiration was an acute rather than chronic event because most acidemic fetuses had abnormally increased partial pressure of carbon dioxide rather than pure metabolic acidemia that could be expected with fetal events leading to the immediate circumstances of birth. There was a significant correlation between infants with meconium aspiration and very low Apgar scores, need for assisted ventilation in the delivery room, neonatal seizures, and death (Table 2).

Conclusion.—The passage of fetal gastrointestinal contents often occurs in conjunction with normal physiologic processes. The meconium becomes a hazard when fetal acidemia supervenes. Prevention of fetal acidemia in the presence of AF meconium is an important obstetric goal. Findings suggest that fetal acidemia occurs acutely and is unpredictable and may be unpreventable.

▶ The YEAR BOOK OF NEONATAL AND PERINATAL MEDICINE should not be permitted to go to press without a few items dealing with meconium and the havoc it may wreak on the lungs. Debates about meconium always generate a high degree of enthusiasm and are invariably punctuated by strong personal opinions, which may or may not be swayed by the prevailing evidence. Meconium analysis gives a profile of the drug or tobacco utilization by the mother and passage of meconium in combination with evidence of fetal jeopardy including fetal heart rate abnormalities (decelerations or tachycardia) and fetal acidosis, identifies the fetus at risk for meconium aspiration syndrome (MAS). Cesarean section or forceps to expedite delivery are additional hazards for MAS.

The title of this review is catchy, but it probably should have concluded with a question mark. The concept of meconium as a fetal environmental hazard has some validity. Meconium in the amniotic fluid does not necessarily mean fetal compromise but could be a maturational phenomenon. The incidence of meconium in amniotic fluid increases with advancing age beyond 36 weeks' gestation. Ramin et al. hypothesized that fetal hypercarbia, in the presence of meconium, stimulates fetal gasping and aspiration of meconium into the alveoli. Parenchymal injury is induced by the combination of hypoxia, acidemia, and meconium. The association between meconium aspiration and fetal acidosis reached statistical significance ($P < 0.001$), but only accounted for half the infants with MAS. What about the other half? A valid hypothesis can't leave out half the subjects at risk. The authors are unable to come up with an "exclusive explanation."

The notion that meconium in and of itself is a minor obstetric hazard is plausible. Meconium complicates 12% to 22% of human labors, with approximately 1 per 1,000 linked to infant mortality.[1, 2] However, as Katz and Bowes[2] vividly commented, MAS is a murky subject with prognostic uncertainty. Ramin and associates, in reviewing an enormous database (almost 8,000 pregnancies with meconium in the amniotic fluid), note significant morbidity including low Apgar scores, seizures, need for mechanical ventilation, and even deaths in the infants with meconium in the amniotic fluid and MAS. We will have to delve deeper into this murky topic to find a unifying explanation for MAS. We conclude that meconium-stained amniotic fluid (MSAF) is common, but MAS is not. Fetal compromise in the face of MSAF may result in MAS; and intrapartum treatment is the key to preventing MAS. Also see Reference 3.

Risk is essential. There is no growth or inspiration in staying within what is safe and comfortable. Once you find out what is best, why not try something else?—Alex Noble.

A.A. Fanaroff, M.B.B.Ch.

References

1. Nathan L, Leveno KJ, Carmody TJ, et al: Meconium: A 1990's perspective on an old obstetric hazard. *Obstet Gynecol* 83:329–332, 1994.
2. Katz VL, Bowes WA: Meconium aspiration syndrome: Reflections on a murky subject. *Am J Obstet Gynecol* 166:171–183, 1992.
3. 1994 Year Book of Neonatal and Perinatal Medicine, pp 123–125.

6 Infectious Diseases and Developmental Immunology

The Effect of Timing of Single-dose Transplacental Ampicillin-Sulbactam Therapy for Prevention of Neonatal Group B Streptococcal Colonization and Bacteremia in a Rabbit Model

McDuffie RS Jr, Blanton SJ, Charland SL, et al (Univ of Colorado, Denver; St Joseph Hosp, Denver)

Am J Obstet Gynecol 175:406–410, 1996 6–1

Introduction.—Intrapartum administration of antibiotics can prevent early-onset neonatal group B streptococcal sepsis, but the precise time before delivery for optimal results has not been determined. The effect of maternal administration of ampicillin-sulbactam on neonatal colonization and bacteremia was evaluated in a rabbit model.

Methods.—Timed-pregnancy New Zealand White rabbits with a 31-day gestation were used in the study. Before the induction of labor with oxytocin, some rabbits received no therapy and others were given ampicillin-sulbactam (50 mg/kg as a single IM dose) 2–8 hours before delivery. The oropharynx of each pup was inoculated after delivery with 10^9 colony-forming units of type Ia group B streptococcus. Cultures were taken from the oropharynx and anorectum of the pups daily and from the heart at death or after 96 hours. Both mothers and pups had ampicillin-sulbactam concentrations measured at delivery.

Results.—Twenty-seven animals were studied, including 14 randomly assigned to receive ampicillin-sulbactam. Whereas all untreated pups had oropharyngeal colonization at 24 hours, those treated with antibiotic were significantly less likely to have positive cultures at 24 (47% vs. 100%) and 48 (68% vs. 91%) hours after birth. Rates of oropharyngeal colonization were similar for treated and untreated pups at 72 and 96 hours. Treated pups were significantly less likely to have positive anorectal cultures and to have positive heart cultures at 48 and 72 hours. The survival rate at 48 hours was 89% for treated pups and 62% for untreated pups. Ampicillin concentrations were highest in both mothers and pups at 3–5 hours after injection. There was a significant polynomial relation between the percentage of pups colonized orally at 24 hours and the length of time from antibiotic injection.

Conclusions.—A single IM dose of ampicillin-sulbactam before delivery significantly decreased neonatal colonization and bacteremia in newborn rabbits inoculated with type Ia group B streptococcus. There was a significant inverse relation between neonatal ampicillin concentrations at delivery and oropharyngeal colonization at 24 hours. The effect of the antibiotic was maximal at 3–5 hours after injection.

► Efforts to eradicate neonatal group B streptococcal disease are in full swing. The recommendations of the Centers for Disease Control and Prevention, American College of Obstetricians, and American Academy of Pediatrics have been widely dispersed and implemented (see Featured Topic in this issue). There remain several contentious issues, one of which is partially addressed in this report by McDuffie and colleagues. This is the importance of the timing of the administration of the antibiotics. Is there something truly significant about the 4-hour period that was chosen, because it represents the timing of the second dose of antibiotics and, hence, is equated with appropriate or complete intrapartum treatment? The results unequivocally demonstrated that the intrapartum antibiotics diminished postnatal positive oropharyngeal cultures as well as blood cultures in the rabbit pups, who then also were more likely to survive. Treatment was effective at least 2 hours before delivery, but appeared to be maximal 3–5 hours after injection. There also was an inverse relation between the rate of colonization and serum ampicillin levels. There is a plea from the authors to interpret the data with caution because the timing of colonization and route of administration of the antibiotics are different in humans. It is tempting, however, to suggest that these data do support the Centers for Disease Control and Prevention recommendations.

Anything a man can perceive and conceive, if his heart can believe, he will achieve.—Unknown

A.A. Fanaroff, M.B.B.Ch.

Nosocomial Infections Among Neonates in High-risk Nurseries in the United States

Gaynes RP, and the National Nosocomial Infections Surveillance System (Ctrs for Disease Control and Prevention, Atlanta, Ga)

Pediatrics 98:357–361, 1996 6–2

Background.—Nosocomial infections are responsible for considerable morbidity and mortality among newborns, particularly in the neonatal ICU setting. There have been few epidemiologic studies of nosocomial infections among newborns. Such a study was performed in newborns treated in level III high-risk nurseries (HRNs).

Methods.—The study included data from 99 HRNs participating in the National Nosocomial Infections Surveillance System of the Centers for Disease Control and Prevention. All of the nurseries used standard surveillance protocols and nosocomial infection site definitions. The analysis included data on 13,179 nosocomial infections from 1986 to 1994.

Findings.—In all birth weight categories, the most common site of nosocomial infection was the bloodstream. This was followed by nosocomial pneumonia, then by infections of the gastrointestinal tract and the eye, ear, nose, and throat. Coagulase-negative streptococci, *Staphylococcus aureus*, enterococci, *Enterobacter* species, and *Escherichia coli* were the most common causative organisms. Viruses—usually rotaviruses—were the most common pathogens in gastrointestinal tract infections. Forty-six percent of maternally acquired bloodstream infections involved group B streptococci. Of the non–maternally acquired bloodstream infections, 58% involved coagulase-negative streptococci, mainly associated with umbilical or central venous catheters.

Conclusions.—Efforts to prevent nosocomial infections in the HRN setting should emphasize bloodstream infections, which are the most common type of nosocomial infections in all birth weight groups. The causative organisms differ for maternally acquired versus non–maternally acquired bloodstream infections. This information may help in preventing group B streptococcal infections outside the HRN. Intravenous catheters are a major source of nosocomial bloodstream infection in the HRN.

▶ Nosocomial infections are a subject near and dear to me. I have spent a considerable part of my career either trying to prevent them or observing their dire consequences. Gaynes and colleagues have gathered a mother lode of information concerning nosocomial infections, but constraints of space have permitted them to publish literally only the tip of the iceberg. They have gathered data diligently from the many participating HRNs and confirmed that bloodstream infections are the most prevalent form of nosocomial infection. Coagulase-negative staphylococci continue to lead the assault on the bloodstream. Nosocomial infections are attributed to the duration of hospitalization and the use of devices, including catheters and ventilators. This is perhaps an oversimplification because the duration of hospitalization is prolonged in low–birth weight infants in whom sepsis develops by an average of almost 3 weeks.[1, 2] The economic consequences of this are surely the focus of many managers of managed care plans.

In my opinion, the manuscript and message contained therein would have been stronger if the early onset infections had been excluded. Early onset infections are relatively uncommon and have a different etiology and pathogenesis. Group B streptococci remain the dominant cause of early onset infections. The combined approach, based on risk identification and intrapartum antimicrobial therapy as recommended by the Centers for Disease Control and Prevention, American College of Obstetricians, and American Academy of Pediatrics, has been implemented broadly in the United States (see this issue's Featured Topic).

The bean counters shortly will inform us whether this aproach has been successful, or they will announce that group B streptococcal disease has been reduced drastically only to be replaced by some other pathogen that is eagerly waiting in the wings.

The manuscript was referenced sparsely, so, for the curious reader (and I know there are many of you), some light reading is appended on the topic. I also am intrigued by the inclusion of all the cases of pneumonia. The diagnosis of pneumonia is challenging, to say the least. Does the presence of a pathogenic organism in the repiratory tract of an infant with an abnormal radiograph constitute pneumonia or merely colonization? That soapbox will be ascended on another occasion.

A.A. Fanaroff, M.B.B.Ch.

References

1. Stoll BJ Gordon T, Korones S, et al: Early-onset sepsis in very low birthweight neonates: A report from the NICHD Neonatal Research Network. *J Pediatr* 129:72–80, 1996.
2. Fanaroff AA, Korones S, Wright LL, et al: A controlled trial of intravenous immune globulin to reduce nosocomial infections in very low birth weight infants. *N Engl J Med* 330:1107–1113, 1994.

Granulocyte Colony-stimulating Factor as a Marker for Bacterial Infection in Neonates

Kennon C, Overturf G, Bessman S, et al (Univ of New Mexico, Albuquerque)
J Pediatr 128:765–769, 1996 6–3

Background.—Bacterial infections in neonates cause significant morbidity and death, especially among preterm infants. The value of granulocyte colony-stimulating factor (G-CSF) as an early marker of bacterial or fungal infection in neonates was determined.

Methods.—One hundred fifty-six infants with gestational ages ranging from 24 to 43 weeks underwent a total of 176 evaluations for sepsis. Half of the patients were less than 35 weeks' gestational age. Three groups of infants were formed: group 1 had a positive bacterial or fungal blood culture result; group 2, negative blood culture result but evidence of clinical sepsis; and group 3, negative blood culture result and no or weak evidence of sepsis.

Findings.—Group 1 and 2 infants had significantly higher mean G-CSF levels than group 3 infants. Mean G-CSF levels were 2,278 pg/mL in group 1, 1,873 pg/mL in group 2, and 280 pg/mL in group 3. Setting the cutoff level at 200 pg/mL, the test had a sensitivity of 95%, specificity of 73%, positive predictive value of 40%, and negative predictive value of 99% (see Table).

Conclusions.—Measurement of G-CSF levels can be used to accurately identify infants with sepsis of any gestational age. In this series, markedly higher mean G-CSF levels were found in infants with a positive blood

TABLE.—Diagnostic Values: Comparison of Complete Blood Cell Count With Granulocyte Colony-stimulating Factor

	Complete blood cell count				
	Total PMN count ↑ ↓ * (%)	I/T ratio >0.20 (%)	Total WBC ↑ ↓ † (%)	Thrombo-cytopenia (<150,000) (%)	G-CSF (>200 pg/ml) (%)
Sensitivity	85	15	25	50	95
Specificity	40	99	87	91	73
PPV	22	60	28	53	40
NPV	93	86	86	90	99

*Greater than 2 SD from normal values, as defined by reference ranges of Monroe, et al. (*J Pediatr* 95:89, 1976.)

†Less than 5,000 or greater than 25,000.

Abbreviations: PMN, polymorphonuclear neutrophil; *I/T,* immature/total neutrophil; *WBC,* white blood cell count; *PPV,* positive predictive value; *NPV,* negative predictive value; *G-CSF,* granulocyte colony-stimulating factor.

(Courtesy of Kennon C, Overturf G, Bessman S, et al: Granulocyte colony-stimulating factor as a marker for bacterial infection in neonates. *J Pediatr* 128:765–769, 1996.)

culture result or in whom infection was strongly suspected compared with infants with minimal evidence of infection.

▶ The list of "candidate markers" of early sepsis in neonates continues to expand. As if manufactured from the same cookie cutter, they all seem to have the same features. Namely, they are sensitive with impeccable negative predictive qualities, moderate specificity, but only weak positive predictive value. Granulocyte colony-stimulating factor appears to be no exception. Assuming a cutoff level of 200 pg/mL, the sensitivity of the test was 95%, specificity was 73%, positive predictive value was 40%, and negative predictive value was 99%.

All studies on neonatal sepsis are hampered by imprecise definitions. A positive blood culture result is the gold standard for the septic group, but a lot of poetic license is required for the diagnosis of pneumonia—the authors' group 2. It was, therefore, not in the least bit surprising to find the wide spectrum of G-CSF values in this group (10–8,000 pg/mL). If there was more than one sepsis risk factor, and these ranged from apnea requiring mechanical ventilation through pneumatosis and hyperglycemia in addition to abnormal white blood cell indices, the mean G-CSF value was 2,737, indistinguishable from that of septic infants.

The authors ran into problems with group 3—infants with negative blood cultures and no risk factors for sepsis. Why were they cultured in the first place? Also, 2 of those infants had markedly elevated G-CSF levels. The G-CSF levels also correlated with maternal preeclampsia and neutropenia, but in contrast to Gessler,[1] these authors found no correlation between G-CSF and gestational age. The G-CSF was not compared with C-reactive proteins and other cytokines, which might have added useful information.[2] The granulocyte colony-stimulating factor offers some promise in the early detection of neonatal sepsis; however, at this stage, it is far-fetched to believe that it will reduce antibiotic usage and shorten hospital stays.

Hold yourself responsible for a higher standard than anybody expects of you. Never excuse yourself. Never pity yourself. Be a hard taskmaster to yourself and be lenient with everybody else.—Henry Ward Beecher

A.A. Fanaroff, M.B.B.Ch.

References

1. Gessler P, Kirchmann N, Kientsch-Engel, R, et al: Serum concentrations of granulocyte colony-stimulating factor in healthy term and preterm neonates and in those with various diseases including bacterial infections. *Blood* 82:3177–3182, 1993.
2. Pourcyrous M, Bada H, Korones S, et al: Significance of serial C-reactive protein responses in neonatal infections and other disorders. *Pediatrics* 92:431–435, 1993.

Infection With *Ureaplasma urealyticum* and *Mycoplasma hominis* and the Development of Chronic Lung Disease in Preterm Infants

Iles R, Lyon A, Ross P, et al (Simpson Mem Maternity Pavilion, Edinburgh, Scotland; Univ of Edinburgh, Scotland)

Acta Paediatr 85:482–484, 1996 6–4

Objective.—Preterm infants at a single center in Scotland were studied prospectively to examine the prevalence of respiratory tract infection with the genital mycoplasmas and its relation to chronic lung disease (CLD).

Methods.—Infants eligible for the study were born at less than 31 weeks' gestation. Tracheal secretions were obtained at hospital admission, before treatment with exogenous surfactant, and weekly thereafter until extubation. Samples were cultured for *Ureaplasma urealyticum, Mycoplasma hominis,* and all other common bacterial pathogens. Culture-positive and culture-negative groups were compared for the development of CLD, defined as a persisting oxygen requirement at 36 weeks of equivalent gestation.

Results.—Forty infants with a median gestational age of 27 weeks were enrolled in the study. Tracheal secretions from 15 (37%) were culture-positive for a genital mycoplasma: *U. urealyticum* was isolated from 9 infants, *M. hominis* from 2, and both organisms from 4. The organism was isolated from the first sample obtained in 11 cases. The development of CLD was significantly more frequent among infants in the culture-positive group than among those in the culture-negative group (87% vs. 41%). The culture-positive and culture-negative groups did not differ significantly in gestational age, birth weight, use of surfactant, or time on ventilator.

Discussion.—Colonization of the female lower genital tract with genital mycoplasmas may occur in up to 70% of pregnancies, and the prevalence of colonization of newborns with these organisms is reported to range from 13% to 47%. Infants born before 30 weeks' gestation are at risk for CLD, and these infants also have a high incidence of colonization of the lower respiratory tract with a genital mycoplasma. The findings of this study suggest a significant association between urogenital mycoplasmas and CLD. Repeated cultures should be performed because some infants may not have positive results until several weeks after birth.

► The circumstantial evidence linking *U. urealyticum* to CLD continues to mount. These data from Scotland can be added to the numbers from Canada and Italy presented in the 1996 YEAR BOOK OF NEONATAL AND PERINATAL MEDICINE.[1, 2] The trends are the same, with more CLD and longer hospital stays for the infants colonized at birth. Iles and colleagues reported that 30% of infants who eventually were culture-positive were culture-negative at the time of admission. Because there is no convincing evidence that nosocomial infection occurs with *U. urealyticum,* it is probable that the organism already was present at birth, but not identified. Use of the polymerase chain reaction or serology may be a better method than culture to detect *U. urealyticum* and identify such infants.

The total experience with *U. urealyticum* remains small, and until a multicenter trial proves its efficacy, caution is warranted with the use of erythromycin because it may be hazardous to the neonate.[3] As noted in Abstract 14–1, the combination of metronidazole and erythromycin reduced the rate of premature delivery in women with bacterial vaginosis and an increased risk for preterm delivery. The antimicrobials were not effective when there was no bacterial vaginosis; hence, indiscriminate use of these agents is not warranted.

A.A. Fanaroff, M.B.B.Ch.

References

1. Alfa MJ, Embree JE, Degagne P, et al: Transmission of *Ureaplasma urealyticum* from mothers to full and preterm infants. *Pediatr Infect Dis J* 14:341–345, 1995.
2. Panero A, Pacifico L, Rossi N, et al: *Ureaplasma urealyticum* as a cause of pneumonia in preterm infants: Analysis of the white cell response. *Arch Dis Child* 73:F37–F40, 1995.
3. 1994 YEAR BOOK OF NEONATAL AND PERINATAL MEDICINE, p 367.

Invasive Candidiasis in Infants Weighing More Than 2500 Grams at Birth Admitted to a Neonatal Intensive Care Unit

Rabalais GP, Samiec TD, Bryant KK, et al (Univ of Louisville, Ky; Kosair Children's Hosp, Louisville, Ky)

Pediatr Infect Dis J 15:348–352, 1996 6–5

Introduction.—Very low birth weight infants—those weighing less than 1,500 g—are vulnerable to acquiring invasive candidiasis in the neonatal ICU (NICU). However, little is known about the risk of invasive candidiasis among NICU infants with greater birth weights. The incidence and clinical features of invasive candidiasis in infants with birth weights of greater than 2,500 g were analyzed.

Methods and Findings.—An 8-year review was performed to identify infants with birth weights of greater than 2,500 g who were admitted to the NICU and acquired invasive candidiasis sometime during their hospitalization. Seventeen such patients were identified, accounting for 0.6% of all infants with birth weights greater than 2,500 g admitted to the NICU during this time. The mean birth weight was 3,434 g, and the mean age at the onset of infection was 47 days. All these infants had underlying conditions necessitating a prolonged NICU stay; three fourths had serious congenital malformations. The urinary tract was the most common site of infection. Sixteen infants were treated with amphotericin B, alone or in combination with other drugs. In the remaining case, invasive candidiasis was identified only after death. Ten of the infants died in the NICU, and 3 of the deaths were related to candidal infection.

Conclusions.—Invasive candidiasis is an uncommon problem among NICU patients with birth weights of greater than 2,500 g. These infants have serious underlying conditions, especially major congenital malformations.

▶ The following commentary was submitted by Dr. Jill E. Baley, Associated Professor, Pediatrics, Division of Neonatology, Rainbow Babies & Childrens Hospital, Case Western Reserve University, Cleveland, Ohio:

▶ The clinical spectrum of larger, or term, infants admitted to an ICU who acquire invasive candidiasis is a topic that has not been totally ignored in the past, but it certainly has not been examined to any real extent recently. Fortunately, because the mortality rate is so high (59% of these infants died, with nearly 20% of the deaths being *Candida*-related), this entity is not seen often in this population (0.6% of the admissions).

There are many commonalities among very low birth weight infants and larger birth weight infants in whom candidiasis develops: it is the disease of infants who have prolonged stays in ICUs and who have endured many days of antibiotic therapy, endotracheal intubation, and parenteral nutrition. In both cases, most infections are caused by *Candida albicans,* and fewer are caused by *Candida parapsilosis, Candida glabrata,* or other species. Infants who are infected often have multiple sites of infection, and infection is common in the urinary tract and bloodstream. The 2 outstanding differences between disseminated disease among infants born weighing more than 2,500 g and very low birth weight infants is that the larger birth weight group is almost exclusively comprised of infants with major congenital malformations. These malformations are very likely related to the extremely high mortality rate.

Of note also is the near absence of infants with meconium aspiration syndrome. These infants represented a large proportion of the term infants in whom invasive candidiasis developed historically, when systemic corticosteroids were used as "therapy" for the aspiration. Also of note is the decreased frequency among these infants, compared with infants in the past, of conditions specifically requiring abdominal surgery. Regardless of the underlying reason for a prolonged stay in an ICU, it is clear that this stay creates the conditions associated with the development of invasive disease and significantly worsens the chances of long-term survival.

J.E. Baley, M.D.

Fetal Pathology in Intrauterine Death Due to Parvovirus B19 Infection

Wright C, Hinchliffe SA, Taylor C (Royal Victoria Infirmary, Newcastle upon Tyne, England)

Br J Obstet Gynaecol 103:133–136, 1996 6–6

Objective.—Fetuses who die in utero of infection with parvovirus B19 are found to be hydropic on autopsy. The clinical, sonographic, serologic, pathologic, and immunohistochemical features of tissue from fetuses who died of such infection were reviewed, and the value of hydrops as a marker for infection was evaluated.

Methods.—Between January 1993 and June 1994, 10 cases of parvovirus infection were identified prospectively in 270 cases of intrauterine fetal death. An additional case of parvovirus infection was discovered retrospectively by immunohistochemical staining using R92F6 antibody.

Results.—The gestational age of the fetuses ranged from 11 to 26 weeks. In 3 fetuses, hydrops was seen at autopsy and on antenatal US. In 2 fetuses, findings included mild nuchal edema in 1 and pleural effusions and ascites in 1. No edema or hydrops was observed in 4 fetuses. One fetus was not assessable. Autopsies on 66 fetuses between 10 and 24 weeks' gestational age revealed 8 with parvovirus infection.

Conclusion.—Hydrops was not a common characteristic of this group of second-trimester fetuses who died of parvovirus infection. Possibly, hydrops develops over time and does not appear until about 18 weeks' gestation. Therefore, parvovirus infection should be considered in all cases of intrauterine death. Immunohistochemical screening may identify some cases of parvovirus infection that were not apparent at autopsy.

► In recent years, parvovirus has received serious consideration in the differential diagnosis of the nonimmune hydropic fetus. Before this report, hydrops was an invariable finding in the fetus, but the search for the parvovirus often was prompted by the presence of hydrops, whereas the current series was unique in that parvovirus was searched for in all the fetal deaths in a region. The authors indicate that hydrops is not an invariable finding; parvovirus was a relatively common cause of midtrimester death; hence, the parvovirus should be contemplated in any case of intrauterine fetal death. The number of early deaths in this series (around 12 weeks) may account for the absence of hydrops. In these cases, the virus was detected easily in the blood cells. Also, the hydrops may resolve in utero, resulting in the birth of an infant with anemia and cardiomyopathy.

Well-recognized features of parvovirus infection in the fetus include hydrops, cardiac dilatation, accumulation of fat in the adrenal cortex, excess hepatic iron deposition, inclusions in the nuclei of the erythroid precursor cells, and increased weight and bulk of the placenta. Clinical manifestations of parvovirus include erythema infectiosum (fifth disease), arthropathy, aplastic crises in susceptible individuals with an underlying hemolytic disorder, and fetal death. The neonatal community should be alerted to epidemics of parvovirus in the area, and blood should be evaluated for parvovirus from any severely anemic infants for whom no other ready explanation is available. The combination of DNA in situ hybridization, DNA amplification by polymerase chain reaction, and the relatively simple immunochemistry should ensure verification of any cases of parvovirus infection.

A.A. Fanaroff, M.B.B.Ch.

Administration of Oral Acyclovir Suppressive Therapy After Neonatal Herpes Simplex Virus Disease Limited to the Skin, Eyes and Mouth: Results of a Phase I/II Trial

Kimberlin D, and the National Institute of Allergy and Infectious Diseases Collaborative Antiviral Study Group (Univ of Alabama, Birmingham; et al)
Pediatr Infect Dis J 15:247–254, 1996 6–7

Objective.—In the newborn, herpes simplex virus (HSV) infection limited to the skin, eyes, and mouth (SEM) can lead to neurologic deficits. The neurologic impairment is directly related to the frequency of cutaneous HSV recurrences. Oral acyclovir therapy was evaluated for its ability to suppress cutaneous recurrence of HSV-2 SEM disease in newborns.

Methods.—The study included 26 infants aged 1 month or less who had virologically confirmed HSV-2 SEM infection. All infants had normal results of CSF tests and neuroradiographic imaging studies. Infants with HSV-1 infection were excluded. The infants received suppressive oral acyclovir therapy, 300 mg/m^2/dose, administered 3 times per day in 21 infants and 2 times per day in 5 infants for 6 months. The patients were followed up by clinical examination and laboratory studies through 6 months of treatment and yearly for 4 years thereafter. Efficacy analysis included 18 infants with SEM disease only.

Results.—Neutropenia of less than 1,000 cells/mm^3 developed in 46% of infants during acyclovir therapy. Eighty-one percent of infants treated 3 times a day remained free of recurrent skin lesions. When recurrences did occur, they were often associated with medication noncompliance. (For comparison, a previous study found that 54% remained free of cutaneous recurrences without treatment.) One patient had HSV DNA detected in the CSF during a cutaneous recurrence. In another patient, recurrence was associated with the development of an acyclovir-resistant HSV isolate. Cutaneous recurrence developed in the 6 months after the end of acyclovir therapy in 44% of patients. All patients who were available for 1-year evaluation were developing normally.

Pharmacokinetic evaluation showed that the mean peak acyclovir concentration with thrice-daily dosing was 1.95 µg/mL, with a mean trough concentration of 1.09 µg/mL. The plasma acyclovir concentration was not obviously related to the presence of neutropenia.

Conclusion.—In infants with HSV-2 SEM infection, oral acyclovir therapy can prevent cutaneous recurrences. Treatment may have to be given 3 times daily, as opposed to 2 times daily, to suppress cutaneous recurrences. Prolonged acyclovir therapy causes transient neutropenia in about half of infants treated. Its effects on neurologic outcome in infants with HSV-2 SEM infection remain to be determined.

▶ Kimberlin and members of the National Institute of Allergy and Infectious Diseases Collaborative Antiviral Study Group have published another in a series of observations dealing with neonatal HSV disease. Although HSV disease that is limited to the skin, eyes, and mouth is the least severe of the 3 forms of neonatal HSV infection, SEM disease can result in neurologic impairment including spasticity, microcephaly, and retinitis. Of the 2 types of HSV disease (HSV-1 and HSV-2), only HSV-2 correlates with the development of neurologic sequelae in infants with SEM disease and, therefore, only infants infected with HSV-2 were included in this study. Although these infants respond to treatment with acyclovir, if treatment is discontinued, recurrence of skin lesions is frequent, and the frequency of these recurrences is directly related to the risk of the development of adverse neurologic sequelae.

These problems are the source of the questions addressed by this study. It is not known how long one should continue to treat these infants with acyclovir, nor has the optimum dosage regimen been determined. Previous studies have shown, however, that normal neurologic outcome is ensured if fewer than 3 cutaneous recurrences occur within the first 6 months of life. It is reassuring, therefore, that when oral acyclovir (300mg/m^2 per dose) was given 3 times per day, it eliminated recurrence of the skin lesions entirely in 81% of infants, and none had 3 or more recurrences. Thirteen of the 18 infants studied were available for evaluation at age 1 year, and all were developing normally. All of these infants were of at least 34 weeks' gestation and weighed at least 2,000 g. Whether oral acyciovir suppressive therapy is as effective in more premature neonates is unknown.

Of particular interest to neonatologists is the observation that almost one third of these neonates had signs of HSV infection *within the first 24 hours of life*, indicating that the infection was congenital rather than infection acquired through the birth canal. In fact, of the 18 infants in this study with SEM disease, signs of infection were present less than 24 hours after birth in 5, between 1 and 5 days after birth in 5, and more than 5 days after birth in 7 (in 1 the timing was unknown). Thus, congenital HSV infection is not as rare as previously reported. The authors refer to some of their recent studies (as yet unpublished) that suggest a similar trend toward an increased number of presumed congenital HSV infections.

In almost half of the treated infants, significant neutropenia developed (absolute neutrophil counts less than 1,000/mm^3), but only 1 infant had a potential complication from this neutropenia—an otitis media when the absolute neutrophil count was less than 500 cells/mm^3. Our understanding of the natural history, risk of perinatal transmission, and management of neonatal HSV disease continues to evolve.

M.J. Maisels, M.B.B.Ch.

Reduced Congenital Cytomegalovirus (CMV) Infection After Maternal Immunization With a Guinea Pig CMV Glycoprotein Before Gestational Primary CMV Infection in the Guinea Pig Model

Harrison CJ, Britt WJ, Chapman NM, et al (Creighton Univ, Omaha, Neb; Univ of Nebraska, Omaha; Univ of Alabama, Birmingham)

J Infect Dis 172:1212–1220, 1995 6–8

Background.—Human cytomegalovirus (CMV) transmission to the developing fetus during pregnancy depends greatly on maternal preconception immunity to the virus. In women lacking preconception seroimmunity to human CMV, the transmission rates range from 35% to 50%, whereas in women with such immunity, they are only 0.2% to 2%. The effects of subunit guinea pig (GP) CMV immunization on congenital infection were investigated.

Methods and Findings.—Two 25-µg doses of an abundant GP CMV glycoprotein, the gp60-90 complex, plus adjuvant were given to guinea pigs before pregnancy. Virus-specific humoral and cellular responses were documented. The rate of offspring loss in nonimmunized dams was significantly greater than in the immunized ones. Fewer than half the pups of nonimmunized infected dams survived, compared with more than 90% of those in the immunized groups. The mean birth weights of the pups of immunized and nonimmunized dams were 99 g and 74 g, respectively. Infection with GP CMV was significantly less frequent in pups of immunized than in nonimmunized dams; the rates were 18.2% and 52.2%, respectively.

Conclusion.—In this GP model, immunized dams had reduced organ involvement and rates of congenital infection and increased mean birth weights. The induction of preconception immunity to CMV by vaccine may be useful in decreasing both the incidence and severity of congenital CMV disease.

► Commenting on this article is William E. Benitz, M.D., Associate Professor of Pediatrics, Clinical Director of Intensive Care Nursery, Division of Neonatal and Developmental Medicine, Stanford University School of Medicine, Palo Alto, California:

► Cytomegalovirus remains the most common intrauterine infection, and the morbidity in these infants is severe. Attempts to treat these infants at diagnosis after delivery have been predictably fruitless.[1] These data suggest, once again, that prevention through immunization is the best strategy. As for hepatitis B, protection of the fetus and newborn is achieved through immunization of the mother. We can only hope that the favorable results seen in these guinea pigs can be extended to our own species!

W.E. Benitz, M.D.

Reference

1. Nigro G, Scholz H, Bartmann U: Ganciclovir therapy for symptomatic congenital cytomegalovirus infection. *J Pediatr* 124:318–322, 1994.

Maternal Viral Load, Zidovudine Treatment, and the Risk of Transmission of Human Immunodeficiency Virus Type 1 From Mother to Infant

Sperling RS, for the Pediatric AIDS Clinical Trials Group Protocol 076 Study Group (Mount Sinai School of Medicine, New York; et al)

N Engl J Med 335:1621–1629, 1996 6–9

Introduction.—The risk of mother-infant transmission of HIV type 1 was reduced dramatically by zidovudine, according to the results of the Pediatric AIDS Clinical Trials Group Protocol 076. The Public Health Service developed guidelines for the use of this drug during pregnancy. It is still unknown how zidovudine therapy reduced the risk of HIV-1 transmission. To determine whether the maternal viral burden predicted either the risk for HIV-1 transmission or the efficacy of zidovudine treatment, the earlier analysis was updated and stored samples of maternal blood collected at study entry were assayed.

Methods.—The initial study was a randomized, double-blind, placebo-controlled study that included HIV-1–infected women between 14 and 34 weeks of pregnancy. They were randomly assigned to receive either placebo or zidovudine. There were 425 mothers (211 in the zidovudine group

TABLE 1.—Median Plasma HIV-1 RNA Levels at Study Entry, According to Whether Mother-Infant Transmission of the Virus Occurred*

Assay and Study Group	HIV-1 Transmission		No Transmission		P Value
	No. of Women Studied	Median (95% CI)	No. of Women Studied	Median (95% CI)	
Reverse-transcription–PCR assay					
Zidovudine	12	19,330 (2100–108,310)	147	4650 (3340–8320)	0.03
Placebo	38	8,320 (4350–26,770)	130	5370 (2890–6770)	0.003
bDNA assay					
Zidovudine	10	2,620 (920–16,310)	136	2770 (1870–3900)	0.45
Placebo	31	4,680 (2200–11,180)	114	1850 (1540–2280)	0.008

*Medians are reported with nonparametric 95% confidence intervals (*CI*). *P* values were calculated by the 2-sample Wilcoxon test.

Abbreviation: PCR, polymerase chain reaction.

(Courtesy of Sperling RS, for the Pediatric AIDS Clinical Trials Group Protocol 076 Study Group: Maternal viral load, zidovudine treatment, and the risk of transmission of human immunodeficiency virus type 1 from mother to infant. *N Engl J Med* 335:1621–1629, 1996,)

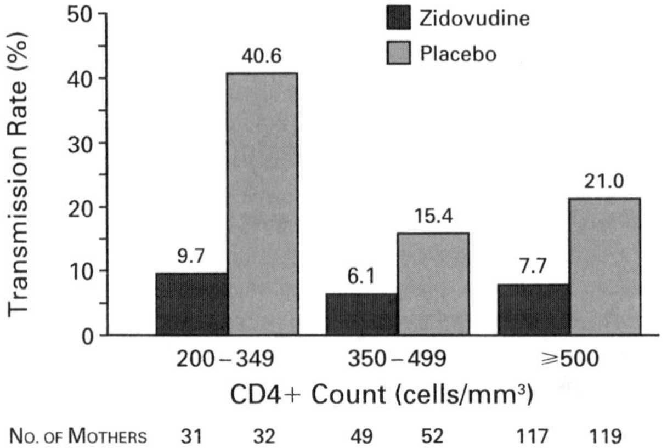

FIGURE 3.—Rates of HIV-1 transmission in the study groups, according to CD4+ cell count at entry. The number of mothers studied in each subgroup is shown below the figure. (Courtesy of Sperling RS, for the Pediatric AIDS Clinical Trials Group Protocol 076 Study Group: Maternal viral load, zidovudine treatment, and the risk of transmission of human immunodeficiency virus type 1 from mother to infant. *N Engl J Med* 335:1621–1629, 1996, Copyright 1996, Massachusetts Medical Society. All rights reserved.)

and 214 in the placebo group) who were included in the present study. They gave birth to 433 infants.

Results.—With zidovudine treatment, the rate of transmission of HIV-1 was 7.6%, whereas with placebo treatment, it was 22.6%. An increased risk of transmission was associated with a large viral burden at entry or delivery or with a positive culture in the placebo group. In the highest quartile of the RNA level, the transmission rate was greater than 40%. There was a wide range of maternal plasma HIV-1 RNA levels, in which transmission occurred in both groups (Table 1). Levels of RNA were reduced somewhat with zidovudine. Regardless of the HIV-1 RNA level, or the CD4+ count, zidovudine was effective (Fig 3). The reduction in viral RNA level from baseline to delivery was not significantly associated with the risk of transmission of HIV-1 when the baseline HIV-1 RNA level and CD4+ count were adjusted in the zidovudine group.

Conclusion.—For the transmission of HIV-1 from an untreated mother to her infant, a high maternal plasma concentration of virus is a risk factor. The reduction in plasma levels of viral RNA partially explains the reduction in such transmission after zidovudine treatment. Regardless of the plasma level of HIV-1 RNA or the CD4+ count, maternal treatment with zidovudine is recommended to prevent HIV-1 transmission.

▶ High maternal plasma concentration of virus is a major risk factor for the transmission of HIV-1 from mother to infant. Nevertheless, in some cases, transmission occurs from mothers who have undetectable plasma viremia. In an editorial comment, Catherine Wilfert, M.D., of Duke University Medical Center, points out that although the relationship between viral burden in the mother and transmission to the infant is clear in untreated mothers, the efficacy of zidovudine in reducing the risk of transmission cannot be explained by this fact alone, as the median reduction in plasma RNA levels was only 0.24 log—a net decrease by a factor of 1.7 and a minimal change in RNA level.[1] The authors suggest that the antiretroviral agent may prevent replication at the time when the infant is exposed to the virus, which could explain their findings. If most mother-infant transmission occurs around the time of delivery, a short course of treatment with antiretroviral agents could be effective. This is very important because, as Dr. Wilfert points out, in the developing nations of Asia and sub-Saharan Africa, it is simply not feasible to expect health care systems to be able to provide zidovudine (or some other agent) to the mother throughout the last trimester and then to the newborn for the first 6 weeks after delivery.

By the year 2000, about 6 million pregnant women and 5–10 million infants and children are expected to be infected with HIV-1. This and other studies show clearly that perinatal transmission of HIV-1 can be reduced significantly by zidovudine and that this intervention is likely responsible for the reported decrease in the incidence of perinatally acquired AIDS in 1995. Dr. Wilfert concludes that "in the developed countries, we now have it in our power to reduce perinatal HIV infection substantially. We must also find efficient and economical ways to reduce these infections in the rest of the world."

M.J. Maisels, M.B., B.Ch.

Reference

1. Wilfert CM: Beginning to make progress against HIV. *N Engl J Med* 335:1678–1680, 1996.

Obstetrical Factors and the Transmission of Human Immunodeficiency Virus Type 1 From Mother to Child

Landesman SH, for the Women and Infants Transmission Study (State Univ of New York, Brooklyn; et al)

N Engl J Med 334:1617–1623, 1996 6–10

Background.—Human immunodeficiency virus type 1 (HIV-1) transmission from mother to infant can occur in the antepartum, intrapartum, or postpartum period. Although increasing evidence suggests that a large percentage of infants are infected at or near delivery, few researchers have reported the role of obstetric factors in HIV-1 transmission.

Methods.—The current study included 525 women participating in the Women and Infants Transmission Study, a prospective, observational study of HIV-1–infected women enrolled during pregnancy and followed up with their infants for 3 years. For all women, HIV-1 infection status was known as of August 31, 1994. All delivered live singleton infants. Obstetric, clinical, immunologic, and virologic data were analyzed.

Findings.—Women with membranes rupturing more than 4 hours before delivery had a 25% HIV-1 transmission rate to their infants, compared with 14% among women with membranes rupturing 4 hours or less before delivery. A multivariate analysis indicated that membrane rupture more than 4 hours before delivery almost doubled the risk of transmission,

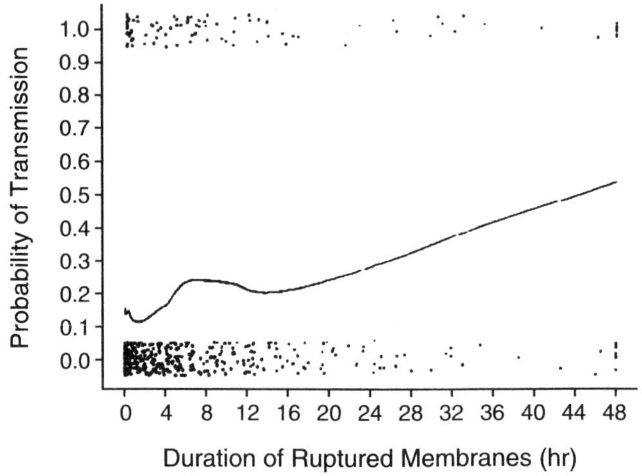

FIGURE 1.—Probability of HIV-1 transmission in relation to the duration of ruptured membranes. The *dots at the top* represent women who transmitted HIV-1 to their infants, and *dots at the bottom* women who did not transmit HIV-1. Data on women whose membranes were ruptured for more than 48 hours are shown at the 48-hour mark. (Reprinted by permission of *The New England Journal of Medicine*, from Landesman SH, for the Women and Infants Transmission Study: Obstetrical factors and the transmission of human immunodeficiency virus type 1 from mother to child. *N Engl J Med* 334:1617–1623, Copyright 1996, Massachusetts Medical Society. All rights reserved.)

regardless of the mode of delivery. Other variables independently associated with transmission were maternal illicit drug use during pregnancy, low antenatal CD4+ lymphocyte count, and birth weight of less than 2,500 g (Fig 1).

Conclusions.—Limiting ruptured membrane duration to 4 hours or less before delivery would reduce the HIV-1 mother-to-infant transmission rate from 18.7% to 13.9%. This would result in 5 fewer perinatal HIV-1 transmissions per 100 deliveries, a decrease of 26%.

► Once again, rupture of the membranes has been linked to the transmission of infection from mother to infant, although in the case of HIV-1, *prolonged* rupture of membranes (greater than 18 hours) apparently is not a factor. Viruses play their game within a narrower window of time, tantalizing obstetricians with shortening the duration of ruptured membranes, perhaps combined with the administration of zidovudine as a means of reducing transmission of HIV-1 further. In a context where the risk of transmission appears particularly high (i.e., in women with a low CD4+ count, a high viral load, or both), a temptation to perform cesarean section seems likely. Importantly, no prospective information can justify such an approach at this time, and cesarean section itself may represent a risk in the context of severely immunocompromised, HIV-1–infected women. Nothing is simple, and it just gets easier and easier to be an obstetrician!

D.K. Stevenson, M.D.

▶ Most instances of perinatal HIV-1 transmission are thought to occur close to the time of delivery. Factors that favor HIV-1 transmission from mother to infant include advanced maternal disease (evidenced by low CD4+ cell count, high viral load, high level of p24 antigenemia), virus phenotype, breast-feeding, and a variety of obstetric factors, such as the use of scalp electrodes and prolonged rupture of membranes (ROM).

The Women and Infants Transmission Study evaluated 525 HIV-1–infected women with live singleton deliveries and found 4 independent risk factors for HIV-1 transmission from mother to infant: ROM for greater than 4 hours (odds ratio [OR] = 1.82, $P = 0.02$), CD4+ level less than 29% (OR = 2.82, $P < 0.001$), birth weight less than 2,500 g (OR = 1.86, $P = 0.04$), and use of illicit drugs (OR = 1.9, $P = 0.01$). The rate of HIV-1 transmission to infants was 25% for women with ROM of greater than 4 hours compared with 14% for those with less than 4 hours' duration of membrane rupture; the observed effect was independent of the mode of delivery. Earlier studies had yielded conflicting results on whether prolonged ROM and/or vaginal delivery were significant risk factors for HIV-1 transmission.[1]

My biggest concern is that the findings of this study may be used to justify the performance of cesarean sections on HIV-1–infected women whose duration of membrane rupture is approaching 4 hours but whose delivery does not appear imminent. Cesarean sections have not been conclusively shown to reduce perinatal HIV-1 transmission but are associated with increased morbidity for these women. Limiting ROM to 4 hours or less would have reduced the *overall* rate of vertical HIV-1 transmission from 19% to 14% (a 26% reduction). This is considerably lower than the benefit derived from zidovudine therapy during pregnancy (a 67% reduction in risk). This study does not address whether there is any added benefit to limiting ROM to 4 hours or less among HIV-1–infected pregnant women being treated with zidovudine.

What is becoming increasingly clear is that the major factor determining the risk of mother-to-infant transmission of viruses such as HIV-1 and hepatitis C is the maternal viral load. The ability to measure HIV-1 viral load in blood is becoming widely available. Reducing maternal HIV-1 viral load appears to be the most promising approach to preventing perinatal transmission. Viral loads of HIV-1 are more effectively reduced to very low or even nonmeasurable levels using antiretroviral drug combinations rather than single agents. Building on the success of zidovudine therapy during pregnancy in reducing the rate of perinatal HIV-1 infection, trials are now under way in the United States to evaluate the effectiveness of various combinations of agents such as zidovudine, didanosine, and lamivudine in further decreasing that risk. The payoff will be greater if we encourage women to undergo antepartum HIV-1 screening and to offer antiretroviral agents to those found to be infected.

B.J. Freij, M.D.

Reference

1. Orloff SL, Simonds RJ, Steketee RW, et al: Determinants of perinatal HIV-1 transmission. *Clin Obstet Gynecol* 39:386–395, 1996.

Human Immunodeficiency Virus Type 1–Infected Cells in Breast Milk: Association With Immunosuppression and Vitamin A Deficiency

Nduati RW, John GC, Richardson BA, et al (Univ of Nairobi, Kenya; Univ of Washington, Seattle; Univ of Manitoba, Winnipeg, Canada)

J Infect Dis 172:1461–1468, 1995 6–11

Introduction.—There is significant risk of mother-to-infant transmission of HIV-1 associated with breast-feeding. However, formula-feeding in developing countries carries substantial risk of high infant mortality because of infectious disease and malnutrition. Therefore, the World Health Organization currently recommends that HIV-seropositive women in areas with high infant mortality rates breast-feed their infants. To investigate the determinants of HIV transmission through breast milk, the prevalence, concentration, and clinical correlates of virus-infected cells in breast milk were studied among HIV-seropositive mothers.

Methods.—Manually expressed samples of colostrum obtained within 1 week of delivery and of breast milk obtained at 6, 14, 26, 39, and 52 weeks after delivery from 107 HIV-seropositive women were analyzed for the presence of HIV DNA using polymerase chain reaction. Correlations were analyzed between clinical variables and the presence or absence of HIV-1 DNA in breast milk and between clinical variables and virus concentrations in breast milk.

Results.—Of the 212 samples, 123 (58%) had detectable HIV-1 DNA. The prevalence of HIV-1 DNA varied from 71% in the samples obtained at 6–9 months to 20% in the samples obtained after 9 months. The prevalence of a high concentration of virus was greatest between 8 and 90 days after delivery and decreased to 0% at 9 months after delivery. Detectable HIV-1–infected cells were significantly correlated with low CD4 cell counts (fewer than 400 cells/mm^3), high CD8 counts (greater than 47%), and low CD4:CD8 ratios (less than 0.5). There was a significant inverse relationship between HIV-1 DNA in colostrum and breast milk and vitamin A levels only among women with fewer than 400 CD4 cells/mm^3.

Conclusions.—Human immunodeficiency virus type 1 DNA was detected in the majority of breast milk samples. The prevalence of infected cells remained high from birth until 9 months after delivery, and some samples contained a very high concentration of infected cells. Both the prevalence and concentration of breast milk HIV-1 DNA were highly correlated with maternal immunosuppression. Women with both advanced HIV disease and prenatal vitamin A deficiency had a particularly high prevalence of infected cells in the colostrum and breast milk, suggesting a particularly high risk of mother-to-infant transmission in these women.

▶ Commenting on this article is William E. Benitz, M.D., Associate Professor of Pediatrics, Clinical Director of Intensive Care Nursery, Division of Neonatal and Developmental Medicine, Stanford University School of Medicine, Palo Alto, California:

▶ This report defines yet another circumstance in which the "breast is best" adage may not be applicable. These authors note that the risk of HIV transmission by breast-feeding may be outweighed by morbidity associated with formula-feeding in developing countries, but neonatologists and pediatricians in developed counties are advised to recommend avoidance of breast-feeding for HIV-seropositive mothers. The relationship between vitamin A deficiency and shedding of virus in breast milk is intriguing and suggests a method for reducing risk in areas where formula-feeding is not an option. Vitamin A sufficiency does not reduce shedding, or presumably risk of transmission, to zero, however, so this is unlikely to be a useful strategy in economically developed regions.

W.E. Benitz, M.D.

Natural History of Human Immunodeficiency Virus Disease in Perinatally Infected Children: An Analysis From the Pediatric Spectrum of Disease Project

Barnhart HX, and the Pediatric Spectrum of Disease Clinical Consortium (Emory Univ, Atlanta, Ga; et al)

Pediatrics 97:710–716, 1996 — 6–12

Introduction.—Largely because of the availability of HIV antibody testing to identify asymptomatic cases, estimates of the time to the development of AIDS and death in children with perinatally acquired HIV infection are longer than initially thought. Using the Centers for Disease Control and Prevention (CDC) 1994 pediatric HIV classification system, it is now possible to classify infected children into 5 mutually exclusive categories based on severity of disease. Those in stage N have no signs or symptoms of HIV infection; those in stages A, B, and C have mild, moderate, and severe signs and symptoms, respectively; and those in stage D are dead. This classification system was used to describe the progression of HIV infection in a large sample of perinatally infected children.

Methods.—The analysis used active surveillance data collected by the Pediatric Spectrum of Disease project, which is coordinated by the CDC. Data were collected every 6 months from participating hospitals in 7 geographic regions. The 1994 CDC pediatric HIV classification system was applied to 2,148 children with perinatal HIV infection, and a 5-stage Markov model was fitted to the data. In an alternative Markov model, the development of AIDS was substituted for stage C of the classification.

Results.—The children spent an estimated mean of 10 months in stage N, 4 months in stage A, 65 months in stage B, and 34 months in stage C. A child born with perinatally acquired HIV infection had an estimated 50% chance of severe signs and symptoms developing by the age of 5 years and a 75% chance of living to 5 years of age. Children in stage B had an estimated 60% chance of severe signs and symptoms developing within the next 5 years and a 65% chance of surviving for 5 more years. The mean duration from birth to the development of stage C was estimated at 6.6 years, and the mean survival from birth at 9.4 years. In the alternative Markov model, the mean duration from birth to the development of AIDS was estimated at 4.8 years.

Conclusion.—In the average child with perinatal HIV infection, moderate signs and symptoms develop in the second year of life. They remain in this moderately symptomatic stage for most of the expected life span, which is about 9 years. These children will, therefore, need clinical care before AIDS develops. The findings of this analysis will be useful in family counseling, health care planning, and clinical trial design.

▶ Although general precautions in nurseries have been routinized by physician and nursing staff, many neonatologists have not kept informed regarding the pediatric spectrum of disease that follows the initial hospitalization of HIV-infected infants, who generally appear to be well newborns. The outcomes may be better than what might have been believed, but it is important to note that among truly infected infants, the chance of severe signs or symptoms developing by 5 years of age is still probably 50%, although 75% have a chance of surviving to 5 years of age. For the later stages of the disease, the risks change.

This information is essential for neonatologists who are counseling families at the time of birth and arranging for proper follow-up. Discharge from the nursery is only the beginning of the story for HIV-infected newborns, not the end of the story, as is the case for most other infants who have benefited from newborn intensive care.

D.K. Stevenson, M.D.

Economic Impact of Treatment of HIV-positive Pregnant Women and Their Newborns With Zidovudine: Implications for HIV Screening

Mauskopf JA, Paul JE, Wichman DS, et al (Glaxo Wellcome Inc, Research Triangle Park, NC)

JAMA 276:132–138, 1996 6–13

Introduction.—As the prevalence of women of childbearing age who are HIV positive increases in the United States, the number of newborns infected by perinatal transmission is also increasing. The majority of these infants have a rapid progression to AIDS. Preventing perinatal transmission of HIV has obvious public health and humanitarian benefits and may have economic benefits as well, as the care of children infected with HIV is very expensive. The AIDS Clinical Trials Group (ACTG) Protocol 076 has demonstrated that treating pregnant women who are HIV positive and their newborns with zidovudine is effective in reducing perinatal transmission of HIV. Estimates of the economic consequences of treating pregnant women who are HIV positive and their newborns with zidovudine were presented. As voluntary screening programs could be used to identify at-risk pregnancies, an economic evaluation of voluntary screening in populations of varying seroprevalence was also presented.

Study Design.—Health care costs associated with the treatment of pregnant women who are HIV positive and their newborns were estimated as the costs of administration of zidovudine and the reduction in cost of treating pediatric HIV infection. The lifetime costs of treatment of pediatric HIV infection were derived from published literature. The amount by which maternal–fetal HIV transmission rates were reduced with zidovudine administration was derived from ACTG Protocol 076. The costs of a voluntary screening program were estimated from costs of screening tests and counseling. Sensitivity and threshold analyses were performed to determine the impact of changes in input parametric values on the estimates of costs.

Results.—When the transmission reduction rates from ACTG Protocol 076 were used, treatment costs per 100 pregnant women who were HIV positive and their newborns of $104,502 are more than offset by the $1,701,333 reduction in the cost of treating pediatric HIV infection; the net savings is $1,596,831. Cost savings were achieved over a wide range of possible parametric values. Voluntary screening programs achieved cost savings when the HIV prevalence rate among pregnant women was greater than 5 in 1,000. This threshold prevalence rate is sensitive to changes in parametric values.

Conclusion.—Existing data on the cost of HIV screening, zidovudine treatment, expected seroprevalence of HIV, and the high costs of medical care for pediatric HIV infection all support the conclusion that zidovudine treatment of pregnant women who are HIV positive and their newborns to prevent perinatal transmission provides cost savings. These data also support voluntary screening for pregnant women as being cost-effective, except where prevalence rates are known to be very low. As the incidence of HIV infection in women of childbearing age continues to increase, voluntary screening and zidovudine treatment for these women should become integral parts of HIV prevention programs.

► Here is another article that gives some reason for hope in our battle with this epidemic. In addition to the highly significant reduction in the transmission of HIV from mother to baby, the use of zidovudine is estimated to produce a net savings of about $1.5 million for every 100 pregnant women identified and treated for HIV-positive status.

M.J. Maisels, M.B.B.Ch.

7 The Nervous System and Special Senses

Cerebral Metabolism Within 18 Hours of Birth Asphyxia: A Proton Magnetic Resonance Spectroscopy Study
Hanrahan JD, Sargentoni J, Azzopardi D, et al (Hammersmith Hosp, London)
Pediatr Res 39:584–590, 1996 7–1

Background.—Hypoxic-ischemic injury in the perinatal period is a major cause of death and neurodevelopmental impairment. Although proton MR spectroscopy (MRS) has been performed after asphyxia in studies of such injury, it has not been done before the onset of secondary energy failure, which may clarify the mechanisms of delayed cerebral injury. Such new knowledge may enable clinicians to better predict which infants are likely to have secondary energy failure and subsequent neurodevelopmental impairment and thus to benefit from treatment with neuroprotective agents.

Methods.—Sixteen term infants with clinical features of birth asphyxia underwent proton MRS within 18 hours of birth. Ten infants with no signs of birth asphyxia were also studied. Fifteen infants suspected of asphyxia underwent phosphorus-31 MRS at a median 62 hours of age to detect delayed impairments in cerebral energy metabolism.

Findings.—In all infants, the studies demonstrated choline, creatine, and *N*-acetylaspartate (NAA) in spectra of the basal ganglia. Fifteen of the 16 infants with possible asphyxia showed lactate, compared with only 4 of the 10 control infants. Glutamine and glutamate were also detected in more infants in the asphyxia group, although the between-group difference was nonsignificant. In the asphyxiated group, the ratio of lactate to creatine in the first 18 hours of life was negatively correlated with phosphocreatine/inorganic phosphate (PCr/P_i) at 33–106 hours. In 5 severely asphyxiated infants, the PCr/P_i was less than 0.75, indicating a poor developmental prognosis. Another infant died before PCr/P_i could be determined. Median lactate/creatine was 1.47 in the 6 infants with severe asphyxia, 0.38 in the 10 infants with PCr/P_i exceeding 0.75, and 0 in the control group.

Conclusions.—Cerebral energy metabolism appears to be abnormal after birth asphyxia, in the period when ^{31}P MRS usually yields normal findings. Proton MRS may be useful for predicting which infants are likely to have a decrease in cerebral high-energy phosphate levels and subsequent neurodevelopmental impairment.

▶ This comment has been provided by William D. Rhine, M.D., Assistant Professor of Pediatrics, Stanford University School of Medicine; Co-director of ECMO, Lucile Salter Packard Children's Hospital at Stanford, Palo Alto, California:

▶ Noninvasive technologies to study brain metabolism and injury continue to be developed, improved, and applied to clinical situations; such a development and application is described in this article. Proton MRS was able to measure early changes in basal ganglia metabolism in infants with birth asphyxia. The details of these asphyxial insults are a little sketchy, and neuroradiographic follow-up was limited to cranial US. Neurodevelopmental follow-up was only up to 3–12 months of age. It would be interesting to see the follow-up of brain MRI and neurodevelopmental studies at 2–3 years of age in this cohort of patients. For now, the authors provide powerful evidence that cerebral metabolism can be measured locally in deep structures such as the basal ganglia and that elevated lactate in this region reflects the severity of injury. As the authors point out, it is important and feasible to distinguish systemic lactate from more focal brain lactate concentrations. It may be impractical to use this technology in very sick neonates who are at highest risk for asphyxial brain injury, as MR scanning is difficult to perform in ventilated patients, who normally have lots of monitoring and IV equipment. The challenge continues to be selecting patients who might benefit from the rapidly emerging field of neuroprotective therapeutics, such as those that inhibit or decrease secondary injury associated with apoptosis.

W.D. Rhine, M.D.

Early [^{18}F]FDG Positron Emission Tomography in Infants With Hypoxic-Ischaemic Encephalopathy Shows Hypermetabolism During the Postasphyctic Period

Blennow M, Ingvar M, Lagercrantz H, et al (Karolinska Hosp, Stockholm)
Acta Paediatr 84:1289–1295, 1995 7–2

Background.—Current techniques for predicting neurologic outcome after severe perinatal asphyxia are not sufficiently accurate. The potential of positron emission tomography (PET) in predicting neurologic outcomes in such patients was investigated.

Methods and Findings.—Six full-term infants with perinatal asphyxia and moderate or severe hypoxic-ischemic encephalopathy underwent PET. [2-^{18}F]2-fluoro-2-deoxy-D-glucose ([^{18}F]FDG) PET scans were obtained at a median age of 2.5 days, and regional cerebral metabolic rates of glucose ($rCMR_{gl}$) were determined. In 5 infants, localized $rCMR_{gl}$ were visually noted. Findings on PET studies showed good agreement with those of neuroradiologic, neurophysiologic, and clinical studies. With PET, information on pathophysiologic events could be obtained earlier than with conventional morphologic imaging methods.

Conclusion.—Positron emission tomographic scans can be included in a clinical research protocol for severely asphyxiated infants, even in the first days of life. Such scans, performed with [^{18}F]FDG, provide useful information regarding neurologic outcomes in this patient population.

► We asked Robert Vannucci, M.D., Professor of Pediatrics at the Pennsylvania State University College of Medicine, Hershey, Pennsylvania, to comment:

► This experimental study by Blennow et al. in asphyxiated newborns raises 2 major questions, one of which is scientific and the other clinical. The first question relates to the origin of the hypometabolic and hypermetabolic areas of brain seen on the PET scans. It is likely that the hypometabolic areas represent the cores of areas of brain infarction. The hypermetabolic areas might represent areas of tissue peripheral to the infarct core that are struggling to remain viable by increasing their metabolic activity to maintain energy status as normal as possible. The hypermetabolic areas might also represent tissue in which low-grade infarction has already occurred, with evolving gliosis. In this regard, activated astrocytes and microglia are capable of incorporating glucose as a metabolizable substrate. An unlikely cause of delayed hypermetabolism is a rebound ischemia secondary to hypoperfusion caused by evolving cerebral edema.

The clinical question relates to the usefulness of PET as a method of ascertaining cerebral metabolic alterations that occur in previously asphyxiated newborns. Positron emission tomography scanners are available at only a few medical centers in the United States and abroad. The major clinical usefulness of PET has been for the diagnosis and surgical management of patients with focal epilepsy. Accordingly, it is unlikely that PET will gain widespread use in newborns, at least in the foreseeable future. In this regard, MRI has gained widespread use in ascertaining early regional anatomical abnormalities that occur after perinatal asphyxia. Given the ready availability of MRI scanners, it is likely that this technique will supersede any availability of PET.

R. Vannucci, M.D.

Posthypoxic Cooling of Neonatal Rats Provides Protection Against Brain Injury

Thoresen M, Bågenholm R, Løberg EM, et al (Univ of Oslo, Norway; Göteborg Univ, Sweden; Ullevål Univ, Oslo, Norway)

Arch Dis Child 74:F3–F9, 1996 7–3

Background.—Severe hypoxia-ischemia continues to cause injury to neonates during labor and delivery. No interventions have been found to

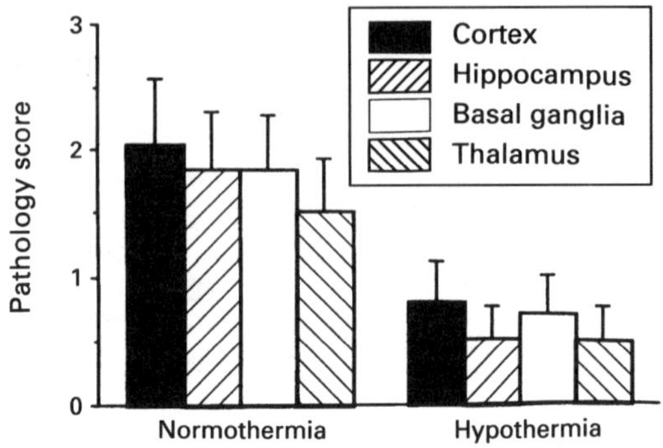

FIGURE 4.—The mean (SEM) values of the pathology score obtained for each of the 4 regions in the left hemisphere. (Courtesy of Thoresen M, Bågenholm R, Løberg EM, et al: Posthypoxic cooling of neonatal rats provides protection against brain injury. *Arch Dis Child* 74:F3–F9, 1996.)

improve the outcomes of encephalopathy after initial cardiorespiratory resuscitation. The possibility of decreasing cerebral injury by cooling after a cerebral insult has not been thoroughly investigated. The effects of 3 hours of moderate hypothermia in an immature rat model were reported.

Methods and Results.—Unilateral hypoxic-ischemic brain damage was induced in 7-day-old rats by left carotid ligation. This was followed by 120 minutes of normothermic exposure to 8% oxygen and random assignment to 3 hours of hypothermia or normothermia. Thirty sections from each brain were assessed histologically, and the distribution and pattern of damage were scored on a scale of 0 to 4. Rats treated with hypothermia were found to have significantly less damage than those in the normothermia group (Fig 4).

Conclusions.—In this neonatal rat model, a 6°C decrease in rectal temperature for 3 hours after the insult substantially protected all regions of the brain. Hypothermia immediately after resuscitation may allow time for drugs to enter the brain and work at an earlier stage of the posthypoxic cascade of the injury process. Further experimental studies are needed to define the best duration and "time window" for this treatment before clinical trials of hypothermia after birth asphyxia can be initiated.

▶ We asked Dr. Charles Palmer, Associate Professor of Pediatrics, Pennsylvania State University School of Medicine, Hershey, to comment:

▶ This important study shows that hypoxic-ischemic brain injury in the neonatal rat can be reduced by lowering brain temperature from 38.5°C to 32.5°C, during the first 3 hours of recovery. During the past few years, there has been a flurry of experiments in more mature animals that support resuscitative hypothermia as an effective, long-lasting brain "rescue" strategy.[1–6] Brain protection can be achieved even if hypothermia is started between 1 and 2 hours after resuscitation. Indeed, an important preliminary report suggests that prolonged focal brain cooling protects against cerebral ischemia in fetal sheep.[7] Just how long does hypothermia need to be maintained? It appears that longer is better; certainly more than 3 hours of hypothermia was needed in all previous studies and, in 1, benefit was obtained by extending hypothermia from 12 to 24 hours.[5, 6, 8]

It is therefore remarkable that only 3 hours of hypothermia offered so much protection in this study, especially because other investigators failed to show protection in a similar model.[9] It must be noted that the control, normothermic rats, were maintained at a core body temperature of 38.5°C, which is higher than most other investigators use with this immature rat model. This difference could be significant because mild hyperthermia during the cerebral ischemia or early recovery worsens brain injury.[10–12]

With this insight, maternal pyrexia has important implications for the fetus in distress, and utmost care should be taken not to overheat the asphyxiated neonate during the first few days after resuscitation. Radiant heat to the infant's head is particularly hazardous. Although pharmacologic approaches continue to make exciting but slow progress toward clinical trials, the most valuable neuroprotective modality, "resuscitative hypothermia," is already part of our therapeutic arsenal. With reference to the asphyxiated neonate, it is now time to step out from the "thermoneutral zone" and explore the clinical application of resuscitative hypothermia.

C. Palmer, M.B., Ch.B.

References

1. Coimbra C, Wieloch T: Moderate hypothermia mitigates neuronal damage in the rat brain when initiated several hours following transient cerebral ischemia. *Acta Neuropathol* 87:325–331, 1994.
2. Coimbra C, Drake M, Boris-Möller F, et al: Long-lasting neuroprotective effect of postischemic hypothermia and treatment with an anti-inflammatory/antipyretic drug: Evidence for chronic encephalopathic processes following ischemia. *Stroke* 27:1578–1586, 1996.
3. Colbourne F, Corbett D: Delayed postischemic hypothermia: A six-month survival study using behavioral and histological assessments of neuroprotection. *J Neurosci* 15:7250–7260, 1995.
4. Sirimanne ES, Blumberg RM, Bossano D, et al: The effect of prolonged modification of cerebral temperature on outcome after hypoxic-ischemic brain injury in the infant rat. *Pediatr Res* 39:591–597, 1996.
5. Markarian GZ, Lee JH, Stein DJ, et al: Mild hypothermia: Therapeutic window after experimental cerebral ischemia. *Neurosurgery* 38:542–550, 1996.
6. Yanamoto H, Hong SC, Soleau S, et al: Mild postischemic hypothermia limits cerebral injury following transient focal ischemia in rat neocortex. *Brain Res* 718:207–211, 1996.
7. Gunn TR, Gunn AJ, deHaan HH, et al: Prolonged selective cerebral cooling prevents cytotoxic edema and improves recovery after cerebral ischemia in fetal sheep. *Pediatr Res* 39:212A, 1996.
8. Colbourne F, Corbett D: Delayed and prolonged post-ischemic hypothermia is neuroprotective in the gerbil. *Brain Res* 654:265–272, 1994.
9. Yager J, Towfighi J, Vannucci RC: Influence of mild hypothermia on hypoxic-ischemic brain damage in the immature rat. *Pediatr Res* 34:525–529, 1993.
10. Dietrich WD, Busto R, Valdes I, et al: Effects of normothermic versus mild hyperthermic forebrain ischemia in rats. *Stroke* 21:1318–1325, 1990.
11. Chen H, Chopp M, Welch KMA: Effect of hyperthermia on the ischemic infarct volume after middle cerebral artery occlusion in the rat. *Neurology* 41:1133–1135, 1991.

12. Dietrich WD, Alonso O, Halley M: Delayed posttraumatic brain hyperthermia worsens outcome after fluid percussion brain injury: A light and electron microscopic study in rats. *Neurosurgery* 38:533–541, 1996.

The Effect of Prolonged Modification of Cerebral Temperature on Outcome After Hypoxic-Ischemic Brain Injury in the Infant Rat

Sirimanne ES, Blumberg RM, Bossano D, et al (Univ of Auckland, New Zealand; Royal Postgraduate Med School, London)

Pediatr Res 39:591–597, 1996 7–4

Introduction.—Pathophysiologic and histopathologic data of hypoxic-ischemic (HI) injury suggest that further neuronal death may occur even days after the primary injury. The first phase is loss of energy failure, followed by loss of membrane function. Cerebral temperature during and immediately after the injury is important in determining outcome. Hypoxic-ischemic brain injury may be prevented or retarded by hypothermia during the period of the insult because it protects the brain by reducing metabolic demands. The injury can be exacerbated by mild hyperthermia. The effects of prolonged environmental temperature modification after a moderate HI injury were examined during the period when delayed damage may occur.

Methods.—In 21-day-old rats, HI injury was induced by unilateral ligation of the right carotid artery followed by exposure to 15 minutes of hypoxia of 8% 0_2 at 34°C. By modifying environmental temperature, cerebral temperature changes were induced. The rats were divided into 4 treatment groups: 15 rats were at 34°C for 72 hours; 14 rats were at 34°C for 6 hours and then at 22°C for the remaining 66 hours; 17 rats were at 22°C for 6 hours and 34°C for the next 66 hours; and 16 rats were at 22°C for 72 hours. Cortical temperatures of 35.5° ± 0.1°C were found for rats kept at 22°C. Cortical temperatures of 37.9° ± 0.2°C were found for rats kept at 34°C. An assessment of histologic outcome was made 72 hours after hypoxia.

Results.—In the group kept at 22°C for 72 hours, the area of cortical infarction was reduced when compared with the other 3 groups (Fig 3). In this same group, striatal damage was reduced. There was no significant alteration of hippocampal neuronal loss. At 21 days after the injury, the area of cortical infarction was 12.1 ± 3 mm^2 in the group kept at 34°C for 72 hours, compared with 3.4 ± 1.5 mm^2 in the group kept at 22°C for 72 hours.

Conclusions.—To improve outcome, hypothermia must be given during the first 6 hours and from 6 to 72 hours after injury. Injury is exacerbated by exposure to a thermoneutral environment. To suppress the cytotoxic processes that occur after HI injury, prolonged moderate cerebral hypothermia can be used. Questions are raised regarding the routine management of temperature in asphyxiated term newborn infants, because current

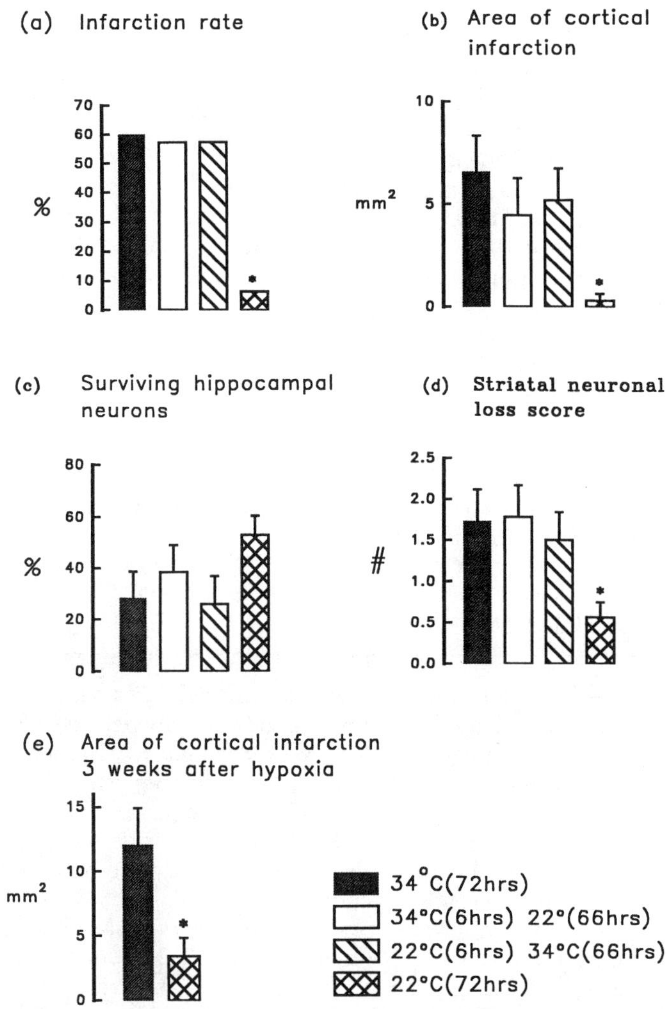

FIGURE 3.—The effect of environmental temperature on histologic outcome after hypoxic ischemic injury. **A,** incidence of cortical infarction (group 4, $P < 0.05$). **B,** area of cortical infarction (group 4, $P < 0.05$). **C,** number of surviving CA1–CA3 hippocampal neurons. **D,** striatal loss (group 4, $P = 0.05$). **E,** area of cortical infarction from rats kept 21 days ($P < 0.01$). (Courtesy of Sirimanne ES, Blumberg RM, Bossano D, et al: The effect of prolonged modification of cerebral temperature on outcome after hypoxic-ischemic brain injury in the infant rat. *Pediatr Res* 39:591–597, 1996.)

practice aims at maintaining thermoneutrality. To evaluate the relevance of these observations, further investigations are needed.

► We are indebted to our colleagues from New Zealand, who have outlined the pathophysiologic sequencing of HI brain injury. They have emphasized the progression of the injury, with neuronal death continuing for hours and days after the initial insult. Hypothermia during the insult can retard or prevent HI brain injury. The clinical implications are profound as we strive to maintain thermoneutrality for all infants. Their data, admittedly obtained in rats, suggest that exposure to the thermoneutral environment in the hours after HI injury can "markedly worsen neurologic outcome." In contrast, prolonged and mild cerebral hypothermia of about 2°C is protective. Is this sufficient evidence to change practice? Hardly. Yet maintaining term asphyxiated infants below the neutral thermal environment is unlikely to be harmful and is something that is relatively easy to accomplish. Hall and colleagues recently demonstrated excellent outcomes for asphyxiated infants treated with large doses of phenobarbital. Perhaps cooling and phenobarbital are a reasonable first step in the management of severe HI encephalopathy.

If it were done when 'tis done, then 'twere well/It were done quickly.—William Shakespeare, Macbeth

A.A. Fanaroff, M.B.B.Ch.

Insulin-like Growth Factor-1 Is a Potent Neuronal Rescue Agent After Hypoxic-Ischemic Injury in Fetal Lambs

Johnston BM, Mallard EC, Williams CE, et al (Univ of Auckland, New Zealand)

J Clin Invest 97:300–308, 1996 7–5

Objective.—Recognition of the secondary or delayed phase of neuronal death in infants with acute hypoxic-ischemic or asphyxial brain injury has raised the possibility of using some type of neuronal rescue therapy in the hours after acute injury. The peptide growth factor insulin-like growth factor-1 (IGF-1) may, through unknown mechanisms, play a key role in the rescue of injured neurons of the adult brain. A fetal sheep model of hypoxic-ischemic encephalopathy was used to study the potential effects of IGF-1 as a neuronal rescue agent.

Methods.—In the models, cerebral ischemia was induced in unanesthetized, late-gestation fetal sheep by inflation of carotid artery occluder cuffs. The cuffs were deflated after 30 minutes. Two hours after the onset of cerebral ischemia, the fetus received recombinant human (rh)IGF-1 in a dose of 0.1, 1, or 10 µg or vehicle only by 1-hour infusion into a lateral cerebral ventricle. The animals were killed for histologic analysis after 5 days.

Results.—Fetuses treated with 0.1 or 1 µg of rhIGF-1 had significant reductions in overall neuronal loss, but those receiving the 10-µg dose did not. Fetuses receiving the 1-µg dose had significantly lower neuronal loss scores in various regions of the brain, including the cortex, hippocampus, and striatum. In comparison, the fetuses receiving the 0.1-µg dose had no improvement in the parietal cortex and thalamus and had less improve-

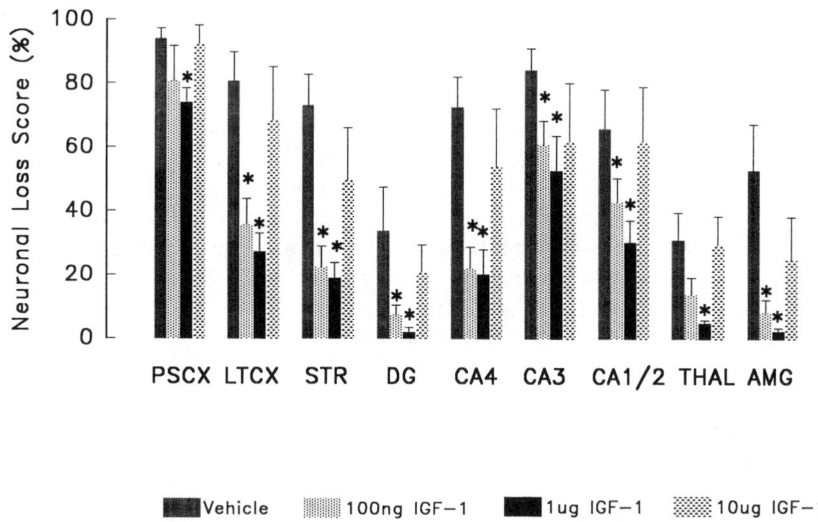

FIGURE 6.—Effect of recombinant human insulin-like growth factor-1 (*rhIGF-1*) treatment on histologically assessed neuronal loss in 9 brain regions at 5 days after 30 minutes of cerebral hypoxia-ischemia. A significant reduction in neuronal loss was seen in all regions in those given 1 µg of rhIGF-1 and a lesser, but significant, reduction in neuronal loss in fetuses treated with 0.1 µg of rhIGF-1. # $P < 0.05$; *$P < 0.01$. *Abbreviations: PSCX,* parasagittal cortex; *LTCX,* lateral cortex; *STR,* striatum, *DG,* dentate gyrus; *CA1/2, 3, 4,* cornu ammonis of hippocampus; *THAL,* thalamus; *AMG,* amygdala. (Reproduced from *The Journal of Clinical Investigation,* courtesy of Johnston BM, Mallard EC, Williams CE, et al: Insulin-like growth factor-1 is a potent neuronal rescue agent after hypoxic-ischemic injury in fetal lambs. *J Clin Invest* 97:300–308, 1996. By copyright permission of The American Society for Clinical Investigation.)

ment in other areas (Fig 6). The 1-µg dose was also associated with a reduced incidence and delayed onset of seizures and with reduced and delayed secondary cytotoxic edema. The same dose also delayed the secondary peak in systemic blood glucose concentration and delayed and attenuated the secondary peak in blood lactate level.

Conclusion.—Treatment with low-dose rhIGF-1 appears to reduce neuronal death after cerebral hypoxic-ischemic injury in fetal sheep in dose-dependent fashion. If given within 2 hours after the onset of ischemia, rhIGF-1 therapy appears to be effective and nontoxic. With further study, IGF-1 treatment could be considered for use in asphyxiated infants who are identified before the start of the secondary phase of brain injury.

▶ We asked Dr. Robert Vannucci, Professor of Pediatrics, Pennsylvania State University College of Medicine, Hershey, Pennsylvania, to comment:

▶ Throughout the past decade, animal research has been conducted to ascertain the efficacy of specific pharmacologic agents in preventing or reducing the brain damage that results from perinatal cerebral hypoxia-ischemia. Drugs under investigation have included oxygen-free radical inhibitors and scavengers, excitatory amino acid antagonists, calcium channel blockers, and nitric oxide synthase inhibitors. These drugs are helpful in ameliorating perinatal hypoxic-ischemic neuronal injury when administered either before, or shortly after, the hypoxic-ischemic insult. The "therapeutic window"—the interval after resuscitation from hypoxia-ischemia during which a specific drug is efficacious—appears to be no more than 2 hours in the perinatal experimental animal.

More recently, specific growth factors, including IGF, have been found useful in reducing the severity of perinatal hypoxic-ischemic brain damage. Johnston, et al have shown in late-gestation fetal sheep that the infusion of IGF into the lateral ventricle of the brain at 2 hours of recovery is associated with a reduction in the severity of neuronal loss in selected regions of the brain. The beneficial effect is dose dependent. The precise mechanism whereby growth factors promote neuronal rescue after cerebral hypoxia-ischemia is unknown. Unfortunately, all growth factors are large molecules and cross the blood-brain barrier poorly. Accordingly, systemic administration of the factors would have little effect on the brain, which minimizes their potential as neuroprotective agents in perinatal cerebral hypoxia-ischemia.

R. Vannucci, M.D.

Nerve Growth Factor Protects the Neonatal Brain Against Hypoxic-Ischemic Injury

Holtzman DM, Sheldon RA, Jaffe W, et al (Washington Univ, St Louis; Univ of California, San Francisco)

Ann Neurol 39:114–122, 1996 7–6

Background.—Research has shown that nerve growth factor (NGF) protects specific neurons that express its signaling receptor, trkA, from various insults. Some studies show that NGF has neuroprotective actions beyond cells expressing trkA. The ability of NGF to protect against brain injury in a neonatal model of hypoxia-ischemia was determined.

Methods.—On postnatal day 7, a right carotid ligation was performed in rat pups, which then were exposed to hypoxic conditions. Before and 48 hours after carotid ligation, the pups were given an intracerebroventricular injection of NGF, denatured NGF dissolved in vehicle, or vehicle alone. On postnatal day 21, the pups were killed and their brains examined.

Findings.—Significant damage to the striatum and cortex ipsilateral to the carotid ligation was observed in pups receiving vehicle and denatured NGF. A volume loss of 30% to 40% was documented in these animals. Most NGF-treated pups, however, had only a 10% volume loss. In NGF injection studies, NGF was found to have stimulated tyrosine phosphorylation of trkA in multiple brain regions (Fig 4).

Conclusions.—In this neonatal model of hypoxia-ischemia, NGF appeared to be globally neuroprotective to the developing brain. There may

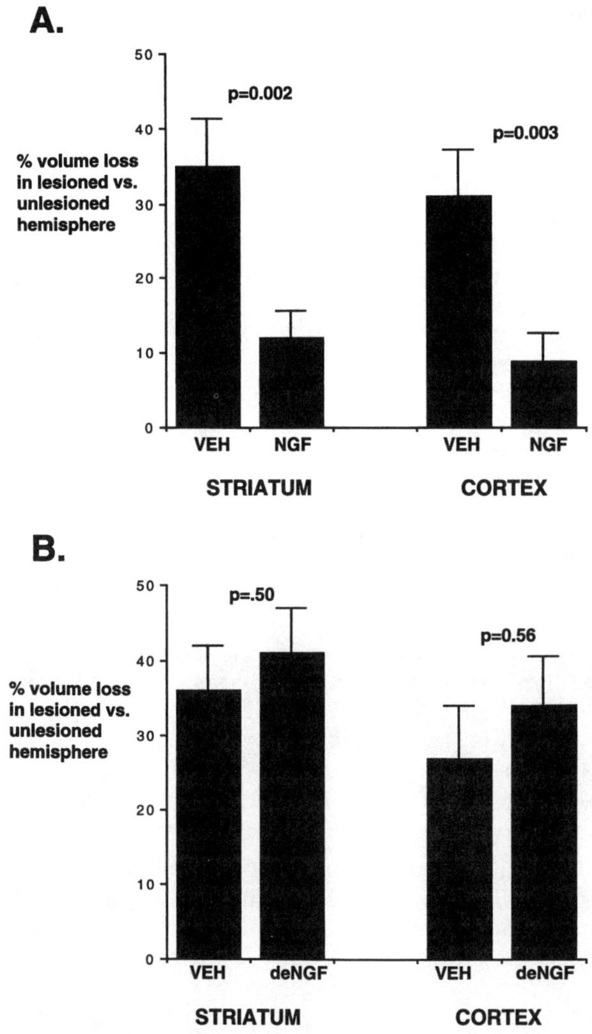

FIGURE 4.—Nerve growth factor (*NGF*) significantly protected against hypoxic-ischemic damage to both the striatum and the cortex, but denatured NGF (*deNGF*) had no significant effect. The volume of tissue in the striatum and cortex ipsilateral to the carotid ligation (lesioned hemisphere) was compared in each animal to the volume of tissue remaining in the striatum and cortex contralateral to the carotid ligation (unlesioned hemisphere). The percentage (96%) of volume loss in each structure then was determined in each animal, and the data are presented as mean plus or minus standard error of the mean for each group, as follows: **A**, striatum-vehicle (35 ± 6.4, n = 23), striatum-NGF (11.9 ± 3.8, n = 22), cortex-vehicle (30.9 ± 6.2 n = 23), cortex-NGF (8.8 ± 4, n = 22); and **B**, striatum-vehicle (36 ± 6.2, n = 17), striatum-denatured NGF (41 ± 6, n = 17), cortex-vehicle (27 ± 7, n ± 17), cortex-denatured NGF (34 ± 6.5, n = 17). The Mann-Whitney rank sum test was used to compare groups. *Abbreviation: VEH,* vehicle. (Courtesy of Holtzman DM, Sheldon RA, Jaffe W, et al: Nerve growth factor protects the neonatal brain against hypoxic-ischemic injury. *Ann Neurol* 39:114–122, 1996. By permission of Little, Brown and Company.)

be novel mechanisms in vivo through which NGF exerts its protective actions.

▶ The mechanisms that underlie neonatal hypoxic-ischemic brain injury have now been fairly well defined. Several theories have emerged regarding how to protect the brain against such injury, and these can be tested in animal models. But (and this is a big but) it is a far cry from experimenting with animals, in which the neuroprotective agent can be administered before the insult, and working with human fetuses, in whom the timing of the insult usually is undetermined and the therapy predominantly will have to be administered after the insult. Hence, there is evidence that blockade of *N*-methyl-D-asparate receptors in the rat model is neuroprotective. Neurotrophic factors, including NGF (as demonstrated in this study) and insulin-like growth factor, also may be neuroprotective. It will be important to determine whether NGF administration still will be effective if it is given after the hypoxic-ischemic insult. There is still much basic science and molecular biology to be studied before any of these potential therapies arrive at the clinical arena. Until then, we must strive to recognize the fetus in distress and prevent a major cause of neonatal morbidity, distress to the family, and potential burden for society. (See also Abstracts 5–1 and 7–4.)

A.A. Fanaroff, M.B.B.Ch.

Nitric Oxide Synthase Inhibition Attenuates Delayed Vasodilation and Increases Injury After Cerebral Ischemia in Fetal Sheep

Marks KA, Mallard CE, Roberts I, et al (Hammersmith Hosp, London; Univ of Auckland, New Zealand)

Pediatr Res 40:185–191, 1996 7–7

Background.—In fetal sheep, transient cerebral ischemia is followed by delayed cerebral injury associated with cerebral vasodilation. Because nitric oxide mediates vasodilation and neuronal death, the ability of nitric oxide synthesis inhibition to attenuate vasodilation and reduce cerebral injury was explored.

Methods.—Eleven fetal sheep were studied late in gestation. Two hours after 30 minutes of transient cerebral ischemia in utero, 5 received a continuous infusion of N^G-nitro-L-arginine, 50 mg/hr for 4 hours followed by 20 mg/hr for the subsequent study period; and 6 fetuses received PBS.

Findings.—The delayed increase in cerebral blood volume began at 13.1 hours after ischemia in the control group and at 12.7 hours in the treatment group. The maximum increases at 30–36 hours were 0.5 and 1.2 mL/100g, respectively, in the treatment and control groups. Final cerebral blood volume was depressed to less than pre-ischemic values in the treatment group only. Also, the treatment group had increased cerebral injury.

Conclusion.—The inhibition of nitric oxide synthesis attenuates the delayed increase in cerebral blood volume after transient cerebral ischemia in fetal sheep. However, it does not reduce the extent of cerebral injury.

► This comment has been provided by William D. Rhine, M.D., Assistant Professor of Pediatrics, Stanford University School of Medicine; Co-director of ECMO, Lucile Salter Packard Children's Hospital at Stanford, Palo Alto, California:

► Nitric oxide is everywhere these days, including the brain. The authors carefully investigated the premise that inhibition of nitric oxide synthesis would decrease reperfusion *and* injury after cerebral ischemia. They were only halfway correct in their original suppositions. N^{G}-nitro-L arginine did indeed decrease cerebral blood volume after cerebral ischemia. However, reduced cerebral blood volume in either treated or control animals was associated with a worse physiologic and pathologic outcome. The authors therefore had to recognize the relative benefit of cerebral blood flow after an ischemic insult. Perhaps Mother Nature is wise in having more blood flow to a damaged brain. These experiments do not completely rule out the possibility that excessive reperfusion might still be bad. We are left with even more unanswered questions regarding the possible local cellular effects of nitric oxide that are independent of its effects on cerebral circulation.

W.D. Rhine, M.D.

Effect of Hyperglycemia on Ischemic Brain Damage During Hypothermic Circulatory Arrest in Newborn Dogs

Vannucci RC, Rossini A, Towfighi J (Pennsylvania State Univ, Hershey)
Pediatr Res 40:177–184, 1996 7–8

Background.—Hypothermic circulatory arrest is now an established method in the surgical correction of congenital heart anomalies in infants. However, some infants sustain brain damage, even when the duration of cardiac arrest is within the therapeutic window. Hyperglycemia may contribute to this complication. A canine model was used to further investigate this possibility.

Methods.—Newborn pups were anesthetized with halothane, paralyzed, ventilated artificially to maintain normoxia and acid-base balance, then surface-cooled to 20°C. Cardiac arrest was induced with IV potassium chloride. Before surface cooling, 12 pups received a bolus injection of 50% glucose to increase plasma glucose levels to about 33 mmol/L. Another 12 pups received an equivalent volume of 1 N saline. The animals were resuscitated after being asystolic for 1.75 hours. All pups survived and were given time to recover from anesthesia. After 8 hours, their brains were perfusion-fixated for pathologic assessment.

Findings.—The 2 groups had no significant differences in severity of neuronal necrosis in the cerebral cortex or caudate nucleus. Greater brain damage was apparent in the amygdaloid nucleus and in the brain stem of the hyperglycemic pups. Severity of the brain damage was positively associated with plasma glucose levels for the caudate nucleus and amygdaloid nucleus but not the cerebral cortex.

Conclusion.—Hyperglycemia with hypothermic circulatory arrest in newborn pups appears to accentuate brain damage in certain brain regions. The caudate and amygdaloid nuclei and brain stem are particularly affected, whereas the cerebral cortex is not.

▶ Just when you thought that glucose was good for you, Vannucci, et al. point out that if a little bit is good, a lot more may not always be, depending on the circumstances. The circumstance in this case is hypothermic circulatory arrest, a procedure often used for surgical correction of congenital heart anomalies in human infants. To be fair, Vannucci, et al. limit their comments to the newborn dog undergoing hypothermic circulatory arrest, concluding that glucose supplementation and associated hyperglycemia are certainly not protective and appear to be deleterious, at least for selective structures of the dog brain.

The relevance of these data to the human circumstance remains unclear, but we are left wondering whether cardiac arrest at normothermia complicated by hyperglycemia might be more damaging as well as more frequently encountered in the postnatal period by neonatologists. Can't something just be "good" for once and not qualified by the phrase "it depends"?

D.K. Stevenson, M.D.

The Correlation of Elevated Levels of an Index of Lipid Peroxidation (MDA-TBA) With Adverse Outcome in the Very Low Birthweight Infant

Inder TE, Darlow BA, Sluis KB, et al (Christchurch School of Medicine, New Zealand; Univ of Otago, New Zealand)

Acta Paediatr 85:1116–1122, 1996 7–9

Background.—Free oxygen radicals appear to be mediators of the tissue damage that results in bronchopulmonary dysplasia, retinopathy of prematurity, and intraventricular bleeding in very low birth weight (VLBW) infants. However, there is little direct evidence of their role in such processes. Increased lipid peroxidation has been associated with poor outcomes in ill, VLBW infants. The relationship between malondialdehyde-thiobarbituric acid (MDA-TBA) concentrations and outcomes in VLBW infants was investigated.

Methods.—Sixty-one VLBW infants in 2 level III neonatal units in New Zealand were enrolled in the prospective, observational, longitudinal study. Concentrations of MDA-TBA were measured in maternal plasma within 48 hours of parturition, in cord plasma, and in infants' plasma on days 2, 7, 14, and 28 of life. These measures were then correlated with antenatal and postnatal factors.

Findings.—At 7 days, increased plasma MDA-TBA levels in the infants were correlated with adverse respiratory and ophthalmologic outcomes. Increased MDA-TBA levels were recorded at sample times close to the time of death in the nonsurvivors.

Conclusion.—These data are consistent with the hypothesis that oxidative injury, especially in the first 7 days of life, is related to the development of long-term complications in preterm infants. Concentrations of MDA-TBA seem to be a useful measurement in the investigation of the role of free radical–mediated disease in VLBW infants.

▶ In this study, the authors examine the relationship between MDA-TBA levels and outcome of VLBW infants. Plasma samples were obtained throughout the neonatal course in infants assessed as having or not having chronic lung disease (CLD) defined as an oxygen requirement at 36 weeks' gestational age. The MDA-TBA levels correlated with values for forced inspiratory oxygen fraction of inspired oxygen at all sample times. The MDA-TBA levels and MDA-TBA levels at 7 days were significantly higher in infants who died or in whom CLD developed. The MDA-TBA value was higher in infants who died than in survivors with CLD.

This article raises important questions regarding the role of oxidant injury in the development of complications of prematurity. Oxidative stress has been mentioned as playing a theoretical role in CLD by others investigators in recent years. In this article, a direct, valid measurement of oxidant injury is shown to correlate with the outcome. Using high performance liquid chromatography to evaluate MDA-TBA adducts gives a very specific index of lipid peroxidation, unlike the TBA assay.

It is still perplexing that oxidative injury seems to peak by 7 days but remains correlated with long-term survival. Perhaps the authors' explanation that the beginning of steroid therapy results in a subsequent fall in the MDA-TBA level is correct. Alas, the abatement of TBA-MDA by steroids does not appear to result in a better outcome, suggesting that critical injury to developing lung cells has occurred in the interim. Therefore, this study raises questions as to whether our interventions for the prevention of CLD (i.e., steroids) are too late, even if done by the seventh day of life. Nonetheless, the clinical trial by Shinwell, et al[1] reminds us that the jury is still out regarding use of early postnatal dexamethasone in preventing CLD in our smallest preterm infants.

Reference

1. Shinwell ES, Karplus M, Zmora E, et al: Failure of early postnatal dexamethasone to prevent chronic lung disease in infants with respiratory distress syndrome. *Arch Dis Child Fetal Neonatal Ed* 74:F33–37, 1996.

D.K. Stevenson, M.D.

Bilateral Cystic Periventricular Leukomalacia in the Premature Infant: Associated Risk Factors

Perlman JM, Risser R, Broyles RS (Univ of Texas, Dallas)
Pediatrics 97:822–827, 1996 7–10

Background.—A major cause of neurodevelopmental delay in premature infants is bilateral cystic periventricular leukomalacia (PVL). Early identification of preterm infants at greatest risk for this lesion is essential. The basic features of symmetric cystic PVL, the relationship between perinatal clinical events and PVL, and the feasibility of early identification of those at greatest risk were investigated.

Methods.—The medical records and cranial US scans of 632 infants with birth weights of less than 1,750 g were reviewed. Periventricular leukomalacia developed in 14 infants (with a mean birth weight of 1,285 and a mean gestational age of 29.4 weeks). Severe intraventricular hemorrhage developed in 21 infants and intraparenchymal echodensity in 12 (with a mean birth weight of 904 and a gestational age of 26.6 weeks). Five hundred eighty-five infants with birth weights of 1,315 g and gestational ages of 29.7 weeks with normal US findings or grade I or II intraventricular hemorrhage comprised a control group.

Findings.—Cystic PVL was found in 2.3% of the infants weighing less than 1,750 g and in 3.2% of those weighing less than 1,500 g. In 10 infants, cysts were found between days 7 and 14 of life; in 4 infants, they were found between days 20 and 46. Seventy percent of the infants had relatively benign clinical courses. Most cases were found by routine US surveillance. Three infants (21%) had overt hypotension in the immediate perinatal period, with late hypotension developing in 1 additional patient. In a univariate analysis, prolonged rupture of the membranes (PROM) and chorioamnionitis significantly predicted PVL. The estimated odds ratio for PROM was 6.6, with a sensitivity of 28.6% and a positive predictive value of 11.5%. For chorioamnionitis, the estimated odds ratio was 6.77, with a 21.4% sensitivity and an 11.5% positive predictive value.

Conclusions.—In this series, most cases of symmetric cystic PVL occurred in infants with relatively benign clinical courses and were detected by routine US screening. Associated postnatal systemic hypotension appears to be uncommon. Preterm infants of mothers with PROM and/or chorioamnionitis seem to have an increased risk of PVL development and require careful evaluation.

▶ This comment has been provided by Phyllis A. Dennery, M.D., Assistant Professor of Pediatrics, Stanford University School of Medicine, Lucile Salter Packard Children's Hospital at Stanford, Palo Alto, California:

▶ Perlman, et al. attempted to identify which preterm infants were at highest risks for development of bilateral cystic PVL. Many previous studies have shown that this lesion is associated with poor neurologic outcome, especially if larger cysts are found.[1] The associated risk factors for the development of PVL were systemic hypotension, prolonged rupture of membranes, PROM, and/or chorioamnionitis. The correlation of PVL and PROM had been made previously by Italian investigators who showed that infants born with PROM were more likely to have severe neurologic impairment than were controls.[2] This further corroboration by Perlman and colleagues should give us a healthy respect for PROM and chorioamnionitis and encourage aggressive detection and treatment. Hopefully, markers such as interleukin-6 [3] could help our obstetric colleagues detect chorioamnionitis early and perhaps obviate the development of PVL in infants at risk. The dilemma will be whether it is safest to deliver early in the face of PROM to prevent potential neurologic sequelae, but risk exposing the neonate to other equally severe complications of prematurity.

P.A. Dennery, M.D.

References

1. Fazzi E, Orcesi S, Caffi L, et al: Neurodevelopmental outcome at 5–7 years in preterm infants with periventricular leukomalacia. *Neuropediatrics* 25:134–139, 1994.
2. Spinello A, Capusso E, Stronati M, et al: Effect of preterm premature rupture of membranes on neurodevelopmental outcome: Follow up at two years of age. *Br J Obstet Gynaecol* 102:882–887, 1995.
3. Yoon BH, Kim CJ, Jun JK: Amniotic fluid interleukin-6: A sensitive test for antenatal diagnosis of acute inflammatory lesions of preterm placenta and prediction of perinatal morbidity. *Am J Obstet Gynecol* 172:960–970, 1995.

Effects of Hypocarbia on the Development of Cystic Periventricular Leukomalacia in Premature Infants Treated With High-frequency Jet Ventilation

Wiswell TE, Graziani LJ, Kornhauser MS, et al (Thomas Jefferson Univ, Philadelphia)

Pediatrics 98:918–924, 1996 7–11

Background.—Cystic periventricular leukomalacia (CPVL) indicates damage to the cerebral white matter. Most neonates with CPVL have cerebral palsy or other neurodevelopmental problems. Most premature infants with CPVL have received mechanical ventilation. Marked hypocarbia in premature infants who are conventionally ventilated during the first 3 days of life is associated with a higher risk of CPVL. It is unclear whether neonates treated with high-frequency ventilation are more likely to have periventricular leukomalacia because the term "periventricular leukomalacia" has been used for both hyperechoic (echodense) and hypoechoic (cystic) findings. High-frequency jet ventilation can effectively lower partial pressure of carbon dioxide in arterial blood ($PaCO_2$) levels. One study reported no differences in the rate of intracranial hemorrhage between neonates treated with high-frequency jet ventilation and neonates treated with conventional ventilation, but this study did not report periventricular leukomalacia findings. Risk factors for CPVL in premature infants receiving high-frequency jet ventilation during the first 72 hours of life were evaluated.

Methods.—There were 63 premature infants born at 33 weeks' gestation or less who were treated with high-frequency jet ventilation as rescue therapy for a mean of 44 hours during their first 3 days of life. Initial treatment was with a conventional ventilator. Indications for rescue therapy were progressive pulmonary interstitial emphysema, pneumothorax or pneumopericardium, needing peak inspiratory pressures of more than 30 cm water to maintain oxygenation while receiving a fraction of inspired oxygen of 1.00, and $PaCO_2$ levels of more than 60 mm Hg in spite of peak inspiratory pressures of more than 30 cm water and 60 breaths or more per minute. The effects of hypotension, acidosis, hypoxemia, and hypocarbia on the development of periventricular leukomalacia were measured. Threshold levels were assigned to specific critical values of these parameters, such as a mean $PaCO_2$ of 20 mm Hg, and an area above the curve between longitudinally connected values of the parameters and threshold levels was calculated.

Results.—Of the 67 infants, 9 died before age 21 days. Of the 58 who survived past 21 days, 18 had large CPVL. The birth weight, gestational age, and nearly all other antepartum, intrapartum, and postpartum parameters were similar in infants with cysts compared with these parameters in the 40 infants who did not have CPVL. In infants who had CPVL, there was a significantly higher risk of moderate or severe periventricular echodensities before the development of CPVL and of periventricular echodensities that persisted longer. No effect of hypotension, acidosis, or hypoxemia on the development of CPVL was detected. At a threshold level of 15 mm Hg, no differences were found in mean $PaCO_2$, absolute low $PaCO_2$ values, or ranges of low $PaCO_2$ values between groups. At a threshold level of 20 mm Hg, no differences were found in mean $PaCO^2$, absolute low $PaCO^{2}$ values, or ranges of low $PaCO^{2}$ in the area above the curve measurements. Logistic regression analysis showed that CPVL was a significant independent risk factor for a greater cumulative hypocarbia below a threshold level of 25 mm Hg during the first 24 hours of life.

Discussion.—In infants treated with high-frequency jet ventilation, the cumulative effect of hypocarbia at levels below 25 mm Hg was associated with CPVL. The presence of CPVL is the best indicator of long-term neurologic problems in premature infants. Comparative studies of the outcome of treatment with conventional ventilation and various high-frequency ventilation devices are needed. The cause of CPVL in preterm infants treated with high-frequency jet ventilation and the role of hypocarbia are unknown.

▶ When considering injury to the nervous system, there has been a tendency to focus on oxygenation and perfusion, with little attention directed at carbon dioxide. Carbon dioxide tension, particularly in the first hours of life, may be of great significance for the development of not only subsequent lung injury, but also white matter injury.[1] Vanucci, et al. suggested that carbon dioxide protects the perinatal brain from hypoxic-ischemic damage.[2] Normocapnic cerebral hypoxia-ischemia was associated with less damage than hypocapnic hypoxia-ischemia, and the least damage was noted with mild hypercapnia. They could not account for the physiologic or biochemical mechanism, whereby carbon dioxide protects the brain. Perlman looked at the associated risk factors for bilateral CPVL, and documented that most of the cases followed relatively benign clinical courses, that prolonged/premature rupture of membranes and/or chorioamnionitis were common antecedents, and that postnatal systemic hypotension was an uncommon event.[3]

Wiswell and colleagues force us to rethink our policies and strategies of ventilation, particularly on the first day of life. With increased use of antenatal steroids and liberal use of surfactant, it is easy to render the infants hypocarbic. Gentle ventilation may be the desirable way to go to prevent brain and lung injury.

...they be blind leaders of the blind. And if the blind lead the blind, both shall fall into the ditch.—Matthew 15:14.

A.A. Fanaroff, M.B.B.Ch.

References

1. Graziani LJ, Spitzer AR, Mitchell DG, et al: Mechanical ventilation in preterm infants: Neurosonographic and developmental studies. *Pediatrics* 90:515–522, 1992.
2. Vanucci R, Towfighi J, Heitjan DF: Carbon dioxide protects the perinatal brain from hypoxic-ischemic damage: An experimental study in the immature rat. *Pediatrics* 95:868–874, 1995.
3. Perlman JM, Risser R: Bilateral cystic-periventricular leukomalacia in the premature infant: Associated risk factors. *Pediatrics* 97:822–827, 1996.

Fetal Sensory Competencies

Lecanuet J-P, Schaal B (Université Paris V-CNRS; INRA-CNRS, Nouzilly, France)

Eur J Obstet Gynecol Reprod Biol 68:1–23, 1996 7–12

Background.—Research on the functioning of fetal sensory systems during gestation is accumulating. Data on the presence of potential sensory stimulation in the fetal milieu, the sequential functional development of the sensory systems, and physiologic and behavioral responses of fetuses to various types of stimulation were reviewed.

Fetal Sensory Competencies.—Most studies have focused on auditory and chemosensory responsiveness in the second half of gestation. Motor and heart rate responsiveness has been shown to depend on gestational age and characteristics of stimulation. In addition, fetal sensory experience apparently has short- and long-term effects at morphologic, functional, and behavioral levels.

To a certain degree, human fetuses can memorize certain sensory properties of their environment, even though they spend much of their time asleep. Extending the Maurer and Maurer hypotheses, full consciousness, defined as the result of the interaction among several brain levels, may gradually develop during brain maturation. Sensory perceptions may initially be organized following "amodal" processes. The polysensorial world of adults may be simplified into a monosensory experience for fetuses.

According to a more classical point of view on consciousness, the poor development of modulatory cortical neurons and the very limited development of associative intrahemispheric and interhemispheric pathways do not allow the conscious processing of sensory inputs. As a result, stored memories in the fetal period and first years of life cannot be retrieved voluntarily, as they have been stored according to a processing mode that is not directly compatible with the functioning of the aroused child or adult brain.

Conclusion.—Research on fetal sensory abilities may have important clinical implications. In fact, almost all studies of fetal response to vibroacoustic stimulation have been done in an attempt to find a fast, practical, reliable method for diagnosing fetal hypoxia. The main limitation to the systematic reliability of analysis of responsiveness to sensory stimulation as a diagnostic tool is cyclic change in fetal behavioral states.

▶ As neonatologists assume care for increasingly immature patients, understanding fetal sensory competencies becomes increasingly important for interpreting the behavioral responses of these displaced fetuses. Increasingly, parents ask questions about how environmental stimuli affect development. In particular, the consequences of the prenatal sensory experience seem of interest to parents, and some understanding of fetal capacities as well as the clinical consequences of external or maternal stimulation—which may include structural, functional, or behavioral effects—should be appreciated by the neonatologist. This review should be added to the meager information available in most standard neonatology textbooks, which deal only cursorily with this topic.

D.K. Stevenson, M.D.

Screening Infants for Hearing Impairment

Vohr BR, Maxon AB (Brown Univ, Providence, RI; Univ of Connecticut, Storrs)

J Pediatr 128:710–714, 1996 7–13

Background.—Sensorineural hearing impairment can have devastating developmental effects in infants, impacting speech and language skills and academic performance. Early identification, habilitation, and amplification can improve the developmental outcome. Screening programs have been designed for both the total population and for high-risk populations. Hearing screening focusing on infants with risk factors can miss up to 50% of the children who ultimately receive a diagnosis of sensorineural hearing loss. Effective programs for the total population have been developed in countries with a national health system. The history of infant hearing screening methods was reviewed.

Screening Methods.—Behavioral observation techniques involve noting physical responses to auditory stimuli. These techniques are time-consuming, only identify infants with bilateral severe hearing loss, and have a high false negative rate. The Crib-o-gram is an objective method of measuring motor response to auditory stimuli, which is also time-consuming, has poor test-retest reliability, and has high false positive rates. The auditory response cradle is another automated device that is limited by its poor sensitivity and specificity and its ability to identify only infants with severe hearing loss. The measurement of brain stem auditory evoked response (BAER) to a click stimulus, using surface electrodes on the skull, has been found to be reliable in the identification of infants with bilateral severe to profound sensorineural hearing loss and has been promising in the identification of unilateral hearing loss. The need for a trained audiologist for testing and interpretation may be obviated by a newer automated BAER technique that requires further testing to confirm its efficacy. Measurement of transient evoked otoacoustic emissions (TEOAE) to a click stimulus indicates when hearing levels are greater than 30 dB but cannot indicate the audiometric threshold. The TEOAE requires less time than the BAER and can be administered, but it may require ear canal dilation and removal of debris.

Conclusions.—The BAER, which is a threshold-specific test, and the TEOAE, which is a frequency-specific test, appear to be the most useful universal hearing screening tools for neonates. It is recommended that all infants be screened for sensorineural hearing loss within the first 3 months of life.

▶ The plea for universal screening for hearing impairment continues to fall on some deaf ears, and only a small proportion of hospitals across the country have universal screening programs in place. As Dr. Vohr points out, the goal of "Healthy People 2000"[1] to reduce the age of identification of hearing impairment in the United States to less than 12 months has not yet been attained. Nonetheless, screening technologies have improved, and cost considerations ultimately play a role in the decision to provide universal screening for hearing impairment. There are some important differences between the most popular technologies, TEOAE and BAER. Studies[2, 3] support the use of either technology for screening with proponents having their references. That the TEOAE represents energy produced by healthy outer hair cells in response to a sound stimulus and is frequency specific and the BAER represents the evoked neurotransmission in the eighth cranial nerve and the brain stem and is threshold specific indicates that information obtained from the 2 kinds of testing may differ. For example, the TEOAE technology might be inappropriate for evaluating certain bilirubin toxicity effects that have been associated with later hearing impairment. If the cost of an automated BAER could be in the same range as TEOAE testing, then the clinician might get more for the money with the BAER.

D.K. Stevenson, M.D.

References

1. U.S. Department of Health and Human Services: Healthy People 2000: National health promotion and disease, prevention objectives. Washington, DC: Public Health Service, 1990.
2. Stevens JC, Webb HD, Hutchins J, et al: Click evoked otoacoustic emissions in neonatal screening. *Ear Hear* 11:128–133, 1990.
3. Kennedy CR, Kimm L, Dees DC, et al: Otoacoustic emissions and auditory brainstem responses in newborn. *Arch Dis Child* 66:1124–1129, 1991.

Neonatal Otoacoustic Emission Screening and the Identification of Deafness

Watkin PM (Whipps Cross Hosp, London)

Arch Dis Child 74:F16–F25, 1996 7–14

Background.—Because the majority of neonates are discharged from the hospital within 48 hours of birth, neonatal identification of deafness is a challenge. A universal transient evoked otoacoustic emission (TEOAE) screening protocol for infants within the first 3 months of life was developed and implemented in a district of London. A 3-year experience with this screening protocol was reported.

Methods.—The infants were initially tested by TEOAE recording in a small dedicated room within the maternity unit. Ears scored as no response, borderline response, or not possible to screen were identified as screen fails. Infants with bilateral failing initial tests were referred for a retest in the audiology department of the hospital. Infants with bilateral retest failures were referred for auditory brain stem response (ABR).

Results.—During the 3-year period, 14,353 infants were screened. There were bilateral failures of the initial test in 13%, including 10% with no response, 2% with borderline responses, and 1% who could not be adequately tested. Both TEOAE screens were failed in both ears in 1.75% of the infants. Of 887 infants with unilateral failures retested by TEOAE recording, 108 (0.9% of the study population) had confirmed unilateral failure. Diagnostic audiologic assessment determined that 23 infants had a permanent hearing impairment, yielding a prevalence of 2 per 1,000 neonates.

Discussion.—The program was highly sensitive in the detection of hearing impairments in infants. The 3-pronged screening protocol also increased the specificity of screening for the identification of deafness. In addition, the cost of implementing the program was reasonable, and the cost per hearing-impaired child was similar to that of other accepted targeted at-risk screening programs.

Infant Hearing Screening With an Automated Auditory Brainstem Response Screener and the Auditory Brainstem Response

Chen S-J, Yang EY, Kwan M-L, et al (Natl Yang-Ming Univ, Taipei, Taiwan; Dalhousie Univ, Halifax, NS, Canada)

Acta Paediatr 85:14–18, 1996 7–15

Background.—Early detection of hearing loss in children enables prompt intervention to maximize treatment benefits. The auditory brain stem response (ABR) procedure is the most objective test in newborns. However, this test requires trained personnel and costly equipment. The usefulness of the newly developed automated ABR screener, the Algo-1 Plus, as a screening tool was assessed.

Methods.—Two hundred sixty of 1,653 infants hospitalized at 1 center from 1993 to 1995 were at risk for hearing impairment. Risk criteria were based on the United States Joint Committee on Infant Hearing 1990 Position Statement recommendations. The infants were screened with the Algo-1 Plus screener at a mean postconceptional age of 40 weeks.

Findings.—Thirty-nine infants (15%) failed the screening in 57 ears. All but 1 infant (who had died) had an ABR test for air- and bone-conducted stimuli and an otologic examination. At the initial ABR test, the case-specific incidence of conductive hearing deficit was 5.4%. The prevalence of sensorineural hearing deficits ranged from 2.3% (confirmed) to 3.1% (including infants who had no follow-up tests). The agreement between Algo-1 and ABR results was 0.64. The overall efficiency of using Algo-1 to identify a pass or fail correctly on the ABR was 83%.

Conclusion.—With a 93% sensitivity and a 95% negative predictive value, the Algo-1 showed a high probability that infants who passed were unlikely to fail the ABR. Consistent with previous studies, this study found a marked discrepancy between the initial and follow-up ABR tests. The reversal probably resulted from a transient conductive deficit.

▶ Betty Vohr, M.D., Professor of Pediatrics, Brown University School of Medicine and Director, Rhode Island Hearing Assessment Program, comments:

▶ The importance of early identification and intervention in infants with permanent hearing loss is well established. The prevalence of newborn and infant hearing loss ranges from 1.5 to 6 per 1,000 births. The 1990s have seen the emergence of important new technological developments pertaining to infant hearing screening. In 1990, the United States Department of Health and Human Services set a Healthy People 2000 goal to reduce the average age at which significant hearing loss is identified to 12 months.[1] The National Institutes of Health consensus report[2] in 1993 recommended screening all infants for hearing loss in the first 3 months of life, preferably before hospital discharge. A 2-stage screening method using TEOAE and ABR was recommended. Finally, the Joint Committee on Infant Hearing issued a statement in 1994 endorsing universal detection of infants with hearing loss.[3]

These statements and recommendations have resulted in the emergence of hundreds of new hearing screening and research programs throughout the United States and abroad. Although some programs continue to screen "at-risk" populations, others have embarked on universal screening. The 2 studies presented here report efforts to address the issue of newborn hearing screening in Taiwan and England.

Chen, et al. (Abstract 7–15) investigated a 2-stage hearing screen protocol using the Algo-1 automated screen followed by standard air- and bone-conduction ABR for infants failing in a population of 1,653 infants with risk factors present. Fifteen percent of infants failed the automated screen. The initial standard ABR test identified a 5.4% incidence of conductive loss and a 2.3% incidence of confirmed sensorineural loss. The use of automated devices such as the Algo-1 are ideal for new universal screen programs because they provide rapid screen results that can be obtained by paraprofessionals.

Watkin (Abstract 7–14) reports the results of a 2-stage hearing screen program using TEOAE screening followed by the ABR test in a population of 11,606 infants screened during a 3-year period. He reports a stage 1 bilateral fail rate of 13%, and a stage 2 fail rate of 1.75%, with an identification rate of 2 in 1,000. Early discharge (less than 48 hours) in the United Kingdom contributed to the stage 1 13% fail rate. Important findings of this study were the clear demonstration of improved program efficiency during a 3-year period and the fact that universal screen program costs were similar to those of a prior program screening only high-risk infants.

It is apparent from these studies that neonatal screening using different methods and protocols is effective and results in the early identification of infants with significant hearing impairment. The continued development of rapid screen methods such as automated ABR and TEOAE to ensure optimal sensitivity, specificity, and cost-effectiveness are needed if all infants are to benefit. Although significant progress has been made in the 1990s, we have not yet achieved universal screening.

B. Vohr, M.D.

References

1. US Department of Health and Human Services (HHS). *Healthy People 2000: National Health Promotion and Disease Prevention Objectives.* Washington, DC, Public Health Service, 1990.
2. National Institutes of Health: Early identification of hearing impairments in infants and young children. NIH Consensus Statement 11, 1–24, 1993.
3. American Speech-Language-Hearing Association: Joint Committee on Infant Hearing 1994 Position Statement. December 1994, pp 38–41.

Retinopathy of Prematurity in Infants of Birth Weight > 2000 g After Haemorrhagic Shock at Birth

Jandeck C, Kellner U, Kössel H, et al (Freie Universität Berlin)
Br J Ophthalmol 80:728–731, 1996 7–16

Objective.—Because infants of low birth weight and low gestational age are at increased risk of retinopathy of prematurity (ROP), screening is recommended for infants with a birth weight of less than 1,500 g or a gestational age less than 32 weeks. Stage 2 or 3 ROP was unexpectedly found in 3 infants with a birth weight greater than 2,000 g and a gestational age of 32 weeks or more who survived severe hemorrhage at birth. The infants were treated surgically with general anesthesia.

Methods.—Records of the 3 infants were evaluated retrospectively and compared with records of 303 premature infants weighing 1,500 g or less and 149 premature infants weighing more than 1,500 g who needed supplemental oxygen or surgery. Infants were examined using an indirect ophthalmoscope at 5–6 weeks after birth. Any retinopathy was treated.

Results.—The 3 infants experienced severe uterine bleeding, fetal blood loss, severe peripartal asphyxia, acidosis, and low to nonmeasurable blood pressure requiring blood transfusions. Packed cell volumes varied from 0.14 to 0.19, whereas the norm is 0.43 to 0.63. All 3 children had an infection, jejunal atresia, cerebral defects, and/or failure of 1 or more organs. All 3 children required surgery with general anesthesia within a few weeks of birth. No other infants weighing more than 1,650 g at birth had ROP. Of 43 other infants requiring surgery, 6 with birth weights between 550 and 1,010 g undergoing surgery progressed to stage 3 ROP. Three of these were treated by cryocoagulation or laser surgery.

Conclusion.—Because premature infants weighing more than 2,000 g may have ROP if they experience severe fetal blood loss or severe illness, it is recommended that all infants weighing more than 1,500 g at birth be screened for ROP.

▶ Although gestational age is the major determinant of the risk for ROP, this set of anecdotes suggests that severe prenatal blood loss requiring blood transfusions and surgery with general anesthesia may be associated with the risk of ROP, even in infants with birth weights exceeding the usual screening criteria. Because screening has become so routine based on gestational age, the need to screen other infants at particularly high risk for environmental reasons may need to be reconsidered. Although such anecdotes do not prove a causal relationship, caretakers should not exclude other severely ill neonates from screening, particularly if they are still premature. Nature does not know the lines that we draw in practice! Moreover, we do not know all of nature's influences.

D.K. Stevenson, M.D.

Observer Sensitivity to Retinal Vessel Diameter and Tortuosity in Retinopathy of Prematurity: A Model System

Freedman SF, Kylstra JA, Capowski JJ, et al (Duke Univ, Durham, NC; Univ of North Carolina, Chapel Hill)

J Pediatr Ophthalmol Strabismus 33:248–254, 1996 7–17

Purpose.—"Plus disease," characterized by increased diameter and tortuosity of the retinal blood vessels in the posterior pole, is associated with a poor outcome in infants with retinopathy of prematurity (ROP). Plus disease is diagnosed by examination of the retinal blood vessels. However, there have been no studies of the examiner's ability to recognize the relevant abnormalities of blood vessel diameter and tortuosity. Examiner accuracy in recognizing these changes was evaluated using a simple model system.

Methods.—The investigators made black-and-white tracings of posterior pole blood vessels for fundus photographs of eyes with ROP of varying severity. Twelve ophthalmologists and 23 "naive" examiners (college graduates with no ophthalmologic training) were asked to study the tracings and rank them according to vessel diameter and tortuosity. The study model was designed to simulate 3 clinical situations: sequential study over time for progression of ROP, comparison of different eyes with ROP at the same time, and comparison of a standard fundus with a group of distinct fundi.

Results.—Assessments of vessel diameter were more often correct than assessments of vessel tortuosity. This was true for both similar and distinct fundus tracings. Compared with a standard image, the observers correctly ranked 25 different images for mean vessel diameter and tortuosity 89% of the time. There was no relation between the observers' assessments of increasing vessel diameter and increasing tortuosity. There was no difference between the test performance of the ophthalmologists and that of the naive observers.

Conclusions.—Human examiners can identify the increments in blood vessel diameter and tortuosity that constitute plus disease in ROP. Increasing vessel diameter and tortuosity can be recognized even by nonophthalmologists. The ability to recognize these changes may aid in the development of standardized diagnostic techniques for plus disease.

▶ Retinopathy of prematurity still blinds several hundred infants yearly in the United States. Major efforts are under way to define the population at risk and the optimal timing for intervention. Plus disease has emerged as a powerful predictor of poor outcome and a trigger for active intervention.[1] The diagnosis of plus disease is dependent on the observer's ability to recognize abnormalities in the diameter and tortuosity of retinal blood vessels. Participants in the major retinopathy trials all have undergone rigorous certification to standardize intervention and optimize communication between investigators.

I found it fascinating to follow the model that Freedman and colleagues developed to simulate sequential examinations of fundi with and without disease. It was somewhat reassuring to note that "human observers were quite accurate at recognizing and comparing increments in retinal blood vessel diameter and tortuosity, regardless of prior ophthalmologic training." That does not translate into an inexperienced observer being able to assess a fundus, because it is a far cry from leisurely studying a still, focused drawing or picture to the transient, barely focused glimpse of the infant's fundus. I have been impressed with the patience and endurance necessary to achieve a thorough examination of the immature infant's fundus. Retinal photography is still unreliable, but if image acquisition improves, more precise classification of the vascular abnormalities and the recognition of "pre-plus" disease may facilitate even earlier intervention and save more sight.

A.A. Fanaroff, M.B.B.Ch.

Reference

1. Cryotherapy for Retinopathy of Prematurity Cooperative Group: Multicenter trial of cryotherapy for retinopathy of prematurity: Preliminary results. *Arch Ophthalmol* 106:471–480, 1988.

Multicenter Trial of Cryotherapy for Retinopathy of Prematurity: Snellen Visual Acuity and Structural Outcome at 5½ Years After Randomization

Palmer EA, and Cryotherapy for Retinopathy of Prematurity Cooperative Group (Univ of Portland, Ore)

Arch Ophthalmol 114:417–424, 1996 7–18

Background.—The Multicenter Trial of Cryotherapy for Retinopathy of Prematurity (ROP) has shown that cryotherapy substantially decreases the incidence of blindness and poor visual acuity outcomes in patients with threshold ROP. However, it does not increase the chance of normal recognition visual acuity. Outcomes at 5.5 years after randomization to cryotherapy or no treatment were reported.

Methods.—Two hundred ninety-one children born preterm, with birth weights of less than 1,251 g, were studied. Two hundred forty had bilateral threshold ROP and received cryotherapy in 1 eye but not the other. The 51 patients with threshold ROP in only 1 eye were assigned randomly to treatment or no treatment.

Outcomes.—Unfavorable outcomes were reduced in the treated eyes, compared with those in the untreated eyes. The outcomes of visual acuity were poor in 61.7% of untreated eyes and in 47.1% of treated eyes. Fundus status was unfavorable in 45.4% of the untreated group and 26.9% of the treated group. Forty-eight percent of the untreated eyes were blind, compared with 31.5% of treated eyes. However, there was a slight trend toward fewer eyes with a visual acuity of 20/40 or better in the treated than in the untreated eyes.

Conclusions.—Caution is warranted in using cryotherapy in the treatment of eyes with retinopathy less severe than threshold ROP. Most eyes with ROP less severe than threshold have good structural outcomes and will probably have good function.

Early Retinal Vessel Development and Iris Vessel Dilatation as Factors in Retinopathy of Prematurity

Kivlin JD, for the Cryotherapy for Retinopathy of Prematurity (CRYO-ROP) Cooperative Group (Med College of Wisconsin, Milwaukee; et al)

Arch Ophthalmol 114:150–154, 1996 7–19

Background.—Whether the degree of vessel development found on early screening tests helps predict the occurrence of retinopathy of prematurity

(ROP) has been difficult to determine. However, sufficient prospective data to determine the prognostic value of early screening for ROP are now available from the Multicenter Trial of Cryotherapy for Retinopathy of Prematurity.

Methods.—Zone I vessel development was defined as vessels extending from the disc to less than twice the distance from the disc to the macula. Zone II development included vessels extending beyond zone I but not to the nasal ora serrata. Eyes with vessels partly in zone I and partly in zone II were classified as transitional. Forty-eight eyes were categorized as zone I, 245 as transitional, and 1,847 as zone II.

Findings.—The chance of having threshold ROP develop was correlated inversely with the early degree of vessel development, being 54% for zone I, 25% for transitional, and 8% for zone II eyes. Prominent iris vessels observed at 34–35 weeks' postmenstrual age were associated with an increased risk in all 3 groups. Ninety-four percent of zone I eyes with this finding needed treatment. The chance of an unfavorable anatomical change in the posterior fundus or poor vision at 1 and 3.5 years of age also was correlated inversely with the degree of early vessel development.

Conclusions.—The need for ablative treatment is more likely in infants with retinal vessels only in zone I on early assessment. If vessels remain in zone I on 2 or more examinations done 2 weeks apart, there is a 54% chance of the development of threshold disease. If the retinal vasculature has progressed into any part of zone II at the the second examination, this risk is decreased to 25%. When vessels end entirely in zone II, there is only an 8% chance of threshold disease. However, the findings of prominent iris vessels at 34–35 weeks of postmenstrual age diminishes the safety for zone II eyes, and more frequent assessments may be necessary.

▶ Two reports provide us with further important data from the massive collaborative, multicenter cryotherapy study. The information from this study has already extended well beyond its main purpose, which was to define the role of cryotherapy in preventing severe ROP. The meticulous, standardized observations and photographic records of this population provide information on the natural history of ROP that is simply not obtainable elsewhere.

In the article by Kivlin (Abstract 7–19), we find that at the 4- to 6-week examination, the degree of retinal vessel development (as measured by the retinal zones) was a significant predictor of ROP outcome and was independent of gestational age, birth weight, and race. This provides important guidance for the ophthalmologist regarding the frequency of future examinations and reduces the likelihood that threshold disease will be missed.

The Cooperative Group's 5½-year outcome (Abstract 7–18) confirms that blindness in the treated eyes (31.5%) was much less common than in the untreated eyes (48%). However, 17% of *control* (untreated) eyes had a visual acuity of 20/40 or better, compared with only 13% of treated eyes ($P = 0.19$). This suggests that although cryosurgery prevents blindness, *in those who will see* it does so at a significant cost to visual acuity. This disappointing finding raises important questions about the adverse effects of cryotherapy on visual acuity. The initial enthusiastic reports of the structural and visual outcomes of cryotherapy must now be tempered somewhat, particularly if there is any movement in the direction of using cryotherapy (or laser therapy) on less severely involved eyes than those defined as "threshold" for the CRYO-ROP study. As the authors point out, the "overwhelming majority of eyes with ROP less severe than threshold have good structural outcome and will very likely have good function." The message is: Intervene at threshold (5 contiguous or 8 cumulative clock hours of stage 3 + ROP in zone II), but no sooner.

M.J. Maisels, M.B., B.Ch.

Postnatal Development of Somatosensory Evoked Potential in Jaundiced Gunn Rats and Effects of Sulfadimethoxine Administration
Silver S, Sohmer H, Kapitulnik J (Hebrew Univ of Jerusalem)
Pediatr Res 40:209–214, 1996 7–20

Background.—The homozygous recessive jj (jaundiced) Gunn rat provides a useful model for studying the kinetics of bilirubin-induced neurotoxicity. The somatosensory evoked potential (SEP), an additional evoked response modality that reflects both peripheral and central activity of the somatosensory pathway, has been found to be a sensitive marker of motor impairment. The postnatal development of the SEP was investigated in young jj rats.

Methods and Findings.—Recordings of the SEP were obtained from jj and nonjaundiced (Jj) rats. Although jaundice did not affect the SEP in young jj rats, adult jj rats had prolonged latencies and reduced amplitudes of the P2 component of the SEP, compared with adult Jj rats. These SEP changes may reflect a synaptic lesion in these rats, possibly because of cumulative and/or progressive damage induced by bilirubin in the first 3 months of life. Sulfadimethoxine administration markedly prolonged the latency periods in the early components of the SEP in young jj, but not Jj, rats as early as 2 hours after injection. These changes became more severe with time and seemed to be mostly peripheral.

Conclusion.—The SEP may be a sensitive marker for the massive entry of bilirubin into the nervous system. It may serve as part of an evoked potential battery in the evaluation of bilirubin-induced neurotoxicity in jaundiced infants.

► If you provide a sensory stimulus (e.g., repetitive clicks into the ear of an infant), you can record the average electrical responses from peripheral and central aspects of the nervous system. These are the evoked potentials that are obtained in response to auditory, visual, or somatosensory repetitive stimuli and reported as brain stem auditory evoked potentials (BAEP, BAER, ABR), visual evoked potentials (VEP), and somatosensory evoked potentials. These measurements permit a noninvasive evaluation of the integrity of the CNS.

Because the SEP is a relatively sensitive measure of motor impairment and because motor impairment is a common finding in infants with bilirubin encephalopathy, these authors measured the SEP in jaundiced Gunn rats and evaluated the effects of sulfadimethoxine administration. This drug is a potent displacer of bilirubin from albumin. We now have another evoked potential measurement to add to those that have already been studied (ABR, VEP) in relationship to hyperbilirubinemia in the newborn, but exactly how these tests can be used in a clinical setting has yet to be defined. For an excellent review of the use of evoked potentials in preterm neonates, please refer to a paper by Taylor, et al.[1]

M.J. Maisels, M.B., B.Ch.

Reference

1. Taylor MJ, Saliba E, Laugier J: Use of evoked potentials in preterm neonates. *Arch Dis Child* 74:F70–F76, 1996.

Intraoperative Vesical Pressure Measurements as a Guide in the Closure of Abdominal Wall Defects

Rizzo A, Davis PC, Hamm CR, et al (Univ of South Alabama, Mobile)
Am Surg 62:192–196, 1996 7–21

Introduction.—In newborns, primary closure of omphalocele and gastroschisis may result in complications such as hemodynamic compromise, respiratory embarrassment, necrotizing enterocolitis, renal insufficiency, and intestinal ischemia. Reduced blood flow secondary to a significant increase in intra-abdominal pressure is the pathogenesis of these complications. Surgical techniques to minimize an increased intra-abdominal pressure include use of synthetic silos with staged reductions, nonoperative coverage with a polymer membrane, and closure with skin flaps leaving a large ventral hernia. As a guide in determining which type of closure to perform, intraoperative vesical pressure measurements can be used, which would improve postoperative care and clinical outcomes. Outcomes with and without vesical pressure measurements in abdominal wall defects were compared.

Methods.—The charts of patients who had undergone abdominal wall closure were reviewed. Recordings were taken of type of defect and closure, weight, gestational age, age at operations, ventilator requirements, urinary output and fluid requirements, days to first and total feeding, hospital days, total parenteral nutrition, hospital charges, morbidity, and mortality. Paired and unpaired Student's *t* tests or Fisher's exact test were used to analyze the results.

Results.—Vesical pressure measurements were not taken for 27 infants, but they were taken for 13 infants. In the parameters recorded in these 2 diverse groups, no significant difference occurred. On postoperative day 2, a significant decrease in IV fluid requirements in the vesical measurement group was found when patients with gastroschisis only were compared

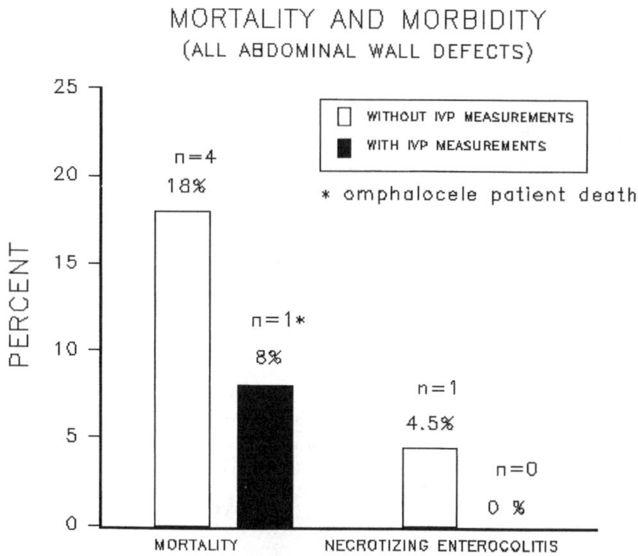

FIGURE 5.—Mortality and morbidity of all patients with abdominal wall defects. Among the 22 infants with gastroschisis and omphalocele who were not monitored with intravesical pressures, 4 (18%) died; 3 of these had omphalocele and 1 (4.5%) had necrotizing enterocolitis. Of the 12 total infants who were monitored with intravesical pressures, 1 infant (8%) with omphalocele died and there were no cases of necrotizing enterocolitis. There were no deaths among patients with gastroschisis who were monitored. *Abbreviation: IVP*, intravesical pressure. (Courtesy of Rizzo A, Davis PC, Hamm CR, et al: Intraoperative vesical pressure measurements as a guide in the closure of abdominal wall defects. *Am Surg* 62:192–196, 1996.)

(155.3 ± 37.5 vs. 109.6 ± 34.3). On postoperative day 3, there was a significant decrease in urinary output for these infants (4.2 ± 112 vs. 3.1 ± 1.1). In the vesical measurement group, ventilatory support, total parenteral nutrition days, and oral feeding data were all lower, but there was no statistical significance. In the vesical measurement group, there was a trend toward lower values for hospital days and hospital charges. In the vesical measurement group, there was 1 death (8%), compared with 4 deaths in the nonmeasured group (18%) (Fig 5).

Conclusions.—To guide the closing of abdominal wall defects, intraoperative vesical pressure measurements represent a simple, effective, and safe method. This may result in less cost and lower morbidity and mortality. Bladder pressure monitoring resulted in good clinical results, and this technique is recommended in the operative repair of all congenital abdominal wall defects.

▶ Improved anesthesia, intraoperative monitoring, surgical instrumentation, and surgical technique have resulted in a rosy outlook for infants with major abdominal wall defects (see Abstract 18–1). However, one must not overlook the many and significant potential complications attendant on primary closure of omphalocele and gastroschisis. These include respiratory failure, hemodynamic compromise, intestinal ischemia, necrotizing enterocolitis, and renal failure. These complications result from increased intra-abdominal pressure on return of the viscera to their rightful place. Monitoring of intra-abdominal pressure, either by vesical pressure measurements as recommended by these authors or by intragastric pressures, is both prudent and the implied standard of care.[1] The critical value is evidently 20 cm H_2O. Pressures less than 20 cm H_2O indicate that primary closure should not be hazardous, whereas pressures greater than 20 cm H_2O call for operative modification and skin flap placement or the use of a Silastic silo. Rizzo and colleagues found a trend toward a more benign postoperative course in the monitored group. There is no reason all infants should not have their intra-abdominal pressure monitored.

A.A. Fanaroff, M.B.B.Ch.

Reference

1. Lacey SR, Carris LA, Beyer AJ III, et al: Bladder pressure monitoring significantly enhances care of infants with abdominal wall defects: A prospective clinical study. *J Pediatr Surg* 28:1370–1375, 1993.

8 Behavior and Pain Management

Breastfeeding, Dummy Use, and Adult Intelligence
Gale CR, Martyn CN (Univ of Southampton, England)
Lancet 347:1072–1075, 1996 8–1

Purpose.—There is evidence that breast-fed infants go on to have better scores on intelligence and language tests than do their bottle-fed peers, although the significance of this link is uncertain. It could result from the nutritional content of breast milk, from some psychological advantage of breast-feeding, or from some factor in the home environment affecting the decision to breast-feed. The association between breast-feeding and higher social class makes it difficult to assess the influence of breast-feeding on intellectual development. The relation between feeding method in infancy and adult intelligence was studied among individuals born when the social connotations of breast-feeding were different.

Methods.—The follow-up study included 994 British men and women born during the 1920s, when breast-feeding was more likely to be practiced by the lower rather than the higher social classes. For each subject, information on feeding method during infancy was available from records of health visits. All subjects took the computerized AH4 intelligence quotient (IQ) test, the results of which were evaluated for relations with method of infant feeding.

Results.—Two thirds of the subjects were breast-fed exclusively, and only 5% were bottle-fed exclusively. Intelligence quotients were somewhat higher in the subjects who had been breast-fed exclusively than in those who had been both breast- and bottle-fed or bottle-fed exclusively. Subjects who had used a pacifier as infants, whose fathers were manual laborers, and whose mothers were young when the subjects were born had lower IQs. Having more older siblings also was associated with lower IQ scores. After adjustment for other variables on multivariate analysis, feeding method was no longer related to IQ. Pacifier use, number of older siblings, maternal age when the subjects were born, and father's occupational class were still significant predictors of adult intelligence, however.

Conclusions.—The higher IQ scores of adults who were breast-fed at birth do not appear to result from the nutritional qualities of breast milk per se but rather from the child's social environment. Other factors, such as maternal age, father's occupation, and number of siblings, are better predictors of adult intelligence than is breast-feeding. There are several possible explanations for the link between pacifier use and lower intelligence.

▶ The debate between nurture and nature, and genetics and environment, is always fun to observe from the sideline. Throw "dummy use," a synonym for "pacifier," into the equation, correlate feeding methodology with adult intelligence, set the scene in Hertfordshire circa 1920–1930 where, according to Eliza Doolittle in *My Fair Lady*, "hurricanes hardly happen," and you have the trappings for a manuscript filled with conjecture. The reader will have to sift through the established facts and decide how best to interpret the data.

Long before there were computers, there were databases, only they were hidden in the county archives. It is a credit to the investigators that they were able to delve through these old records and establish the feeding methodology, pacifier use, and IQ scores of this large cohort born between 1920 and 1930. They also were able to reconstruct the social environment and to establish, beyond a reasonable doubt, that the dummy was regarded as a hazard to the babies' health in that era; hence, health visitors were advised to instruct mothers against its use. The inference is that those who used dummies (pacifiers) were "less educated, less intelligent or had poorer child rearing skills." Even today, in the era of the controlled trial, when comparing breast- and bottle-feeding, there are many confounding factors that cannot be controlled. Causality of differences thus remains an eternal problem.

There are few who dispute that the method of feeding affects early life. There also is a substantial body of evidence denoting superior intellect and language development in breast-fed infants when compared with those who were artificially nourished. Credence to the hypothesis that the apparent relation between IQ and breast-feeding may be genetic or determined by other factors that influence both the choice of feeding methodology and the child's cognitive development are provided in Gale and Martyn's provocative manuscript. Because use of the dummy adversely affected intellect, they suggest that "subsequent intelligence may have more to do with the child's social environment than with the nutritional qualities of the mind." Further, they query whether infants who are willing to accept these counterfeit nipples are destined to be less intelligent that those who refuse them; alternatively, the whole environment of infants presented with the pacifier may be less stimulating.

More questions have been raised and the debate will simmer on. I will continue to express my bias for the belief that the breast-fed baby will not turn out to be the dummy.[1]

A.A. Fanaroff, M.B.B.Ch.

Reference

1. Lucas A, Morley R, Cole TJ, et al: Breast milk and subsequent intelligence quotient in children born preterm. *Lancet* 339:261–264, 1992.

Effect of Non-sucrose Sweet Tasting Solution on Neonatal Heel Prick Responses

Ramenghi LA, Griffith GC, Wood CM, et al (Univ of Leeds, England)

Arch Dis Child 74:F129–F131, 1996 8–2

Background.—Although painful procedures such as heel pricks may seem minor, recent research suggests that infants' early pain experience may adversely affect their pain response later in infancy. Concentrated sucrose solution significantly decreases infants' duration of crying when given immediately before a heel prick blood sampling for serum bilirubin. This response may be mediated by the release of endogenous opiates. Because this sucrose solution has high tonicity and cariogenic effects on erupted teeth, a sweet-tasting, sugar-free solution was tested as a vehicle for paracetamol (Calpol) to reduce pain response after heel prick blood sampling.

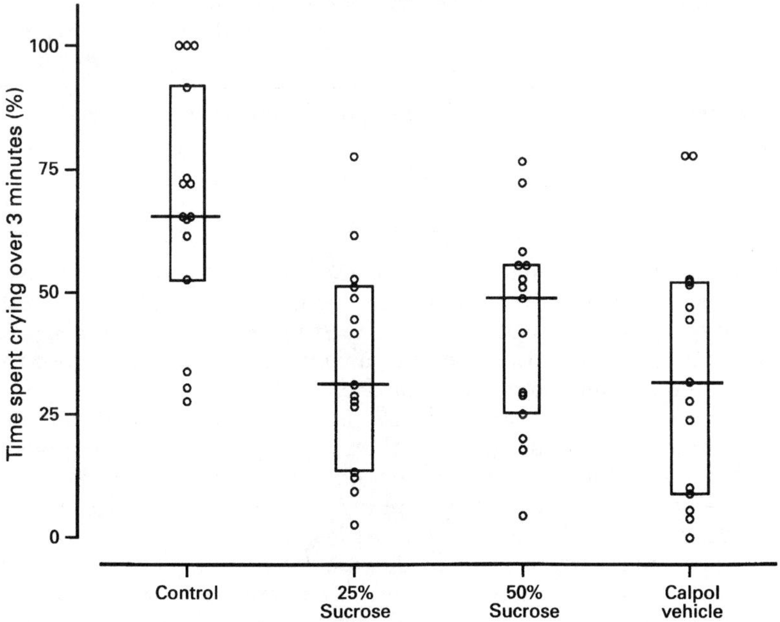

FIGURE 2.—Percentage time spent crying in the first 3 minutes after heel prick in 60 infants. (Courtesy of Ramenghi LA, Griffith GC, Wood CM, et al: Effect of non-sucrose sweet tasting solution on neonatal heel prick responses. *Arch Dis Child* 74:F129–F131, 1996.)

Methods and Findings.—Sixty healthy term newborn infants were assigned randomly to receive sterile water, 25% or 50% sucrose, or the sweet-tasting solution. Solutions were syringed into the infants' mouths for 1 minute, mainly to the anterior part of the tongue. One observer recorded changes in facial expressions and crying. Compared with infants in the control group, infants in the other 3 groups had a significant decrease in duration of crying and pain scores 3 minutes after the painful stimulus was applied (Fig 2).

Conclusions.—The sweet-tasting solution tested has analgesic effects as potent as those of concentrated sucrose solutions. The speed of the Calpol solution response is consistent with a preabsorptive mechanism that stimulates endogenous opiate release.

► We should all be thinking about ways to reduce pain and discomfort in our infants, and now considerable evidence exists that oral sucrose solutions increase the release of endogenous opiates and significantly reduce pain perception. In this study, we find out that this effect can also be achieved by a sweet-tasting, non–sucrose-containing solution (it contained hydrogenated glucose). The 2 mL of the test solution was applied mainly to the anterior part of the tongue to promote taste perception. Dozens of heel sticks are obtained every day in every nursery, and some infants could be stuck 50–100 times during their hospital stay. I can't think of any reason not to make this form of pain relief a routine part of our newborn care.

M.J. Maisels, M.B., B.Ch.

Premature Infant Pain Profile: Development and Initial Validation

Stevens B, Johnston C, Petryshen P, et al (Univ of Toronto; McGill Univ, Montreal; St Michael's Hosp, Toronto)

Clin J Pain 12:13–22, 1996 8–3

Introduction.—In premature infants, there is inadequate assessment of pain, which is an unresolved clinical problem. There is a need for a valid measure that is clinically useful. Using existing research on the responses of premature infants to painful events, a pain measure was developed that could be implemented in clinical practice.

Methods.—To develop and validate the Premature Infant Pain Profile (PIPP), infants of varying gestational ages (32–34 weeks, 28–30 weeks, and 37–40 weeks) undergoing different painful procedures (heel lance and circumcision) were studied in a prospective and retrospective design. Clinical experts and the literature were used to develop indicators of pain: physiologic indicators, such as cardiovascular and respiratory measures (heart rate, vagal tone, respiratory rate, blood pressure, oxygen saturation, intracranial pressure), and endocrine and metabolic indicators (catecholamines, corticosteroids, growth hormone, and glucagon). There also were behavioral indicators, such as facial actions, acoustical and temporal cry characteristics, and body activity and movement. The modifying factors included gestational age, behavioral state, and health status.

Results.—The PIPP had 15 indicators initially, 2 physiologic factors (heart rate and oxygen saturation), 11 behavioral factors (facial actions of brow bulge, eye squeeze, nasolabial furrow, open lips, vertical and horizontal mouth stretch, and taut tone), 4 cry characteristics, and 2 modifying factors (gestational age and behavioral state). An indicator had to be present at least 50% of the time after tissue-damaging stimuli to be considered sensitive. Thus, cry characteristics were not considered sensitive because only 47% of premature infants cried during a painful procedure. The indicators were reduced to 7: brow bulge, eye squeeze, nasolabial furrow, heart rate, oxygen saturation, and behavioral state. Each indicator had a 4-point scale.

Conclusions.—More prospective research in the clinical setting is necessary to determine the practicality and feasibility of this method. The pain experience of premature infants is reflected most heavily by upper facial activity, physiologic activity, and behavioral state.

▶ A pain profile suitable for the assessment of premature infants has been slow to emerge. In commenting on another article from the same collaborators,[1] Linda Franck observed that 1995 did not bring us the definitive clinical pain assessment tool. The development of the PIPP has now reached the advanced phase and requires clinical evaluation and validation. The goal was to develop a measure that "would identify most, but not all, infants in pain." The profile must be multidimensional and incorporate physiologic indicators, behavioral indicators, and modifying factors such as gestational age and behavioral state.

The latest iteration of the PIPP has been achieved by pilot-testing many variables and eliminating the least sensitive and least specific factors. Three factors (upper facial activity, including brow bulge, eye squeeze, and nasolabial furrow; physiologic activity, including heart rate and oxygen saturation; and behavioral state) appear to contribute most heavily to the pain experience in premature infants. Unfortunately, the study population includes very few extremely immature infants, and the validation was done only on infants beyond 28 weeks' gestation.

I have not been a great proponent of scoring systems. However, there appears to be a sound basis for the derivation of the PIPP, and if the end result is a sound measurement instrument to evaluate the efficacy of analgesics in premature infants, it will serve a very useful purpose. Establishing the realiability, practicality, feasibility, and validity of the PIPP will not be pain-free for the investigators. (Please also see Abstract 8–4.)

A.A. Fanaroff, M.B.B.Ch.

Reference

1. Johnston CC, Stevens BJ, Yang F, et al: Differential response to pain by very premature neonates. *Pain* 61:471–479, 1995. (1996 Year Book of Neonatal and Perinatal Medicine, p 216.)

Experience in a Neonatal Intensive Care Unit Affects Pain Response

Johnston CC, Stevens BJ (Royal Victoria Hosp, Montreal; Mt Sinai Hosp, Toronto; McGill Univ, Montreal; et al)

Pediatrics 98:925–930, 1996 8–4

Background.—The stress of pain can be harmful to preterm newborns who are already struggling to maintain homeostasis. Physiologic and behavioral disorganization after experiencing a heel stick has been reported in preterm infants born at 26 weeks' gestation. Younger preterm infants may experience more pain than older preterm infants. Responsiveness to pain increases with gestational age. The pain behaviors of infants of the same postconceptual age, but different postnatal age, have not been studied. Postnatal age may be a key factor in the development of pain response. An infant's exposure to painful events between 28 and 32 weeks' gestation, when many invasive procedures are performed, may affect the pain response later. Differences in response to a painful event in infants born at 32 weeks' postconceptual age who were of different postnatal ages were investigated, and factors explaining those differences were sought.

Methods.—A heel stick procedure was performed in thirty-six 4-week-old infants and in fifty-three 4-day-old infants. All infants were born at a mean postconceptual age of 32 weeks. The mean gestational age of the older infants was 27.3 weeks, and the gestational age of the younger infants was 32.3 weeks. Outcome measures were maximum heart rate, minimum oxygen saturation, and facial actions. The number of invasive procedures for each infant was recorded.

Results.—Different responses to the heel stick were seen in the 2 groups of infants. The 4-week-old infants had fewer behavioral displays of pain than did the 4-day-old infants. These differences were chiefly explained by the number of invasive procedures the infants had undergone. Apgar score was a secondary factor. Before and during the heel stick, higher heart rates and lower oxygen saturation were noted in older infants than in younger infants. These differences were explained by age at birth and birth weight.

Discussion.—Infants of 32 weeks' postconceptual age born at 28 weeks' gestational age had decreased pain responses. This was associated with the number of painful invasive procedures they had undergone. Further research should examine the effect of painful procedures on the pain response in preterm newborns for a longer period and study this association and its underlying mechanism in different patient samples.

▶ These Canadian investigators are leading the charge to better understand pain responses in premature infants. The article abstracted represents a sequel to last year's YEAR BOOK feature on differential responses to pain by very premature neonates.[1] The authors have also been the principal investigators on the Premature Infant Pain Profile (see Abstract 8–3). The comparison of infants delivered at 32 weeks' gestation with a cohort born at 28 weeks' gestation, who have had a month in the intensive care nursery to achieve the same postconceptual age, demonstrated the blunting effects of multiple painful experiences on behavioral maturity. At the time the study data were collected, clustering of invasive procedures, time-out periods, and minimal handling were not part of nursery procedures. Furthermore, the nursery environment, including noise and light, which may have modified responses, was not recorded.

Nursery personnel have become more attuned to soothing behaviors, the need to cluster painful procedures, and the analgesic requirements of sick premature infants. Control of the nursery environment and responding to the infants' cues, together with the above behavioral modification, may enhance the healing process.

A.A. Fanaroff, M.B.B.Ch.

Reference

1. Johnston CC, Stevens BJ, Yang F, et al: Differential response to pain by very premature neonates. *Pain* 61:471–479, 1995. (1996 YEAR BOOK OF NEONATAL AND PERINATAL MEDICINE, pp 215–216.)

Effectiveness of Individualized Developmental Care for Low-risk Preterm Infants: Behavioral and Electrophysiologic Evidence

Buehler DM, Als H, Duffy FH, et al (Children's Hosp, Boston; Harvard Med School, Boston; Boston Univ)

Pediatrics 96:923–932, 1995 8–5

Introduction.—More than 10% of infants born in the United States are low birth weight (less than 2,500 g), with the number of infants born between 30 and 35 weeks after the last menstrual period increasing. These infants frequently experience long-term effects such as reduced intelligence, learning disabilities, attention deficit disorder, speech and visual impairment, and emotional difficulties. It is thought that the extrauterine environment during the time of rapid brain development may affect brain differentiation and subsequent brain development. The effect of an individualized approach to care on the brain development of healthy preterm infants was evaluated.

Methods.—Premature infants were randomly assigned to 1 of 2 groups: one group received standard care, whereas those in the second group were given individualized developmental care. A group of full-term infants were used as a comparison group. Thirty-six infants were included in the study, with 12 infants in each group. Medical, behavioral, and electrophysiologic outcomes were assessed at 2 weeks after the expected delivery date. During the individualized developmental care approach, infant behavior was regularly evaluated and suggestions made for support of development by a developmental psychologist and a specially trained nurse.

Results.—The 3 groups were similar in age at the time of assessment. The 2 preterm groups were comparable, with the exception that the preterm group assigned to individualized care had lower Obstetric Complications Scale Scores and higher oxygen requirements, as indicated by

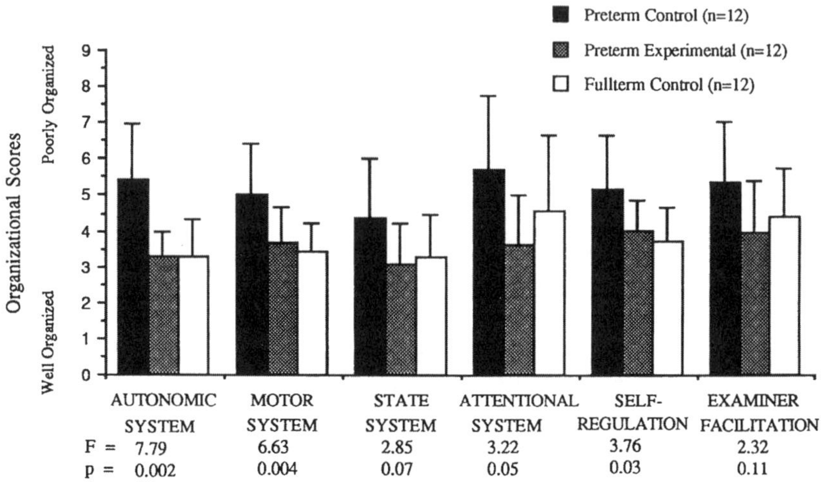

FIGURE 1.—Means and standard deviations of the Assessment of Preterm Infants' Behavior subsystem scores for the preterm control, preterm experimental, and full-term comparison groups derived from the behavioral examination at 2 weeks post–expected date of confinement. Behavioral systems are the autonomic system, the motor system, the state organizational system, the attentional system, the self-regulatory system, and the degree of examiner facilitation necessary in the course of the examination. All system scores are scaled from 1 to 9, with 1 representing well-organized performance and 9 representing poorly organized performance. The 6 system scores are based on means of 18 scores per system obtained in the course of an examination for each child on the autonomic, motor, state, and self-regulation system; the means of 3 scores are obtained on the attentional system; and the means of 6 scores are used on the variable examiner facilitation. (Courtesy of Buehler DM, Als H, Duffy FH, et al: Effectiveness of individualized and developmental care for low-risk preterm infants: Behavioral and electrophysiologic evidence. Reproduced by permission of *Pediatrics* vol 96, pp 923–932. Copyright 1995.)

mean daily pulmonary index. Medical outcomes did not differ between the 2 preterm groups. Significant differences in behavioral outcomes were found among the 3 groups. Infants in the preterm control group had significantly higher Assessment of Preterm Infants' Behavior (APIB) measures, indicating the least well-organized behavioral performance of the 3 groups (Figs 1 and 2). There were no significant differences in APIB scores between the preterm treatment group and the full-term comparison group. Electrophysiologic testing found many similarities between the preterm treatment group and the full-term comparison group. Findings for the preterm control group were significantly different. Areas that were significantly different with the preterm control group included the frontal lobe (18 features); the temporal region (12 features); and the central, occipital, and parietal regions (11 features total). Twenty-eight of these 41 features correlated significantly with APIB behavioral outcomes. Of the 28 significant correlations, 13 were between frontal lobe features and APIB behavioral measures for attentional control and state organization.

Conclusion.—Individualized, developmental care for preterm infants resulted in significant better neurobehavioral functioning at 2 weeks post term as compared with preterm infants who received standard care. This type of approach seemed to especially support frontal lobe development and attentional control and state organization.

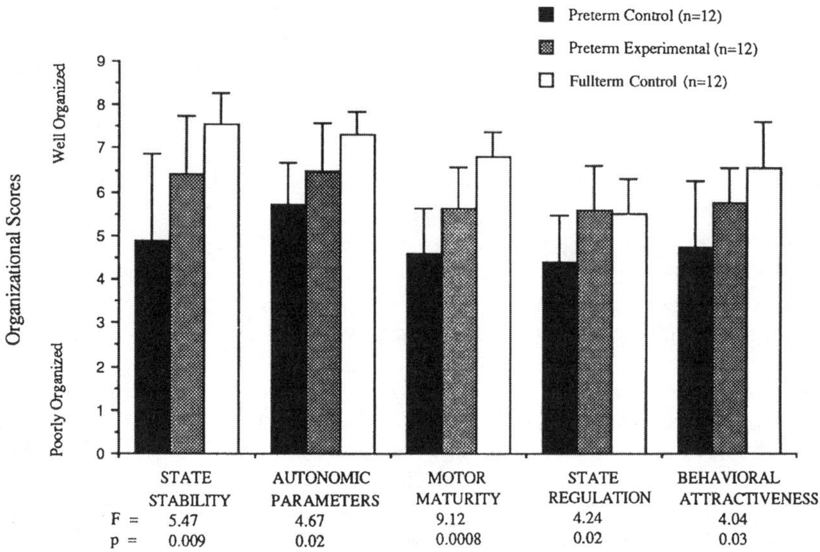

FIGURE 2.—Mean and standard deviations of the Assessment of Preterm Infants' Behavior summary scores showing significant differences between the preterm control, preterm experimental, and full-term comparison at 2 weeks post–expected date of confinement. Summary scores are scaled from 1 to 9, with 1 representing poorly organized performance and 9 representing well-organized performance. State stability measures a combination of indices that include lability of states, ability to quiet when motorically aroused, ability to be consoled when motorically aroused, rapidity of buildup to motoric arousal, peak of motoric arousal, and degree of discharge smiles vs. stimulus-related smiles in alertness. Autonomic indices include the degree of tremulousness, startles, skin color lability, and the threshold to color change. Motor maturity measures the degree of flaccidity vs. hypertonicity and the degree of smoothness and control of limb movements. State regulation consists of the range of flexibility of states, irritability, robustness in handling the examination, control over-input, and improvement with facilitation. Behavioral attractiveness measures the overall organization and modulation paired with social responsiveness and engagement. (Courtesy of Buehler DM, Als H, Duffy FH, et al: Effectiveness of individualized and developmental care for low-risk preterm infants: Behavioral and electrophysiologic evidence. Reproduced by permission of *Pediatrics* vol 96, pp 923–932, Copyright 1995.)

► Ernest F. Krug, M.D., Director of Developmental Pediatrics, William Beaumont Hospital, Royal Oak, Michigan, provided this comment:

► When we talk to parents in the neonatal ICU, we tend to be quite optimistic about the likely outcome for a newborn between 30 and 35 weeks' gestation who has never been ventilated and who has a normal cranial US examination. As Buehler et al. point out, however, these apparently normal infants do not always emerge unscathed. They have a significant incidence of learning disabilities, attention deficit hyperactivity disorder, language and speech problems, emotional difficulties, and lower intelligence quotients. Not everything important for the fetus occurs in the first 2 trimesters. The last trimester is a particularly active period of brain development, so premature infants between 30 and 34 weeks' gestation have brains that are still organizing and differentiating and are therefore subject to the environment found in many neonatal ICUs—bright lights, loud noises, alarms, cool environments, frequent heel sticks, gavage feeding, etc.

During the past 15 years, Dr. Als and her colleagues have shown us how premature infants behave, how they respond to the environment, and how changes in the environment can have profound effects on outcomes. Thus, we are at a point in the history of neonatal care when we can no longer focus our attention solely on the prevention and/or treatment of organ failure. We must pay attention to the infant's neurobehavioral organization and, as Buehler et al. show in this remarkable study, individualized developmental care actually has protective and facilitative effects on neurobehavioral organization, largely mediated by the frontal lobes of the brain.

This care has to do with being responsive to infant cues about their needs; reducing sensory assaults (e.g., bright lights and noise); supporting the infant's capacity to relax, recuperate, and self-regulate; and assisting parents to feel competent in caring for their infants. It is particularly striking that these behavioral and electrophysiologic effects were seen in healthy premature infants, a forceful reminder that how we nurse these infants affects their neurobehavioral organization. Furthermore, it is becoming clear that self-regulatory capacities in infancy can have a profound impact on regulation of mood and attention later in life. Promoting infant competence in self-regulation and parent competence in supporting that process may have a significant impact on the ultimate psychological and emotional health of individuals who are born prematurely.

E.F. Krug, M.D.

9 Gastroenterology and Nutrition

A Prospective Randomized Trial Comparing Continuous Versus Intermittent Feeding Methods in Very Low Birth Weight Neonates
Silvestre MAA, Morbach CA, Brans YW, et al (Wayne State Univ, Detroit, Mich)
J Pediatr 128:748–752, 1996 9–1

Introduction.—In preterm infants, various regimens have been used for enteral nutrition, but the optimal feeding method still has not been determined. Little has been done in comparing continuous vs. intermittent feeding methods. In very low birth weight infants (less than 1,500 g), the effects of continuous vs. intermittent feedings were compared to study physical growth, gastrointestinal tolerance, and macronutrient retention.

Methods.—There were 82 neonates with birth weights between 750 and 1,500 g who were born between 27 and 34 weeks' gestation and who were randomly assigned to an intermittent feeding group (n = 40) or a continuous feeding group (n = 42). (see Table 6) Between days 2 and 3, feedings with half-strength Similac Special Care formula were initiated and advanced isoenergetically to goal. Data collections were taken of daily weights, volume-caloric intakes, weekly anthropometric and dynamic skinfold thickness measurements, feeding milestones, and clinical complications. On a subset of 30 male infants, nitrogen, carbohydrate, and fat balance studies were performed.

Results.—There were no differences in baseline demographics and severity of respiratory distress between the 2 groups, and no differences in days to regain birth weight, days to discharge, days to full enteral feedings, and discharge anthropometric measurements. In the 17 continuously fed and 13 intermittently fed male neonates, retention rates of nitrogen, fat, total carbohydrate, and lactose were comparable. Feeding-related complications were not found among very low birth weight neonates who were fed continuously.

Conclusion.—Whether they are fed with continuous or intermittent feedings, very low birth weight infants achieve similar growth and macronutrient retention rates and have comparable lengths of hospital stay. Continuous feedings were better tolerated in the individual very low birth weight infant who had feeding problems. In continuously fed infants,

TABLE 6.—"Intent-to-Treat" Analysis by Weight Groups*

	750–999 gm		1000–1249 gm		1250–1499 gm	
	Continuous (n = 12)	Intermittent (n = 18)	Continuous (n = 17)	Intermittent (n = 14)	Continuous (n = 16)	Intermittent (n = 16)
Time to full feeds (days)	17 ± 12	21 ± 12	10 ± 5	12 ± 7	15 ± 10	10 ± 5
Time to regain BW (days)	23 ± 10	25 ± 9	15 ± 4	19 ± 8	16 ± 6	16 ± 4
Time to discharge (days)	68 ± 14	79 ± 16	48 ± 9	50 ± 11	36 ± 7	35 ± 7
Daily ΔW (gm/day)	15 ± 2	13 ± 2	16 ± 2	14 ± 3	14 ± 3	14 ± 2
Daily ΔL (cm/day)	0.13 ± 0.03	0.12 ± 0.03	0.15 ± 0.03	0.15 ± 0.03	0.17 ± 0.04	0.15 ± 0.05
Daily ΔHC (cm/day)	0.12 ± 0.02	0.11 ± 0.02	0.12 ± 0.02	0.12 ± 0.14	0.11 ± 0.02	0.11 ± 0.02

*Values are means plus or minus standard deviations. All comparisons between intermittent and continuous groups in the 3 birth weight categories were not significant.

Abbreviations: ΔBW, change in birth weight; *ΔHC*, change in head circumference; *ΔL*, change in length; *ΔW*, change in weight.

(Courtesy of Asuncion A, Silvestre MAA, Morbach CA, Brans YW, et al: A prospective randomized trial comparing continuous versus intermittent feeding methods in very low birth weight neonates. *J Pediatr* 128:748–752, 1996.)

pulmonary function was less compromised. In intermittently fed infants, there were significant decreases in tidal volume, minute ventilation, and dynamic compliance, and an increase in pulmonary resistance. The endocrine milieu may be altered by the marked cyclical surges of enteroinsular hormones that occur with intermittent feedings and may affect nutrient metabolism.

► It was with more than a twinge of sadness that I reviewed this article, because one of the authors, Yves Brans, died before its publication. He had made significant contributions to our understanding and management of nutrition and fluid and electrolyte disturbances in the sick newborn. The topic of intermittent vs. continuous feeding crops up mainly when there are difficulties in establishing enteral feeding in low–birth weight infants. Most infants with birth weights of less than 1,500 g require gavage feeding and, in the United States, the preferred route is intragastric. For the few centers that still use the transpyloric route, continuous feeding is mandatory.

These authors, acknowledging that there are still wide gaps in our knowledge of how best to feed small infants, compare continuous vs intermittent feeding with the null hypothesis that there will be equivalent rates of growth, macronutrient accretion, progression to full oral enteral feeding, and lengths of hospital stay. The sample size was sufficient to detect a 10% or greater rate of weight gain, defined as ([weight at discharge − birth weight]/length of stay) in continuously fed vs. intermittently fed infants. Similar growth and macronutrient retention rates were found in the 2 groups. The authors reported no feeding-related complications in the continuously fed group, and suggested that this method may have been more suitable for "the individual very low birth weight infant with feeding problems." This study will not drastically change feeding practices for low–birth weight infants.

When you can't have what you want, it's time to start wanting what you have.—Kathleen A. Sutton

A.A. Fanaroff, M.B.B.Ch.

Esophageal Body and Lower Esophageal Sphincter Function in Healthy Premature Infants

Omari TI, Miki K, Fraser R, et al (Women's and Children's Hosp, North Adelaide, Australia; Royal Adelaide Hosp, Australia; Kure Natl Hosp, Hiroshima, Japan)

Gastroenterology 109:1757–1764, 1995 9–2

Introduction.—Premature infants frequently experience problems with gastroesophageal reflux, but little is known about the esophageal motor mechanisms responsible for competence at the gastroesophageal junction or subsequent clearance of refluxate in this population. A new manometric device was used to examine the lower esophageal sphincter (LES) and

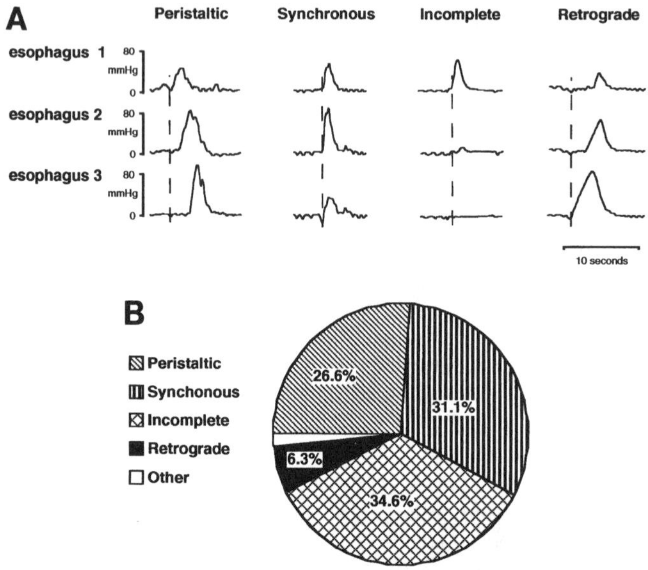

FIGURE 2.—A, example tracings of the predominant esophageal motor patterns observed in the esophageal body of healthy premature infants. B, the expression of the different motor patterns relative to the total number of pressure wave sequences recorded. (Courtesy of Omari TI, Miki K, Fraser R, et al: Esophageal body and lower esophageal sphincter function in healthy premature infants. *Gastroenterology* 109:1757–1764, 1995.)

esophageal pressure in normal premature infants before and after swallowing.

Methods.—Twenty-seven premature infants underwent 49 studies using micromanometric feeding assemblies (outer diameter, 2 mm or less) that incorporated 4–9 manometric channels. A total of 20 standardized puffs of air to the face were administered by using a neonatal compression bulb ventilator to stimulate Santmyer swallowing at a rate of 1 per minute. Primary (swallow-related) and secondary (nonswallow-related) esophageal pressure waves were classified. After feeding, esophageal body motility was recorded at 3 different sites. The LES pressures were recorded for 15 minutes before and after feeding in 32 studies.

Results.—The procedure was well tolerated by all neonates. The mean infant weight was 2,118 g. Nonperistaltic esophageal pressure waves were significantly more frequent than peristaltic esophageal pressure waves (73.4% vs. 26.6%). The nonperistaltic motor patterns were 31.1% synchronous, 34.6% incomplete, and 6.3% retrograde (Fig 2). Reflex swallowing was elicited more often in neonates older than 34 weeks' postconceptional age compared with younger neonates. The mean LES pressure was 20.5 mm Hg before feedings and 13.7 mm Hg after feedings. The difference was significant.

Conclusion.—More than 70% of esophageal body contractile sequences in healthy premature infants are nonperistaltic. In these infants, the motor mechanisms responsible for tonic contraction of the LES are well developed, and LES pressure appears to be adequate for maintaining esophagogastric competence. The decrease in esophageal body peristalsis could allow refluxed material to remain in the esophagus and increase the risk for subsequent complications.

► Almost every neonatologist is dealing with gastroesophageal reflux in premature infants on a daily basis. Drugs like cisapride are becoming more common than furosemide. However, there has been little systematic study of the electric/mechanical behavior of the esophagus. There is a great need to understand the behavior of the esophagus and its response to drugs so that our treatment of this very common condition can improve. Until the mechanisms of the dysfunction are elucidated, a targeted solution is probably not possible. It is amazing that there are as few problems as there are in view of the esophageal behavior described in Figure 2.

D.K. Stevenson, M.D.

Lack of Intestinal Pacemaker (C-KIT–positive) Cells in Infantile Hypertrophic Pyloric Stenosis

Yamataka A, Fujiwara T, Kato Y, et al (Dokkyo Univ, Tochigi, Japan; Juntendo Univ, Tokyo)

J Pediatr Surg 31:96–99, 1996 9–3

Introduction.—The pathogenesis of infantile hypertrophic pyloric stenosis (IHPS) is not clearly understood. Theories include an abnormality of hormonal control of the pylorus, loss of peptide-containing nerve fibers, marked reduction of nitric oxide, and axonal degenration in the myenteric plexus. What is known is that the proto-oncogene *c-kit* encodes a transmembrane tyrosine kinase receptor. The ligand for the *c-kit* receptor is the *Sl* factor. It has been shown in mice that *c-kit* is important in the development of a component of the pacemaker system required for the generation of autonomic gut motility. It also has been shown that the *c-kit* gene protein product (C-KIT)–positive cells in the mammalian gut are responsible for intestinal pacemaker activity. Full-thickness muscle biopsy specimens were obtained during pyloromyotomy in 16 infants treated for IHPS to determine whether C-KIT–positive (C-KIT$^+$) cells were present in the smooth muscles of the pylorus.

Methods.—In addition to the biopsies performed, control samples of pyloric tissues were taken from neonatal, infantile, and adult sources at autopsy. All specimens were imbedded in O.C.T. compound and stored until cut into 4-μ-thick cryostat sections. Half were stained with hematoxylin and eosin and the remaining sections underwent immunohistochemical analysis to visualize C-KIT$^+$ cells in the pyloric tissues. Three investigators evaluated the number of C-KIT$^+$ cells semiquantitatively and graded them on a scale of "−" (no C-KIT$^+$ cells visible) to "+++" (many C-KIT$^+$ cells).

Results.—Many C-KIT immunoreactive (IR^+) cells were seen in the muscle layers in the normal pyloric tissue from normal neonatal, infantile, and adult control subjects. The C-KIT–IR^+ cells were either absent or markedly reduced in the pyloric muscles of patients with IHPS. There also were no C-KIT–IR^+ cells observed around the myenteric plexuses.

Conclusions.—Many C-KIT^+ cells were observed in normal pyloric muscle tissue. The expression of *c-kit* was greatly reduced in the pyloric smooth muscle from patients with IHPS. It is possible that C-KIT^+ cells are needed for the development or maintenance of normal gut motility, and that a significant reduction in the expression of *c-kit* in the pyloric muscle may allow the smooth muscle cells to escape from this regulatory mechanism in patients with IHPS. This may cause the pylorospasms that result in hypertrophy. Further investigation is needed to support these findings.

▶ Pyloric stenosis is not a neonatal disorder. However, understanding its cause may unlock the mysteries of gut autonomic function control. This could lead to better management of the frustrating motility problems that characterize the extremely low birth weight and sick newborn. Motor activity, responsible for the aboral movement of nutrients, has characteristic patterns during fasting and after feeding in adults. Immature infants have patterns that differ from those of adults and even term infants. They are quiescent most of the time and may even have depression of motor activity in response to feeding. This is in sharp contrast to the burst of activity observed in fed term infants and adults. There is a rapid maturation of duodenal motor responses in response to feeding.[1] In sick premature infants, it remains to be proven whether poor propulsion reflects a series of slow pacemakers, missing pacemakers, diminished synapses, lack of gene expression, or various permutations thereof. The research presented above supports the hypothesis that a lack of *c-kit* expression (as an indicator of intestinal pacemaker activity) in the hypertrophic smooth muscles may be an improtant factor in the pathogenesis of idiopathic hypertrophic pyloric stenosis. The receptor for the *c-kit* is structurally similar to platelet-derived growth factor and the colony-stimulating factor-1 receptors that may be important in the pathogenesis of necrotizing enterocolitis. Further evaluation of the intestinal motility pacemakers and their hormonal and genetic control may soon permit clinicians to enhance autonomic gut motility and improve the outcome for these infants. In the meantime, the uncontrolled use of unproven propellants will no doubt continue.

What I hear, I forget. What I see, I remember. What I do, I know.—Chinese proverb

A.A. Fanaroff, M.B.B.Ch.

Reference

1. Al Tawil Y, Berseth CL: Gestational and postnatal maturation of duodenal motor responses to intragastric feeding. *J Pediatr* 129:374–381, 1996.

Gastric Emptying in Pre-term Infants: The Effect of Breast Milk Fortifier
Ewer AK, Yu VYH (Monash Med Centre, Melbourne, Australia)
Acta Paediatr 85:1112–1115, 1996 9–4

Background.—Early enteral nutrition in preterm infants can fail because of inadequate gastric emptying. The effect of adding breast milk fortifier on gastric emptying has not been established. Clinical experience suggests that it is less well tolerated by some infants. Gastric emptying rates associated with breast milk and fortified breast milk in preterm infants were compared.

Methods and Findings.—Eleven infants were assessed using an ultrasonography technique on 22 occasions. The median gestational age was 28 weeks; the median birth weight was 1,090 g. The infants received the human milk fortifier FM-85. Unfortified breast milk had a half-emptying time of less than half that of fortified breast milk. The mean half-emptying times were 21 and 48 minutes for unfortified and fortified milk, respectively. In 10 of 11 infants, breast milk emptied faster than fortified breast milk.

Conclusion.—Adding fortifier to human milk can significantly slow gastric emptying times, which has important implications for the management of infants with feed intolerance. Withholding fortifier until expressed breast milk is well tolerated or discontinuing its use temporarily in such infants is recommended.

▶ This study examined the tolerance of either expressed breast milk (EBM) or fortified breast milk in preterm infants with a median gestational age of 28 weeks who averaged a postnatal age of 44 days. Using a technique in which the emptying time of the stomach was estimated by looking at the antral cross-sectional area, the authors noted that unfortified EBM was digested at twice the rate of fortified breast milk. This was consistent with previous studies of feeding tolerance of infants receiving fortifier. Obviously, addition of fortifier to breast milk has advantages in improving growth and bone mineralization and diminishing electrolyte imbalances such as hyponatremia. In fact, a recent study by Lucas et al.[1] shows that when breast milk intake exceeds 50% of total intake, fortification promotes faster weight gain and higher plasma calcium.

However, in this same study fortification was associated with a significant increase in clinical infection, both suspected and proven, and a trend toward increased incidence of necrotizing enterocolitis. Also, no specific benefits to developmental outcome were found when looking at long-term development at 18 months. Therefore, for the small, preterm infant, fortifying EBM is not a panacea as it can be associated with feeding intolerance as well as other potentially important consequences such as increased infection. Future research is needed to develop an ideal feeding regimen for such small newborns. Perhaps use of infant formulas with immunity-enhancing antibodies or antigens that are genetically engineered, as suggested by Lo and Kleinman,[2] will be the way of the future.

D.K. Stevenson, M.D.

References

1. Lucas A, Fewtrell MS, Morley R, et al: Randomized outcome trial of human milk fortification and developmental outcome in the pre-term infant. *Am J Clin Nutr* 64:142–151, 1996.
2. Lo CW, Kleinman RE: Infant formula, past and future: Opportunities for improvement. *Am J Clin Nutr* 63:646S–650S, 1996.

Nucleotide Supplementation and the Growth of Term Small for Gestational Age Infants

Cosgrove M, Davies DP, Jenkins HR (Univ of Wales, Cardiff)
Arch Dis Child 74:F122–F125, 1996 9–5

Background.—The intestinal mucosae of infants who are small for gestational age (SGA) are functionally impaired by fetal undernutrition. Such infants may benefit from nucleotide supplementation of milk formulas with improved catch-up growth.

Methods.—Seventy-four infants were included in a double-blind, randomized, controlled trial. In all infants, intestinal mucosae were shown to be functionally impaired. Thirty-nine infants were randomly assigned to a nucleotide supplemented group and 35 to a standard formula group.

Findings.—At 2 months of age, infants receiving supplementation had significantly greater mean rates of weight and length gain than the infants receiving the standard formula. Mean rates of weight gain in the 2 groups were 106.3 and 94.7 g/kg of baseline weight/wk, respectively, and mean rates of length gain, 21.8 and 19.7 mm/m of baseline length/wk. During the entire 6 months of the study, the supplemented group had significantly greater mean rates of weight, length, and head circumference gain.

Conclusion.—Nucleotide supplementation of infant formula improves catch-up growth in SGA infants. The addition of the 5 nucleotide monophosphates, which contributed extra nitrogen and phosphate to the formula, may have contributed to a positive growth effect. The improved growth rates observed were probably the result of trophic effect of nucleotides on the intestinal mucosa previously damaged by intrauterine malnutrition.

► We asked Gilberto Pereira, M.D., Professor of Pediatrics, University of Pennsylvania Medical School, Philadelphia, to comment:

► Nucleotide and related compounds are abundant in human milk, accounting for up to 20% of the total nonprotein nitrogen. Experimental studies have suggested that exogenous nucleotides play a role in the modulation of immune function and gastrointestinal tract development and this controlled trial shows that if you give nucleotide-supplemented formulas to SGA infants during the first 6 months of life, they grow better.

The authors suggest that the nucleotides exerted a trophic effect on a gastrointestinal mucosa previously affected by in utero malnutrition; this, in turn, produced more efficient nutrient absorption. Intestinal biopsies could not be obtained, and there were no measurements of gut hormone levels or absorption studies to confirm the suggested mechanism of improved gastrointestinal function and growth. It is also debatable whether the observed differences in growth between the 2 study groups, although statistically significant, are clinically important. Clinical trials continue to suggest that the presence of nucleotides in human milk is not coincidental and that these compounds have important biological properties. Nevertheless, further studies are needed before the routine supplementation of nucleotides to infant formulas can be recommended.

G. Pereira, M.D.

Randomised Trial of Effect of Delayed Intravenous Lipid Administration on Chronic Lung Disease in Preterm Neonates

Alwaidh MH, Bowden L, Shaw B, et al (Liverpool Maternity Hosp, England; Univ of Liverpool, England)

J Pediatr Gastroenterol Nutr 22:303–306, 1996 9–6

Background.—Chronic neonatal lung disease (CNLD) occurs in as many as 44% of very low birth weight neonates, and the incidence of the condition may be increasing. The wide variation in rates of CNLD at different neonatal units has been attributed to differences in ventilatory practices. In one neonatal ICU, a recent sevenfold increase in the annual incidence of CNLD was linked to early administration of IV lipid in ventilated preterm neonates. The association between early IV lipid use and an increased incidence of CNLD was examined in a prospective study.

Patients and Methods.—The study population included 64 infants with a birth weight of less than 1,500 g who were admitted to the ICU and required parenteral nutrition. After consent of the parents was obtained, infants were randomly assigned to begin receiving IV lipid on day 5 (early) or day 14 (late). Randomization was stratified by weight (less than 1,000 g or 1,000 g or more) and ventilation status (ventilated or not on day 5). Parenteral nutrition was administered to all neonates starting at 48 hours of age.

Results.—The early and late lipid groups did not differ significantly in birth weight, gestational age, or number requiring ventilation. Age at regaining birth weight and age at starting milk feeds also were similar for the 2 groups. Thirteen infants in the late IV lipid group did not receive the treatment because parenteral nutrition had been discontinued by day 14. The relative risk of oxygen dependency at postnatal day 28 was 1.5 in the early lipid group as compared with the late lipid group, not a significant difference. Duration of ventilation was not significantly different for early and late IV lipid groups. One infant in each group died between 5 and 28 days of age.

Discussion.—The risks of delaying IV lipid therapy in sick preterm neonates would have to be weighed against the potential benefits of this course of action, and most neonatologists believe that early administration of IV lipid can prevent energy and essential fatty acid deficiency. Findings in this series of infants do not indicate that starting IV lipid at 5 days of age is associated with a higher incidence of CNLD. Because of its important neurodevelopmental advantages, early IV lipid is recommended in all parenterally fed neonates.

▶ The modern era of neonatology has witnessed dramatic improvements in the survival of smaller, less mature infants. This has been attributed to increased use of antenatal steroids, the advent of surfactant therapy, and better anticipation and management of a host of other problems. Nonetheless, the prevalence of CNLD has not wavered. Chronic neonatal lung disease remains a perplexing problem, with culpability apportioned by various investigators to ventilator strategies, oxygen, inflammation, and nutritional practices. Cooke[1] reported a 63% incidence of CNLD when the infants were delivered before 30 weeks' gestation and were placed on a ventilator for 4 days. He found a sevenfold increase in the incidence of CNLD in a subgroup of ventilated infants who had received IV intralipid, which prompted the present study. Sosenko[2] reported an increased mortality rate in infants weighing between 600 and 800 g who received early lipid supplementation.

The hypothesis of the current study was that delaying IV intralipid would reduce the incidence of CNLD by 50%. After weighing the risks, no compelling reason not to perform the study emerged. The risks of delaying IV fat were minimal and included reduced caloric intake, the possibility of essential fatty acid deficiency, and the remote possibility that vision and intellect could be affected. On the other hand, the risks of IV lipid infusion included thromboxane generation leading to pulmonary hypertension, lipid peroxidation, and free radical generation; impairment of pulmonary diffusion; and increased risk of infection with coagulase-negative staphylococci.

The sample size was based on the presumption that 85% of infants with birth weights of less than 1 kg and 40% of those with birth weights between 1 and 1.5 kg would be oxygen-dependent at 28 days of life. The results revealed no significant effect of delaying IV lipid therapy, refuting the hypothesis.

A.A. Fanaroff, M.B.B.Ch.

References

1. Cooke RWI: Factors associated with chronic lung disease in preterm infants. *Arch Dis Child* 66:776–779, 1991.
2. Sosenko IRS, Rodriguez-Pierce N, Bancalari E: Effect of early initiation of intravenous lipid administration on the incidence and severity of chronic lung disease in premature infants. *J Pediatr* 123:975–982, 1993.

Effect of Parenteral Amino Acids on Leucine and Urea Kinetics in Preterm Infants

Battista MA, Price PT, Kalhan SC (Case Western Reserve Univ, Cleveland, Ohio; Rainbow Babies and Childrens Hosp, Cleveland, Ohio)

J Pediatr 128:130–134, 1996 9–7

Objective.—Ten preterm infants receiving all of their calories by the parenteral route were studied to determine the effect of 2 commonly used amino acid mixtures on whole-body leucine and urea kinetics.

Methods.—All infants were healthy and medically stable at the time of the study; none were receiving supplemental oxygen, nor had they been given corticosteroids at any time. Prescribed nutrient regimens included parenteral nutrition in the form of glucose, amino acids, and IV infusions of lipid emulsions. Six infants were randomly assigned to receive Trophamine (a mixture containing higher branched-chain amino acids, lower glycine, and added dicarboxylic acids) and 4 to receive Aminosyn (a standard amino acid mixture). Stable isotopic tracers were used to examine the effect of these mixtures on whole-body protein turnover and protein oxidation. Infants received their last enteral calorie intake 5–6 hours before the tracer isotope study.

Results.—The 2 groups were similar in clinical characteristics, with the exception of mean postnatal age, which was 12 days in the Trophamine group and 30 days in the Aminosyn group. Although the rate of appearance of leucine, an indication of whole-body protein turnover, did not differ significantly in the 2 groups, the fraction of leucine oxidized and the total rate of oxidation of leucine were higher in the Trophamine group. The additional branched-chain amino acids in the Trophamine mixture caused increased decarboxylation and thus a higher contribution of carbon-1 of leucine to CO_2. There were no significant differences in the mean rate of urea nitrogen synthesis (2.92 mg of nitrogen per kg per hour with Trophamine vs. 2.70 mg of nitrogen per kg per hour with Aminosyn). Rates of urea synthesis and of oxidation of leucine showed no significant correlation.

Discussion.—The amino acid mixture Trophamine was found to normalize the blood amino acid pattern in preterm infants, but it did not appear to improve nitrogen/protein kinetics. Increased oxidation disposes of the solution's additional branched-chain amino acids. Protein oxidation calculated from measured rates of leucine C-1 decarboxylation proved much higher than that calculated from urea synthesis.

Proteolysis and Phenylalanine Hydroxylation in Response to Parenteral Nutrition in Extremely Premature and Normal Newborns

Denne SC, Karn CA, Ahlrichs JA, et al (Indiana Univ, Indianapolis)

J Clin Invest 97:746–754, 1996 9–8

Purpose.—It can be difficult to build up and maintain whole-body protein in premature infants. The available evidence leads to the question of whether complete parenteral nutrition solutions are able to suppress proteolysis, and thus preserve endogenous protein, in newborns regardless of whether they are normal or immature. Immature and normal newborns

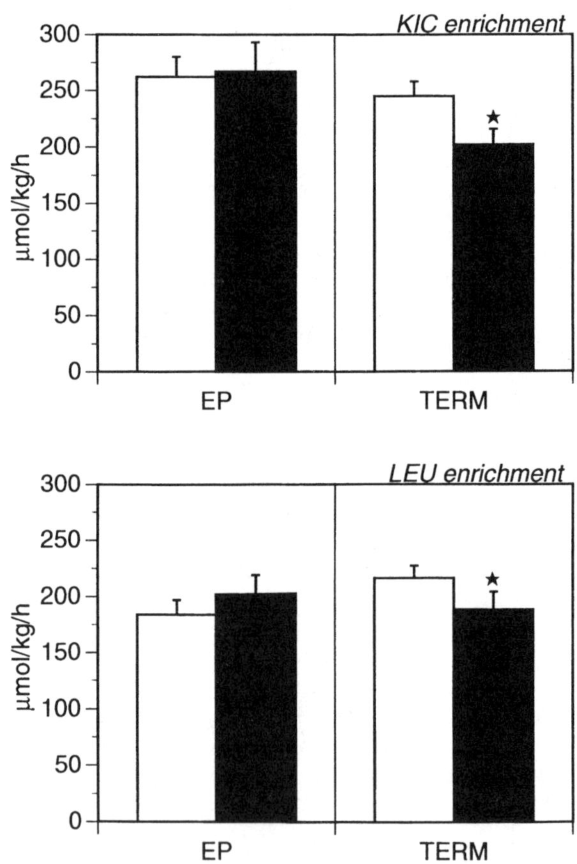

FIGURE 2.—Endogenous leucine (*LEU*) rate of appearance in the basal period (*open bars*) and during parenteral nutrition (*filled bars*) in extremely premature (*EP*) and term infants. Results are presented based on the enrichments of ketoisocaproic acid (*KIC*) and LEU. The *asterisk* indicates $P < 0.01$ basal vs. parenteral nutrition. Endogenous LEU rate of appearance (KIC) during parenteral nutrition is significantly higher in EP compared with term infants (analysis of variance; $P < 0.05$). (Courtesy of Denne SC, Karn CA, Ahlrichs JA, et al: Proteolysis and phenylalanine hydroxylation in response to parenteral nutrition in extremely premature and normal newborns. *J Clin Invest* 97:746–754, 1996. Reproduced by copyright permission of the American Society for Clinical Investigation.)

TABLE 4.—Leucine, Phenylalanine, and Tyrosine Rate of Appearance in the Basal Period and During Parenteral Nutrition

	EP		Term	
	Basal	PN	Basal	PN
Leucine Ra (KIC)	262 ± 18	363 ± 26*‡	243 ± 13	297 ± 14*‡
Leucine Ra (Leu)	184 ± 13	297 ± 17*‡	216 ± 11	283 ± 16*‡
Phenylalanine Ra	88 ± 5*‡	194 ± 5*‡	75 ± 3	83 ± 3*
Tyrosine Ra	115 ± 13‡	102 ± 8‡	69 ± 5	64 ± 5†

Note: Leucine Ra is reported based on both the enrichment of KIC and leucine.
**P* <0.001 basal vs. PN.
†*P* <0.05 basal vs. PN.
‡*P* <0.05 EP vs term.
Abbreviations: EP, extremely premature; *KIC*, ketoisocaproic acid; *PN*, parenteral nutrition; *Ra*, rate of appearance.
(Courtesy of Denne SC, Karn CA, Ahlrichs JA, et al: Proteolysis and phenylalanine hydroxylation in response to parenteral nutrition in extremely premature and normal newborns. *J Clin Invest* 97:746–754, 1996. Reproduced by copyright permission of the American Society for Clinical Investigation.)

were compared for phenylalanine hydroxylation and tyrosine rate of appearance under basal conditions and during parenteral nutrition.

Methods.—The study included 8 extremely premature (EP) newborns, born at about 26 weeks' gestation and in clinically stable condition, and 10 normal term newborns. In both groups, the ability to convert phenylalanine to tyrosine and the kinetics of phenylalanine and leucine were studied at baseline and during parenteral nutrition. The study hypothesis was that the EP infants would have a reduced capacity to convert phenylalanine to tyrosine under basal conditions and in response to the phenylalanine given during parenteral feeding.

Results.—Compared with the term infants, the EP group showed significantly less suppression of endogenous leucine and of phenylalanine rate of appearance in response to parenteral nutrition (Fig 2 and Table 4). In both groups, the use of phenylalanine for protein synthesis increased by about 15%. The rate of conversion of phenylalanine to tyrosine was significantly higher for the EP group, under both baseline and parenteral nutrition conditions.

Conclusions.—Both EP and term infants have the capacity to convert phenylalanine to tyrosine; in EP infants, the rate of conversion increases during parenteral nutrition. There is no evidence of immaturity of the phenylalanine hydroxylation pathway. Protein synthesis increases to a similar extent in response to parenteral nutrition in EP and term infants. However, for reasons that remain unclear, EP infants show less suppression of proteolysis.

Relative Kinetics of Phenylalanine and Leucine in Low Birth Weight Infants During Nutrient Administration

van Toledo-Eppinga L, Kalhan SC, Kulik W, et al (Vrije Universiteit, Amsterdam; Case Western Reserve Univ, Cleveland, Ohio)

Pediatr Res 40:41–46, 1996 9–9

Objective.—Because the effectiveness of nutrient administration on the growth rate of low–birth weight (LBW) infants depends on the efficiency of protein metabolism, nonradioactive essential amino acid tracers have been used to measure protein kinetics by following the turnover of the amino acid. Whether labeled leucine and phenylalanine give similar estimates of protein turnover has not been evaluated in small infants. The relative kinetics of phenylalanine and leucine metabolism in LBW infants during enteral feeding with preterm formula (PF), parenteral nutrition (PN), or fortified human milk (HM) were compared.

Methods.—Three groups of 10 LBW infants received either PF (117 kcal/kg/day), HM (106 kcal/kg/day), or PN (80 kcal/kg/day and 1.8 g of protein per kg per day) labeled with L-[1-^{13}C]leucine, L-[$^{2}H_5$]phenylalanine, and L-[$^{2}H_2$]tyrosine. Breath gas and blood samples were analyzed for enrichment by labeled amino acids. The rate of appearance of each amino acid was calculated using the equation, $Ra = Ox + NOD = I + ARP$, where Ra is the rate of appearance, Ox is the oxidative disposal rate of leucine or the hydroxylation rate of phenylalanine to tyrosine, and NOD is the nonoxidative disposal rate.

Results.—The rate of appearance of leucine was significantly greater in the PF group (434 µmol/kg/hr) than in either the HM or PN group (377 or 359 µmol/kg/hr, respectively). The rate of appearance of endogenous phenylalanine was significantly higher in the PF group (115 µmol/kg/hr) than in the HM group (94 µmol/kg/hr), whereas the rate in the PN group was intermediate (108 µmol/kg/hr). Ratios of phenylalanine hydroxylation to leucine decarboxylation were 0.202 in the PF group, 0.212 in the HM group, and 0.161 in the PN group, suggesting that the oxidation of leucine proceeds faster than the hydroxylation of phenylalanine.

Conclusion.—Leucine turnover is higher than phenylalanine turnover in LBW infants, and their relative rates are different from those of adults. These variations may be the result of different nutrient regimens. Turnover of a single amino acid tracer does not satisfactorily characterize whole-body protein metabolism.

► This commentary was contributed by Satish C. Kalhan, M.D., Professor, Department of Pediatrics, Case Western Reserve University School of Medicine, Cleveland, Ohio:

► Protein turnover (i.e., the breakdown and synthesis of body proteins) is a continuous process occurring throughout the day. Rates of protein turnover have been estimated to be higher during periods of growth, as in the fetus and neonates, and to decline with age, so that they are much lower in older as compared with younger individuals. Because protein turnover is an energy-consuming process requiring adenosine triphosphate, it is responsible for a significant component of the basal metabolic rate. A close relation has been demonstrated between basal energy consumption and the whole-body rate of protein turnover. The whole-body pool of proteins consists of a large number of different proteins that are broken down (proteolysis) and resynthesized at different rates. Because the amino acid compositions of these proteins vary, differences in breakdown rates of the proteins will lead to differences in release rates of amino acids.

Studies like the one done by Denne and colleagues (Abstract 9–8) assume the whole-body protein mass to be a uniform pool (i.e., all the body proteins are represented by a single pool) so that the breakdown rate of protein (proteolysis) can be estimated by the appearance of essential amino acids such as leucine and phenylalanine into the circulation. By knowing the rate of irreversible loss (catabolism) of these amino acids, the rate of nonoxidative exit of these amino acids from the amino acid pool or their entry into protein pool, and therefore the rate of protein synthesis, can be calculated. In the present study, the authors also have examined the response of rates of protein breakdown and synthesis to parenteral nutrition. In addition, by measuring the rate of conversion of phenylalanine to tyrosine using an isotope trace method, they have demonstrated that even very LBW premature infants have a significant ability to hydroxylate phenylalanine to tyrosine. This latter finding is significant because of the suggestion in the literature that newborn infants cannot convert phenylalanine to tyrosine, with the result that tyrosine is considered to be an essential amino acid, particularly for prematurely born infants.

The authors are to be applauded for their conduct of this very carefully designed study. For the uninitiated, this study also shows that complex studies of this type can be performed safely, even on the smallest of infants. Like any good research investigation, the data from this study raise more exciting questions than answers. For example, why, in the presence of substantial phenylalanine hydroxylation, did not the rate of appearance of tyrosine in the circulation change during parenteral nutrition in the extremely preterm infant? In relation to proteolysis, why was there a difference in response to parenteral nutrition in preterm versus full-term infants? Is it because the preterm infants were under "stress," resulting in a different state of metabolic and hormonal homeostasis? Even though clinically stable, these infants have been shown to have higher levels of circulating "stress" hormones. We eagerly await the answers to these and many other questions.

The paper by Battista and associates (Abstract 9–7) points to the inadequacies of the currently used amino acid mixtures for parenteral nutrition. Because these amino acid mixtures were formulated to maintain normal blood amino acid patterns and do not necessarily reflect the amino acid composition of the whole-body proteins, the exogenously administered amino acids cannot all be used to synthesize proteins. As shown in their study, the excess amino acids were oxidized for energy production. In addition, the use of a specifically prepared balanced amino acid mixture for the neonate did not result in any advantage in whole-body protein dynamics. An ideal amino acid mixture perhaps would reflect the amino acid composition of the body protein; however, such a mixture may not be able to maintain a normal blood amino acid pattern and acid-base homeostasis.

The Dutch study abstracted here (Abstract 9–9) emphasizes that the newborn infant is not the same as an adult, even in terms of protein dynamics. As suggested above, the whole-body protein is a dynamic mixture of thousands of proteins, each turning over at a different rate. Thus, if a certain group of proteins with different amino acid compositions has a high rate of turnover (i.e., breakdown and synthesis) in infants as compared with adults, the appearance of essential amino acids in the blood will reflect the amino acid compositions of these proteins. Thus, van Toledo-Eppinga and colleagues observed a higher rate of appearance of leucine compared with phenylalanine in infants as compared with adults, or even as compared with the amino acid compositions of their nutrients. Their data suggest a higher rate of breakdown and synthesis of protein rich in leucine as compared with phenylalanine.

These types of studies, by using multiple amino acid tracers, should help us better define and examine the response to nutrient intake during periods of nitrogen accretion as well as during catabolic states.

S.C. Kalhan, M.D.

Parenteral Nutrition–related Cholestasis in Postsurgical Neonates: Multivariate Analysis of Risk Factors

Beath SV, Davies P, Papadopoulou A, et al (Univ of Birmingham, England; Children's Hosp, Birmingham, England)

J Pediatr Surg 31:604–606, 1996 9–10

Introduction.—Parenteral nutrition has aided in the management of neonates with major intestinal anomalies, but the infusions are associated with various complications. Cholestasis leading to liver failure is the most common cause of death among neonates dependent on parenteral nutrition after abdominal surgery. To better understand the pathogenesis of cholestasis in this setting, the medical records of 74 neonates were retrospectively reviewed.

Methods.—Eligible infants had received parenteral nutrition within 2 weeks of abdominal surgery, and infusions were continued for at least 21 days. Data analyzed included birth weight, gestational age at birth, the composition and total duration of parenteral nutrition, the duration of enteral starvation (less than 2 mL per hour of feeding), septic episodes, and plasma bilirubin measurements.

Results.—Cholestatic jaundice developed in 27 infants within 28 days of the start of parenteral nutrition. All but 2 were weaned from parenteral nutrition within 4 months, and the cholestasis resolved within 1–4 months after weaning. One infant continued receiving parenteral nutrition and died of liver failure at the age of 2 years; the other became independent of parenteral nutrition at 18 months and his cholestasis resolved. All 47 infants who were free of jaundice on day 28 remained so, and only 1 received parenteral nutrition for more than 2 months. Cholestatic infants differed significantly from noncholestatic infants in birth weight, gestational age at birth and at the start of parenteral nutrition, early sepsis, and total number of septic episodes. The 2 groups had received almost identical solutions. In multiple regression analysis, the best predictors of elevated log bilirubin were a short interval between birth and the initiation of parenteral nutrition, young gestational age at the start of parenteral nutrition, and a large number of septic episodes.

Conclusion.—Prematurity was the most important factor in the development of jaundice, suggesting a link between cholestasis and immaturity of the hepatobiliary system. Because early surgery usually is unavoidable, prevention of IV catheter–related sepsis is the most important factor in reducing the rate of cholestasis.

▶ Parenteral nutrition has saved the lives of many neonates with major gastrointestinal anomalies. There also may be major complications, including sepsis, metabolic disorders, cholestasis, and thromboembolism, directly attributable to its use. Beath and colleagues reviewed the medical records of 74 neonates who were dependent on parenteral nutrition for at least 3 weeks to identify the risk factors for cholestasis. Septicemia, lack of enteral stimulation, and intestinal bacterial overgrowth previously had been recognized as risk factors. The most important factor in the development of jaundice was prematurity, closely followed by sepsis. Surprisingly, lack of enteral nutrition and the nature of the parenteral fluid were not significant risk factors. Thus, avoidance of catheter sepsis becomes the top priority. Nosocomial infections remain a monumental problem in the hospital setting, and infections in ICUs account for more than 20% of all nosocomial infections, even though ICUs account for only 5% of hospital beds. We should never ignore an opportunity to remind personnel of the importance of washing their hands before and after every patient contact.[1]

A.A. Fanaroff, M.B.B.Ch.

Reference

1. Brown J, Froese-Fretz A, Luckey D, et al: High rate of hand contamination and low rate of hand washing before infant contact in a neonatal intensive care unit. *Pediatr Infect Dis J* 15:907–910, 1996.

Meconium Obstruction in the Markedly Premature Infant

Greenholz SK, Perez C, Wesley JR, et al (Univ of California, Sacramento)

J Pediatr Surg 31:117–120, 1996 9–11

Background.—Traditionally, small-bowel obstruction caused by inspissated meconium in the ileum and colon has been associated with cystic fibrosis. However, with increased survival of markedly premature infants, the number of infants with bowel obstruction from inspissated meconium who do not have cystic fibrosis is rising. One clinical experience with such infants was reported.

Methods and Findings.—Thirteen infants with a mean birth weight of 760 g were treated for intestinal obstruction caused by inspissated meconium between 1990 and 1994. Prenatal and postnatal risk factors included intrauterine growth retardation, maternal hypertension, prolonged administration of tocolytics, patent ductus arteriosus, hyaline membrane disease, and intraventricular bleeding. In the first 2 weeks of life, stools were absent or infrequent. Distension and/or perforation occurred between 2 and 17 days of life. Operation was needed in 12 infants. One or more obstructing meconium plugs with proximal distention and frequent necrosis of the dilated segments were documented. Resection or enterotomy, accompanied by primary closure or distal irrigation and exteriorization, was done. In 2 patients, irrigation caused iatrogenic bowel injury. Treatment with oral and rectal gastrograffin and oral acetylcysteine was successful in 1 patient. Ten infants with normal stools and negative findings on cystic fibrosis testing were discharged. Three infants died; the primary disease was the cause of death in 2.

Conclusions.—Markedly premature infants are at risk for obstruction and eventual perforation from meconium plugs. These plugs probably are formed in conjunction with intestinal dysmotility. Prompt diagnosis and timely intervention rely on a high index of suspicion, attention to stool patterns, abdominal testing, and screening radiographs when indicated.

▶ Add meconium obstruction to the already comprehensive list of gastrointestinal disorders in markedly premature infants. These infants already are vulnerable to necrotizing enterocolitis and upper gastrointestinal perforations, which may occur spontaneously or secondary to tocolytics such as indomethacin or postnatal steroids.

Greenholz and associates draw attention to meconium obstruction, in the absence of cystic fibrosis, as a distinct entity in low–birth weight infants. They are unable to step beyond the descriptive phase, shedding no light on the etiology, which is described as "conjectural and possibly multifactorial." The associated risk factors, including maternal hypertension, prolonged use of tocolytics, intrauterine growth retardation, and the neonatal morbidities respiratory distress, patent ductus, arteriosus and intraventricular hemorrhage, are nonspecific. The clinical presentation is distinctive, but the plea to follow up the stool pattern is self-evident but not necessarily helpful. Delayed and irregular stool patterns appear to be the norm in most extremely immature infants. Hence, there may be little warning of the impending obstruction. The cost-benefit ratio of the gastrograffin enema is tilted in favor of such an examination, with due precautions. However, irrigation of the bowel at the time of operation is fraught with danger.

None of the infants subsequently were confirmed to have cystic fibrosis; however, with 4 deaths during the neonatal period, this is a very serious entity.

More than 40% of the references were to manuscripts published before 1975. It seems, therefore, appropriate and timely to draw attention to meconium obstruction in premature infants. Forewarned is forearmed.

A.A. Fanaroff, M.B.B.Ch.

Limited Fat Digestion in Infants With Bronchopulmonary Dysplasia

Boehm G, Bierbach U, Moro G, et al (Maternity Hosp Macedonio Melloni, Milan, Italy; Univ of Leipzig, Germany)

J Pediatr Gastroenterol Nutr 22:161–166, 1996 9–12

Background.—Although growth failure is common in infants with bronchopulmonary dysplasia (BPD), very little is known about digestive function in such patients. Pancreatic lipase and trypsin activities and the bile acid levels in duodenal aspirates were studied in very low birth weight infants with hyaline membrane disease (HMD) with or without BPD development. The purpose was to determine the effects of different clinical courses of HMD on these parameters.

Methods.—Ten patients with HMD with BPD, 16 with HMD but not BPD, and 12 very low birth weight infants with no major medical problems were included. Lipase activity, trypsin activity, and bile acid concentrations were measured in preprandially aspirated duodenal juice. Fat and nitrogen balances were done in the fifth and sixth weeks of postnatal life.

Findings.—The average duodenal lipase activity was significantly lower in patients with BPD than in those without it. The mean total bile acid level was less than 4 mmol/L, the critical micellar concentration, only in patients with BPD. Patients with BPD had a significantly greater fecal fat excretion rate than the patients without BPD.

Conclusions.—The development of BPD is associated with limited fat absorption. This may be responsible for the inadequate weight gain in infants with BPD.

▶ Gilberto Pereira, M.D., Professor of Pediatrics, University of Pennsylvania School of Medicine, Philadelphia, comments:

▶ Infants with BPD are at great risk for malnutrition because of their high energy requirements and poor nutritional intake. Thus, recommended nutritional support includes (1) high energy intake (120–140 kcal/day per kilogram) to compensate for high metabolic demands for catch-up growth; (2) feedings of high calorie density (24–30 kcal/30 mL) to provide high energy intake without the risk of fluid overload and respiratory decompensation; and (3) the administration of high-fat formula or fat supplements to reduce the respiratory quotient and the rate of carbon dioxide elimination by their compromised lungs.

In this study, Boehm et al. showed that small premature infants with BPD who received pasteurized human milk had a limited intestinal phase of fat digestion when compared with 2 other groups of premature infants without

BPD. The infants with BPD received more parenteral nutrition and had lower caloric intakes than the other infants, and the authors attribute their findings to a combination of cholestatic liver disease and poor nutritional status. They remind us to consider these limitations of fat digestion when prescribing high-fat nutritional supplements to premature infants with BPD.

However, we should interpret the results of this study with some caution. The infants were fed pasteurized human milk, which may not be entirely appropriate for the study of fat absorption. The process of pasteurization inactivates the bile-salt stimulated lipase, thus significantly reducing the absorption of dietary fat. If the babies had been fed fresh human milk or premature infant formulas that contained 50% of their fat calories in the form of medium-chain triglyceride oil, they would likely have shown less impairment of fat digestion. Second, the limitation of fat digestion may not be related to BPD per se, but could simply be the result of total parenteral nutrition–induced cholestasis, poor nutritional status, or both.

G. Pereira, M.D.

Orally Administered Lactoferrin Increases Hepatic Protein Synthesis in Formula-fed Newborn Pigs

Burrin DG, Wang H, Heath J, et al (Baylor College of Medicine, Houston, Tex)
Pediatr Res 40:72–76, 1996 9–13

Background.—Lactoferrin, a 78-kd single-chain polypeptide initially isolated from bovine and human milk, is especially abundant in human, porcine, and bovine colostrum, with concentrations of 1–5 mg/mL. The in vivo biological significance of colostrum-borne lactoferrin in the newborn is not clear. The mitogenic effect of relatively high lactoferrin levels in porcine colostrum may contribute to the marked stimulation of gastrointestinal protein synthesis previously observed in colostrum-fed newborn pigs. The potential anabolic effect of oral lactoferrin on visceral organ growth and protein synthesis in newborn pigs was determined.

Methods.—Three pigs from each of 6 litters were randomly assigned to 1 of 3 dietary treatment groups. Six each were bottle-fed formula, formula containing physiologic levels of added bovine lactoferrin (bLF), or colostrum. Visceral organ protein synthesis was measured after 24 hours of feeding. In addition, visceral organ protein and DNA mass, intestinal hydrolase activities, and villus morphology were assessed.

Findings.—Hepatic protein synthesis in pigs fed formula with bLF or colostrum was comparable and significantly higher than in pigs fed formula. Splenic protein synthesis did not differ in pigs fed formula or bLF-containing formula but was significantly greater in pigs given colostrum. All 3 groups had similar small intestinal growth, protein synthesis, and hydrolase activity (Fig 1).

Conclusion.—In newborns pigs, formula containing physiologic levels of bLF increases hepatic protein synthesis. Thus, colostrum-borne lactoferrin appears to serve an anabolic function in newborns.

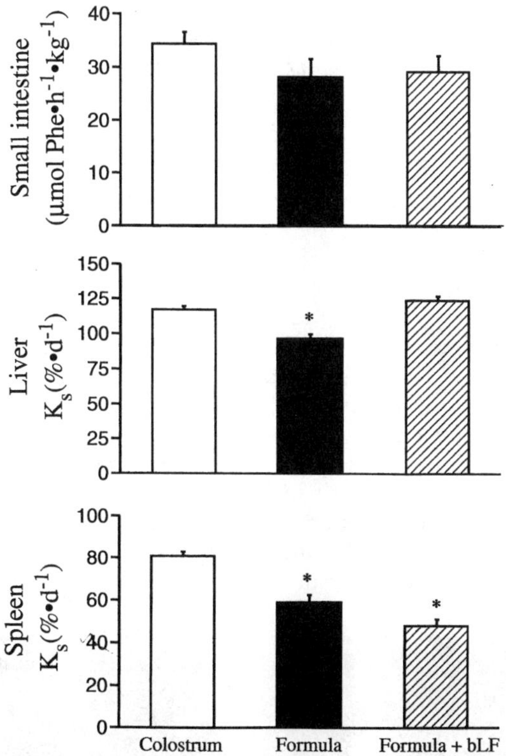

FIGURE 1.—In vivo protein synthesis rates in the small intestine, liver, and spleen of newborn pigs fed colostrum (*open bars*), formula (*solid bars*), or formula plus bovine lactoferrin (*bLF*) (*hatched bars*). Liver protein synthesis was different in formula-fed pigs vs. colostrum and formula + bLF–fed pigs, $^*P < 0.05$. Spleen protein synthesis was different in colostrum-fed pigs vs. formula and formula + bLF–fed pigs, $^*P < 0.05$. Values are means + standard error of the means, $n = 6$. *Abbreviation: Phe,* phenylalanine. (Courtesy of Burrin DG, Wang H, Heath J, et al: Orally administered lactoferrin increases hepatic protein synthesis in formula-fed newborn pigs. *Pediatr Res* 40:72–76, 1996.)

▶ There seems no end to the benefits of human milk for human infants, and this study demonstrates another salutary role for the lactoferrin found in colostrum. The newborn pigs fed additional bLF or simply colostrum (which contains an abundance of lactoferrin) had increased protein synthesis in the liver. Those fed colostrum also showed increased protein synthesis in the spleen. This is just one of the manifold blessings that human milk bestows on infants. Unfortunately, not every infant can nurse, and many mothers do not wish to, or cannot, breast-feed their infants. Surely, the future of mankind lies in a genetically engineered cow that will produce human milk. Given the latest news about cloning, this does not seem at all far-fetched.

M.J. Maisels, M.B., B.Ch.

Interrupted Air Column in the Large Bowel on Plain Abdominal Film: A New Radiological Sign of Intussusception

Lazar L, Rathaus V, Erez I, et al (Meir Hosp, Kfar-Saba, Israel; Tel Aviv Univ, Israel)

J Pediatr Surg 30:1551–1553, 1995 9–14

Background.—Small-bowel obstruction in infants and toddlers is often caused by intussusception. Early diagnosis and treatment are essential. A fairly consistent radiologic finding on plain abdominal radiographs was reported for the first time.

Methods.—Sixty children, 2–22 months of age, were brought to an emergency department with colicky abdominal pain, restlessness, and vomiting. Thirty-two patients (group 1) were subsequently found to have ileocolic intussusception or ileoileal intussusception. Twenty-eight patients (group 2) had other causes for their symptoms, such as gastroenteritis, constipation, otitis, and viral illness. Plain abdominal supine and upright radiographic views were obtained in all children.

Findings.—The children in group 1 had a longer duration of symptoms than did those in group 2. The plain abnormal radiographs of 21 of the 32 children in group 1 were interpreted as abnormal. In a review of the 11

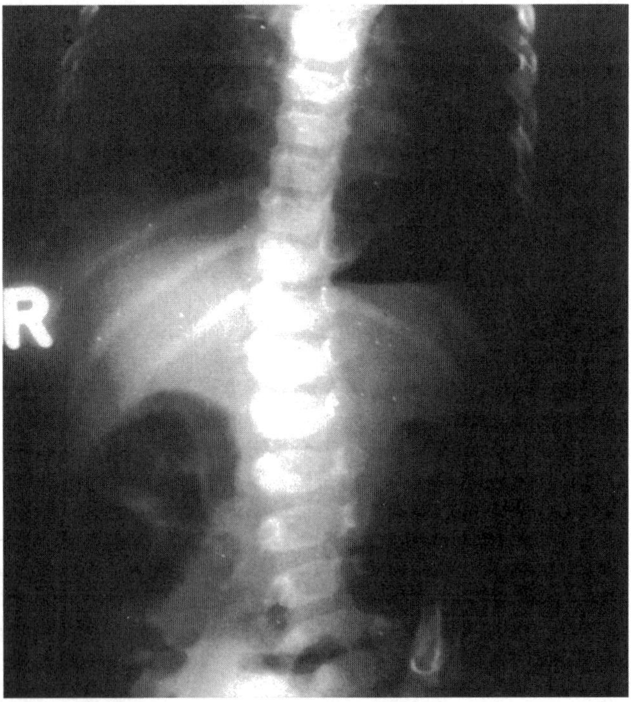

FIGURE 1.—Plain abdominal radiograph. Note the interruption of the air column at the tranverse colon. (Courtesy of Lazar L, Rathaus V, Erez I, et al: Interrupted air column in the large bowel on plain abdominal film: A new radiological sign of intussusception. *J Pediatr Surg* 30:1551–1553, 1995.)

radiographs interpreted as normal, an interruption of the colonic air column was identified in 8 patients (Fig 1). The discontinuity of gas occurred in the transverse colon in 5 patients and in the right colon in 3. The location of the discontinuity was well correlated with barium enema findings. None of the radiographs in group 2 suggested intussusception.

Conclusions.—The finding of an "interrupted air column" in the large bowel should alert clinicians to the possibility of intussusception. The recognition of this, along with other well-known radiologic signs of intussusception, may facilitate diagnosis and successful nonoperative treatment of intussusception in infants and toddlers.

▶ Commenting on this article is Phillip Sunshine, M.D., Professor of Pediatrics, Division of Neonatal and Developmental Medicine, Stanford University Medical Center; Co–Medical Director, Mid-Coastal California Perinatal Outreach Program, Palo Alto, California:

▶ These authors have described a unique finding in patients with intussusception who had previously been described as having normal or nonspecific findings on plain abdominal radiographs. In a review of radiographs of 32 patients with intussusception, definite abnormalities were found in 21 of the infants. In a second review of the 11 "normal patients," the authors found "interruption of the colonic air column" in 8. In 5, discontinuity was in the transverse colon; in 3, it was in the right colon. They compared these findings with those of a group of 28 patients who had similar clinical manifestations as intussusception with colicky abdominal pain and vomiting. These latter patients had gastroenteritis, constipation, otitis, or viral illnesses. None of the latter group had any abnormalities of their abdominal radiographs. Through the use of this finding, the authors have increased the accuracy of their diagnosis of intussusception on plain abdominal radiographs from 66% to 91%.

This is a neat radiograph sign that would lead clinicians to think more of intussusception than other causes of colicky abdominal pain and would lead to earlier use of an air or barium enema in the diagnosis and treatment of patients with intussusception.

P. Sunshine, M.D.

Gastrointestinal Perforation and Peritonitis in Infants and Children: Experience With 179 Cases Over Ten Years

Grosfeld JL, Molinari F, Chaet M, et al (Indiana Univ, Indianapolis; James Whitcomb Riley Hosp for Children, Indianapolis, Indiana)

Surgery 120:650–656, 1996 9–15

Introduction.—In spite of advances in neonatal intensive care and perioperative and postoperative management, premature, very low birth weight infants continue to have a high death rate after gastrointestinal perforation. The outcome of infants and older children with gastrointestinal perforation and peritonitis. was examined in a retrospective study. Etiologic factors, causes of death, and mortality rates were evaluated.

Methods.—The medical records of 179 infants and children with gastrointestinal perforation and peritonitis were reviewed. There were 139 neonates and 40 children between 2 months and 17 years of age; 113 patients were boys and 66 were girls. Neonates were divided into groups that included those with necrotizing enterocolitis and those with perforation from other causes.

Results.—The site of perforation was small bowel in 105 patients, colon in 37, stomach in 16, duodenum in 9, and undesignated in 12 patients. Multiple perforations were present in 18 patients. In infants younger than 2 months, the 2 most common causes of perforation were necrotizing enterocolitis and isolated perforation of the ileum (Fig 2). In older children, causes of perforation were trauma, Meckel's diverticulum, intussusception, pseudomembranous colitis, adhesions, stomal leak, duodenal ulcer, cytomegalic viral ulcer, volvulus, and lymphoma. Mortality was 48% for infants with necrotizing enterocolitis, 27.2% for infants without necrotizing enterocolitis, 15.1% for older children, and 25% for infants with gastric perforation (Fig 3). Deaths of infants were associated with overwhelming sepsis, immaturity of systems, and multiorgan failure. Deaths of older children were associated with sepsis, multiorgan failure, and immunodeficiency.

Discussion.—Gastrointestinal perforation is more common in premature infants. Premature, very low birth weight infants, especially those

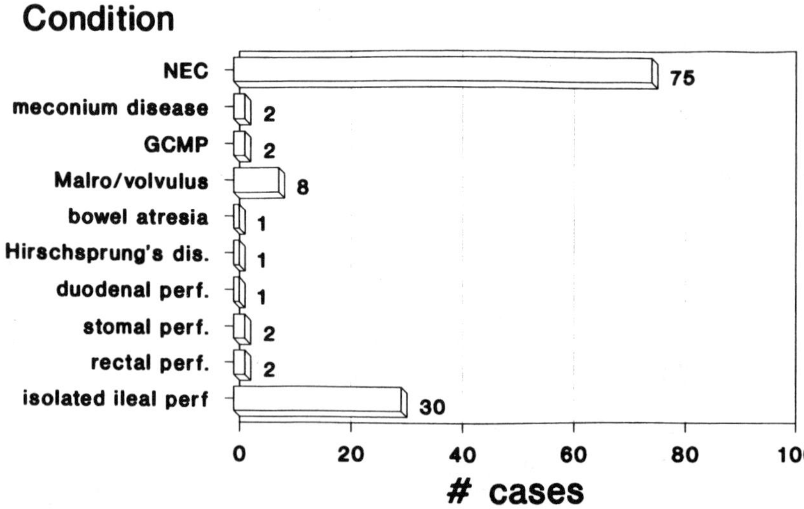

FIGURE 2.—Horizontal bar graph shows causes of perforation in infants younger than 2 months. Necrotizing enterocolitis (n = 75) and spontaneous isolated perforation of the ileum (n = 30) were the 2 most common causes of perforation. *Abbreviations*: *dis.*, disease; *GCMP*, giant cystic meconium peritonitis; *NEC*, necrotizing enterocolitis; *perf.*, perforation. (Courtesy of Grosfeld JL, Molinari F, Chaet M, et al: Gastrointestinal perforation and peritonitis in infants and children: Experience with 179 cases over ten years. *Surgery* 120:650–656, 1996.)

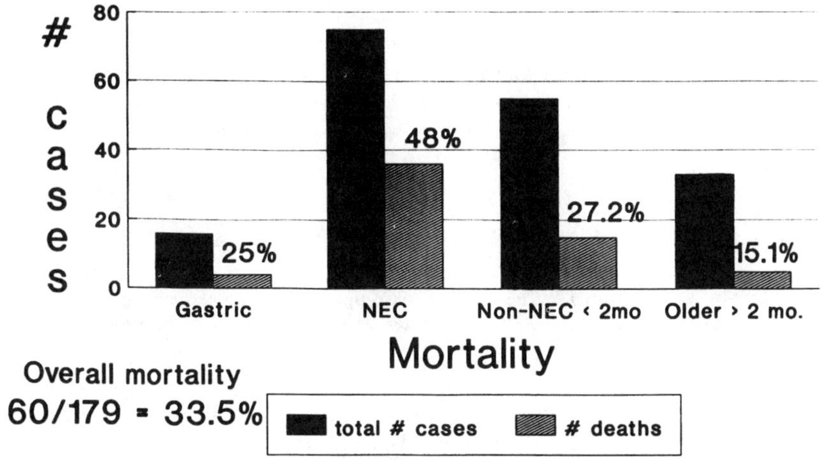

FIGURE 3.—Bar graph shows mortality for various study groups. Highest mortality was observed in premature infants with necrotizing enterocolitis, 36 of 75 (48%). This was significantly higher mortality than infants without necrotizing enterocolitis younger than 2 months, 15 of 55 (27.2%), and older children, 5 of 33 (15.1%) ($P < 0.05$ necrotizing enterocolitis vs. both other groups). *Abbreviation*: NEC, necrotizing enterocolitis. (Courtesy of Grosfeld JL, Molinari F, Chaet M, et al: Gastrointestinal perforation and peritonitis in infants and children: Experience with 179 cases over ten years. *Surgery* 120:650–656, 1996.)

with necrotizing enterocolitis, continue to have a high death rate after necrotizing enterocolitis. It may be possible to improve outcome with adjunctive therapy to counteract the immaturity of organ function and immune status.

► This large series of gastrointestinal perforations accumulated at a single center over a prolonged period provides some perspective on the quandary. The high mortality rates, even in the postneonatal period, attest to the gravity of the situation. Unfortunately, even this experience provides little insight into the pathogenesis. Figure 1 and the table in the original article paint the portrait of the disorder, but the reader will come away frustrated by the conspicuous absence of any strategy to prevent the perforations. Determining the prognosis from the site of the perforation and the underlying etiologic factor is no consolation.

The time frame covered in this review precedes the more liberal use of prenatal and postnatal steroids as well as indomethacin. The discussion emphasized multiorgan immaturity and the poor prognosis when there is multiorgan failure. Although the equivalent of the Acute Physiology and Chronic Health Evaluation scoring systems in adults and children is still under review in the neonatal period, the imagination needs no stretching to realize that an immature infant with a gastrointestinal perforation, sepsis, renal failure, and pulmonary insufficiency has a poor outlook.

The prognosis is often determined by the site of the perforation; this is well and good, but what determines the site? There is a growing body of experimental evidence demonstrating the cascade of events interrelating ischemia and infection, together with formula. The end result is bowel ischemia and perforation. The various cytokines, including platelet activating factor and tumor necrosis factor-α, and the activation of the prostaglandin metabolites play a pivotal role. However, what turns on the cascades and how to prevent progression to gastrointestinal perforation remains, for the moment, beyond our grasp.[1] (See also Abstract 9–16.)

A.A. Fanaroff, M.B.B.Ch.

Reference

1. Horwitz JR, Lally KP, Cheu HW, et al: Complications after surgical intervention for necrotizing enterocolitis: A multicenter review. *J Pediatr Surg* 30:994–999, 1995.

Focal Intestinal Perforation in Preterm Infants Is an Emerging Disease

Raghuveer G, Speidel B, Marlow N, et al (Southmead Hosp, Westbury on Trym, Bristol, England; St Michaels Hosp, Bristol, England)

Acta Paediatr 85:237–239, 1996 9–16

Introduction.—The clinical picture of focal intestinal perforation has been contrasted with that of necrotizing enterocolitis, but there has been no previous attempt to isolate factors that specifically antedate the former. Focal intestinal perforation has been considered to be linked to indomethacin therapy, mechanical ventilation by face mask or nasal prongs, and congenital defects of the intestinal musculature. Antecedent factors of focal intestinal perforation were evaluated in 8 infants.

Methods.—Two gestation-matched control infants were selected for comparison with the 8 infants with focal intestinal perforation. Several variables were compared between groups.

Results.—All infants with focal intestinal perforation had birth weights between 630 and 1,050 g, and were ventilated immediately after birth. Seven were still being ventilated at the time of perforation. Seven infants underwent laparotomy. All infants recovered, and 6 were alive at follow-up and had no gastrointestinal complications. Infants with focal intestinal perforation had significantly lower birth weights for gestational age, more frequent ductus arteriosus, and intraventricular hemorrhage, than did control subjects (Table 1). Although not reaching statistical significance, infants with focal intestinal perforation had higher frequencies of fetal distress, surfactant use, and umbilical arterial catheterizations than control subjects. There were no between-group differences in Apgar scores at 1 and 5 minutes, the need for mechanical ventilation, the prevalence and type of feeds, the presence of *Staphylococcus epidermidis* on blood culture, and the use of indomethacin.

Conclusions.—Three antecedents were associated with focal perforation: low weight for gestation, presence of a patent ductus, and intraventricular hemorrhage. All other perinatal variables tested failed to reach significance.

TABLE 1.—Profile of Antecedents Among Cases and Controls

	Index cases (*n* = 8)	Controls (*n* = 16)	*P*
Gestational age (weeks): median (range)	27.5 (24–31)	27.5 (24–32	
Birthweight (g): median (range)	900 (630–1050)	1025 (645–1740)	—
SDS of weight for gestational age: median (range)	−1.02 (−2.06 to 0.90)	−0.08 (−2.12 to 1.17)	0.013
Fetal distress	4 (50%)	3 (19%)	0.27
Umbilical arterial catheter	6 (75%)	7 (44%)	0.31
Indomethacin	3 (38%)	4 (25%)	0.86
Surfactant	7 (88%)	7 (44%)	0.10
Intraventricular haemorrhage	5 (63%)	1 (6%)	0.014
Patent ductus arteriosus	7 (88%)	4 (25%)	0.012
Ventilated	7 (88%)	15 (94%)	1.00
Positive blood culture for *S. epidermidis*	6 (75%)	9 (56%)	0.67

Abbreviation: SDS, standard deviation score.
(Courtesy of Raghuveer G, Speidel B, Marlow N, et al: Focal intestinal perforation in preterm infants is an emerging disease. *Acta Paediatr* 85:237–239, 1996.)

▶ This is a short and sweet analysis of a very specific entity that strikes without warning. True, the case analysis reveals that growth retardation, patent ductus, and intraventricular hemorrhage are common antecedents, but then again, hundreds of premature infants with these complications will not have isolated gastrointestinal perforations. The unifying theory is intestinal ischemia, but there must be some other factor that renders these infants particularly vulnerable to intestinal perforation yet protects them from the more severe necrotizing enterocolitis. Neither steroids nor indomethacin were factors in this small, but well-analyzed, series. Grosfeld (see Abstract 9–15) adds sheer weight of numbers but brings us no closer to the cause.

We should derive some comfort from the good prognosis, be alert to promptly diagnose and treat the disease, and keep searching for the cause.

A man must not swallow more beliefs than he can digest.–Havelock Ellis

A.A. Fanaroff, M.B.B.Ch.

10 The Respiratory Tract

Randomized Trial of Antenatal Dexamethasone in Surfactant-treated Infants Delivered Before 30 Weeks' Gestation

Silver RK, Vyskocil C, Solomon SL, et al (Evanston Hosp, Ill; Northwestern Univ, Chicago)

Obstet Gynecol 87:683–691, 1996 10–1

Background.—Corticosteroid administration to the mother has been the main treatment approach to the prevention of respiratory distress syndrome (RDS). Exogenous surfactant replacement administered postnatally has also been found to be effective in preventing RDS. It is unclear whether both antenatal and postnatal treatments in the same mother-infant pair have an advantage over either treatment alone.

Methods.—One hundred twenty-four pregnant women at risk for delivery at 24–29 weeks' gestation were enrolled in the randomized, double-blind trial. Fifty-four women were given dexamethasone in 4 doses of 5 mg each every 12 hours, and 42 were given placebo. All infants received prophylactic surfactant at birth. Seventy-five women gave birth to a total of 96 infants between 24 and 29 weeks' gestation.

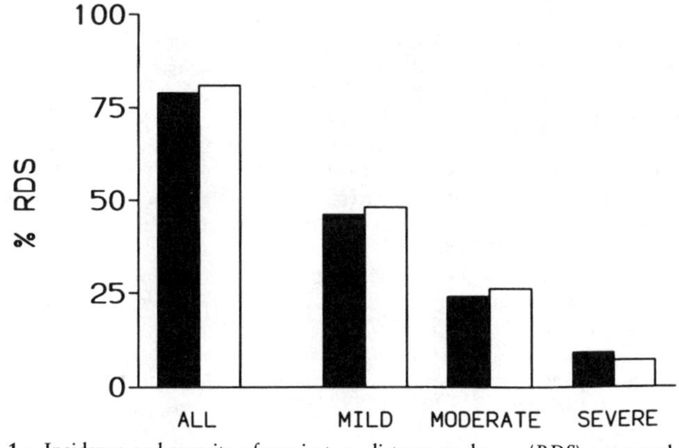

FIGURE 1.—Incidence and severity of respiratory distress syndrome (*RDS*) compared between dexamethasone- (*solid bars*) and placebo- (*open bars*) exposed neonates receiving prophylactic surfactant. (Courtesy of Silver RK, Vyskocil C, Solomon SL, et al: Randomized trial of antenatal dexamethasone in surfactant-treated infants delivered before 30 weeks' gestation. *Obstet Gynecol* 87:683–691, 1996. Reprinted with permission from The American College of Obstetricians and Gynecologists.)

Findings.—The infants given dexamethasone or placebo did not differ significantly in the occurrence or severity of RDS or in any of the secondary clinical end points, including bronchopulmonary dysplasia, pneumothorax, patent ductus arteriosus, necrotizing enterocolitis, retinopathy, intraventricular bleeding, and death. However, the neonates exposed to dexamethasone had significantly fewer grade 3 and 4 intraventricular hemorrhages (Fig 1).

Conclusions.—Antenatal dexamethasone treatment apparently does not reduce the incidence or severity of RDS in surfactant-treated neonates at 24–29 weeks' gestation. However, the severity of intraventricular bleeding in surfactant-treated singletons delivered in this age range may be reduced by the maternal treatment.

▶ This is the second controlled trial that has reached this conclusion for infants at less than 30 weeks' gestation (the first was by Garite, et al.[1]), and it is certainly disappointing for those of us who champion antenatal steroid use. However, the data appear to be unassailable. Nevertheless, there was a significant reduction in the risk of grade 3 and 4 intraventricular hemorrhage in the neonates who had been exposed to dexamethasone. Thus, although the data supporting the efficacy of antenatal corticosteroids in reducing the incidence of RDS in infants less than 29 weeks' gestation is slim, the evidence for their efficacy in reducing intraventricular hemorrhage is compelling.[2-6] In 1997, virtually every mother in preterm labor at 23–34 weeks who does not have obvious chorioamnionitis should receive steroids.

M.J. Maisels, M.B., B.Ch.

References

1. Garite TJ, Rumney DJ, Briggs GG, et al: A randomized, placebo-controlled trial of betamethasone for the prevention of respiratory distress syndrome at 24 to 28 weeks' gestation. *Am J Obstet Gynecol* 166:646–651, 1992.
2. NIH Consensus Development Conference on the Effect of Corticosteroids for Fetal Maturation on Perinatal Outcomes: Effect of corticosteroids for fetal maturation on perinatal outcomes. *JAMA* 273:413–418, 1995.
3. Wright L, Horbar JD, Gunkel H: Evidence from multicenter network on the current use and effectiveness of antenatal corticosteroids in low birth weight infants. *Am J Obstet Gynecol* 173:263–269, 1995.
4. Garland JS, Buck R, Leviton A: Effect of maternal glucocorticoid exposure on risk of severe intraventricular hemorrhage in surfactant-treated preterm infants. *J Pediatr,* 126:272–279, 1995.
5. Kari MA, Hallman M, Eronen M: Prenatal dexamethasone treatment in conjunction with rescue therapy of human surfactant: A randomized placebo-controlled multicenter study. *Pediatrics* 93:730–736, 1994.
6. Leviton A, Kuban KC, Pagamo M, et al: Antenatal corticosteroids appear to reduce the risk of postnatal germinal matrix hemorrhage in intubated low birth weight newborns. *Pediatrics* 91:1083–1088, 1993.

Influence of Early Postnatal Dexamethasone Therapy on Ventilator Dependency in Surfactant-substituted Preterm Infants

Suske G, Oestreich K, Varnholt V, et al (Univ Children's Hosp, Mannheim, Germany)

Acta Paediatr 85:713–718, 1996 10–2

Background.—The effect of early postnatal dexamethasone combined with surfactant replacement therapy in preterm infants with respiratory distress syndrome (RDS) has not yet been reported in the literature. Whether early postnatal dexamethasone therapy in preterm infants with surfactant-substituted RDS would facilitate extubation, improve response to surfactant treatment, and decrease acute barotraumatic complications and bronchopulmonary dysplasia was determined.

Methods.—Twenty-six infants were enrolled in the randomized, controlled, prospective study. Fourteen infants were given dexamethasone, 0.5 mg/kg per day for 5 days, in addition to surfactant substitution. Treatment and control groups were similar in birth weight, gestational age, prenatal characteristics, and initial respiratory and blood gas values.

Findings.—One infant in each group died. Those receiving dexamethasone responded better to surfactant, were extubated earlier, and spent less time receiving supplemental oxygen. Pulmonary complications and the frequency of retinopathy were lower in the infants given dexamethasone.

Conclusion.—Early postnatal dexamethasone treatment improves response to surfactant replacement. Arterial oxygenation is enhanced and weaning is facilitated. Also, extubation and ambient air breathing can be achieved sooner. A double-blind study involving more infants is now needed to verify these findings.

▶ Commenting on this article is Louis P. Halamek, M.D., Professor of Pediatrics, Division of Neonatal and Developmental Medicine, Stanford University Medical Center, Palo Alto, California:

▶ Although this is a small study with all of the limitations thereof, the results are intriguing and add to a growing body of data indicating that relative hypoadrenalism in the premature neonate plays a role in the pathophysiology of several neonatal diseases. Much remains to be determined regarding the following:

The corticosteroid of choice. Although dexamethasone is most frequently used in neonatal ICUs across the United States, other corticosteroids, alone or in combination, may turn out to be better choices.

Optimal dose and dosing interval. Supraphysiologic doses are commonly used in studies, but lower doses may be just as efficacious and without the frequency and severity of undesired side effects, such as glucose intolerance and hypertension.

Timing of therapy. Experience with the use of hydrocortisone in the treatment of neonatal hypotension in the first days of unresponsiveness to volume and inotropes has shown promise.[1] Early treatment with physiologic doses in the first days of life, guided by monitoring of serum levels and weaning of therapy as the neonatal hypothalamic-pituitary-adrenal axis begins to function normally, may prove to be useful in treating and/or ameliorating both acute and chronic conditions such as hypotension and bronchopulmonary dysplasia.

L.P. Halamek, M.D.

Reference

1. Helbock HJ, Insoft RM, Conte FA: Glucocorticoid-responsive hypotension in extremely low birth weight newborns. *Pediatrics* 92:715–717, 1993.

Failure of Early Postnatal Dexamethasone to Prevent Chronic Lung Disease in Infants With Respiratory Distress Syndrome

Shinwell ES, Karplus M, Zmora E, et al (Soroka Med Ctr, Beersheva, Israel; Ha'emek Med Ctr, Afula, Israel Carmel Med Ctr, Haifa, Israel; et al)

Arch Dis Child 74:F33–F37, 1996 10–3

Background.—Despite the introduction of surfactant treatment for respiratory distress syndrome (RDS), the incidence of chronic lung disease (CLD) in premature infants continues to be disturbingly high. Steroid treatment given just after birth may prevent inflammatory insult to lungs, thus reducing the likelihood of CLD. The efficacy of dexamethasone administered 1–3 days after birth in preterm infants with RDS was investigated.

Methods.—Two hundred forty-eight infants at 18 neonatal ICUs in Israel were enrolled in a randomized, placebo-controlled, blinded trial. One hundred thirty-two received dexamethasone, and 116 were given placebo. Outcome measures were survival to discharge with no need for supplemental oxygen treatment past 28 days of life, need for mechanical ventilation at 3 and 7 days, duration of ventilation or oxygen treatment, need for subsequent steroids for established CLD, and incidence of major morbidities.

Findings.—The only between-group difference in outcome variables was a decrease in the requirement for mechanical ventilation at 3 days of age in treated infants. Although gastrointestinal hemorrhage, hypertension, and hyperglycemia were more common in the treated infants, no life-threatening complications occurred.

Conclusion.—These findings do not support the routine use of early postnatal steroid therapy for preventing CLD. However, a much larger multicenter trial of early prolonged dexamethsaone therapy is warranted.

► Lu-Ann Papile, M.D., Professor of Pediatrics, of the University of New Mexico School of Medicine, comments:

► It has been 13 years since Mammel et al. reported that dexamethasone improved pulmonary function and decreased ventilator dependence in a select group of infants with established CLD.[1] Since then, the use of corticosteroid therapy not only to ameliorate, but also to prevent, CLD has gained widespread acceptance in clinical neonatology. Although there are adequate data to support steroid use to wean infants with CLD from intermittent ventilation, the efficacy of steroids in preventing the disease is, as yet, unknown.[2] In the only published trial that had a sample size sufficient to evaluate the risks and benefits of early steroid treatment, Shinwell et al. report that a short course of early steroid treatment is not beneficial in lowering the frequency of CLD among premature infants at highest risk.

I suspect knowing nods among opponents and shouts and murmurs among proponents of steroid use after reading the report. Steroid naysayers will point out that it just may be that postnatal steroid treatment at any age is not an effective therapy for the prevention of CLD and that the significantly higher reported incidence of gastrointestinal hemorrhage among the steroid-treated infants ($P = 0.001$) does not warrant exposing these infants to a doubtful therapy. Conversely, steroid mavens will quickly point out that the duration of steroid therapy (3 days) was too short and that a longer course is needed to adequately suppress the inflammatory response in the lungs and allow enough time for repair. The observation that the need for ventilatory support was significantly less after 3 days of steroid treatment, but insignificant several days after treatment was stopped, buttresses this point of view.

Because many neonatologists who advocate early steroids to prevent CLD utilize a treatment period longer than 3 days, the reported trial, despite its magnitude, will not vastly change clinical practice. In fact, the results of a recent small trial by Rastogi et al, suggest that using a longer course of early steroids is beneficial.[3] Although these preliminary data are promising, at least one more large, multicenter trial of early steroid treatment using a longer duration of therapy will be needed before there are sufficient data to resolve the controversy of early steroid use in the prevention of CLD.

L. Papile, M.D.

References

1. Mammel MC, Green TP, Johnson DE, et al: Controlled trial of dexamethasone therapy in respirator-dependent infants with bronchopulmonary dysplasia. *Lancet* 1:1356–1358, 1983.
2. Collaborative Dexamethasone Trial Group. Dexamethasone therapy in neonatal chronic lung disease: An international placebo-controlled trial. *Pediatrics* 88:421–427, 1996.
3. Rastogi A, Akintorin SM, Bez ML, et al: A controlled trial of dexamethasone to prevent bronchopulmonary dysplasia in surfactant-treated infants. *Pediatrics* 98:204–210, 1996.

Partial Liquid Ventilation With Perflubron in Premature Infants With Severe Respiratory Distress Syndrome

Leach CL, for the LiquiVent Study Group (State Univ of New York, Buffalo; et al)

N Engl J Med 335:761–767, 1996 10–4

Objective.—Ventilation with perfluorocarbon liquids has been used successfully to treat lung dysfunction in premature neonates with surfactant deficiency. The safety and efficacy of partial liquid ventilation, in which perfluorocarbon liquid is introduced into the lungs during continuous positive-pressure gas ventilation, in premature infants with severe respiratory distress syndrome were evaluated and compared with those of other treatments.

Methods.—Perflubron was instilled at a rate of 1 mL/kg/min into the lungs of 13 premature infants, less than 5 days old, at risk of death, with

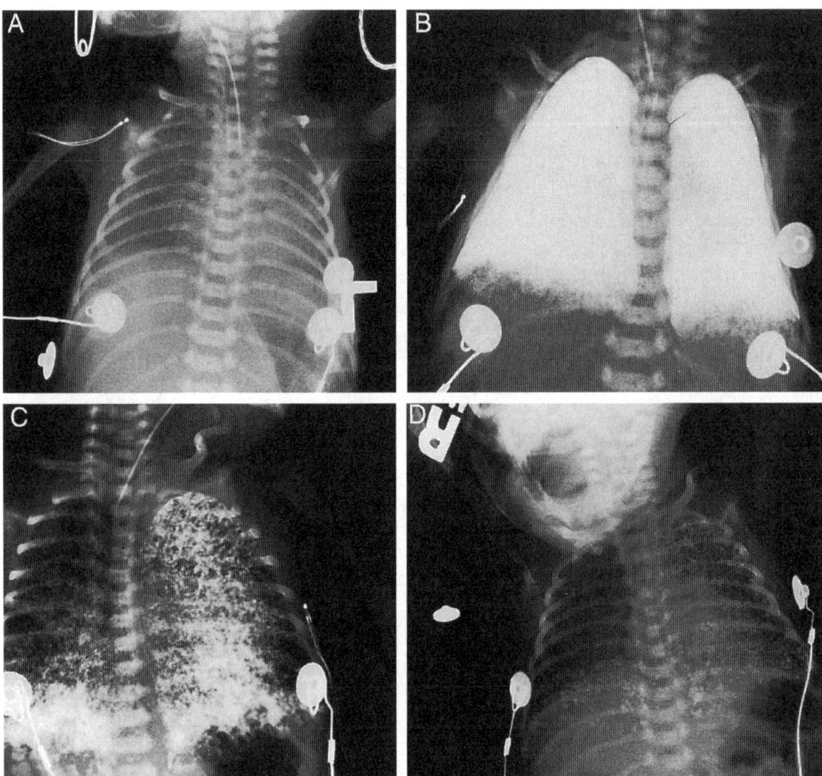

FIGURE 1.—Chest radiographs in 1 infant during treatment with gas ventilation (**A**), 1 hour after the initation of partial liquid ventilation with perflubron (**B**), and 48 hours (**C**) and 3 weeks (**D**) after the last dose of perflubron. (Courtesy of Leach CL, for the LiquiVent Study Group: Partial liquid ventilation with perflubron in premature infants with severe respiratory distress syndrome. *N Engl J Med* 335:761–767, Copyright 1996, Massachusetts Medical Society. All rights reserved.)

arterial oxygen tension of less than 60 mm Hg or arterial carbon dioxide tension of greater than 60 mm Hg. Mechanical ventilation maintained at an end-expiratory pressure of 4 cm H_2O was continued throughout the instillation, and partial liquid ventilation was continued for a minimum of 24 hours. New medical conditions, developmental progress, changes in arterial tension, dynamic compliance, ventilatory requirements, oxygenation index ([fraction of inspired oxygen × mean airway pressure × 100]÷ arterial oxygen tension), and survival were monitored.

Results.—The 10 infants who completed the study were ventilated for an average of 42 hours. Gas exchange and lung mechanics improved, and arterial oxygen tension increased from 60 mm Hg at baseline to 143 mm Hg after 1 hour of ventilation. Within 24 hours, the fraction of inspired oxygen was significantly reduced, and the arterial carbon dioxide tension normalized. The oxygenation index decreased sigificantly from 49 at baseline to 9 at 24 hours. The procedure was well tolerated. Adverse events included endotracheal tube obstruction ($n = 5$), hypoxic episode ($n = 2$), intracranial hemorrhage ($n = 3$), pneumothorax ($n = 1$), and upper gastrointestinal hemorrhage ($n = 1$). There were 5 deaths, 2 from respiratory distress syndrome, 2 from intracranial hemorrhage, and 1 from pneumonia and sepsis. Largely gas-filled lungs with some remaining perflubron were seen on chest radiographs 48 hours and 3 weeks after the final dose of perflubron (Fig 1).

Conclusion.—Partial liquid ventilation results in clinical improvement and increases survival in premature neonates with respiratory distress syndrome.

► The commentary below was provided by Dr. Eileen K. Stork. Dr. Stork is Director of the ECMO Center at Rainbow Babies & Childrens Hospital in Cleveland, Ohio, and Associate Professor of Pediatrics, Case Western Reserve University School of Medicine:

► Few topics have generated as much interest among pediatricians in the past year as the study of liquid ventilation in preemies with respiratory failure. This was a safety and efficacy study conducted by a multi-institutional research group (the Liquid Ventilation Group) of 13 premature infants between 24 and 34 weeks' gestation who still required 100% inspired oxygen and significant ventilator support after surfactant therapy. Perflubron was instilled gradually into the infants' lungs to a volume corresponding to functional residual capacity (about 15 mL/kg). The liquid-filled lungs then were ventilated with a standard positive-pressure gas ventilator. The perflubron lost through evaporation in the upper airways was replaced periodically to maintain a meniscus of the trachea. This technique is known as "partial liquid ventilation," and it is relatively easy to perform without any special equipment in the neonatal ICU. This contrasts with the original technique of tidal (or total) liquid ventilation, in which a fixed volume of perflubron ultimately is instilled and expelled from the lungs several times each minute. Tidal liquid ventilation requires a special liquid ventilator to cycle the perflubron in and out of the lungs and is, therefore, more technically demanding than the process used in this study.

Ten of the 13 infants completed the study with impressive improvement in arterial oxygen, dynamic compliance, and oxygenation index. Several infants suffered episodic endotracheal obstruction with thick mucoid material necessitating frequent, and sometimes vigorous, suctioning with saline. However, no life-threatening events were attributed to liquid ventilation.

On the downside, however, 3 of the 13 infants were removed from the study because their ventilation was deemed superior with high-frequency oscillatory ventilation. In the infants who completed this study, there were measurable levels of perflubron in the blood 4 hours after initiation of liquid ventilation. This concentration doubled after 24 hours. There still were measurable levels of perflubron in the blood of these infants 20–28 days after the last dose. The significance of this persistent blood/tissue level is unknown, but it certainly warrants a cautionary note for the use of such chemicals in the immature neonate.

Ultimately, if liquid ventilation is to prove useful in the respiratory support of neonates, it must be shown to be superior to all current modes of gas ventilation with regard to survival or the incidence of chronic lung disease. Outcome data no doubt will define the efficacy of this novel respiratory technique. To answer this question, expensive, multicenter, randomized trials will be required down the road.

On a final note, I hope that studies will continue with tidal liquid ventilation in the neonate because this technique lavages the lung of debris and inflammatory agents in a way that partial liquid ventilation can never achieve. A tidal liquid ventilator is no more complicated than extracorporeal membrane oxygenation, and heaven knows many intensivists have mastered this technique with unbridled enthusiasm!

E.K. Stork, M.D.

► Commenting on this article is Louis P. Halamek, M.D., Professor of Pediatrics, Division of Neonatal and Developmental Medicine, Stanford University Medical Center, Palo Alto, California:

► Although therapies such as administration of artificial and modified natural surfactants, high-frequency ventilation (jet, flow interruption, and oscillation), and inhaled nitric oxide have proven effective in various subpopulations of neonates with respiratory failure, they are neither uniformly efficacious nor without sequelae. The ideal mode of mechanical ventilation in the neonate is unknown, and any therapy using gas ventilation of the lung carries a risk of barotrauma and oxygen toxicity. Liquid ventilation is a novel therapeutic modality that holds tremendous promise as a treatment for neonatal respiratory failure. The history of liquid ventilation is marked by numerous firsts: the groundbreaking submersion experiments of Clark[1]; the development of mechanical systems to effectively deliver perfluorochemicals into the lung by Shaffer and Wolfson[2, 3]; the initial human trial by Greenspan and colleagues[4, 5]; and the combination of conventional mechanical gas ventilation with perfluorochemical delivery by Fuhrman and associates.[6] This paper, authored by many of the leaders in the field of liquid ventilation, is a seminal work and ushers in a new era in neonatal-perinatal medicine.

L.P. Halamek, M.D.

References

1. Clark LC, Gollan F: Survival of mammals breathing organic liquids equilibrated with oxygen at atmospheric pressure. *Science* 152:1755–1756, 1966.
2. Shaffer TH, Moskowitz GD: Demand-controlled liquid ventilation of the lungs. *J Appl Physiol* 36:208–213, 1974.
3. Wolfson MR, Tran N, Bhutani VK, et al: A new experimental approach for the study of cardiopulmonary physiology during early development. *J Appl Physiol* 65:1436–1443, 1988.
4. Greenspan JS, Wolfson MR, Rubenstein SD, et al: Liquid ventilation of preterm babies. *Lancet* 2:8671–1095, 1989.
5. Greenspan JS, Wolfson MR, Rubenstein SD, et al: Liquid ventilation of human preterm neonates. *J Pediatr* 117:106–111, 1990.
6. Fuhrman BP, Paczan PR, DeFrancisis M: Perfluorocarbon-associated gas exchange. *Crit Care Med* 19:712–722, 1991.

Liquid Assisted Ventilation: An Alternative Ventilatory Strategy for Acute Meconium Aspiration Injury

Foust R III, Tran NN, Cox C, et al (Temple Univ, Philadelphia; Jeanes Hosp, Philadelphia; Bryn Mawr Hosp, Pa; et al)

Pediatr Pulmonol 21:316–322, 1996 10–5

Background.—Meconium aspiration syndrome (MAS) is a cause of serious morbidity in the neonatal ICU. Surfactant dysfunction appears to play a key role in the pathophysiology of MAS, leading to the use of exogenous surfactant therapy in its management. Previous studies have shown improved cardiopulmonary function after liquid-assisted ventilation in lungs with high surface tension. An animal study of acute meconium aspiration injury was performed to compare exogenous surfactant therapy with liquid-assisted ventilation.

Methods.—Thirty-two newborn lambs were anesthetized and intubated. They were placed on mechanical ventilation, with a peak inspiratory pressure of 13–16 cm H_2O, a positive end-expiratory pressure of 3–4 cm H_2O, and a fractional inspired oxygen concentration of 1.0. The respiratory rate was 30–35 breaths/min. After arterial blood gases, pulmonary function, and arterial blood pressure were measured, the animals were given unfiltered 25% meconium solution, 2–3 mL/kg. The animals were then randomly assigned to 4 hours of treatment with surfactant or partial liquid ventilation (PLV) or total liquid ventilation (TLV) with liquid perfluorocarbon; a control group received gas ventilation only. The results were assessed by repeated arterial blood gas and pulmonary function studies and by histologic examination of the lungs.

Results.—Arterial oxygenation improved significantly in animals treated with either surfactant or perfluorocarbon. For lambs in the surfac-

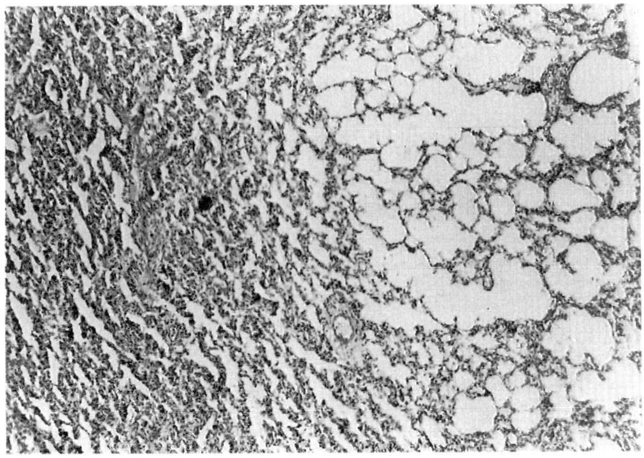

FIGURE 5.—Photomicrograph of meconium control conventional mechanical ventilation lung. Areas of atelectasis juxtaposed to regions of overexpansion are evident; hematoxylin-eosin; original magnification, ×10. (Foust R III, Tran NN, Cox C, et al: Liquid assisted ventilation: An alternative ventilatory strategy for acute meconium aspiration injury. *Pediatr Pulmonol* 21:316–322, 1996. Reprinted by permission of John Wiley & Sons, Inc.)

tant and PLV groups, arterial partial pressure of carbon dioxide was significantly reduced as well. All 3 treatment groups had increased compliance, but the greatest improvement was seen in the TLV group. On histologic examination, the alveolar epithelium was intact and the alveoli were homogeneously expanded only in animals treated with TLV (Figs 5 through 8).

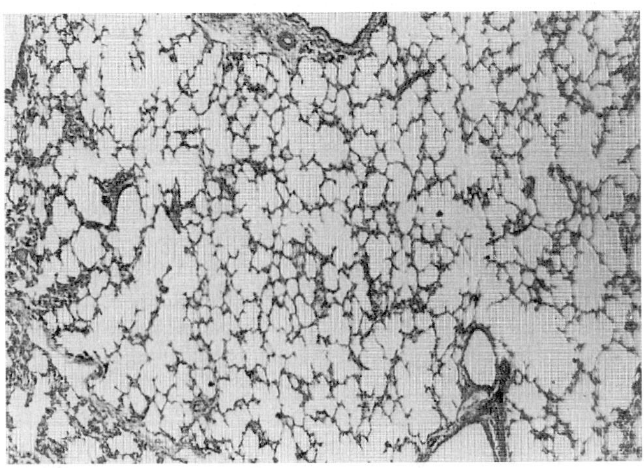

FIGURE 6.—Photomicrograph of meconium-injured, surfactant-treated lung. Well-expanded regions with slightly thickened alveolar membranes; hematoxylin-eosin; original magnification, ×10. (Foust R III, Tran NN, Cox C, et al: Liquid assisted ventilation: An alternative ventilatory strategy for acute meconium aspiration injury. *Pediatr Pulmonol* 21:316–322, 1996. Reprinted by permission of John Wiley & Sons, Inc.)

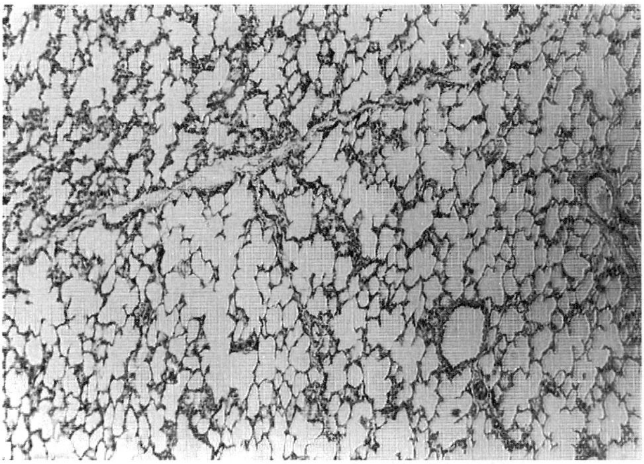

FIGURE 7.—Photomicrograph of meconium-injured, partial liquid ventilation–treated lung. Nonhomogeneous aeration of alveoli. Partial atelectasis; hematoxylin-eosin; original magnification, ×10. (Foust R III, Tran NN, Cox C, et al: Liquid assisted ventilation: An alternative ventilatory strategy for acute meconium aspiration injury. *Pediatr Pulmonol* 21:316–322, 1996. Reprinted by permission of John Wiley & Sons, Inc.)

Conclusion.—Experimental evidence suggests that exogenous surfactant therapy and partial or total liquid-assisted ventilation are potentially useful treatments for infants with MAS. The physiologic and histologic improvements observed with TLV may be related to improved ventilation/perfusion matching resulting from alveolar recruitment and débridement, abolition of surface tension at the air-liquid interface, and elimination of underlying diffusion impairment. The use of surfactant therapy for MAS

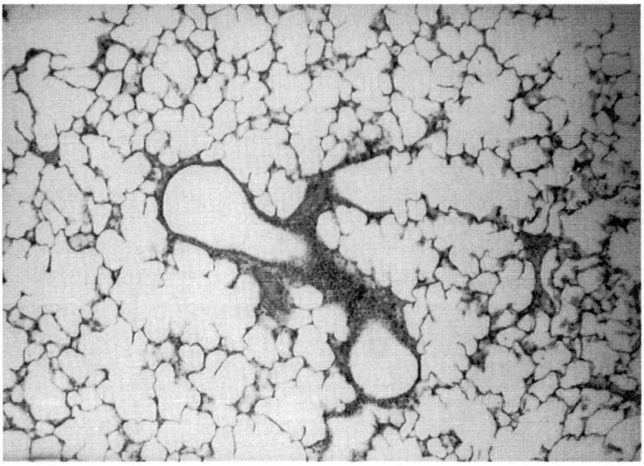

FIGURE 8.—Photomicrograph of meconium-injured, total liquid ventilation–treated lung. Alveolar spaces are uniformly expanded, clear, and unobstructed; hematoxylin-eosin; original magnification, ×10. (Foust R III, Tran NN, Cox C, et al: Liquid assisted ventilation: An alternative ventilatory strategy for acute meconium aspiration injury. *Pediatr Pulmonol* 21:316–322, 1996. Reprinted by permission of John Wiley & Sons, Inc.)

should continue, and PLV and TLV should receive further consideration for this purpose.

▶ Commenting on this article is Louis P. Halamek, M.D., Professor of Pediatrics, Division of Neonatal and Developmental Medicine, Stanford University Medical Center, Palo Alto, California:

▶ Although total (or tidal) liquid ventilation is still very much an experimental therapy requiring equipment that is still in the development phase, PLV is being used successfully to treat various causes of respiratory failure in humans. The potential benefits of using a perfluorochemical to achieve gas exchange in the human neonate are many, including reduction in surface tension, improvement in ventilation-perfusion matching, recruitment of atelectatic alveoli, and lavage of substances such as meconium and other debris. It is also becoming apparent that these chemicals, although inert, act to modulate the inflammatory cascade and, therefore, protect the immature lung; this may prove to have an impact on the incidence of bronchopulmonary dysplasia. It is possible that the delivery room of the future will be a place where premature neonates are intubated before drawing their first breath, their lungs immediately filled with perfluorochemical, never allowing for an air-liquid interface to develop. After a course of liquid ventilation, during which their lungs would be allowed to reach anatomical and functional maturity—perhaps with the delivery of a cocktail of growth factors and steroids—they would then be extubated to room air.

L.P. Halamek, M.D.

The Provo Multicenter Early High-frequency Oscillatory Ventilation Trial: Improved Pulmonary and Clinical Outcome in Respiratory Distress Syndrome

Gerstmann DR, Minton SD, Stoddard RA, et al (Utah Valley Regional Med Ctr, Provo; Mem Hosp, Colorado Springs, Colo; Clinique Saint Vincent, Rocourt, Belgium; et al)

Pediatrics 98:1044–1057, 1996 10–6

Introduction.—Studies in primate models of hyaline membrane disease report clear advantages for using early high-frequency oscillatory ventilation (HFOV) strategies in respiratory distress syndrome (RDS), but randomized clinical trials involving premature infants have raised questions about the efficacy of HFOV as a primary treatment modality for RDS. In a multicenter trial, the clinical course and outcomes of preterm infants with RDS given surfactant and randomized to ventilator care with HFOV were comparred with those given conventional mechanical ventilation (CV).

Methods.—Eligible infants were 35 weeks or less estimated gestation and less than 12 hours old at study entry. All required intubation and mechanical ventilation and had an arterial-to-alveolar oxygen ratio less than 0.50. Sixty-one were randomized to continue CV and 64 to be

NO POSTAGE
NECESSARY
IF MAILED
IN THE
UNITED STATES

BUSINESS REPLY MAIL
FIRST CLASS MAIL PERMIT No. 762 CHICAGO, IL

POSTAGE WILL BE PAID BY ADDRESSEE

Chris Hughes
Mosby-Year Book, Inc.
161 N. Clark Street
Suite 1900
Chicago, IL 60601-9981

NO POSTAGE
NECESSARY
IF MAILED
IN THE
UNITED STATES

BUSINESS REPLY MAIL
FIRST CLASS MAIL PERMIT No. 762 CHICAGO, IL

POSTAGE WILL BE PAID BY ADDRESSEE

Chris Hughes
Mosby-Year Book, Inc.
161 N. Clark Street
Suite 1900
Chicago, IL 60601-9981

changed to HFOV. Infants at each of the 3 study centers were treated with bovine-derived surfactant and received routine neonatal ICU care. Pulmonary outcomes recorded included suctioning frequency, surfactant dosing, air leak, oxygenation, ventilation, oxygen use, ventilator use, chronic lung disease, and need for oxygen at discharge.

Results.—The 2 treatment groups were similar in demographic features. The mean gestational age was 30.9 weeks and the mean birth weight was 1.51 kg; all infants were entered in the study at age 2–3 hours. Compared with CV-treated infants, those randomized to HFOV required less intensive vasopressor support and less frequent surfactant redosing. Fewer infants in the HFOV group required prolonged supplemental oxygen or ventilator support and more survived without chronic lung disease at 30 days. Oxygenation improved more rapidly and remained higher during the first 7 days with HFOV than with CV. Other advantages associated with HFOV were fewer abnormal hearing test results and fewer episodes of necrotizing enterocolitis illness (Table 3). Although length of hospital stay was similar for the 2 groups, hospital costs were lower for HFOV- vs. CV-treated infants (Fig 4). The 2 groups were similar in the rate of survival

TABLE 3.—Clinical Outcomes

		HFOV Group	CV Group
Vasopressor support	Patients on vasopressors	42.2% (27/64)	42.6% (26/61)
	Use index >120 h	16.6% (4/27)*	42.3% (11/26)
PDA	Treated PDA	45.4% (20/44)	40.4% (19/47)
NEC illness	No symptoms	60	49
	Suspected	2	9
	Medically treated	2	2
	Surgically treated	0	1
	Suspected or treated	6.2% (4/64)*	19.7% (12/61)
Retinopathy	No eye exam	17	16
	No ROP	35	32
	Stage 1 ROP	6	3
	Stage 2 ROP	3	3
	Stage 3 ROP	2	6
	≥Stage 3 + ROP	1	1
	Any grade ROP	25.6% (12/47)	28.9% (13/45)
	ROP > stage 2	6.4% (3/47)	15.6% (7/45)
Intracranial morbidity	No craniosonography	8	6
	Normal exams	41	36
	Grade 1 IVH	8	8
	Grade 2 IVH	1	2
	Grade 3 IVH	2	1
	Grade 4 IVH	0	5
	Periventricular leukomalacia (PVL) (with/without IVH)	4	3
	Abnormal study	26.8% (15/56)	32.7% (18/55)
	Grade 3–4 IVH or PVL	10.7% (6/56)	16.4% (9/55)
Hearing screen	Abnormal brain stem audio-evoked response	1.9% (1/52)†	16.0% (8/50)

*$P < 0.05$.
†$P < 0.01$; values are mean ± SD or median (5, 95% confidence limits).
(From Gerstmann DR, Minton SD, Stoddard RA, et al: The Provo multicenter early high-frequency oscillatory ventilation trial: Improved pulmonary and clinical outcome in respiratory distress syndrome. *Pediatrics* 98:1044–1057, 1996. Reproduced by permission of *Pediatrics*, Copyright 1996.)

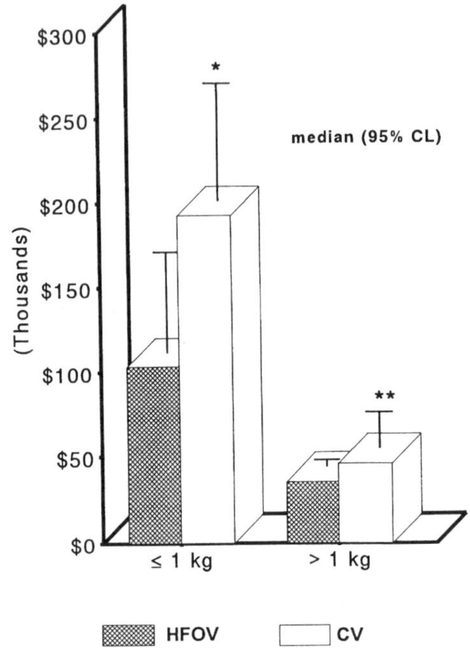

FIGURE 4.—Hospital cost. HFOV, *filled bar;* CV, *open bar.* The values shown are median and 95% confidence limits. Illustrated are total hospital cost information for the 83 patients at site 1. Lower total health care costs were seen in HFOV-treated patients, both less than or equal to 1 kg (*P = 0.044) and greater than 1 kg (**P = 0.030). *Abbreviations: HFOV,* high-frequency oscillatory ventilation; *CV,* conventional mechanical ventilation. (From Gerstmann DR, Minton SD, Stoddard RA, et al: The Provo multicenter early high-frequency oscillatory ventillation trial: Improved pulmonary and clinical outcome in respiratory distress syndrome. *Pediatrics* 98:1044–1057, 1996. Reproduced by permission of *Pediatrics,* Copyright 1996.)

to discharge and in the frequency and severity of patent ductus arteriosus, air leak, retinopathy of prematurity, and intraventricular hemorrhage.

Discussion.—The use of exogenous surfactant and CV has improved pulmonary management for premature infants, but additional benefits can be gained by early HFOV treatment. Both acute and chronic lung injury are reduced, as well as overall morbidity, with the protocol of surfactant replacement, early HFOV, and a lung recruitment strategy.

High-frequency Jet Ventilation in the Early Management of Respiratory Distress Syndrome Is Associated With a Greater Risk for Adverse Outcomes

Wiswell TE, Graziani LJ, Kornhauser MS, et al (Thomas Jefferson Univ, Philadelphia)
Pediatrics 98:1035–1043, 1996 10–7

Introduction.—Respiratory distress syndrome (RDS) requiring ventilatory support remains a common condition among small premature infants.

A new method of high-frequency jet ventilation (HFJV) was compared with conventional mechanical ventilation for its ability to safely reduce pulmonary morbidity in premature infants with RDS.

Methods.—Eligibility criteria were gestational age less than 33 weeks, birth weight greater than 500 g and less than 2,000 g, younger than 24 hours at randomization, chest roentgenographic findings consistent with RDS, and need for assisted ventilation with peak inspiratory pressure of more than 16 and fraction of inspired oxygen more than 0.30. Thirty-six infants were randomly assigned to conventional ventilation and 37 to HFJV. Infants were to be treated for at least 7 days until they could be extubated or met crossover criteria. Neurosonographic studies were obtained at regular intervals and reviewed by 2 radiologists unaware of the infants' clinical course or ventilator assignment.

Results.—The 2 groups of infants were comparable in obstetric and perinatal characteristics and in neonatal clinical and demographic features. Infants were randomly assigned to ventilation method at similar ages (mean, 7.2 hours of life), and the 2 groups had nearly identical prerandomization ventilator settings and arterial blood gases. Pulmonary outcomes, based on the occurrence of air leaks and the need for oxygen or ventilation at 36 weeks post conception, were comparable in HFJV and conventional ventilation groups. The 2 groups were also similar in mean number of days oxygen was required, number of days ventilated, and length of hospital stay. Certain adverse effects, however, were associated with HFJV. Cystic periventricular leukomalacia developed in 10 infants ventilated with HFJV but in only 2 infants in the conventional group. A poor outcome, defined as either grade IV intracranial hemorrhage, cystic periventricular leukomalocia, or death, was significantly more likely in the HFJV-managed group (17 vs. 7 infants).

Conclusion.—Use of HFVJ in the management of premature infants with RDS led to significantly more adverse outcomes than the use of conventional mechanical ventilation. The HFJV should be used only as a rescue device, not as a primary device for managing RDS or other neonatal respiratory disorders.

▶ The following commentary was submitted by Donald M. Null, Jr., M.D., Professor of Pediatrics and Director of Neonatology, Allegheny General Hospital, Pittsburgh, Pennsylvania:

▶ The HiFi Study by the NIH[1] was thought by many individuals to have dealt a death blow to high-frequency ventilation. However, many individuals, because of animal data and rescue data in humans, continued to pursue this technology. The article by Gerstmann et al. (Abstract 10–6), along with other earlier articles,[2, 3] demonstrates the efficacy of high-frequency oscillatory ventilation in the management of newborns with RDS.

There were fundamental differences between the HiFi study strategies and those used by Clark et al.[2] and Gerstmann et al. These included (HiFi vs. Clark/Gerstmann) initially a lower-volume strategy vs. a high-volume strategy, a frequency of 15 Hz vs. 10 Hz, a device that had a 1:1 i.e. ratio vs. a device being used at a 1:2 i.e. ratio, and once inflation occurred, a more rapid weaning of the mean airway pressure. Whether these differences were the sole reason for the different outcomes is not certain.

As with all technologies, there are risks and benefits. To minimize the risks, one must apply the technologies in an appropriate manner (strategy). A thorough understanding of not only the device and how it functions but also the pathophysiology of the pulmonary disease being treated is necessary for a favorable outcome. Additionally, an understanding of the specific risks the device may impart to patients, be they the micro preemie, term infant, or child, is imperative.

The article by Wiswell and colleagues (Abstract 10–7) nicely points out the problem that new technologies may pose. Each day, neonatologists face the problem that a therapy may work superbly for one organ system (the lungs), but may have adverse effects on other organ systems (brain) that can be lifelong.

High-frequency ventilation has proven itself to be a technology that offers advantages in specific pulmonary problems over conventional ventilatory techniques. However, as the article by Wiswell, et al. demonstrates, we need to understand more about the interaction of this therapy with organ systems of the patient to ensure the optimal outcome for our patients. Whether the adverse outcomes are device-specific, strategy-specific, or a combination of the two needs to be researched.

Philosophically, the art of the application of the technology, rather than the technology itself, may have the most to do with its successful use.

D.M. Null, Jr., M.D.

References

1. HiFi Study Group: High-frequency oscillatory ventilation compared with conventional mechanical ventilation in the management of respiratory failure in preterm infants. *N Engl J Med* 320:88–93, 1989.
2. Clark RH, Gerstmann DR, Null DM Jr, et al: Prospective randomized comparison of high-frequency oscillatory and conventional ventilation in respiratory distress syndrome. *Pediatrics* 89:5–12, 1992.
3. Durand DJ, Asselin JM, Courtney SE, et al: Randomized study of high-frequency oscillatory ventilation in infants with severe respiratory distress syndrome. *J Pediatr* 122:609–619, 1993.

Randomized Multicenter Trial Comparing Synchronized and Conventional Intermittent Mandatory Ventilation in Neonates

Bernstein G, Mannino FL, Heldt GP, et al (Univ of California, San Diego; Callahan Associates, San Diego; Univ of California, San Francisco; et al)
J Pediatr 128:453–463, 1996 10–8

Background.—Conventional intermittent mandatory ventilation (IMV) in neonates commonly results in asynchrony between spontaneous breathing and mechanical ventilation, which can lead to poor gas exchange, agitation, and increased risk of barotrauma and intraventricular hemorrhage. This asynchrony can be prevented by administering sedative/analgesic drugs or muscle relaxants, which abolish spontaneous breathing. However, the technology is now available to deliver patient-triggered ventilation, or synchronized intermittent mandatory ventilation (SIMV), with sensors to detect spontaneous breathing. Synchronized intermittent mandatory ventilation was compared with IMV in a prospective, randomized, multicenter trial.

Methods.—At 6 centers during a 2-year period, infants with a birth weight of at least 500 g and significant lung disease related to respiratory distress syndrome, pneumonia, or meconium aspiration pneumonitis were stratified by birth weight and randomly assigned to continue with IMV or change to SIMV. The infants were evaluated for oxygenation, sedative/analgesic drug requirements, incidence of air leaks, and duration of ventilation.

Results.—A total of 350 infants were studied. The 2 groups had similar birth weight, gestational age, sex, 5-minute Apgar score, and duration of ventilator support and degree of respiratory insufficiency at the time of randomization. The groups also were similar for surfactant administration, use of dexamethasone, and incidence of sepsis, necrotizing enterocolitis, seizures, and secondary pneumonia. Among infants with a birth weight exceeding 2,000 g, the SIMV group had a shorter duration of mechanical ventilation than the IMV group. Among infants with a birth weight of 1,000–1,499 g, the 2 groups had a similar number of infants receiving sedative/analgesic drugs, but the total dose was lower in the SIMV group. All of the infants had a lower mean airway pressure if they were in the SIMV group. A lower inspired fraction of oxygen was required by the infants receiving SIMV in the 1,000- to 1,499-g–birth weight group; these infants also had better oxygenation at 1 hour than the infants in the IMV group. There were no differences between the IMV and SIMV groups at any birth weight in the incidence of pharmacologic paralysis, air leak, or grade III or IV intraventricular hemorrhage. The mortality rates also were similar, both when analyzed as total mortality and as cause-specific mortality. Infants receiving SIMV regained their birth weights more quickly than did infants receiving IMV.

Conclusions.—Synchronized intermittent mandatory ventilation is at least as effective as IMV in treating neonates who require mechanical ventilation. Certain outcomes are improved with SIMV in birth weight–specific patterns. There are no deleterious effects of SIMV.

► The commentary outlined below was submitted by Dr. Waldemar A. Carlo, Director of Neonatology at the University of Alabama School of Medicine, Birmingham, Alabama:

► Bernstein and collaborators should be commended for their remarkable effort in completing such a large multicenter study of ventilatory management. Six excellent clinical centers enrolled 327 of 875 neonates who underwent mechanical ventilation. This well-designed study compared a state-of-the-art, commercially available, synchronized intermittent mandatory ventilator to the same type of ventilator used in the IMV mode. The triggering system used has a fast response time (55 msec) and is free of the many problems of earlier SIMV systems.

The primary outcome measures included acute effects on oxygenation, use of sedation or analgesia, air leaks, and duration of mechanical ventilation. Analysis of all patients revealed that the only difference in primary outcomes was that mean airway pressure was 0.5 cm H_2O lower in the SIMV group. An expanded analysis of 12 outcome measures in infants from the different weight subgroups (a total of 48 comparisons) revealed statistically significant benefits of SIMV in only 4 of these comparisons. Further, the outcome measures improved were affected inconsistently across the various weight subgroups. More importantly, major outcome measures (e.g., death, air leaks, and intraventricular hemorrhage) were not improved by SIMV. Thus, until further data are available, SIMV should be considered to be as good as, but not superior to, conventional mechanical ventilation.

W.A. Carlo, M.D.

Patient-triggered Ventilation in Neonates: Comparison of a Flow- and an Impedance-triggered System

Hummler HD, Gerhardt T, Gonzalez A, et al (Jackson Mem Med Ctr, Miami, Fla)

Am J Respir Crit Care Med 154:1049–1054, 1996 10–9

Background.—In ventilated neonates, asynchrony between mechanical and spontaneous breaths may result in ventilation and gas exchange impairment or barotrauma. Although several ventilator systems capable of synchronized mechanical ventilation are now available, only a few have been assessed systematically. The performances of an impedance-triggered ventilator with a flow-triggered infant ventilator were compared by measuring response time, rate of autotriggered breaths and trigger failure, minute ventilation, and gas exchange.

Methods and Findings.—The 2 systems were used in random order in 10 preterm infants. Ventilator settings were identical. Median response times for the impedance and flow/volume systems were 169 and 115 msec, respectively. The response time of the impedance system was longer and more variable because of a phase lag of the impedance signal caused by chest wall distortion. Although 13.1% of mechanical breaths were autotriggered with the impedance system, no autotriggered breaths occurred using the flow/volume system. The rate of trigger failures in the 2 systems did not differ significantly. Because the number of breaths triggered late in inspiration or during expiration was greater, the impedance system was associated with smaller minute ventilation.

Conclusions.—The flow/volume–triggered system is less prone to autotriggering than is the impedance-triggered system. The former also has a shorter, more consistent response time. Artifacts and chest wall distortion occurred more often with the impedance-triggered system.

► This comment has been provided by William D. Rhine, M.D., Assistant Professor of Pediatrics, Stanford University School of Medicine; Co-director of ECMO, Lucile Salter Packard Children's Hospital at Stanford, Palo Alto, California:

► This report is similar to comparing a Mercedes Benz and a BMW. One may have distinct advantages, but they are both much better than the "Volkswagen Beetle generation" of ventilators that many of us continue to use on newborns. They will usually all get you there, but newer technology can make the ride to extubation quicker and safer. The impedance flow system tested had a longer response time and higher autotriggering, but the latter still occurred rarely. As the authors point out, variable chest electrode placement might further impact impedance-based performance. It would be nice to see a similarly detailed study of the other synchronized systems so that we can make more informed comparisons, especially when it comes time to buy these newer and more expensive ventilators.

W.D. Rhine, M.D.

Intratracheal Pulmonary Ventilation *versus* Conventional Mechanical Ventilation in a Rabbit Model of Surfactant Deficiency

Makhoul IR, Kugelman A, Garg M, et al (Univ of Southern California, Los Angeles)

Pediatr Res 38:878–885, 1995 10–10

Background.—Intratracheal pulmonary ventilation (ITPV) enhances CO_2 clearance from dead space and lungs by a bias flow of gas delivered to the distal trachea (Figs 1 and 2). Compared with conventional mechanical ventilation (CMV), ITPV may increase minute CO_2 clearance, decrease the partial pressure of CO_2 in arterial gas ($Paco_2$, and reduce distal tracheal peak inspiratory pressure (dPIP).

Methods.—Surfactant deficiency was induced in 15 adult rabbits, which were ventilated through a double-lumen 4 endotracheal tube inserted through a tracheostomy incision. In phase 1 of the study, CO_2 clearance and $Paco_2$ with ITPV and CMV were compared using similar ventilatory pressures. In phase 2, the efficacy of ITPV in reducing dPIP and tidal volume was compared with that of CMV while eucapnea was maintained.

Findings.—In phase 1, ITPV resulted in a mean percentage reduction of $Paco_2$ of 31.4% at a respiratory rate of 30 breaths/min; by 37.1% at 45 breaths/min; and by 38.3% at 70 breaths/min. The mean percentage increases in minute CO_2 clearance were 61.3%, 56%, and 98%, respectively. In phase 2, ITPV resulted in mean percentage reductions of dPIP of 35.5%, 38%, and 37.2%, respectively. The mean percentage reductions in tidal volume were 34.7%, 36.4%, and 52.7%, respectively. Oxygenation and pH did not differ significantly between ITPV and CMV (Figs 3 and 4).

Conclusions.—In this rabbit model of surfactant deficiency, ITPV was an efficient mode of assisted ventilation, increasing CO_2 clearance and

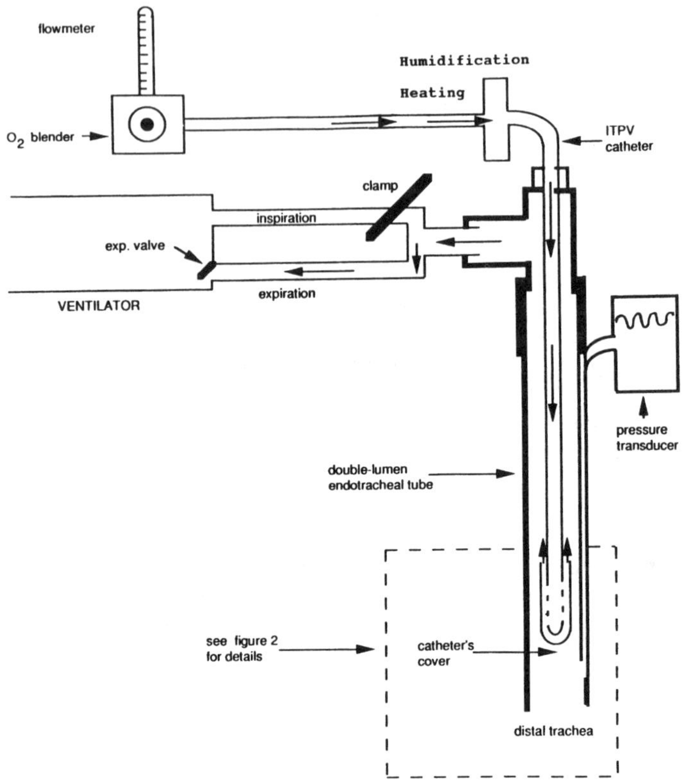

FIGURE 1.—The intratracheal pulmonary ventilation (*ITPV*) system. The inspiratory flow from the ventilator is blocked (*clamp*). Gas flows to the patient exclusively through the ITPV catheter (*continuous flow*). The ventilator serves for setting the respiratory rate, inspiratory: expiratory ratio, positive end expiratory pressure, and for timed exhalations via its expiratory valve. (Courtesy of Makhoul IR, Kugelman A, Garg M, et al: Intratracheal pulmonary ventilation *versus* conventional mechanical ventilation in a rabbit model of surfactant deficiency. *Pediatr Res* 38:878–885, 1995.)

decreasing ventilator pressures needed for adequate ventilation. Lung barotrauma associated with mechanical ventilation may be minimized by ITPV.

▶ Dr. Wally Carlo, Professor of Pediatrics, University of Alabama School of Medicine, Birmingham, comments:

▶ This study of an innovative technique developed by Kolobow and associates[1] demonstrates that ITPV clearly improves CO_2 elimination and decreases $Pa{CO_2}$. Distal displacement of the site of gas exchange from the connector to the tip of the endotracheal tube reduces anatomical dead space. Because endotracheal tube dead space may account for from 25% to 50% of the tidal volume, it makes perfect sense that ITPV should improve CO_2 elimination. Neonatal studies have confirmed that ITPV improves CO_2 elimination.[2, 3] Dassieu et al[3] recently presented their preliminary results

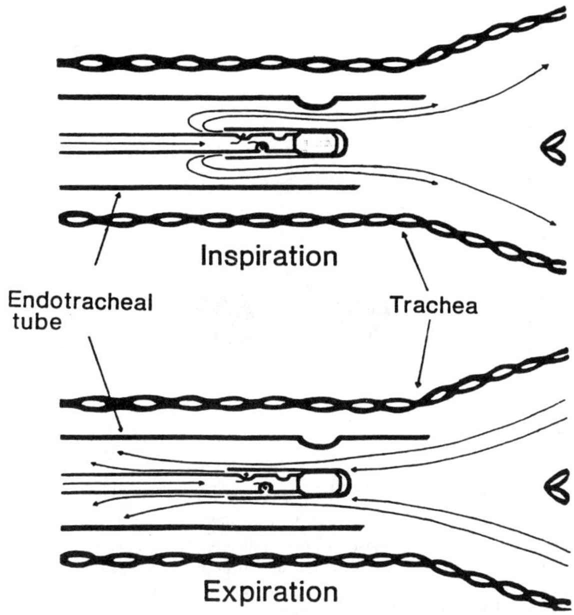

FIGURE 2.—Direction of intratracheal gas flow during inspiration and expiration in the intratracheal pulmonary ventilation system. (Printed with permission from Kolobow T, 1991. Introduction to Intratracheal Pulmonary Ventilation (ITPV), in: *ITPV Training Manual*, unpublished.) (Courtesy of Makhoul IR, Kugelman A, Garg M, et al: Intratracheal pulmonary ventilation *versus* conventional mechanical ventilation in a rabbit model of surfactant deficiency. *Pediatr Res* 38:878–885, 1995.)

regarding 28 neonates with respiratory failure and observed that $Pa{CO_2}$ decreased by a mean of 21%.

Recent data suggest that the deleterious effects of mechanical ventilation are more related to volume (volutrauma) than to pressure (barotrauma). Large tidal volumes are particularly harmful to the developing lung.[4, 5] With the use of ITPV, the decrease in dead space will allow a reduction of the tidal volume, which may prevent lung injury.

However, important limitations of ITPV must be overcome before it can be used in clinical practice. A pressure-release or pop-off valve is necessary to servocontrol the flow. Second, care must be exercised to minimize proximal obstruction of expiratory flow or gas trapping that may be caused by plugs, a suction catheter, or the catheter itself. Gas trapping will be more prominent with the use of smaller endotracheal tubes (a 4F, rarely used in neonates, was used in this study). Dr. Kolobow's ingenious development, the reversed-thrust catheter, will minimize gas trapping. However, if the reversed-thrust catheter reduces positive and expiratory pressure and decreases functional residual capacity, impairment of oxygenation and atelectasis may occur. Finally, in the study abstracted here, 3 of 15 animals died when high flow rates were used, although in 1 case the cause of death (accidental venous air embolism) was not related to the ventilatory treat-

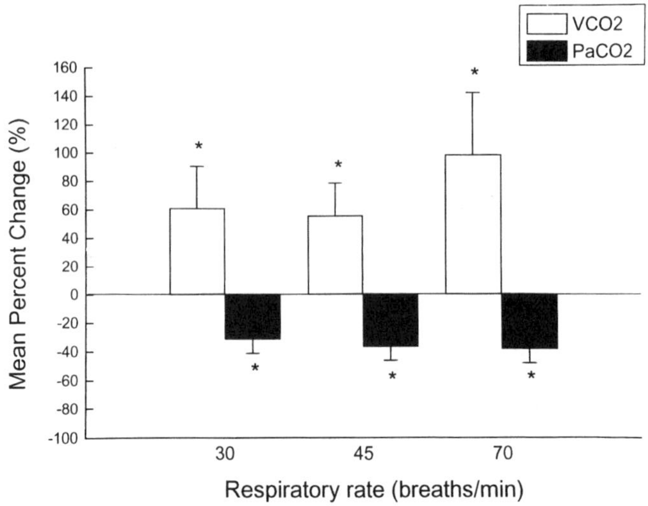

FIGURE 3.—Percent changes (mean ± standard deviation) in minute CO_2 clearance (CO_2) and partial pressure of arterial CO_2 (*Pa*CO_2) during phase 1 of the study: comparison of step 2 intratracheal pulmonary ventilation (*ITPV*)and step 1 conventional mechanical ventilation (*CMV*), at respiratory rates of 30, 45, and 70 breaths/min. *Asterisk* indicates $P < 0.05$ compared with a change of 25%. The mean percent changes of V_{CO_2} with ITPV compared with CMV, at respiratory rates of 30, 45, and 70 breaths/min, respectively; 61.3 ± 29, 56.4 ± 23.5, and 98.4 ± 40.7. The mean percent changes of Pa_{CO_2} with ITPV compared with CMV, at respiratory rates of 30, 45, and 70 breaths/min, respectively; −31.4 ± 10, −37.1 ± 9.7, and −38.3 ± 9.9. (Courtesy of Makhoul IR, Kugelman A, Garg M, et al: Intratracheal pulmonary ventilation *versus* conventional mechanical ventilation in a rabbit model of surfactant deficiency. *Pediatr Res* 38:878–885, 1995.)

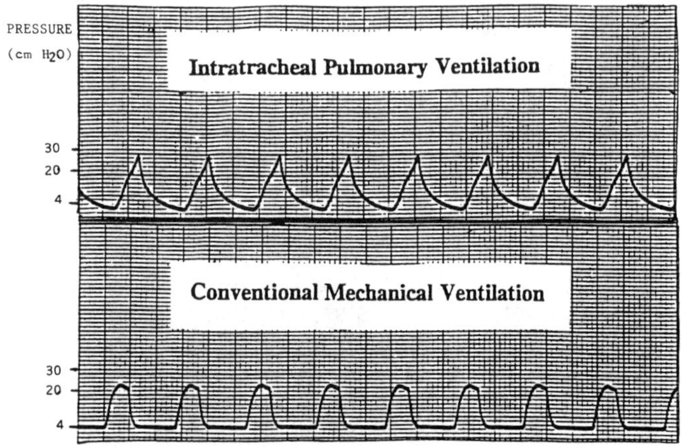

FIGURE 4.—Distal tracheal pressure tracing during phase 1 of the study; (step 2) intratracheal pulmonary ventilation (*ITPV*) vs. step 1 conventional mechanical ventilation (*CMV*), Hewlett Packard 78304A: speed = 10 mm/sec, distal peak inspiratory pressure (*dPIP*) = 24 cm H_2, distal positive end expiratory pressure (*dPEEP*) = 4 cm H_2O, distal mean airway pressure = 11 cm H_2O, inspiratory: expiratory ratio, 1:2, respiratory rate = 45 breaths/min. and $ITPV_{flow}$ = 7 L/min. Note the gradual increase of distal peak inspiratory pressure and the decelerating pattern of dPEEP with ITPV, compared with CMV. (Courtesy of Makhoul IR, Kugelman A, Garg M, et al: Intratracheal pulmonary ventilation *versus* conventional mechanical ventilation in a rabbit model of surfactant deficiency. *Pediatr Res* 38:878–885, 1995.)

ment. Thus, further animal studies are necessary to ensure that ITPV is as safe as CVM before we embark on large clinical trials.

W. Carlo, M.D.

References

1. Kolobow T, Giacomini M, Reali-Forster C, et al: The current status of intratracheal-pulmonary ventilation (ITPV). *Int J Artif Organs* 18:670–673, 1995.
2. Danan C, Dassieu G, Janaud JC, et al: Efficacy of dead-space washout in mechanically ventilated premature newborns. *Am J Respir Crit Care Med* 153:1571–1576, 1996.
3. Dassieu G, Brochard L, Janaud JC, et al: Instrumental dead-space washout by continuous tracheal gas insufflation (CTGI) increases the efficacy of the conventional ventilation. *Pediatr Res* 39:1210A, 1996.
4. Peevy KJ, Hernandez LA, Moise AA, et al: Barotrauma and microvascular injury in lungs of nonadult rabbits: Effect of ventilation pattern. *Crit Care Med* 18:634–639, 1990.
5. Parker JC, Hernandez LA, Peevy KJ: Mechanisms of ventilator-induced lung injury. *Crit Care Med* 21:131–143, 1993.

A Multicenter, Randomized Trial Comparing Synthetic Surfactant With Modified Bovine Surfactant Extract in the Treatment of Neonatal Respiratory Distress Syndrome

Soll RF, for the Vermont-Oxford Neonatal Network (Univ of Vermont, Burlington; et al)

Pediatrics 97:1–6, 1996 10–11

Background.—Surfactant preparations have proven successful in treating respiratory distress syndrome (RDS) of neonates. Clinical outcomes were compared between the 2 types of surfactant, synthetic and bovine.

Methods.—In a consortium of 38 neonatal ICUs, 1,296 small (501- to 1,500-g) infants with RDS who required ventilatory support by 6 hours of age received either synthetic surfactant (Exosurf Neonatal) or modified bovine surfactant (Survanta), up to 4 doses, under standard protocols. The combined incidence in the first 28 days of either death or development of chronic pulmonary disease was recorded for each surfactant. Secondary outcomes, including the course of RDS and various concurrent diagnoses, also were recorded.

Results.—Significantly more Survanta-treated infants had a 5-minute Apgar score of less than 3 (8%) than Exosurf-treated infants (4%). Otherwise, the 2 groups were similar. More infants required a second dose with Exosurf (68%) than Survanta (61%), but more infants required all 4 doses with Survanta (22%) than Exosurf (9%). There was no overall difference in death or chronic lung disease at 28 days between Exosurf- (57%) and Survanta-treated infants (54%). However, among infants weighing 1,001 to 1,500 g, Survanta yielded a significantly better outcome. Overall, Survanta-treated infants experienced more rapid improvement in RDS and significantly fewer pneumothoraces (9%) than Exosurf-treated infants (15%).

Conclusions.—The outcome of surfactant therapy in small infants is about the same, whether synthetic or modified bovine surfactant is used. The bovine product, however, leads to better secondary outcomes, such as more rapid improvement in RDS.

▶ The clinical trials leading to the Food and Drug Administration approval of surfactant heralded a new era in neonatology. By the early 1990s, most of these multicenter, randomized trials had been published and surfactant therapy was firmly entrenched as a therapeutic modality. Surfactant has been credited with significantly reducing the neonatal mortality rates. It is now used in about half the infants weighing less than 1,500 g. Clinicians have become comfortable with the use of surfactant and will reluctantly change "their brand" only if there is compelling clinical reason to do so. This enormous clinical trial does not generate such data, so little behavioral change can be anticipated. The results tend to favor the modified bovine surfactant, but there were no statistically significant differences in the combined incidence of death or chronic lung disease, the primary outcome variable. Air leaks developed in fewer infants who received the natural surfactant, in keeping with the meta-analysis on this topic.

When there is no major outcome difference, even the best-conducted trials will not muster much enthusiasm—such is the case with this manuscript. There have been rumblings about a new, improved surfactant, so we will keep a lookout for any breakthrough in this important field. In the meantime, surfactant is used not only for preterm infants with RDS, but also for term infants with RDS or meconium aspiration syndrome. In neonates with pulmonary hypertension and respiratory distress, surfactant may avert the need for extracorporeal membrane oxygenation.[1]

A.A. Fanaroff, M.B.B.Ch.

Reference

1. Soll RF, Sinclair JC, Bracken MB: Natural surfactant extract vs synthetic surfactant, meta-analysis of randomized controlled trials. *Pediatr Res* 37:374A, 1995.

Inactivation of Surfactant in Rat Lungs

Bruni R, Fan BR, David-Cu R, et al (UCLA School of Medicine, Los Angeles)
Pediatr Res 39:236–240, 1996 10–12

Introduction.—Surfactant replacement therapy decreases the severity of neonatal respiratory distress syndrome (RDS) and subsequently reduces infant mortality. A sustained clinical response is observed in only about two thirds of treated premature infants. Nonresponse to surfactant replacement therapy may be a result of extreme lung immaturity and surfactant inactivation secondary to aspecific biophysical events. It is not known which surfactant properties are needed to function under adverse conditions, such as serum leakage and surfactant inactivation. Existing surfactants offer limited resistance to inactivation and require the presence of SP-A, a large hydrophilic oligomeric glycoprotein, to restore lung function. An excised rat lung model was used to compare the susceptibility of various surfactants to serum inactivation.

Methods.—Exosurf (a protein-free synthetic surfactant), Survanta (a surfactant containing proteins B and C [SP-B and SP-C]), and a porcine surfactant (containing SP-A, SP-B, and SP-C) were evaluated by pressure-volume determinations as an in situ measure of surfactant activity. The same preparations were retested after mixing with human serum, which acts as a nonspecific surfactant inactivator.

Results.—Porcine surfactant was inactivated to a smaller degree by human serum compared with Survanta, Exosurf, or synthetic phospholipids. Temperature caused a significant effect on deflation stability as evidenced by a greater lung compliance in untreated, normal lungs and a larger improvement in compliance after treating lavaged lungs with synthetic phospholipids at 37°C rather than 22°C.

Conclusion.—Surfactant containing SP-A, SP-B, and SP-C is moderately susceptible to inactivation with whole serum and may produce a greater clinical response than protein-free surfactants or those containing only SP-B and SP-C. Pressure-volume deflation curves were useful in determining the extent of serum inactivation of surfactant in situ.

▶ The surfactant story is becoming increasingly sophisticated. Now investigators are trying to understand surfactant inactivation and suggest that a surfactant containing SP-A, SP-B, and SP-C may be less susceptible to inactivation with whole serum than some of the protein-deficient artifical surfactants and may, therefore, have a greater clinical efficacy under conditions of universal protein leakage in the lung. A limitation of the study is acknowledged by the authors; that is, measures of gas exchange need to be related to changes in lung mechanics. Also, the amount of protein that was used was based on previous in vitro studies and may not reflect what actually occurs under clinical conditions. If such behavior of the surfactant preparations can be confirmed by others, these data would serve as the rationale for introducing genetically engineered proteins back into the artificial surfactants for use in premature infants. Surfactant preparations in general work quite well, although RDS obviously has not been eliminated and there is more to pulmonary insufficiency than surfactant deficiency. Whether the expense of creating new surfactants will be worth the additional benefit is not only a scientific issue but also a commercial issue.

D.K. Stevenson, M.D.

Antioxidant-Surfactant Liposomes Mitigate Hyperoxic Lung Injury in Premature Rabbits

Walther FJ, David-Cu R, Lopez SL (Charles R Drew Univ, Los Angeles; Univ of California, Los Angeles)

Am J Physiol 269:L613–L617, 1995 10–13

Objective.—Surfactant liposomes with antioxidant activity protect against hyperoxic cell damage by metabolizing superoxide anions. Premature infants whose lungs are deficient in surfactant and antioxidant enzymes are subject to respiratory distress syndrome. The effect of intratracheal instillation of liposomal superoxide dismutase (SOD) and catalase in premature and term rabbit pups after exposure to hyperoxia for 24 hours was investigated.

Methods.—Preterm (28 and 29 days) and term rabbit pups, divided into 4 groups of 12–15 pups each, received 0.1 mL per 15 g of body weight of antioxidant-surfactant liposomes by intratracheal injection, surfactant liposomes without antioxidants, 0.1 mL per 15 g of body weight of air placebo, or no treatment. The first 3 groups were subjected to hyperoxia (greater than 95% oxygen) for 24 hours and killed. The fourth group was killed. Lung homogenates were assayed for SOD and catalase activity, and for DNA content.

Results.—In the untreated pups, SOD activity increased with the age of the pups. Before hypoxia, SOD activity in both term and premature pups was lowest in the untreated pups and the pups given air placebo, intermediate in the liposome-only–treated pups, and highest in the pups treated with the antioxidant-surfactant liposomes. Catalase activity mirrored SOD activity. Differences between treatment groups were significant.

Conclusions.—Antioxidant-surfactant liposome treatment provides premature and term rabbit pups with significant protection against hyperoxic lung injury. Lung antioxidant capacity increases significantly with increasing maturity in both treated and untreated pups.

► In view of the high incidence of bronchopulmonary dysplasia in premature infants with respiratory distress syndrome requiring ventilatory assistance, a closer look at pulmonary oxygen toxicity and the antioxidant defense systems is warranted. Antenatal steroids increase lung antioxidant enzyme activity but have not substantially affected the incidence of chronic lung disease. In adult animals, pulmonary oxygen toxicity can be ameliorated by augmenting the intracellular antioxidant capacity through preexposure to hyperoxia or hypoxia, and by administering endotoxin or exogeneous antioxidant enzymes. These include SOD, catalase, and glutathione peroxidase. In many mammals, surfactant has been used as the vehicle to deliver these antioxidants. Surfactant liposomes encapsulating SOD and catalase sharply increase antioxidant activity in type II cells.

The purpose of this study was to verify whether exogenous antioxidant enzymes would protect the fetal lung against exposure to hyperoxia for 24 hours. They did. Indeed, the authors demonstrated that intratracheal instillation of the surfactant liposomes boosted antioxidant activity. The effect was amplified when the surfactant liposomes encapsulated SOD and catalase. The authors speculated that the addition of surfactant protein A, which was not present in the surfactant used, would enhance the antioxidant activity even further. The natural question is how to translate these animal data to the human fetus. Should the surfactants be modified to incorporate the antioxidants? The physiology appears to be sound, but where is the clinical relevance?

A.A. Fanaroff, M.B.B.Ch.

Effects of Oxygen, Positive End-expiratory Pressure, and Carbon Dioxide on Oxygen Delivery in an Animal Model of the Univentricular Heart

Riordan CJ, Randsbaek F, Storey JH, et al (Univ of Louisville, Ky)

J Thorac Cardiovasc Surg 112:644–654, 1996 10–14

Background.—Respiratory manipulations are commonly used in the treatment of infants with univentricular hearts, although little experimental information on this treatment has been available until recently. In an animal model of a univentricular heart, the physiologic effects of a number of commonly used ventilatory treatments were characterized.

Methods and Findings.—Neonatal pigs were used. Treatments performed included altering inspired oxygen tension, adding positive end-expiratory pressure, and adding supplemental carbon dioxide to the ventricular circuit. The ratio of pulmonary to systemic flow declined when inspired oxygen tension was lowered. At an inspired oxygen tension of 100%, this ratio was 1.29; at 0.61, it was 21%; and at 15%, 0.42. Adding high-concentration supplemental carbon dioxide reduced inspired oxygen tension from 1.29 to 0.42. The pulmonary/systemic flow ratio was not significantly affected by 95% oxygen and 5% carbon dioxide. These 3 interventions had an effect on systemic oxygen delivery, which was a function of the pulmonary/systemic flow ratio. As the pulmonary/systemic flow ratio declined from its initially high levels, oxygen delivery increased, peaking at a flow ratio of slightly less than 1. As the pulmonary/systemic flow ratio further declined to less than 0.7, oxygen delivery dropped. In an assessment of the ability of systemic arterial and venous oxygen saturations to predict pulmonary/systemic flow ratio, venous oxygen saturation was found to correlate well with both pulmonary/systemic flow ratio and systemic oxygen delivery. By contrast, arterial oxygen saturation did not accurately predict pulmonary/systemic flow ratio or oxygen delivery.

Conclusions.—Estimating the pulmonary/systemic flow ratio before treatment initiation is useful. When initial ratios exceed about 0.7, interventions that reduce the ratio increased oxygen delivery. When this ratio was less than 0.7, interventions that reduced the ratio decreased oxygen delivery.

▶ This comment has been provided by William D. Rhine, M.D., Assistant Professor of Pediatrics, Stanford University School of Medicine, Co-director of ECMO, Lucile Salter Packard Children's Hospital at Stanford, Palo Alto, California:

▶ A pig is not a human, a univentricular prep is not complex congenital heart disease, and a few hours of altering shunts is not the same as a few days. These caveats aside, the authors have a lot to tell us about what we really are doing when we alter some of the respiratory parameters in patients with mixing cardiac lesions. One of the primary take-home messages is the importance of pulmonary/systemic shunt ratios in such patients. Also noteworthy is that mixed venous saturations can be quite helpful in evaluating shunts and oxygen delivery. All too often, we focus on arterial saturations and ignore venous saturation. Although oxygen delivery was maximal at 50% and fell significantly when the fraction of inspired oxygen (FIO_2) was reduced to 15%, the accompanying decrease in left-to-right shunt ratio at the lower FIO_2 could possibly be beneficial over hours to days by reducing pulmonary circulation and edema. Thus, the clinician will continue to have to balance adequate oxygen delivery with optimal cardiorespiratory circulation.

W.D. Rhine, M.D.

Postnatal Treatment With Retinoic Acid Increases the Number of Pulmonary Alveoli in Rats

Massaro GD, Massaro D (Georgetown Univ, Washington, DC)
Am J Physiol 270:L305–L310, 1996 10–15

Objective.—Among prematurely born infants, those with bronchopulmonary dysplasia have rewer alveoli and a smaller gas exchange surface area (SA) than those without this condition. The ability of retinoic acid, administered to postnatal rats, to prevent the inhibition of the number of alveoli formed and the low body mass–specific SA produced by treatment with dexamethasone, a glucocorticosteroid hormone that inhibits the formation of alveoli, was determined.

Methods.—Three-day-old male Sprague-Dawley rats were entered into 4 treatment groups: diluent, dexamethasone, retinoic acid, and retinoic acid and dexamethasone. The animals were injected intraperitoneally with diluent (cottonseed oil) or with all *trans*-retinoic acid in diluent (500 μg/kg). On the next day, half of the rats in each group were started on treatment with dexamethasone (0.25 μg/day subcutaneously). Treatment continued through the age of 13 days, and the rats were killed the next day. Serial lung sections were prepared for analysis.

Results.—The 4 groups did not differ in lung volume at 14 days, but body mass–specific lung volume was greater in dexamethasone-treated rats and in rats treated with retinoic acid and dexamethasone than in diluent-treated rats. Retinoic acid prevented the low number of alveoli and the low body mass–specific SA caused by treatment with dexamethasone. The number of alveoli increased by 50% with retinoic acid treatment, but no increase in SA was seen. This finding suggests the action of a regulatory mechanism to prevent unneeded SA.

Discussion.—Retinoic acid causes an increase in alveolar number and a rise in body mass–specific SA in dexamethasone-treated rats. This increase is greater than that present in rats treated with dexamethasone only. The ability of retinoic acid to induce the formation of alveoli offers hope for remedial treatment of the common chronic lung diseases of prematurity. Support is provided for the preventive or remedial treatment of patients who have too few alveoli for adequate gas exchange.

► Vitamin A compounds are fat-soluble micronutrients that are critical for visual function and for promotion of the epithelial cell growth and differentiation that are important to many physiologic processes. Vitamin A supplementation may lower the frequency of chronic lung disease in infants with birth weights of less than 1.5 kg. The Massaros provide elegant experimental evidence to demonstrate the actions of vitamin A on the lung. In rats exposed to steroid therapy, retinoic acid prevented, to a large degree, reduction of the number of alveoli. Perhaps of more importance was the observation that retinoic acid caused a 50% increase in the number of alveoli in rats that were not receiving other medications.

The National Institute of Child Health and Human Development Neonatal Research Network Trial of vitamin A supplementation to infants with birth weights of less than 1,000 g, to reduce the incidence of chronic lung disease and perhaps even nosocomial infections, has enrolled 75% of the projected cohort. The results should be available for the 1998 YEAR BOOK OF NEONATAL AND PERINATAL MEDICINE. At that time, it will be apparent whether vitamin A supplementation is justified. Let us pray that the wonderful data generated by the Georgetown scientists can be replicated in the low–birth weight infants.

A.A. Fanaroff, M.B.B.Ch.

Apparent Life-threatening Events in Presumed Healthy Neonates During the First Three Days of Life

Grylack LJ, Williams AD (Columbia Hosp for Women, Washington, DC)

Pediatrics 97:349–351, 1996 10–16

Background.—Little is known about sudden infant death syndrome and apparent life-threatening events (ALTEs) in mature infants during the first few days of life. The historical, clinical, and pneumographic correlates of ALTEs were studied in a term newborn nursery population during the first 3 days of life in a maternity hospital.

Methods and Findings.—During a 3-year period, 20 of about 15,000 newborns had ALTEs. The most common initial symptom was apnea, usually accompanied by cyanosis. Treatment most often consisted of tactile stimulation and oxygen. Airway clearance, intermittent positive-pressure ventilation, and cardiac massage was performed less commonly. The causes were potentially identifiable in 40% of the events. These included CNS abnormality, airway obstruction, and persistent fetal cardiovascular shunt. Analysis of the multichannel recordings done after the ALTEs showed desaturation of less than 85% in 11 infants, apneic pauses of more than 15 seconds in 10 infants, and bradycardia of less than 80 beats/min in 4 infants (Table 3). Eighteen infants were discharged with home monitors. Medication was prescribed for 4 infants. Four infants had recurrent ALTEs before discharge and 1 infant, after discharge. None of the infants died.

Conclusions.—Apparent life-threatening events can occur in low-risk, term neonates during the first 3 days of life. In most infants, the causes of these events are not discovered. Multichannel recordings may show ab-

TABLE 3.—Results of Initial Multichannel Recordings (n = 20)

Median day of life for initial study	day 3
Findings	
Apnea greater than 15 s	12
16–20 s	8
>20 s	4
Bradycardia	4
Desaturations	11
Apnea and hypopnea	5

(Courtesy of Grylack LJ, Williams AD: Apparent life-threatening events in presumed healthy neonates during the first three days of life. *Pediatrics* 97:349–351, 1996. Reproduced by permission. Copyright 1996.)

normalities. The likelihood of an ALTE recurring is higher in the first week than over the next 2 months.

▶ The following commentary is submitted by Dr. Richard J. Martin, Co-director of neonatology, Rainbow Babies & Childrens Hospital, Cleveland, Ohio:

▶ Although it is widely known that the sudden infant death syndrome rate in North America approximates 1 in 1,500, the current report coincidentally finds that there is a comparable rate of ALTEs in term infants during the first 3 days of life. This is not widely known, although we have all heard anecdotes of such events in very early postnatal life. A diverse series of etiologies is reported for the current 20 patients and, interestingly, documented sepsis is not on the list.

Cardiorespiratory recordings in these infants did reveal evidence of desaturation to less than 85% and apnea of more than 15 seconds' duration in more than half of the infants. This raises a new question: what are "normal" apnea and desaturation rates for such infants? These data are not easy to come by in a healthy population, although normative data are becoming available. The ongoing National Institutes of Health–sponsored CHIME study will allow the frequency of such events to be correlated with various types of apnea (central, mixed, and obstructive) in both preterm and term infants. Of interest are recent reports by Barrington and colleagues[1] and by the CHIME study group[2] that preterm infants have persistent apnea and desaturation events documented by monitoring for many days after hospital discharge. The latter observation may require us to reexamine the relevance of the so-called 5- or 7-day apnea-free countdown for preterm infants before hospital discharge.[3]

R.J. Martin, M.D.

References

1. Barrington KJ, Finer N, Li D: Pre-discharge respiratory recordings in very low birth weight newborn infants. *J Pediatr* 129:934–940, 1996.
2. Hunt CE, Hufford DR, Bourguignon C, et al: Home documented monitoring of cardiorespiratory pattern and oxygen saturation in healthy infants. *Pediatr Res* 39:216–222, 1996.

3. Ramanathan R, Corwin MJ, Hunt CE, et al: Preterm infants have prolonged apneas with obstruction and associated oxygen desaturation at home. *Pediatr Res,* in press.

Predominant Role of Peripheral Chemoreceptors in the Termination of Apnea in Maturing Newborn Lambs

Delacourt C, Canet E, Bureau MA (Sherbrooke Univ, Quebec, Canada)
J Appl Physiol 80:892–898, 1996 10–17

Objective.—Apnea is common and even normal in newborns; most such breathing stoppages end within a few seconds. However, when the episode does not end, it can be life-threatening. The mechanisms of these apneas, the inducing factors, and the mechanisms of resumed breathing are unknown. Factors involved in prolonged apnea could include low peripheral chemoreceptor activity and a central depressant effect of hypoxia. Factors affecting the termination of apnea were studied in fetal lambs.

Methods.—Apnea was induced in awake, intubated, newborn lambs by passive hyperventilation at differing levels of inspired O_2 fraction. The arterial PCO_2 value at which a lamb took its first breath was considered to be the apnea termination threshold ($PATT_{CO_2}$). One group of lambs was studied on the 1st and 15th days of life, and another was studied after central tissue hypoxia had been induced by breathing carbon dioxide. A third group of lambs that underwent carotid body denervation (CBD) was studied on the 1st day of life.

Results.—The analysis detected a PO_2–PCO_2 response curve that determined whether an individual instance of apnea would terminate. The curve was operative at both ages studied and regardless of whether CBD had been performed. At both 1 and 15 days, increasing arterial PO_2 was associated with increasing $PATT_{CO_2}$. The $PATT_{CO_2}$ was significantly lower under conditions of hypoxia and normoxia in the lambs studied at 15 days than in those studied at 1 day; during hyperoxia, there was no difference. Lambs in the CBD group had significantly higher $PATT_{CO_2}$values. However, even in the CBD lambs, hypoxia did not lower the $PATT_{CO_2}$.

Conclusions.—Apnea terminates at a different PCO_2 level for fetal lambs at 1 day of age than at 15 days. The function of the carotid bodies plays a key role in lowering the PCO_2 threshold value at which apnea terminates, helping to prevent prolonged apnea. In addition, even after CBD, hypoxia does not act to depress the newborn's recovery from apnea.

► The commentary below was submitted by Dr. Richard J. Martin, Professor of Pediatrics, Co-director of Neonatology, Rainbow Babies & Childrens Hospital, University Hospitals of Cleveland, Case Western Reserve University School of Medicine, Cleveland, Ohio:

► Ventilatory responses to hypoxia have been characterized extensively in both human infants and neonatal animals of several species. Invariably, hypoxia is associated with a transient increase in ventilation, followed by respiratory depression beyond about 2 minutes of hypoxic exposure. It is assumed that the latter is secondary to central inhibition of respiratory neural output, which overrides hypoxic stimulation, induced by peripheral chemoreceptors. Interestingly, there are no available data to indicate that neonates who exhibit apnea are predisposed to hypoxic respiratory depression (or the reverse) when compared with nonapneic infants. Further, although hypercapnic and hypoxic ventilatory responses have been characterized extensively during postnatal maturation, their interactions are less well understood. This is an important line of investigation because neonatal apnea causes simultaneous elevation in $Paco_2$ and decline in Pao_2.

The current observation in unanesthetized newborn lambs indicates that hypoxia lowers the $Paco_2$ threshold at which apnea is terminated; in other words, hypoxia enhances recovery from apnea. This apparent absence of a depressant effect of hypoxia on hypercapnic responsiveness is in disagreement with the only available study in newborn infants, performed more than 20 years ago,[1] which demonstrated a depressant effect of hypoxia on CO_2 responses in early postnatal life. The current study questions whether hypercapnic responses (and recovery from apnea) are impaired by hypoxia, and suggests the opposite, namely that there is enhanced responsiveness to CO_2 during hypoxia. Because apnea of prematurity remains a ubiquitous and troublesome neonatal problem, it is important to unravel the underlying physiology in human infant and animal models and to relate such findings to the rapid advances being made in developmental neurobiology.

R.J. Martin, M.D.

Reference

1. Rigatto H, De La Torre Verduzco R, Gates DB: Effects of O_2 on the ventilatory response to CO_2 in preterm infants. *J Appl Physiol* 30:896, 1975.

Prone Sleep Position and the Sudden Infant Death Syndrome in King County, Washington: A Case-Control Study

Taylor JA, Krieger JW, Reay DT, et al (Univ of Washington, Seattle; Seattle King County Dept of Public Health)
J Pediatr 128:626–630, 1996 10–18

Objective.—A meta-analysis of several non-US sudden infant death syndrome (SIDS) studies has established as a risk factor for SIDS an odds ratio (OR) of 2.72 for the prone sleep position. The risk for SIDS in American infants posed by the prone sleep position was compared in infants who died of SIDS and in similarly aged, living infants in King County, Washington.

Methods.—Sleep position data were obtained by telephone survey for 47 infants who died of SIDS within 1 month after death and for 142 matched controls.

Results.—Infants with SIDS had a significantly lower birth weight than control infants (3,095 vs. 3,397 g). Mothers of infants with SIDS were significantly younger (26.3 years vs. 30.1 years), were significantly more likely to smoke during pregnancy (52.3% vs. 12.7%), and were less likely to be married (55.3% vs. 13.5%) than were mothers of control infants. Infants with SIDS were significantly more likely to sleep prone than control infants (57.4% vs. 24.6%). Control infants who slept prone were significantly more likely to be born to single mothers and significantly more likely to be born to black mothers than were infants who did not sleep in the prone position. Sleeping in the prone position was a significant risk factor for SIDS (unadjusted OR, 4.69). The adjusted OR was 3.02.

Conclusion.—Sleeping in the prone position carries a significant risk for SIDS in American infants.

Face-straight-down and Face-near-straight-down Positions in Healthy, Prone-sleeping Infants

Waters KA, Gonzalez A, Jean C, et al (McGill Univ, Montreal, Canada; Montreal Children's Hosp, Canada)

J Pediatr 128:616–625, 1996 10–19

Objective.—Face-straight-down (FSD) sleeping postures can increase the risk of asphyxia from rebreathing or airway obstruction in prone-sleeping infants, 2 mechanisms thought to be responsible for sudden infant death syndrome. The frequency and consequences of spontaneous FSD episodes were investigated by monitoring the cardiovascular measurements of 10 healthy prone-sleeping infants overnight in their homes.

Methods.—From a questionnaire soliciting sleeping habit information for 151 infants aged 1–7 months, 10 of the 33% who slept prone were studied using cardiorespiratory monitoring and infrared video for 3 consecutive nights. Infants slept in the prone position on nights 1 and 3, and in the lateral position on night 2.

Results.—Infants maintained the prone position all night in 17 of 19 measurements and assumed the FSD position 27 times during these periods for an average duration of 3.3 minutes. Four of 9 infants maintained the lateral position all night. Infants assumed the face-near-straight-down (FNSD) position 130 times (an average of 5.3 times per night) for an average duration of 22.4 minutes. Partial or complete airway obstruction was observed in 3 FSD and 4 FNSD episodes that initiated spontaneous arousal and head turning.

Conclusions.—Healthy prone-sleeping infants frequently spontaneously assume FSD and FNSD positions that can result in airway obstruction. Sudden infant death syndrome may occur in infants who do not have appropriate arousal and head-turning responses or who are unable to do so because of something in their environment. Infants should not sleep in the prone position.

Prone Sleeping in Healthy Infants and Victims of Sudden Infant Death Syndrome

Hunt CE (Med College of Ohio, Toledo)

J Pediatr 128:594–596, 1996 10–20

Background.—In 1994, a "Back to Sleep" campaign was begun in the United States to inform parents about the hazards of prone sleeping in early infancy. In that year, the U.S. sudden infant death syndrome (SIDS) mortality rate declined by 13.7%, compared with earlier annual decreases of 2%. However, there are no data quantifying the extent to which this reduced rate can be attributed to a reduction in the prevalence of prone sleeping.

Discussion.—A retrospective case-control study of the relation of sleep position to SIDS rate was performed in King County, Washington. Fifty-seven percent of the infants who died of SIDS and only 25% of those who did not usually slept prone in the preceding 2 weeks. After adjusting for potential confounders, the odds ratio for the prone sleeping position was 3.1. However, this study has many potential limitations. Although it is important in extending our knowledge of the increased risk of SIDS in U.S. infants who sleep prone, further studies are needed. A better understanding of the complex and dynamic interactions between sleep position and other major sociodemographic factors associated with SIDS is necessary. Observed changes in national SIDS rates need to be related further to changes in infant care practices, including sleep position. Adapting hospital-based physiologic observations to the home environment should enable a better understanding of the interactions between epidemiologic risk factors, such as prone sleeping, and biological risk factors, such as deficient asphyxial arousal responsiveness.

► Richard J. Martin, M.D., Co-director of Neonatology at Rainbow Babies & Childrens Hospital, is a Professor of Pediatrics at Case Western Reserve University in Cleveland, Ohio. His commentary is detailed below:

► North America has now joined the ranks of worldwide geographic locations in which prone sleeping has been associated with a higher risk for SIDS. Earlier studies from around the world revealed that avoidance of prone sleeping could reduce SIDS rates in settings where the underlying SIDS rate was severalfold higher than in the United States, and maybe such a reduction was not relevant to North America. This issue should now be resolved, as Abstracts 10–18 through 10–20 showed prone sleep position as a risk factor for SIDS with an OR of 3:4 in a geographic area with a SIDS death rate of only 1.4 per 1,000 live births. The dilemma as to potential mechanisms underlying this relationship is addressed creatively by a series of home videos from Montreal on healthy term neonates from 1 to 7 months of age. The investigators have documented that the face-down position does occur in prone infants, may be accompanied by signs of airway obstruction, and is presumably terminated by arousal-related mechanisms. Several interesting questions remain to be answered. For example, how much of the SIDS risk associated with prone sleeping (and possibly the face-down position) can be eliminated by avoidance of all soft bedding? What is the optimal sleep position for former preterm infants, many of whom have residual lung disease? It is tempting to speculate that timing of postnatal neural development is critical in determining an infant's ability to adapt to a vulnerable body and face position and then eliciting the appropriate arousal mechanisms to avert disaster.

R.J. Martin, M.D.

Correction of Congenital Diaphragmatic Hernia In Utero VIII: Response of the Hypoplastic Lung to Tracheal Occlusion

Harrison MR, Adzick NS, Flake AW, et al (Univ of California, San Francisco)

J Pediatr Surg 31:1339–1348, 1996 10–21

Objective.—When congenital diaphragmatic hernia (CDH) is diagnosed before 24 weeks' gestation, the fetus usually dies, even with optimal postnatal care. Prenatal repair is difficult or impossible when the liver is herniated into the chest because reducing the liver back into the abdomen produces acute obstruction of umbilical venous return. Animal studies have suggested that obstructing the normal outflow of fetal lung fluid causes the developing lungs to grow larger. This reduces the herniated viscera, hastens lung growth, and improves pulmonary function after birth. The authors, who have tested this tracheal obstruction technique in fetal animals, have now applied it to human fetuses with CDH and liver herniation.

Methods.—The families of 20 fetuses with CDH and liver herniation were counseled regarding their treatment options (i.e., standard postnatal care or experimental tracheal occlusion). Eight families chose experimental fetal surgery. The procedures were performed at 25–28 weeks' gestation. Initially, tracheal occlusion was achieved with an internal plug (Fig 1). In the latter 6 patients, an external clip was placed on the trachea. The authors also developed a technique for unplugging the trachea at birth, called "ex utero intrapartum tracheoplasty." This allowed the infant to be maintained on the umbilical circulation until the airway was established.

Results.—One of 2 fetuses with a foam plug implanted in the trachea had dramatic lung growth and subsequently survived. In the other fetus, a smaller plug was used to avoid tracheomalacia. This patient had no significant lung growth and died at birth. Two fetuses were managed with external spring-loaded aneurysm clips on the trachea. One fetus was aborted because of tocolytic failure. The other patient had no lung growth, presumably because of a leak in the trachea, and died after 3 months.

Placement of a metal clip on the trachea produced dramatic lung growth in 4 of 4 cases. All of these fetuses had reversal of pulmonary hypoplasia after birth. All died of nonpulmonary causes, including an umbilical cord

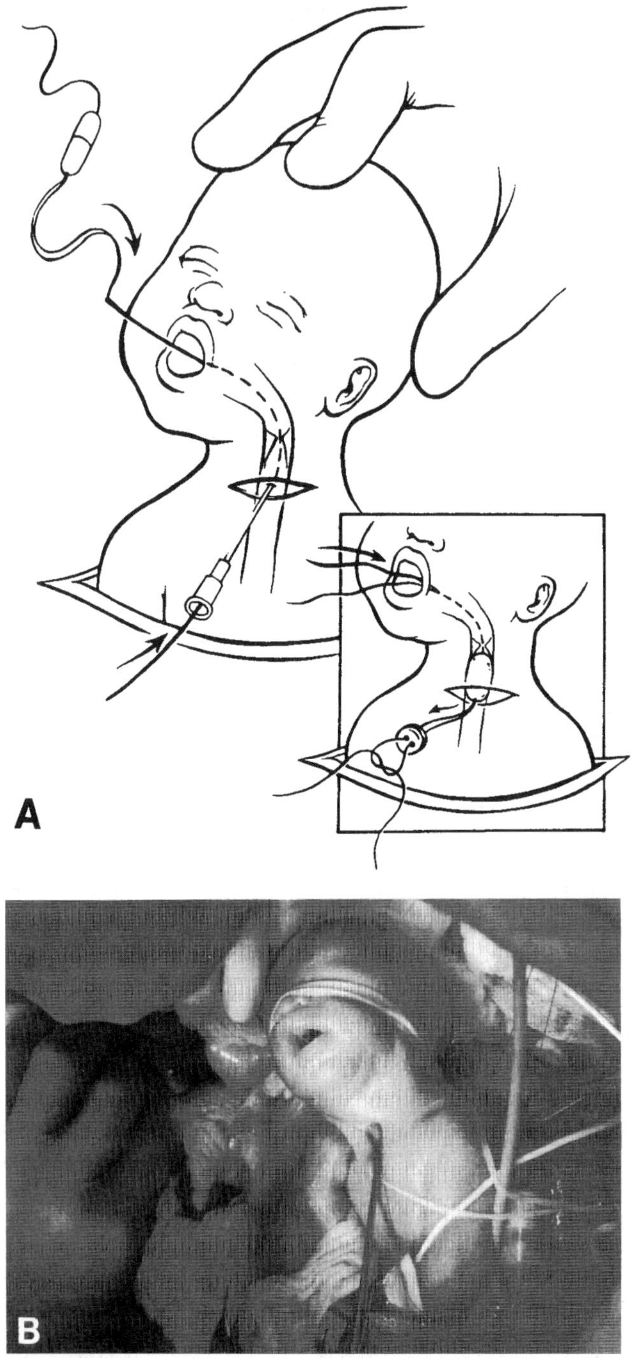

FIGURE 1.—**A,** the procedure used in the first 2 cases to place an internal foam "plug" in the trachea of a fetus with diaphragmatic hernia. A flexible guide wire is passed retrograde up the trachea and out the mouth. A suture attached to the leading end of the plug is fixed to the wire and pulled through the larynx. The plug is secured in the upper trachea by tying the suture to a button. **B,** the plug being pulled into the trachea through the mouth of the fetus. (Courtesy of Harrison MR, Adzick NS, Flake AW, et al: Correction of congenital diaphragmatic hernia in utero VIII: Response of the hypoplastic lung to tracheal occlusion. *J Pediatr Surg* 31:1339–1348, 1996.)

accident, intracranial hemorrhage, unrelated bowel necrosis, and CNS damage.

Conclusion.—Occlusion of the trachea in fetuses with CDH and liver herniation into the chest can accelerate development of the fetal lung while improving associated pulmonary hypoplasia. However, because of complications—most related to the hysterotomy rather than the fetal problem—survival has been poor. Further development of this experimental procedure will be needed before it can be recommended as a treatment for fetal pulmonary hypoplasia.

► Whereas technical approaches to temporary fetal tracheal occlusion are being improved through research involving animal models like the fetal lamb,[1] the human experience to date, using a variety of techniques of tracheal occlusion, reflects the complicated circumstance of the neonate with CDH, which often involves other incapacities. That occlusion of the trachea can sometimes impact favorably on fetal lung growth has been established. It has been demonstrated as well that some infants can survive tracheal occlusion procedures in utero and can survive the immediate postnatal period.

What is also absolutely clear is that the procedure should be considered experimental and, at this point, probably still offers a less desirable alternative to traditional, or even experimental, postnatal therapies. The authors themselves acknowledge that "Prenatal treatment is ... expensive and may prove unsuccessful. Temporary tracheal occlusion currently is promising but thus far has been a largely unsuccessful therapy."

D.K. Stevenson, M.D.

Reference

1. Skarsgard ED, Meuli M, Vander-Wall KJ, et al: Fetal endoscopic tracheal occlusion (Fetendo-PLUG) for congenital diaphragmatic hernia. *J Pediatr Surg* 31:1335–1338, 1996.

Effect of Very Delayed Repair of Congenital Diaphragmatic Hernia on Survival and Extracorporeal Life Support Use

Reickert CA, Hirschl RB, Schumacher R, et al (Univ of Michigan, Ann Arbor; Henry Ford Hosp, Detroit)

Surgery 120:766–773, 1996 10–22

Background.—Extracorporeal life support (ECLS), inhaled nitric oxide, administration of surfactant, high-frequency oscillatory ventilation, and permissive hypercapnia have been used to treat infants with congenital diaphragmatic hernia (CDH). Traditional mortality of these infants is 50%, but there have been recent reports of 30% mortality or less. Currently, CDH is not treated as a surgical emergency; surgical repair is now often delayed 3–108 hours. At the University of Michigan Medical Center, all newborns with CDH are managed by stabilization with conventional mechanical ventilation and very delayed repair. The outcomes of delayed repair and immediate repair of CDH in newborns were compared in a retrospective analysis.

Methods.—The medical records of all infants with CDH treated during a period of 7.5 years were reviewed: 66 infants had immediate repair and 33 had very delayed repair. The outcomes of the 2 groups of infants were compared. All patients were considered for ECLS. Delayed repair was performed when respiratory insufficiency resolved with a mean airway pressure of 8 cm water or less and fraction of inspired oxygen of 0.4 or less or had been maintained for 72 hours.

Results.—At repair, mean patient age was 8.9 days. Extracorporeal life support was used in 11 patients. Of those 11 patients, 6 survived. Of the survivors, 1 underwent repair while receiving ECLS and the other 5 underwent repair after decannulation from ECLS. The remaining 20 candidates for repair of CDH survived without ECLS. Overall survival was 79% in patients who had delayed repair and 56% in patients who had immediate repair.

Conclusions.—In these neonates, delayed repair of CDH was associated with better overall survival and less use of ECLS than immediate repair. Very delayed repair of CDH is safe and may improve outcome. Weaning from life support and maintenance with conventional mechanical ventilation before repair was tolerated by most of these infants.

▶ The commentary below was provided by Dr. Eileen K. Stork. Dr. Stork is Director of the ECMO Center at Rainbow Babies & Childrens Hospital in Cleveland, Ohio, and Associate Professor of Pediatrics, Case Western Reserve University School of Medicine, Cleveland, Ohio:

▶ In this retrospective review, survival was improved and the need for ECLS reduced by 50% by delaying surgical repair of CDH 1–2 weeks after birth. No adverse events (such as bowel infarction) were reported in the delayed surgery group either. The authors readily admit, however, that the use of newer technologies such as high-frequency oscillatory ventilation, inhaled nitric oxide, and surfactant available to the delayed surgical group may also have been instrumental in improving outcome.

I can remember rushing these infants to surgery within minutes of delivery, operating under the theory that alleviating a mass effect of bowel impinging on the contralateral lung might somehow attenuate the inevitable pulmonary hypertension that kills so many of these patients. The problem was, survival did not improve with this heroic gesture. Later, the introduction of extracorporeal membrane oxygenation (ECMO) into the management of infants with CDH also produced mixed reviews. Bleeding complications among postoperative patients undergoing bypass, especially those repaired while receiving ECLS, makes avoidance of ECMO a very desirable goal. Delaying surgery in infants with CDH until the respiratory insufficiency and persistent pulmonary hypertension have abated is a simple concept that makes powerful sense. If these data hold up in expanded trials, both neonatologists and pediatric surgeons will have to relearn that patience is, indeed, a virtue.

E.K. Stork, M.D.

Plasminogen Activator Activity in Preterm Infants With Respiratory Distress Syndrome: Relationship to the Development of Bronchopulmonary Dysplasia

Singhal KK, Parton LA (State Univ of New York at Stony Brook)

Pediatr Res 39:229–235, 1996 10–23

Background.—Respiratory distress syndrome (RDS), caused by a pulmonary surfactant deficiency, is histologically characterized by fibrinous exudates and fibrin-rich hyaline membranes lining the alveoli. Excessive alveolar deposition of fibrin and its degradation products may hinder surfactant function, damage vascular endothelium, act as chemotactic

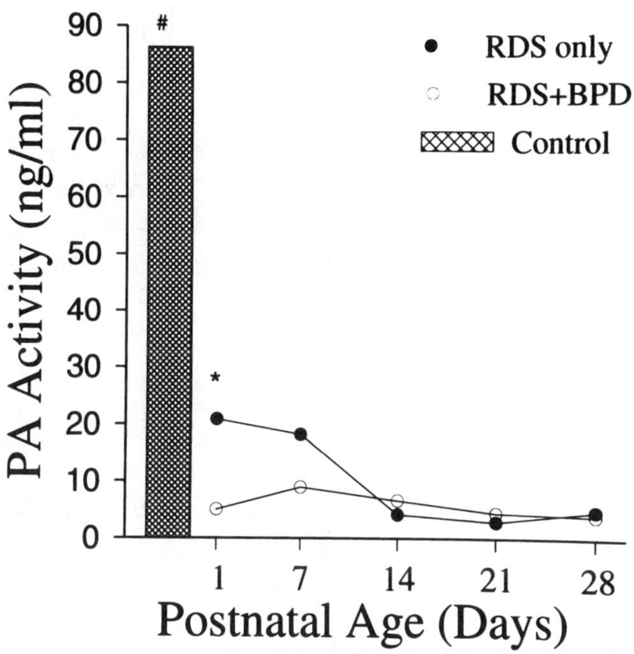

FIGURE 4.—Plasminogen activator (*PA*)/plasmin activity in tracheal aspirate (*TA*) samples over the first month of life. PA/plasmin activity for the group with self-resolved respiratory distress syndrome (*RDS*) (median values, *closed circles*) is compared with the PA/plasmin activity for the group with RDS who progressed to bronchopulmonary dysplasia (*BPD*) (median values, *open circles*). Tracheal aspirate samples obtained from intubated neonates without RDS (controls) on day 1 are shown as a *hatched bar.* A significant difference (*number symbol*) between the neonates without RDS and both the self-resolved RDS group ($P < 0.05$) and the RDS group who progressed to BPD ($P < 0.001$) was noted. A significant difference (*asterisk*) between the self-resolved RDS group and the RDS group that progressed to BPD was noted on day 1 ($P < 0.001$). (Courtesy of Singhal KK, Parton LA: Plasminogen activator activity in preterm infants with respiratory distress syndrome: Relationship to the development of bronchopulmonary dysplasia. *Pediatr Res* 39:229–235, 1996.)

factors for neutrophils, and function as immunoregulatory peptides. In addition, fibrin deposition and inadequate breakdown may accelerate the inflammatory cascade, which may play a role in the pathogenesis of bronchopulmonary dysplasia (BPD). It was hypothesized that preterm neonates with RDS have depressed alveolar fibrinolytic activity and that infants with RDS progressing to BPD have an even greater impairment of alveolar fibrinolysis.

Methods and Findings.—Forty-six intubated infants with RDS and 9 control infants were studied. Serial tracheal aspirate samples were obtained and analyzed for fibrinolytic activity. In the infants with self-resolved RDS and in those with RDS progressing to BPD, net PA/plasmin activity in tracheal aspirate was significantly depressed on the first day of life compared with that of control patients. In neonates with disease progressing to BPD, plasminogen activator (PA)/plasmin activity was significantly lower on the first day of life compared with that of neonates with self-resolved RDS (Fig 4).

Conclusion.—Depressed fibrinolytic activity may place preterm infants at risk for RDS. The degree of this depression may predict progression to BPD. In infants of 30 weeks' gestation or younger with RDS, a PA/plasmin activity of 10 ng/mL or less on the first day of life had positive and negative predictive values of 80% and 82%, respectively, for progression to BPD.

► We asked Dr. Jonathan Davis, Associate Professor of Pediatrics, State University of New York at Stony Brook's School of Medicine, to comment:

► One of the most common pathologic features of RDS is the presence of fibrin-rich hyaline membranes lining the alveolar surface. These membranes are broken down and cleared from the alveoli when RDS resolves normally. However, if not degraded properly, they can organize and obliterate the alveolar space. This particular histologic finding can be seen in the early phases of BPD. The pathogenesis of BPD is complex and not completely understood. It is thought to begin as early as the first day of life as an acute inflammatory response caused by exposure of the neonatal lung to hyperoxia (even 21% O_2 is supraphysiologic) and mechanical ventilation. The influx of inflammatory cells into the lung causes further damage by releasing oxygen-free radicals and proteases, such as elastase and collagenase. This amplification phenomenon leads to acute lung injury, which subsequently progresses to chronic lung disease (i.e., BPD).

This study by Singhal and Parton is important because it shows that neonates with RDS in whom BPD subsequently develops have markedly impaired fibrinolytic activity in their lungs on day 1 of life. Excessive fibrin deposition and incomplete breakdown can accelerate the inflammatory cascade and accentuate lung injury. This also may help to explain why the hyaline membranes are not cleared from the alveoli. This is another example of lung damage caused by an imbalance between proteases and antiproteases. The results of this study also reinforce the concept that the early inflammatory changes are a major determinant in the pathogenesis of BPD, and for potential therapeutic interventions such as corticosteroids or antioxidants to be effective, they must be initiated soon after birth.

Finally, the study is important in demonstrating that urea can be accurately measured and used as an effective marker to correct for the dilution of epithelial lining fluid that occurs when tracheal aspirates are obtained. If further studies can confirm these findings, tracheal aspirate analyses can be performed more accurately and efficiently.

J. Davis, M.D.

Changes in Intubation Rates and Outcome of Very Low Birth Weight Infants: A Population-based Study

Poets CF, Sens B (Hannover Med School, Germany; Lower Saxony Perinatal Working Group, Hannover, Germany)

Pediatrics 98:24–27, 1996 10–24

Introduction.—The practice of intubating and mechanically ventilating very low birth weight (VLBW) infants has never been tested in a large, randomized, controlled investigation. Many neonatologists started reconsidering this practice after a presentation at a major session of the 1993 annual meeting of the German-Austrian Society of Neonatology and Pediatric Intensive Care. Dr. Marcovich, a neonatologist from Vienna, Austria, presented her findings of low mortality and low rate of chronic lung disease in VLBW infants who were not intubated or mechanically ventilated. The changes in intubation rates and outcomes during the last 3 years were evaluated for VLBW infants in northern Germany.

Methods.—Population-based data on the treatment and outcome of VLBW infants discharged from a statewide quality assurance program in Lower Saxony, North were examined. From 1992 to 1994, data were gathered on 2,001 VLBW infants who weighed 500 to 1,499 g at birth and were admitted to a neonatal care unit.

Results.—The incidence of infants weighing less than 1,000 g who were not intubated and mechanically ventilated rose from 7% in 1992 to 14% in 1994. The respective figures in infants weighing 1,000 g or more were 28% and 44%. There was a 35% reduction in the mean duration of ventilation, from 23 days in 1992 to 15 days in 1994, in infants weighing less than 1,000 g. This trend toward decreased utilization of intubation and mechanical ventilation in VLBW infants was not associated with significant increases in adverse outcomes, such as death, intraventricular hemorrhage, periventricular leukomalacia, or bronchopulmonary dysplasia (BPD). There was a significant increase, from 38% in 1992 to 48% in 1994, in the proportion of infants weighing less than 1,000 g who survived without BPD and a decrease in the proportion of infants weighing 1,000 g or more in whom BPD developed.

Conclusions.—Findings indicate a reduction in the aggressiveness of the treatment of VLBW infants in a geographically defined area. The change was not associated with increased mortality or short-term morbidity. It should not be inferred from these findings that a more selective approach to the intubation of VLBW infants will result in improved outcome.

▶ The following commentary is submitted by Dr. Richard J. Martin, Co-director, Division of Neonatology, Department of Pediatrics, Rainbow Babies & Childrens Hospital, Cleveland, Ohio:

▶ It is interesting, but not surprising, to note that intubation rates for VLBW infants may fluctuate over time, without obvious favorable or detrimental effects or adverse outcomes. One is reminded of the postnatal use of corticosteroids, in which an enhanced ability to extubate has yet to have an obvious effect on the incidence of either BPD or neurodevelopmental outcome.

The question of whether intubation is good or bad is a very complex one. Regional differences must be called into play. For example, the intricacies of ventilator management vs. delivery of supplemental oxygen by a hood, nasal prongs, or continuous positive airway pressure are a function of clinical expertise, individual staff training, and other idiosyncracies. The German experience described in this report is of interest because of their good outcomes with less invasive treatment.

It is regional, but is it generalizable? The approach has been subjected to much debate but not to a controlled trial, and I do not suspect it will be. Regional preferences and center differences will prevail!

R.J. Martin, M.D.

Passive Smoking and Respiratory Function in Very Low Birth Weight Children

Doyle LW, Ford GW, Olinsky A, et al (Royal Women's Hosp, Melbourne, Australia; Royal Children's Hosp, Melbourne, Australia)

Med J Aust 164:266–269, 1996 10–25

Objective.—Although depressed respiratory function has been linked to maternal smoking in low–birth weight children, the effects of passive smoking have not been examined. The effects of passive smoking on respiratory function in low–birth weight children at age 11 years were examined.

Methods.—Respiratory function of 120 children aged 11 years, who weighed less than 1,501 g at birth, was measured. Smoking habits of other household members during the child's lifetime were determined. The relationship between respiratory function variables and number of cigarettes smoked by household members per day was tested by regression analysis.

Results.—Most airflow respiratory function variables were significantly decreased and air trapping variables increased with increasing exposure to passive smoking.

Conclusion.—Passive smoking is associated with reduced respiratory function in very low birth weight children at age 11 years. Respiratory function continues to be adversely affected with increasing exposure to passive smoking.

▶ This comment was co-authored by Daniel S. Seidman, M.D., of The Sheba Medical Center, Tel-Hashomer, Israel:

▶ The danger of secondhand smoke has received growing recognition during the past few years. One of the first health outcomes shown to be associated with passive smoking was asthma in children of parents who smoke. The magnitude of the risk presented by exposure to environmental tobacco smoke remains unclear, as the degree of exposure depends not only on the number of cigarettes smoked by each household member, but also on room ventilation and the proximity to the smoker. These factors are often influenced by the weather, with a lower degree of ventilation during the winter months. Although the exact magnitude of the damage caused by passive smoking remains the subject of intensive research, the need for maximal protection of innocent children from the risks of tobacco smoke remains beyond dispute. The present report demonstrates the irony in that children of parents who smoke are not only at higher risk of lower birth weight and premature delivery, but they also may be victims of a secondary assault by a continuing exposure to tobacco smoke.

D. Seidman, M.D.
D.K. Stevenson, M.D.

Congenital Stridor
Lis G, Szczerbinski T, Cichocka-Jarosz E (Polish American Children's Hosp, Krakow, Poland)
Pediatr Pulmonol 20:220–224, 1995 10–26

Background.—Stridor is a common indication for direct visual assessment of the upper airway in infants and children. Fiberoptic bronchoscopic findings in children with stridor were evaluated, and the characteristics of laryngomalacia were interpreted.

Methods.—Fifty-two children whose median age was 5 months were examined. The ratio of boys to girls was 2:1. In all patients, the origin of stridor could not be identified without fiberoptic bronchoscopy.

Findings.—Laryngomalacia was the most common cause of stridor, identified in 65%. Most commonly, laryngomalacia was caused by large, floppy arytenoid cartilages. Boys had this abnormality more than twice as often as girls. Compared with the normal population, the children with laryngomalacia had significant weight and height deficits of 24% and 7.7%, respectively. Blood gas values were normal in all but 4 children. In the 18 children without laryngomalacia, the causes of stridor varied substantially (Table 2).

TABLE 2.—Major Diagnostic Findings in 52 Children With Stridor

Finding	Patients No.	%
Laryngomalacia	34	65
Tracheal compression by an innominate artery	4	8
Subglottic stenosis	3	6
Tracheomalacia	3	6
Tracheal torsion* and stenosis	1	2
Tracheal stenosis	1	2
Subglottic hemangioma	1	2
Laryngeal web	1	2
Subglottic cyst	1	2
Laryngeal papillomatosis	1	2
Adenoidal hypertrophy	1	2
Subglottic edema	1	2

*Tracheal twisting along the long axis.

(Courtesy of Lis G, Szczerbinski T, Cichocka-Jarosz E: Congenital stridor. *Pediatr Pulmonol* 20:220–224. Copyright 1995, Wiley-Liss, Inc. Reprinted by permission of John Wiley & Sons, Inc.)

Conclusions.—In about two thirds of these children, laryngomalacia was the cause of stridor. Many children with laryngomalacia had weight and height deficits, probably because inspiratory efforts require more energy, calorie intake is reduced because of swallowing problems, and gas exchange may be compromised, leading to hypoxemia. Identifying the cause of stridor in children without laryngomalacia is important, because prognosis depends on the type and cause of the anatomical and functional abnormality.

▶ Fiberoptic bronchoscopy is in vogue and is a major component of the pulmonologist's armamentarium. It has revealed a lot about the airway that we never knew before. In this study, the fiberoptic bronchoscope produced a definitive diagnosis in the minority of hoarse infants who did not have laryngomalacia or tracheomalacia and could be treated. We all see noisy breathers from time to time, and it is useful to recall the differential diagnosis and epidemiology. Laryngomalacia remains the most common cause and, for unknown reasons, is twice as common in boys as in girls. Although we have tended to regard laryngomalacia as a relatively benign condition that infants "grow out of," it is worrisome to learn that a significant number of these infants fail to thrive.

M.J. Maisels, M.B., B.Ch.

11 The Heart and Blood Vessels

Haemodynamic Features at Presentation in Persistent Pulmonary Hypertension of the Newborn and Outcome

Skinner JR, Hunter S, Hey EN (Freeman Hosp, Newcastle upon Tyne, England; Princess Mary Maternity Hosp, Newcastle upon Tyne, England)

Arch Dis Child 74:F26–F32, 1996 11–1

Background.—Estimation of the prognosis of neonates with persistent pulmonary hypertension of the newborn (PPHN) is difficult and usually based on ventilatory requirements and oxygenation ratios, despite the knowledge that this is a circulatory problem.

Purpose.—Doppler echocardiography was used to examine circulatory parameters in neonates with PPHN and to determine whether any had prognostic significance.

Methods.—From April 1989 to September 1991, 34 neonates with evidence of PPHN were referred from 2 regional hospitals for Doppler echocardiography, including measurement of pulmonary arterial pressure, left ventricular function, and left ventricular output (LVO). The results were compared with those of 51 healthy neonates. Four neonates in the study group were excluded because of transposed great arteries in 1, a large left-to-right shunt without PPHN in 1, and diffuse skeletal myopathy in 2.

Results.—The pulmonary-to-systemic arterial pressure ratio range was 0.7:1 to 1.83:1. The time-to-peak velocity of the pulmonary valve/right ventricular ejection time was in the normal range in most patients. It was not correlated with other measurements of pulmonary arterial pressure. Left ventricular function was below the 10th centile in only 11% of these neonates, whereas LVO was below the 10th centile in 41%, and left ventricular stroke volume index (LSVI) was below the 10th centile in 66%. When 18 survivors were compared with 10 nonsurvivors, there were no significant differences in pulmonary arterial pressure or left ventricular function, but LVO and LSVI were significantly lower in the nonsurvivors. All 4 neonates with LVO of less than 100 mL/kg/min died, and 6 of 7 neonates with LSVI of less than 1 mL/kg died.

Conclusions.—In a Doppler echocardiographic analysis of 30 patients with PPHN, clinical diagnosis was difficult and the hemodynamic findings were diverse. The only Doppler echocardiographic parameters with prognostic implications were low LVO and stroke volume, which were associated with increased risk of mortality. The term PPHN is misleading and should be replaced with "neonatal pulmonary hypoperfusion" or "persistent transitional circulation." Further study is required to evaluate the predictive power of Doppler measurements of LVO and LSVI and their potential for therapeutic monitoring.

▶ Thomas Riggs, M.D., Director of Pediatric Cardiology, William Beaumont Hospital, Royal Oak, Michigan, comments:

▶ Neonates with PPHN are notorious among neonatologists and cardiologists for their critically ill, labile clinical condition and extreme sensitivity to environmental stress. The challenge has been to separate these neonates from those with cyanotic congenital heart disease in an accurate, noninvasive, and expeditious manner. Even in the best of hands, diagnoses are occasionally missed, as was the case with 1 patient in this series who was later found to have transposition of the great arteries.

There was right-to-left shunting at both atrial and great artery levels in many patients, although 17% had no patent ductus arteriosus present. No measure of pulmonary artery hypertension was useful as a predictor of survival, but poor outcome was associated with poor LVO and stroke volume, perhaps implying poor pulmonary blood flow and therefore diminished pulmonary venous return.

The authors have done us a service by providing echocardiographic measurements that are associated with poor outcome. These prognostic features are important because, in the past, we have had to rely entirely on ventilatory measurements such as oxygen ratios and so on to determine prognosis. This is rather unsatisfactory because we are dealing with a circulatory, rather than a ventilatory, problem. In addition, it is interesting that measurements of pulmonary arterial pressure, although important in making the diagnosis, were not a useful guide to disease severity and did not have an inverse relation to pulmonary arterial blood flow.

The authors would have us replace the term PPHN with a term that they believe is a more appropriate descriptor for low pulmonary blood flow. Having gone from PFC to PPHN, are we ready for NPH (neonatal pulmonary hypoperfusion) or PTC (persistent transitional circulation)?

T. Riggs, M.D.

Plasma Immunoreactive Endothelin-1 Concentrations in Infants With Persistent Pulmonary Hypertension of the Newborn

Kumar P, Kazzi NJ, Shankaran S (Wayne State Univ, Detroit)

Am J Perinatol 13:335–341, 1996 11–2

Background.—Studies have shown that plasma endothelin-1 (ET-1) levels are increased in children and adults with pulmonary hypertension. Infants with persistent pulmonary hypertension of the newborn (PPHN) may also have elevated plasma ET-1 concentrations.

Methods.—Twenty infants with PPHN and 20 normal-term infants of comparable birth weight and gestational age were studied. Plasma levels of immunoreactive–ET-1 (ir–ET-1) were measured using a radioassay.

Findings.—The infants with PPHN had significantly higher mean plasma ir–ET-1 levels than normal-term infants. In a linear regression analysis, ir–ET-1 concentrations were significantly correlated with alveolar-arterial oxygen gradient and mean airway pressure. In addition, ir–ET-1 levels were significantly associated with duration of extracorporeal membrane oxygenation (ECMO) in infants with PPHN.

Conclusions.—Plasma ir–ET-1 levels are increased in infants with PPHN. The current findings suggest that ET-1 may be a useful marker of disease severity in such neonates. Further research is needed to determine the role of ET-1 in the pathophysiology of PPHN.

► This comment has been provided by William D. Rhine, M.D., Assistant Professor of Pediatrics, Stanford University School of Medicine; Co-director of ECMO, Lucile Salter Packard Children's Hospital at Stanford University, Palo Alto, California:

► We now have further confirmation that ET-1 plays a part in the drama of pulmonary hypertension. But is this role *good* (through vasodilation at low concentrations), *bad* (via vasoconstriction and smooth muscle cell induction), or *indifferent* (with levels secondarily affected by changes in pulmonary blood flow)? These investigators replicate many of the results of previous studies, such as those of Rosenberg et al.[1] A notable exception is that the currently reported assays have twofold to tenfold lower levels of ET-1, presumably the result of technical differences. Even with these differences, we are again shown that higher ET-1 levels in newborns correlated with worse pulmonary disease. It would be nice to see how their ET-1 levels changed with time and clinical improvement, with or without ECMO. It is also curious that the 3 patients with PPHN who died had ET-1 levels much closer to normal infants than those of PPHN survivors. Assays of ET-1 seem unlikely to be helpful in clinical decisions to use new therapies for PPHN such as high frequency, ECMO, inhaled nitric oxide or liquid ventilation, especially when such measurements currently require more than 24 hours to perform. Perhaps, with additional understanding of ET-1 and other factors affecting pulmonary blood flow, we will have the scientific basis necessary to improve our therapeutic approaches to PPHN.

W.D. Rhine, M.D.

Reference

1. Rosenberg AA, Kennaugh J, Koppenhafer SL, et al: Elevated immunoreactive endothelin-1 levels in newborn infants with persistent pulmonary hypertension. *J Pediatr* 123:109–114, 1993.

Inhaled Nitric Oxide for Avoidance of Extracorporeal Membrane Oxygenation in the Treatment of Severe Persistent Pulmonary Hypertension of the Newborn

Müller W, Kachel W, Lasch P, et al (Kinderklinik, Neonatal ICU, Mannheim, Germany)

Intensive Care Med 22:71–76, 1996 11–3

Background.—Persistent pulmonary hypertension of the newborn (PPHN), occurring as a primary idiopathic disease or caused by various underlying conditions, is the most common cause of conventional respiratory therapy failure in neonates. Inhaled nitric oxide (NO) is thought to be a noninvasive treatment alternative to extracorporeal membrane oxygenation (ECMO) in the treatment of PPHN in neonates. The value of inhaled NO in this setting was investigated.

Methods.—Ten candidates for ECMO with clinical and echocardiographic evidence of PPHN were given NO treatment. Nitric oxide gas was delivered by conventional intermittent positive-pressure ventilation ventilation, with concentrations increasing incrementally from 20 to 80 ppm.

Findings.—At NO levels ranging from 30 to 60 ppm, 5 infants had a significant increase in mean partial pressure of arterial oxygen. Three patients had transient improvement, and 2 had prolonged improvement. In these latter 2 infants, ECMO was avoided. Five infants did not respond to treatment. Mean respiratory tidal volume differed between responders and nonresponders, being 8.9 and 4.18 mL/kg, respectively.

Conclusion.—Inhalation of NO obviated the need for ECMO treatment in only 2 of the 10 infants. Thus, clinicians should not be overoptimistic in their expectations for NO therapy in this setting. Still unknown is whether earlier intervention with inhaled NO and/or NO combined with an exogenous surfactant—and possibly with high-frequency oscillatory ventilation—for improving alveolar ventilation may be useful for PPHN treatment.

▶ Dr. Robert Schumacher, Associate Professor of Pediatrics, University of Michigan Medical Center, Ann Arbor, Michigan, comments:

▶ Initial reports of success with NO seemed to presage obituaries for ECMO programs. The message of this paper is "Don't sell your ECMO pumps just yet!" These German investigators have long been active in the field of "ECMOlogy" and related "high-tech" treatments of newborn respiratory failure, and studies such as this are important because they address the initial question, "Will any infant respond to therapy with NO?" If selective response to NO occurs, the clinically important follow-up questions are "How do clinicians identify responders?" and "Which therapy (ECMO or NO) should one choose?"

"Avoidance of ECMO" is used by many investigators as a primary outcome measure of success of efficacy. Although survival with any therapy except ECMO is assumed to produce the best, least costly, most beneficial outcome, I am unaware of any study suggesting that, on a per-survivor basis, ECMO is more or less costly. The problem becomes one of defining and refining specific clinically meaningful outcomes, (e.g., long-term intact survival in patients with diaphragmatic hernia or meconium aspiration or ______________________ (enter your disease here) and then assigning a value to each of the various outcomes (alive without handicap, alive with handicap, dead, hospital days, dollars spent, etc.). Of course, these are much more difficult questions to answer, and accurate probability estimates require many more patients than the authors present in this paper.

R. Schumacher, M.D.

Four Patterns of Response to Inhaled Nitric Oxide for Persistent Pulmonary Hypertension of the Newborn

Goldman AP, Tasker RC, Haworth SG, et al (Great Ormond Street Hosp for Children, London)

Pediatrics 98:706–713, 1996 11–4

Background.—Recent research suggests that the endogenous vasodilator nitric oxide (NO) may be an important factor in the decline of pulmonary vascular resistance at birth and that endothelial dysfunction causing a reduction in endogenous NO production may play a critical role in the evolution of persistent pulmonary hypertension of the newborn (PPHN). Inhaled NO (iNO) is therefore an attractive treatment possibility. The clinical role of iNO in patients with PPHN was investigated prospectively.

Methods.—Twenty-five consecutive neonates born at more than 35 weeks of gestation were given a trial iNO, 20 ppm for 20 minutes, in the treatment of severe PPHN. Response was defined as a greater than 20% improvement in partial pressure of oxygen in arterial blood and a reduction in the oxygenation index to less than 40. Responders received continued treatment.

Findings.—Four patterns of response were noted. Pattern 1 was no response, occurring in 2 neonates. One of these patients survived. Pattern 2, occurring in 9 patients, was initial iNO response with a failure to sustain the response for 36 hours (as defined by an increase in the oxygenation index to more than 40). Six neonates in this group survived, 5 with

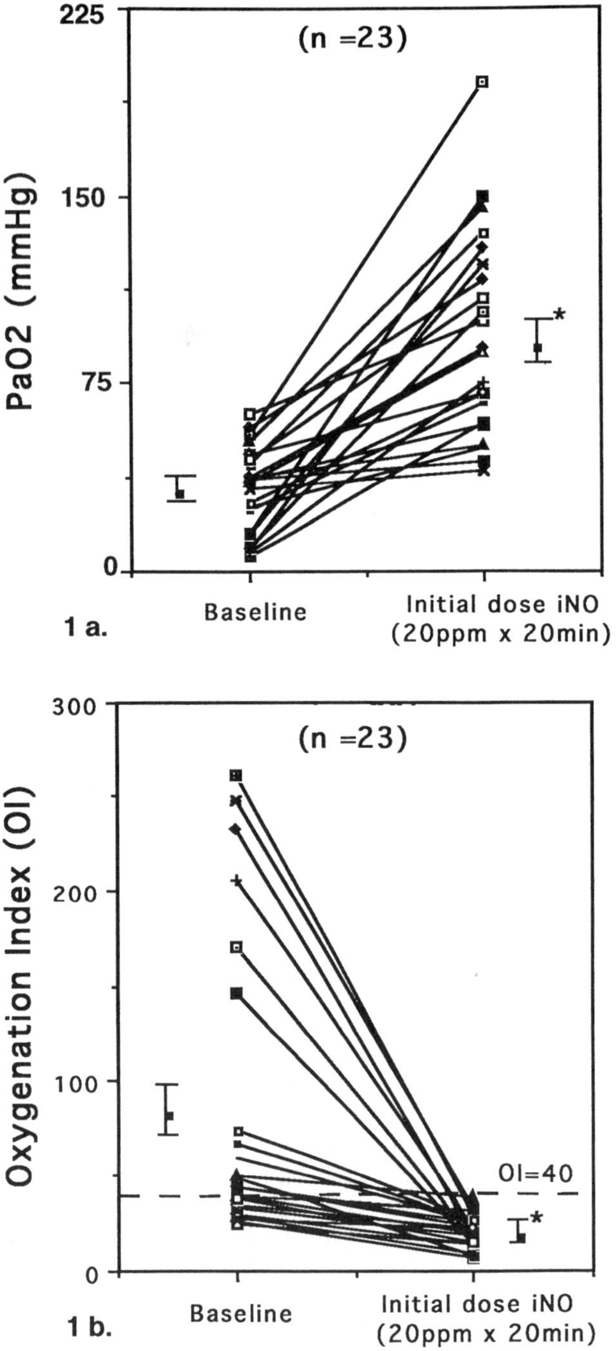

FIGURE 1.—Changes in PaO_2 (**A**) and OI (**B**) from baseline with the initial trial of iNO in the responders (n = 23). Values are expressed as mean ± SEM *PaO_2, OI; baseline compared with initial trial iNO, $P < 0.001$. *Abbreviations: iNO,* inhaled nitric oxide; *OI,* oxygenation index; PaO_2, partial pressure of arterial oxygen. (From Goldman AP, Tasker RC, Haworth SG, et al: Four patterns of response to inhaled nitric oxide for persistent pulmonary hypertension of the newborn. *Pediatrics* 98:706–713, 1996. Reproduced by permission of *Pediatrics*. Copyright 1996).

extracorporeal membrane oxygenation. Pattern 3 was an initial and sustained response with successful weaning from iNO within 5 days. All 11 neonates in this group survived to discharge. Pattern 4, observed in 3 patients, was an initial response, with the development of a sustained dependence on iNO for 3 to 6 weeks. All 3 of these neonates died, and histologic assessment of the lungs showed severe pulmonary hypoplasia and dysplasia. Neonates with a pattern 4 response needed iNO for a longer time than did those with a pattern 3 response and also required significantly greater iNO doses in the first 5 days of iNO treatment (Fig 1).

Conclusions.—Early responses to iNO treatment for severe PPHN may not be sustained. Infants with pulmonary hypoplasia and dysplasia may have a lower sensitivity than patients with PPHN in fully formed lungs. The time course of iNO response may also differ between these groups.

▶ Persistent pulmonary hypertension (PPHN) is a complex disorder that occurs in 1–2 per 1,000 live births. Most commonly, PPHN is associated with conditions that increase pulmonary vascular reactivity, such as meconium aspiration syndrome, sepsis or pneumonia (especially group B streptococcal disease), respiratory distress syndrome, and pulmonary hypoplasia with or without a congenital diaphragmatic hernia. Pulmonary vascular disease, with an onset before birth characterized by precocious extension of smooth muscle into the smallest arterioles, may follow in utero hypoxia or premature closure of the ductus arteriosus with maternal salicylate ingestion. A significant percentage of cases of PPHN are designated as idiopathic, and a number of these follow repeat elective cesarean section. Given the wide array of conditions with PPHN as the end result, it is not surprising that there are variable responses to iNO.

In the piglet model, endogenous NO is important in the regulation of pulmonary vascular tone during normoxia and hypoxia.[1] Inhaled nitric oxide completely reversed the elevations in pulmonary vascular resistance caused by inhibition of endogenous NO and may normalize pulmonary vascular resistance in diseases in which the production of NO is compromised.[1] Nitric oxide is but one of many variables involved in the control of pulmonary vascular tone. Thus, it is not surprising to find unpredictable responses. Inhaled nitric oxide diffuses through smooth muscle cells. Cyclic quanosine monophosphate levels are raised, leading to a decrease in intracellular calcium and smooth muscle relaxation. In different disease states, the diffusion capacity may differ or inadequate ventilation results in inadequate delivery of NO, which could account for the variable efficacy.

This report from Goldman and associates, and the companion article by Day[2] in the same journal provide some perspective on the response to iNO. They separate the responders from the nonresponders and indicate that infants with a clear chest radiograph are more likely to respond. It should be apparent that there are a number of unanswered questions currently being investigated in clinical trials and in the molecular laboratories (Abstracts 9–7, 11–5). These include the dosing and safety issues as well as the key adjunctive therapies. Is iNO more effective with high-frequency ventilation or are conventional ventilators satisfactory? What about surfactant, liquid ventilation, or phosphodiesterase inhibitors? Can they enhance iNO therapy?

As the presses started to roll, or the computers started to whir, on this edition of the YEAR BOOK OF NEONATAL AND PERINATAL MEDICINE, the Neonatal Inhaled Nitric Oxide Study was published, reporting that NO therapy reduced the use of extracorporeal membrane oxygenation but had no apparent effect on mortality in critically ill infants with hypoxic respiratory failure.[3] In a companion article in the same journal, Roberts and associates similarly concluded, "Inhaled nitric oxide improves systemic oxygenation in infants with persistent pulmonary hypertension and may reduce the need for more invasive treatment."[4] These 2 articles will be analyzed in depth in the 1998 YEAR BOOK.

Consider the postage stamp. It secures success by sticking to one thing until it gets there.—Josh Billings

A.A. Fanaroff, M.B.B.Ch.

References

1. Lipsitz EC, Weinstein S, Smerling AJ, et al: Endogenous nitric oxide and pulmonary vascular tone in the neonate. *J Pediatr Surg* 31:137–140, 1996.
2. Day RW, Lynch JM, White KS, et al: Acute responses to inhaled nitric oxide in newborns with respiratory failure and pulmonary hypertension. *Pediatrics* 98:698–705, 1996.
3. The Neonatal Inhaled Nitric Oxide Study Group: Inhaled nitric oxide in full-term and nearly full-term infants with hypoxic respiratory failure. *N Engl J Med* 336:597–604, 1997.
4. Roberts JD, et al: Inhaled nitric oxide and persistent pulmonary hypertension of the newborn. *N Engl J Med* 336:605–610, 1997.

Inhaled Nitric Oxide Injures the Pulmonary Surfactant System of Lambs In Vivo

Matalon S, DeMarco V, Haddad IY, et al (Univ of Alabama, Birmingham; Univ of Florida, Gainesville; Univ of Calgary, Alberta, Canada)

Am J Physiol 270:L273–L280, 1996 11–5

Introduction.—Inhaled nitric oxide (·NO) exerts beneficial effects in pulmonary hypertension and decreases pulmonary arterial pressure and intrapulmonary shunting in patients with adult respiratory distress syndrome. Studies also indicate, however, that ·NO may cause sublethal injury to the mammalian lung. The potential adverse effects of inhaled ·NO on the pulmonary surfactant system were studied in newborn lambs.

Methods.—Thirty-five newborn lambs were prepared for the experimental protocol. The animals were randomly assigned to 1 of 6 treatment groups in which they were exposed to 0, 20, 80, or 200 ppm of ·NO in either 21% or 60% O_2 for 6 hours. Gas was delivered at a constant flow rate of 10 L/min. Changes in the surface-active properties of pulmonary surfactant were measured by using both a captive and a pulsating bubble surfactometer. Surfactant protein A (SP-A) was isolated from the lungs of lambs that breathed 0, 80, or 200 ppm of ·NO for 6 hours to measure SP-A–induced lipid aggregation in vitro. In addition, structural changes in SP-A were assessed by sodium dodecyl sulfate–polyacrylamide gel electrophoresis and Western blot studies.

Results.—After 6 hours of ·NO exposure, values of arterial partial pressures of oxygen (Po_2) and carbon dioxide (Pco_2) and of pH were normal in the lambs, as were levels of total protein concentration in the bronchoalveolar lavage fluid. The air and 60% O_2 groups showed no differences in the surface properties of surfactant. Abnormal surface properties were observed in 36% of surfactant samples isolated from the lungs of lambs that breathed 80 ppm of ·NO and in 60% of the samples from lambs that breathed 200 ppm of ·NO, findings that were confirmed with a pulsating bubble surfactometer. The primary structure of SP-A was not altered in the experiment, but SP-A isolated from the lungs of lambs that breathed the highest concentration of ·NO had decreased ability to aggregate lipids in vitro.

Discussion.—Pulmonary surfactant, by lowering the surface tension of the air–blood gas interface and stabilizing alveoli at low lung volumes, decreases the work of breathing and prevents the transudation of fluid into the alveolar space. Exposure to inhaled ·NO at 80 or 200 ppm for 6 hours resulted in injury to surfactant apoproteins in the lungs of newborn lambs.

► The following commentary has been provided by Dr. Charles F. Potter, Senior Neonatal Fellow, Rainbow Babies & Childrens Hospital, University Hospitals of Cleveland, Cleveland, Ohio:

► This paper by Matalon and colleagues serves as a reminder to all neonatologists that a rush to accept novel therapies without appropriate basic and clinical experimentation runs the risk of harming rather than helping our newborn patients. Although much attention is focused on the success of ·NO in treating persistent pulmonary hypertension of the newborn (PPHN)[1] and reducing the need for extracorporeal membrane oxygenation,[2] the complex biochemical interactions of NO demand the judicious use of ·NO, especially in light of the many different approaches in dealing with PPHN and hypoxic respiratory failure.

One such potentially damaging interaction involves both NO and oxygen. The successful use of ·NO as previously cited required prolonged administration (longer than 6 hours) under hyperoxic conditions.[1] Matalon and colleagues suggest that ·NO at clinically efficacious concentrations (20 ppm) given over 6 hours in 21% or 60% O_2 does not damage surfactant apoproteins. Higher concentrations, however, are deleterious.

To the authors' credit, they question the safety of low-dose ·NO over prolonged periods of hyperoxia. This is extremely relevant because high concentrations of ·NO (100 ppm) during hyperoxic conditions promote both surfactant dysfunction and pulmonary inflammation.[3] Confusion reigns, however, because endogenous NO may have a protective role against pulmonary damage induced by hyperoxia.[4]

The final judgment on the safety or toxicity of ·NO as used in the neonatal ICU will depend on further studies examining its short- and long-term effects under the many different clinical approaches to respiratory failure. Until then, one is reminded by Alexander Pope that "fools rush in where angels fear to tread."

C.F. Potter, M.D.

References

1. Roberts JD Jr, Fineman JR, Morin FC III, et al: Inhaled nitric oxide and persistent pulmonary hypertension of the newborn. *N Engl J Med* 336:605–610, 1997.
2. The Neonatal Inhaled Nitric Oxide Study Group: Inhaled nitric oxide in full-term and nearly full-term infants with hypoxic respiratory failure. *N Engl J Med* 336:597–604, 1997.
3. Robbins CG, Davis JM, Merrit TA, et al: Combined effects of nitric oxide and hyperoxia on surfactant function and pulmonary inflammation. *Am J Physiol* 269:L545–L550, 1995.
4. Capellier G, Maupoil V, Boillot A, et al: L-NAME aggravates pulmonary oxygen toxicity in rats. *Eur Respir* 9:2531–2536, 1996.

Prevention of Ischemia-Reperfusion Lung Injury by Inhaled Nitric Oxide in Neonatal Piglets

Barbotin-Larrieu F, Mazmanian M, Baudet B, et al (Université Paris-Sud; Université Paris V)

J Appl Physiol 80:782–788, 1996 11–6

Background.—The release of nitric oxide (NO) by the pulmonary epithelium is decreased by lung ischemia-reperfusion (IR). A neonatal piglet model of lung oxidant stress induced by IR was used to test the hypothesis that inhalation of NO might compensate for the decrease in endogenous NO and attenuate lung injury by decreasing neutrophil lung accumulation. Neonates with acute lung injury have benefited from inhaled NO, which may selectively decrease pulmonary inflammation.

Methods.—Eighteen 1-day-old piglets were studied. After total pulmonary vascular resistance (RT), coefficient of filtration (K_{fc}), and circulating neutrophil counts were determined at baseline, the isolated neonatal piglet lungs underwent a 1-hour period of ischemia followed by a 1-hour period of blood reperfusion and reventilation. Some piglets had NO added to the breathing circuit (IR-NO group) and others did not (IR control group). A time-control group was used to assess the stability of permeability, hemodynamic variables, and white blood cells in the isolated blood-perfused lung preparation.

Results.—The addition of NO prevented reperfusion-induced increases in RT and K_{fc}, as well as the decrease in circulating neutrophils. In contrast to the IR control group, the IR-NO group had no significant differences between baseline and postreperfusion values. White blood cell populations were markedly reduced in the IR control group, suggesting massive sequestration in the lung. In the IR-NO group, however, this effect was totally prevented, and all white blood cell populations remained virtually unchanged after reperfusion. The addition of NO prevented a reperfusion-induced decrease in endothelium-dependent relaxation on precontracted pulmonary arterial rings.

Discussion.—Inhaled NO was confirmed as having lung-protective effects in this neonatal piglet model of lung oxidant stress induced by IR. Animals treated with NO at reperfusion only did not have IR-induced increases in lung microvascular permeability or in pulmonary vascular resistance. In associated effects, lung neutrophil accumulation was inhibited and endothelium-dependent relaxation was restored in isolated pulmonary arteries.

▶ Dr. Charles F. Potter is a Senior Fellow in the Division of Neonatology at Rainbow Babies & Childrens Hospital, University Hospitals of Cleveland, Cleveland, Ohio. His commentary follows:

▶ It is becoming extremely difficult to limit the physiologic role of inhaled NO in the newborn to pulmonary vasodilation. Evidence suggests that NO can affect many differet forms of normal and pathologic cellular interactions; specifically, it has a major role in mediating oxidation injury.

Barbotin-Larrieu and associates used low-dose (10 ppm) inhaled NO to prevent the pulmonary endothelial injury and inflammation associated with IR. They suggest that normal endothelial function is preserved by supplementing depleted endothelial NO production with inhaled NO. Normal endothelial function thus limits the accumulation of neutrophils and their pathologic production of oxygen radicals. Supporting studies have shown that inhaled NO at 10 ppm protects the lung from oxygen damage.[1] In the brain, on the other hand, blockade of the excessive NO production found after hypoxic-ischemic reperfusion preserves CNS antioxidant capacity and is beneficial.[2]

Within the lung, NO is produced not only by the endothelium, but also by pulmonary neutrophils. Overproduction of NO can promote inflammation and collagen deposition.[3] Peroxynitrate formed from the combination of superoxide and NO also can damage alveolar epithelium and surfactant, suggesting that a newborn's pulmonary superoxide dismutase concentration also may play a role in the lung's response to NO.[4]

Taken together, the protective physiologic vs. pathologic oxidative role that NO performs remains controversial. Preservation of function without excessive pathologic production of NO appears to be crucial to future therapeutic interventions. Until then, we must remember that too much of a good thing can be harmful.

C.F. Potter, M.D.

References

1. Adnot S, Raffestin B, Eddahibi S: NO in the lung. *Respir Physiol* 101:109–120, 1995.

2. Dorrepaal CA, Van Bel F, Moison RMW, et al:Oxidative stress during post-hypoxic-ischemic reperfusion in the newborn lamb: The effect of nitric oxide synthesis inhibition. *Pediatr Res* 41:321–326, 1997.
3. Grisham MB, Specian RD, Zimmerman TE: Effects of nitric oxide synthase inhibition on the pathophysiology observed in a model of chronic granulomatous colitis. *J Pediatr* 271:1114–1121, 1994.
4. Haddad IY, Pataki G, Hu P, et al: Quantitation of nitrotyrosine levels in lung secretions of patients and animals with acute lung injury. *J Clin Invest* 943:2407–2413, 1994.

UK Collaborative Randomised Trial of Neonatal Extracorporeal Membrane Oxygenation

Field DJ, for the UK Collaborative ECMO Trial Group (Univ of Leicester, England; et al)

Lancet 348:75–82, 1996 11–7

Background.—Extracorporeal membrane oxygenation (ECMO) is a technique that oxygenates blood outside the body and can be used to provide temporary support during respiratory failure in mature neonates. The value of this technique has been disputed, because the definitive clinical trial comparing ECMO and conventional support has not been done. A collaborative randomized, blinded clinical trial involving 55 hospitals from the United Kingdom was undertaken. Its objective was to evaluate referral for ECMO vs. conventional management in the treatment of mature infants with severe respiratory failure. The primary outcome measure was survival to 1 year without disability.

Methods.—Between 1993 and 1995, 185 infants who had a gestational age of at least 35 weeks, a birth weight of at least 2 kg, and severe respiratory failure (defined as an oxygenation index of at least 40) were enrolled in a randomized trial of conventional management or referral for ECMO. Conventional management consisted of liberal use of oxygen, correction of acidosis, maintenance of adequate blood pressure, and use of

TABLE 4.—Overall Status at 1-Year Follow-up of 124 Infants Enrolled by December 1, 1994

Outcome	ECMO (n=63)	CM (n=61)
Death		
Before discharge home	18 (29%)	37 (61%)
After discharge home and before age 1 year	2 (3%)	0
Severe impairment and disability	1 (2%)	1 (2%)
Signs of Impairment		
Disability not classified as severe	8 (13%)	2 (3%)
Without disability	2 (3%)	4 (7%)
Number of infants with no signs of impairment or disability	32 (51%)	17 (28%)

Abbreviations: ECMO, extracorporeal membrane oxygenation; *CM*, conventional management.

(Courtesy of Field DJ, for the UK Collaborative ECMO Trial Group: UK Collaborative randomised trial of neonatal extracorporeal membrane oxygenation. *Lancet* 348:75–82, 1996. Copyright by The Lancet Ltd. 1996.)

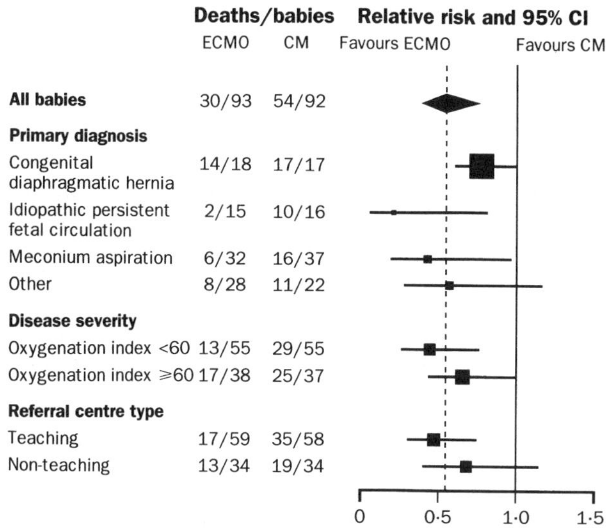

FIGURE.—Effects of extracorporeal membrane oxygenation (*ECMO*) policy on known deaths. Relative risks (*squares*; proportional to amount of information contributed) and 95% confidence intervals (*horizontal lines*) are plotted for various subgroups. Overall results shown by the *diamond*. *Abbreviation: CM*, conventional management. (Courtesy of Field DJ, for the UK Collaborative ECMO Trial Group: UK Collaborative randomised trial of neonatal extracorporeal membrane oxygenation. *Lancet* 348:75–82, 1996. Copyright by The Lancet Ltd. 1996.)

pulmonary vasodilators, high-frequency ventilation, and surfactant, as necessary. The diagnoses were persistent pulmonary hypertension resulting from aspiration of meconium, congenital diaphragmatic hernia, isolated persistent fetal circulation, sepsis, and idiopathic respiratory distress syndrome. Of the 93 infants randomly assigned to ECMO referral, 84% received ECMO support. Infants who survived to 1 year underwent blinded neurologic evaluation.

Results.—Eighty-one infants died before hospital release and 2 died subsequently. A significant difference in the mortality rate between the 2 treatment groups was found—32% in the ECMO group and 59% in the conventional management group. This difference was sustained irrespective of primary diagnosis, disease severity, or type of referral center. The benefit of ECMO was sustained for the primary outcome measure of disability-free survival at 1 year (Table 4). There was 1 infant in each treatment group with severe disability, 10 in the ECMO group with lesser disability, and 6 in the conventional group with lesser disability. The overall death rate was higher in those with more severe respiratory failure, but the death rate for these infants was lower in the ECMO group. There was a lower rate of mortality in all oxygenation index groups for those infants allocated to ECMO (Figure).

Conclusions.—When compared with conventional management in mature infants with severe respiratory failure, ECMO reduced the risk of death and severe disability at 1-year follow-up. Recruitment to the trial was halted early on the advice of an independent committee because of the already clearly demonstrated advantage of ECMO. Because the costs of both types of treatment are roughly similar, ECMO support should be considered for all mature neonates with severe but potentially reversible respiratory failure. Large, rigorous, randomized collaborative trials of treatment for life-threatening conditions can be successfully done.

▶ Although some neonatologists in the United States may think that they already know the answers to the questions posed by these investigators, this is the first and only study of ECMO that satisfies the important principles of research design and is characterized by strict, random allocation, adequate sample size, complete follow-up, and blinded assessment of outcome. The authors are correct when they point out that "no other study of ECMO has these strengths." The result is a resounding vote of confidence for the use of ECMO in the management of appropriately selected infants at 35 weeks' gestation or more with birth weights of 2 kg or more who have severe respiratory failure (oxygen index 40 or greater).

Infants from no less than 55 hospitals throughout the United Kingdom who met the criteria were randomly assigned to receive ECMO or conventional intensive care (which could include nitric oxide, surfactant, and high-frequency ventilation). As has been found in the United States, the outcome for congenital diaphragmatic hernia was poor, no matter what the treatment. Nevertheless, 22% of infants with congenital diaphragmatic hernia who received ECMO survived, compared with none in the conventional group. For diagnoses other than congenital diaphragmatic hernia (persistent pulmonary hypertension resulting from meconium aspiration, isolated persisted fetal circulation, sepsis, and respiratory distress syndrome, the mortality rate in the ECMO group (21%) was less than half that in the conventional management group (49%). Fifty-one percent of those receiving ECMO showed no signs of impairment or disability, compared with 28% of those allocated to conventional management.

Nothing further need be said except that the cost of care for the patients receiving ECMO (~$37,366 per survivor) and those receiving conventional management (~$36,324 per survivor) was virtually identical.

In 1976, Dr. Robert Bartlett first performed ECMO successfully on a neonate with severe respiratory failure.[1] The first properly conducted, randomized, controlled trial showing that such patients are less likely to die or be disabled has been a long time in coming.

M.J. Maisels, M.B., B.Ch.

Reference

1. Bartlett RH: Esperanza. Presidential address. *Trans Am Soc Artif Intern Org* 30:723–726, 1985.

ECMO in Evolution: The Impact of Changing Patient Demographics and Alternative Therapies on ECMO

Wilson JM, Bower LK, Thompson JE, et al (Children's Hosp, Boston)

J Pediatr Surg 31:1116–1123, 1996 11–8

Background.—The incidence of neonatal extracorporeal membrane oxygenation (ECMO) is declining nationally, presumably because of the use of alternative technologies. Changes in ECMO use over time at 1 center were determined.

Methods.—Data on 455 patients receiving ECMO during a 12-year period were analyzed. The 370 neonates included in the study were categorized according to diagnostic group.

Findings.—During the study, the total number of patients receiving ECMO per year declined; this was attributed to a decrease in the total number of neonates treated (except those with congenital diaphragmatic hernia [CDH]). The complexity of each ECMO run increased over time, as evidenced by marked increases in mean ECMO duration per patient and an increase in the incidence of patient complications on ECMO. Overall survival decreased significantly. The patient mix shifted from more straightforward neonatal cases to more complex pediatric and cardiac cases because of improvements in the pre-ECMO management of neonates. However, there was also a worsening of the severity of the condition in each diagnostic group.

Conclusion.—If the above trends continue, ECMO will be increasingly used for pediatric, cardiac, and CDH patients. Existing ECMO centers must be prepared to develop programs that support such patients in addition to neonates. The difficulty of transporting these unstable patients and the likelihood that the number of active ECMO centers will decline may necessitate the development of long-distance transport capabilities at ECMO centers.

► Commenting on this article is Krisa P. Van Meurs, M.D., Assistant Professor of Pediatrics, Co-director of ECMO Program, Division of Neonatal and Developmental Medicine, Stanford University School of Medicine, Palo Alto, California:

► The authors' analysis of the changes in ECMO use, duration, incidence of complications and survival over the past 12 years at Boston Children's Hospital yields some not-too-surprising, but highly interesting, results. It is not unanticipated that the use of surfactant, high-frequency oscillatory ventilation (HFOV), and nitric oxide have resulted in decreased numbers of neonatal ECMO patients, decreased neonatal transports, and increased transports for each ECMO performed. More unexpected is the finding of an increase in bypass days per patient; a decrease in overall neonatal and disease-specific survival rates; and an increase in patient and circuit complications, independent of the length of time on ECMO. Wilson et al. attribute these last changes to an increase in disease severity. Whether this change in severity of illness is a result of selecting for patients unresponsive to surfactant, HFOV, and nitric oxide or a result of delayed referral is an important and unanswered question.

These trends have numerous implications for existing ECMO centers. Smaller, neonatal ECMO centers may have insufficient patient numbers to maintain ECMO expertise. To remain viable, ECMO centers may need to develop programs that support older pediatric and cardiac patients. These recommendations have been made by the University of Michigan ECMO program. The difficulty in transporting from a referring hospital the neonate that has failed HFOV or nitric oxide or the unstable pediatric patient seems to be a valid reason for having ECMO transport available. To date, ECMO transport remains a capability available at only a few selected centers in the United States, and many of us will be happy if it stays that way.

K.P. Van Meurs, M.D.

Oxygen Delivery With a Single Cannula Tidal Flow Venovenous System for Extracorporeal Membrane Oxygenation

Keszler M, Moront MG, Cox C, et al (Georgetown Univ, Washington, DC)

ASAIO J 41:850–854, 1996 11–9

Background.—Although extracorporeal membrane oxygenation (ECMO) is increasingly being accepted, the use of carotid artery ligation for the venoarterial technique limits its usefulness. Venovenous perfusion, in which blood is both drained and reinfused on the venous side, has many advantages, but early attempts using jugular and femoral veins were limited by problems with recirculation, venous insufficiency of the leg, bleeding, and longer cannulation time. A single-cannula system would have the advantages of the venovenous perfusion but eliminate the second cannula and its associated problems. A single-lumen venovenous system was used in an experimental newborn sheep model.

Methods.—Six newborn lambs received ECMO via a single-cannula, single-lumen system with tidal flows directed by alternating tubing occluders. The ratio of drainage to infusion time was 2:1 to prevent excessive reinfusion pressure problems. The total time of the in/out cycle was varied from 2 to 6 sec, with a cycling frequency of 30 to 10 cycles/per minute and a tidal volume of 17–50 mL. Systemic arterial, mixed venous, and preoxygenator and postoxygenator partial pressure and oxygen satu ration were assessed. Recirculation, oxygen delivery, and effective bypass flow were derived.

Results.—As the cycling frequency was decreased, recirculation decreased and effective flow and oxygen delivery were significantly increased. The oxygen delivery was limited by the oxygen-carrying capacity in these animals.

Conclusions.—A tidal-flow venovenous system can provide complete respiratory support in a newborn lamb ECMO model if larger tidal volumes are used. Use of larger tidal volumes decreases recirculation while permitting sufficient effective bypass flow and oxygen delivery. These results should provide a stimulus for the development of a commercial tidal-flow, single-lumen, single-cannula device in the United States. Similar devices are already being used in France and Italy.

▶ This comment has been provided by William D. Rhine, M.D., Assistant Professor of Pediatrics, Stanford University School of Medicine, Co-director of ECMO, Lucile Salter Packard Children's Hospital at Stanford University, Palo Alto, California:

▶ The development of single-cannula tidal-flow venovenous ECMO in America is still in its infancy, especially compared with its already accepted use in France and Italy. This article shows how laboratory evaluation can be helpful in introduction of new clinical technology, with animal data suggesting optimal drainage-to-infusion ratios and cycling frequencies. Comparison to the European systems is guarded because these systems use a nonocclusive roller pump with distensible tubing substituting for venous and reinfusion bladders (which might be potential sites for clot formation) and also use a single alternating clamp rather than 2 separate occluders. Such differences could affect the percentage of recirculation and optimal cycling frequency.

It turns out that the animal data from this article are consistent with current clinical applications; my European ECMO colleagues inform me that cycling frequencies are now usually 10–15/min. Clearly, additional development and testing would be necessary for United States Food and Drug administration device approval of tidal-flow ECMO. In the meantime, more neonates are receiving double-lumen venovenous ECMO with the increased size availability of catheters: 12 and 14 French ones from Kendall and 12 and 15 French ones from Jostra.

W.D. Rhine, M.D.

Haemodynamic Changes During High Frequency Oscillation for Respiratory Distress Syndrome

Laubscher B, van Melle G, Fawer C-L, et al (Centre Hospitalier Universitaire, Lausanne, Switzerland; Institut Universitaire de Médecine Sociale et Préventive, Lausanne, Switzerland)

Arch Dis Child 74:F172–F176, 1996 11–10

Background.—There have been no published studies of cardiac output or left ventricular output (LVO) and cerebral blood flow velocity (CBFV) in preterm infants with respiratory distress syndrome (RDS) during high-frequency oscillation. Animal studies suggest that high-frequency oscillation, when used with a cautious strategy of lung volume recruitment, would not impair LVO or CBFV in such infants.

Methods.—Ten preterm infants with RDS receiving conventional mechanical ventilation were transferred to high-frequency oscillation in a crossover trial. Using Doppler ultrasonography, LVO, CBFV, and resistance index of the anterior cerebral artery were compared.

Findings.—With high-frequency oscillation, LVO was 14% to 18% lower than during conventional mechanical ventilation. No significant changes were seen in CBFV. A trend toward a lower resistance index on high-frequency oscillation was observed on the first day of life. The decline in LVO during high-frequency oscillation was unassociated with lung hyperinflation.

Conclusion.—When compared with conventional mechanical ventilation, high-frequency oscillation appears to significantly reduce LVO without affecting blood pressure and heart rate in premature infants with RDS. In addition, high-frequency oscillation significantly improved oxygenation, consistent with previous research.

▶ We asked Eduardo Bancalari, M.D., Professor of Pediatrics at the University of Miami, to comment:

▶ These data obtained in infants with RDS are similar to those found in piglets.[1] Cardiac output was lower in piglets receiving high-frequency oscillation (HFO) than in those receiving conventional ventilation (IPPV). Unfortunately, some of the comparisons between HFO and IPPV reported in this paper were made shortly after the administration of surfactant, when the mechanical characteristics of the respiratory system were changing rapidly. This can clearly influence the effect of ventilation on hemodynamics.

The other limitation of this study is that the mean airway pressures used during HFO were higher than during IPPV, which could explain the lower LVO found during HFO. It would be important to know whether IPPV and HFO at similar mean airway pressures produced differences in hemodynamic measurements, as it is known that depression of cardiovascular function is related to the mean pressure applied to the airway.

E. Bancalari, M.D.

Reference

1. Osiovich HC, Suguihara C, Goldberg RN, et al: Hemodynamic effects of conventional and high-frequency oscillatory ventilation in normal and septic piglets. *Biol Neonate* 59:244–252, 1991.

Molecular Pathways Controlling Heart Development

Olson EN, Srivastava D (Univ of Texas, Dallas)
Science 272:671–675, 1996 11–11

Introduction.—The greatest number of human birth defects involve malformations of the heart and blood vessels. The recent identification of genes involved in the early stages of heart development and the discovery that these genes are evolutionarily conserved has prompted study of the

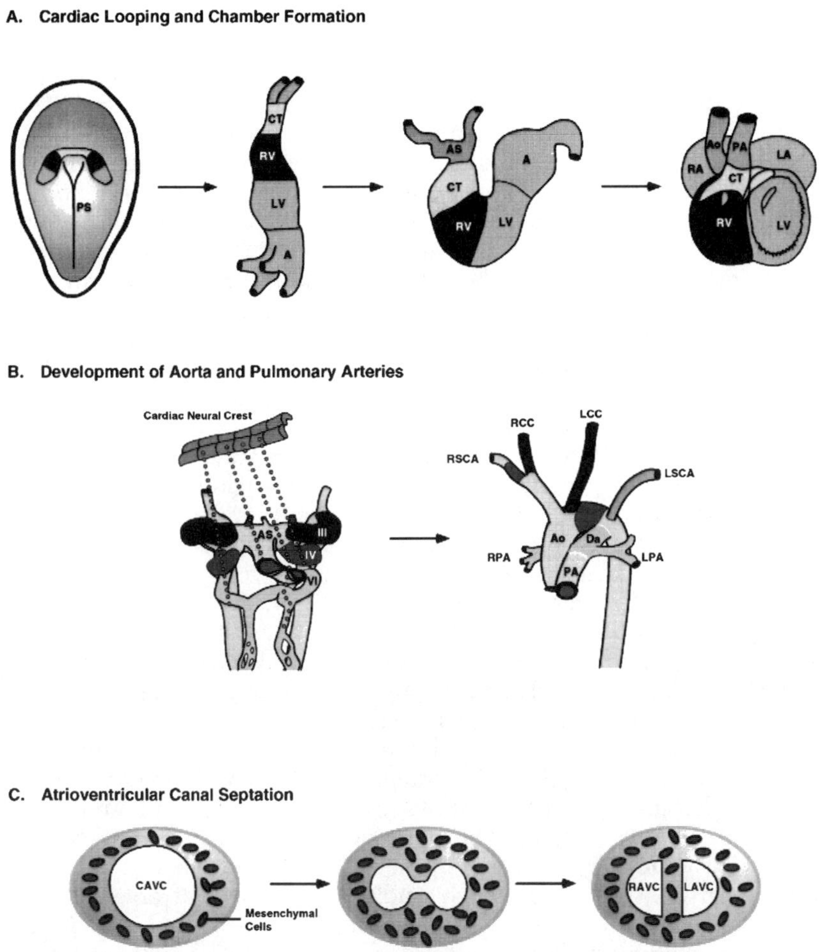

FIGURE 1.—Anatomical events of cardiac morphogenesis. The schematic illustrations depict cardiac development with color coding of morphologically related regions. **A,** cells of the precardiogenic mesoderm, shown in color, are specified at the embryonic primitive streak (*PS*) stage (**leftmost panel**) to form specific regions of the straight heart tube. The straight heart tube is specified in an anteroposterior gradient to form the various regions and chambers of the looped and mature heart. *Abbreviations: AS,* aortic sac; *CT,* conotruncus; *RV,* right ventricle; *LV,* left ventricle; *A,* atria; *RA,* right atrium; *LA,* left atrium; *Ao,* aorta; *PA,* pulmonary artery. **B,** cardiac neural crest cells populate the bilateral aortic arches III, IV, and VI, and the aortic sac. Extensive remodeling of the vasculature results in formation of the left aortic arch and proximal pulmonary arteries. Contributions of the aortic arch arteries to these regions are depicted in color. *Abbreviations: Da,* ductus arteriosus; *LSCA,* left subclavian artery; *LCC,* left common carotid; *RCC,* right common carotid; *RSCA,* right subclavian artery; *LPA,* left pulmonary artery; *RPA,* right pulmonary artery. **C,** separation of the common atrioventricular canal (*CAVC*) into a right (*RAVC*) and left (*LAVC*) atrioventricular canal is accomplished by invasion of ectomesenchymal cells. (Courtesy of Olson EN, Srivastava D: Molecular pathways controlling heart development. *Science* 272:671–675. Copyright 1996, American Association for the Advancement of Science.)

functions of cardiac regulatory genes. Current knowledge of the morphogenetic mechanisms controlling cardiac development as they relate to the anatomical and molecular abnormalities responsible for several congenital cardiac defects was reported.

Morphogenesis.—The heart arises through a complex series of morphogenetic interactions that include cells from several embryonic origins (Fig 1). Looping of the heart to the right occurs in all vertebrate species, implying the existence of an evolutionarily conserved mechanism for this important step in cardiac morphogenesis. The mutant phenotypes of the mechanisms that control the directionality of cardiac looping have been explored by genetic analysis in 2 mouse mutants with abnormalities in left-right orientation of the heart. The asymmetric expression of the morphogen nodal may give clues regarding the defects. Distinct subsets of cardiac muscle genes provide the contractile, electrophysiologic, and pharmacologic properties distinct to the atrial and ventricular chambers. The atrial and ventricular cells arise from different lineages that are specified before looping occurs and differentiate according to their positions along the anteroposterior axis of the embryo. Early myocardial growth is affected by a diversity of genes. These tissues are particularly sensitive to perturbations in early growth stages. Separate genes are responsible for depolarization along the various anatomical sites within the conduction system. The neural crest cells migrate from the neural folds and differentiate into distinct cell types, including melanocytes, neurons, connective tissue, and smooth tissue. A variety of neural crest defects have been observed in chick embryos. The CATCH-22 syndrome encompasses a wide spectrum of clinical manifestations, including cardiac defects, abnormal facies, thymic hypoplasia, cleft palate, and hypocalcemia. These are the result of deletions in chromosome 22. The most common CATCH-22 cardiac defect is persistent truncus arteriosus.

Conclusions.—There are several congenital cardiac defects that arise from abnormalities in cardiac morphogenesis. Some lesions become a subset of defects that are compatible with fetal development, and others result in embryonic lethality. The major defects are those of cardiac looping, arteriovenous septation, and the neural crest. Molecular cardiology is entering an exciting era in which studies of a variety of organisms are providing detailed molecular information about normal and abnormal cardiac development. Genetic screening and counseling will be able to offer more to individuals with congenital heart disease.

► Cardiac malformations account for a high percentage of birth defects. Routine fetal evaluation (see Abstract 4–5) detects anomalies of the cardiovascular system in about 1% of fetuses. Hoffman[1, 2] reported the frequency among stillbirths to approach 10%. "Formation of the heart requires migration, differentiation, and precise interactions among multiple embryonic cell types." The anatomical and physiologic characterization of most cardiac malformations has been chronicled; it is time to direct attention to the genetic bases of these abnormalities.

Olson and Srivastava review the current status of knowledge concerning the genetic control of cardiac development. The fate of the fetus is determined by the nature of the defect, so defects incompatible with the fetal circulation are lethal to the embryo. The hemodynamic alterations also contribute to the phenotype of the developmental defects. Simply classified, there are defects in the looping of the cardiac tube, defects in arteriovenous septation, and neural crest defects. The CATCH-22 syndrome, with microdeletion of chromosome 22q11, includes cardiac defects, abnormal facies, thymic hypoplasia, cleft palate, and hypocalcemia. Truncus arteriosus is the most common cardiac lesion. Other cardiac defects include malalignment of the aorta with respect to the ventricular septum (tetralogy of Fallot; double outlet right ventricle). It seems likely that these clinically diverse abnormalities have a common etiology that is based on cardiac neural tube defects.

As the genetic understanding of cardiac development expands, propsects for genetic screening and counseling emerge. However, the ultimate progress will be to control cardiac myocytes and regenerate injured cardiac muscle.

A.A. Fanaroff, M.B.B.Ch.

References

1. Hoffman JIE: Incidence of congenital heart disease. Part I: Postnatal incidence. *Pediatr Cardiol* 16:103–113, 1995.
2. Hoffman JIE: Incidence of congenital heart disease. Part II: Prenatal incidence. *Pediatr Cardiol* 16:155–165, 1995.

Surgical Management of Hypoplastic Left Heart Syndrome

Bando K, Turrentine MW, Sun K, et al (James W Riley Hosp for Sick Children, Indianapolis, Ind; Indiana Univ, Indianapolis)

Ann Thorac Surg 62:70–77, 1996 11–12

Background.—Many centers perform either palliative operations or transplantation in infants with hypoplastic left heart syndrome (HLHS), but the study institution offers both procedures to the families of affected newborns. A retrospective analysis of 50 newborns with HLHS assessed the operative and intermediate-term results of surgical management and risk factors for early mortality.

Methods.—Fifty of 86 infants referred for treatment of HLHS from January 1989 through June 1995 were eligible for surgical intervention. After the families were informed of potential risks and benefits of the surgical options, 28 chose palliation and 22 chose cardiac transplantation. Those selecting transplantation were told that changes in the infant's condition or lack of a donor heart might make crossover necessary (Fig 1). The palliative procedure in this series consisted of a stage 1 Norwood operation, followed at a median of 9.5 months by a second-stage Semi-Fontan procedure; at a median of 22 months later, the third-stage (fenestrated) Fontan procedure was performed.

Results.—Seven infants whose families had chosen transplantation had to undergo palliative operations because of lack of donors. Ten of the 15 infants who received donor hearts were alive, and all were in New York Heart Association class I. Two infants underwent transplantation after the first-stage Norwood operation and were doing well. One of the 34 infants

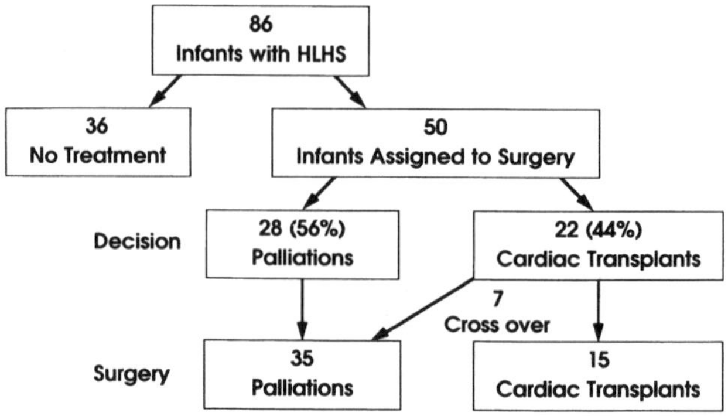

FIGURE 1.—Treatment option and surgical procedure performed as dictated by patient status, family wishes, and donor availability. *Abbreviation: HLHS*, hypoplastic left heart syndrome. (Reprinted with permission from the Society of Thoracic Surgeons, courtesy of Bando K, Turrentine MW, Sun K, et al: Surgical management of hypoplastic left heart syndrome. *Ann Thorac Surg* 62:70–77, 1996.)

who had Norwood procedures had inoperable anatomy and the operation was aborted. Ten infants had the second-stage procedure, and 7 completed the third stage of palliation. The 1-year mortality rate was 50% (17 of 34 newborns) for the Norwood procedure vs. 18% (3 of 18) for heart transplantation. Results of both surgical procedures improved with time: the 1-year survival rate was 75% for those who had the Norwood operation from 1993 to mid-1995, and no infants who received donor hearts since 1992 have died (Fig 2). Risk factors for early mortality in the palliative

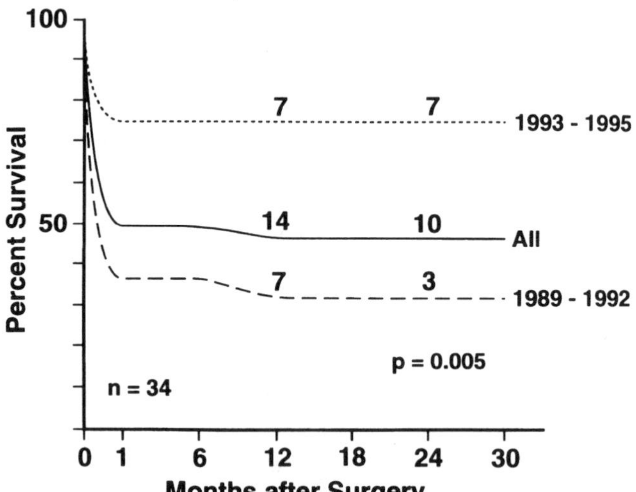

FIGURE 2.—Actuarial survival of infants undergoing palliation. The survival of infants having operations between 1993 and mid-1995 was significantly better than that of patients operated on from 1989 through 1992 ($p = 0.005$). One patient whose palliation was aborted was not included in this analysis. (Reprinted with permission from the Society of Thoracic Surgeons, courtesy of Bando K, Turrentine MW, Sun K, et al: Surgical management of hypoplastic left heart syndrome. *Ann Thorac Surg* 62:70–77, 1996.)

group included circulatory arrest time > 50 minutes, preoperative acidosis, systemic-pulmonary artery shunt 4 mm or greater, an ascending aorta 2 mm or less, and anatomical subtype of aortic and mitral atresia. None of the variables examined were predictive of early death after transplantation.

Discussion.—The management of newborns with HLHS is difficult and controversial. The Norwood procedure has been associated with high operative mortality, and rejection after transplantation is a problem. With a flexible approach and refinements in surgical technique and postoperative management, the results of both staged palliation and cardiac transplantation have improved in the past few years.

Staged Reconstruction for Hypoplastic Left Heart Syndrome: Contemporary Results

Bove EL, Lloyd TR (Univ of Michigan, Ann Arbor)
Ann Surg 224:387–395,1996 11–13

Background.—The use of staged reconstructive procedures has dramatically improved the prognosis of neonates with hypoplastic left heart syndrome (HLHS), which was once uniformly fatal. The improved outlook for such patients is largely the result of refinements in surgical technique and perioperative management. The outcomes in 1 series were reported.

Patients and Findings.—One hundred fifty-eight neonates with classic HLHS underwent stage 1 reconstruction with a Norwood procedure. Classic HLHS was defined as a right ventricular dependent circulation in association with atresia or severe hypoplasia of the aortic valve. One

TABLE 1.—Patient Groups

Group	No.
Standard risk	127
High risk	31
Noncardiac congenital condition	17
Prematurity/low birth weight	4
Chromosomal anomaly	5
Galactosemia	1
Absent corpus callosum	1
Anal atresia	1
Chronic renal failure	1
Multiple limb defects	1
Congenital diaphragmatic hernia	1
Recurrent left atrial tumor	1
Hypothyroidism and portal fibrosis	1
Pulmonary venous obstruction	8
Age > 1 mo at Norwood	6

Note: $n = 158$.

(Courtesy of Bove EL, Lloyd TR: Staged reconstruction for hypoplastic left heart syndrome: Contemporary results. *Ann Surg* 224:387–395, 1996.)

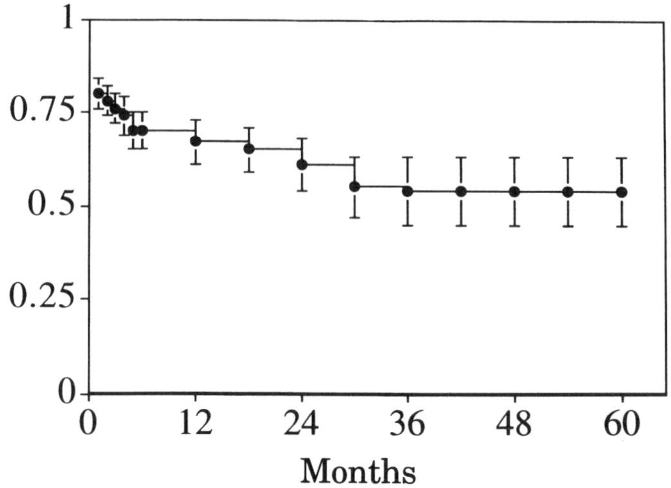

FIGURE 1.—Actuarial survival for the entire study group of 158 patients. (Courtesy of Bove EL, Lloyd TR: Staged reconstruction for hypoplastic left heart syndrome: Contemporary results. *Ann Surg* 224:387–395, 1996.)

hundred twenty patients survived to hospital discharge. Survival was significantly greater among the 127 patients at standard risk than among the 31 with major risk factors (Table 1). Significant related noncardiac congenital conditions and severe preoperative obstruction to pulmonary venous return were associated with lower survival. One hundred six patients underwent second-stage reconstruction with the hemi-Fontan procedure. One hundred three survived to discharge. Of the 62 patients in whom the

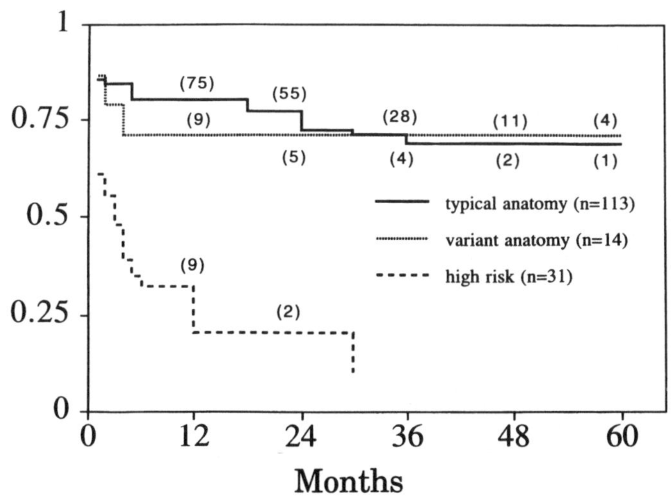

FIGURE 2.—Actuarial survival analyzed for standard and high-risk groups separately. The standard risk group is subdivided further into those with typical anatomy and those with variant anatomy. (Courtesy of Bove EL, Lloyd TR: Staged reconstruction for hypoplastic left heart syndrome: Contemporary results. *Ann Surg* 224:387–395, 1996.)

Fontan procedure has been completed, 53 have survived. Deaths after this procedure occurred early and were mostly caused by left pulmonary artery stenosis or hypoplasia. Patients judged to be at standard risk with typical anatomy had a 5-year actuarial survival of 69%. Patients at standard risk with variant anatomy had a 71% 5-year survival. Overall, the cohort had a survival rate of 58%. Most deaths occurred in the first month of life. Late deaths occurred primarily in the high-risk group (Figs 1 and 2).

Conclusions.—Staged reconstruction in neonates with HLHS yields good intermediate-term outcomes. Current attempts to decrease mortality after the Norwood procedure are focused on providing a more stable circulation and eliminating the risk factors for the Fontan procedure.

▶ We asked Edward L. Bove, M.D., Professor of Surgery at the University of Michigan School of Medicine, Ann Arbor, to comment:

▶ The article by Bando and associates from Indiana University (Abstract 11–12) reviews the authors' experience with the surgical management of HLHS during the past 6½ years. The parents were presented with the treatment options and allowed to make the decision for staged reconstruction, cardiac transplantation, or supportive care. Among the 35 patients submitted to a Norwood procedure, 16 survived (46%). Two of these survivors subsequently underwent a cardiac transplant because of the presence of significant tricuspid regurgitation, whereas the remaining 14 remain alive through various stages of reconstruction.

The authors' results improved during the latter half of their experience secondary to refinements in perioperative care, intraoperative management, and, most probably, patient selection. Of note, patients with significant associated risk factors were not offered staged reconstruction. Among the 22 patients selected for heart transplantation, 7 crossed over to a Norwood (included above) because of the lack of a suitable donor heart. The remaining 15 were transplanted, with 10 late survivors. Therefore, among all 50 patients undergoing surgical therapy at the authors' institution, 26 (52%) remain alive after 1 form of therapy or the other.

Bando and associates have shown that the results of palliative reconstructive surgery for HLHS, in addition to cardiac transplantation, will improve with increasing institutional experience. In many ways, their results mirror those from our own institution. In the most recently reported series from the University of Michigan (Abstract 11–13), the results of 158 consecutive patients with HLHS undergoing a Norwood procedure between 1990 and August of 1995 were analyzed. There were 120 hospital survivors (76%). Among the entire group, 127 patients were considered to be at standard risk and were, presumably, similar to the patients selected for palliation by the Indiana University group. Among this group, actuarial survival through all 3 stages of reconstruction was 70% at 5 years. The vast majority of deaths, in our own experience, occurred within the first month of life. This was similar to that found in the Indiana experience.

A number of similarities can be noted between the Indiana experience and that from our own institution. Survival improved with institutional experience. At the University of Michigan, survival has more than doubled in the years since 1990 when compared with our prior experience.[1] The Indiana group also found that the use of smaller, more centrally positioned shunts improved survival. These modifications—also previously reported by us—help to control pulmonary blood flow and limit the volume overload on the single right ventricle.[1] In contrast to our experience, however, the Indiana University group chose to submit patients with significant tricuspid regurgitation to transplantation rather than continuing with staged reconstruction. We have had excellent late results in a significant number of patients with moderate-to-severe tricuspid regurgitation who have undergone tricuspid valve repair at the time of the hemi-Fontan and/or Fontan procedures.

The risk factors observed by these authors differ from our experience. They noted that longer circulatory arrest time, the presence of preoperative acidosis, the use of a larger shunt, a small ascending aorta, and the morphologic subgroups of aortic and mitral atresia were associated with poor results. None of these factors proved to be significant predictors of increased mortality in our own series. Our risk factor analysis identified significant obstruction of the pulmonary venous return and major associated noncardiac conditions as the 2 most important factors associated with increased mortality. The reasons for the difference between our 2 experiences may be sample size or patient selection. Bando and associates did not offer staged palliation to patients with significant associated anomalies. In contrast, we have been willing to proceed with surgery even when the preoperative condition was extremely poor or in the presence of significant associated morphologic and/or hemodynamic conditions. Although the results clearly are not as good, a number of excellent long-term outcomes have been seen.

Many institutions, initially discouraged by the poor results of palliative reconstructive surgery for HLHS, abandoned this approach in favor of transplantation. However, the lack of available donor hearts, late complications of cardiac transplantation, and the improvements noted with staged reconstruction have again encouraged many centers, both in this country and elsewhere, to reevaluate this form of therapy. Efforts to improve early survival after the Norwood procedure will translate into improved long-term outcome because this remains the highest risk period. Although late results must continue to be analyzed, we have been encouraged by the excellent quality of survival achieved by many of our older patients, a significant number of whom are now entering their second decade of life.

E.L. Bove, M.D.

References

1. Iannettonio MD, Bove EL, Mosca RS, et al: Improving results with first-stage palliation for hypoplastic left heart syndrome. *J Thorac Cardiovasc Surg* 107:934–940, 1994.
2. Bove EL, Mosca RS: Surgical repair of the hypoplastic left heart syndrome. *Prog Pediatr Cardiol* 5:23–35, 1996.

Prophylactic Indomethacin Therapy in the First Twenty-four Hours of Life for the Prevention of Patent Ductus Arteriosus in Preterm Infants Treated Prophylactically With Surfactant in the Delivery Room

Couser RJ, Ferrara TB, Wright GB, et al (Children's Health Care, Minneapolis; Children's Heart Clinic, Minneapolis)

J Pediatr 128:631–637, 1996 11–14

Objective.—For infants with hyaline membrane disease, treatment with surfactant may lead to a more rapid decrease in pulmonary vascular resistance and thus greater susceptibility to the development of hemodynamically significant patent ductus arteriosus (PDA). Previous studies have suggested that prophylactic indomethacin treatment can reduce problems with PDA. Infants receiving prophylactic surfactant therapy were studied to determine whether low-dose indomethacin treatment can decrease the incidence of PDA.

Methods.—The prospective, randomized, placebo-controlled trial included 90 infants with birth weights of 600–1,250 g who received prophylactic surfactant therapy in the delivery room. They were assigned to receive either indomethacin, 0.1 mg/kg per dose, or placebo once within 24 hours and again every 24 hours for 6 doses. The patients underwent echocardiography on the first day of life, before the start of treatment, and again on day 7, 24 hours after treatment. Additional, out-of-study echocardiograms were obtained to evaluate suspected PDA. For patients who did not respond to the study treatment, standard indomethacin therapy or ligation was performed.

Results.—Forty-three infants received indomethacin and 47 received placebo (Table 2). Echocardiography demonstrated a PDA in 86% of infants on the first day of life, before the start of treatment. The PDAs were classified as moderate-sized or large in 84% of indomethacin-treated pa-

TABLE 2.—Patent Ductus Arteriosus (PDA) and Cranial US Data

Variable	Birth weight 600 to 1250 gm Indomethacin (n = 43)	Placebo (n = 47)	*P*	Birth weight <1000 gm Indomethacin (n = 25)	Placebo (n = 32)	*P*
Echocardiographic findings*						
PDA present	37 (86%)	44 (94%)	0.790	23 (92%)	30 (94%)	0.970
PDA moderate/large	31 (72%)	37 (79%)	0.630	20 (80%)	25 (78%)	1.000
PDA nonresponders	9 (21%)	22 (47%)	0.018	7 (28%)	18 (56%)	0.062
PDA clinical†	8	17	0.104	7	14	0.344
Ligation	4	8	0.444	4	8	0.617
IVH (grades 3, 4)	3	4	1.000	2	4	0.686
PVL	3	8	0.325	1	5	0.258
IVH or PVL	6 (14%)	12 (26%)	0.267	3 (12%)	9 (28%)	0.248

Note: Values are expressed as occurrence and/or percentage.
*On postnatal day 1.
†Needing treament (routine indomethacin or ligation).
Abbreviations: IVH, intraventricular hemorrhage; *PVL*, periventricular leukomalacia.
(Courtesy of Couser RJ, Ferrara B, Wright GB, et al: Prophylactic indomethacin therapy in the first twenty-four hours of life for the prevention of patent ductus arteriosus in preterm infants treated prophylactically with surfactant in the delivery room. *J Pediatr* 128:631–637, 1996.)

TABLE 3.—Outcome

Variable	Birth weight 600 to 1250 gm Indomethacin (n = 43)	Birth weight 600 to 1250 gm Placebo (n = 47)	Birth weight <1000 gm Indomethacin (n = 25)	Birth weight <1000 gm Placebo (n = 32)
Survived	42 (98%)	46 (98%)	24 (96%)	32 (100%)
Duration (days)				
Endotracheal intubation	23.3 ± 21	21.4 ± 14	31.2 ± 22	26.7 ± 14
Oxygen therapy	44.5 ± 46	34.0 ± 28	60.4 ± 52	44.6 ± 27
Length of stay at level 3	42.7 ± 25	39.7 ± 19	53.8 ± 23	46.8 ± 15
Total length of stay	86.3 ± 42	79.2 ± 23	101 ± 46	88 ± 20
Regain birth weight	16.3 ± 7	16.4 ± 7	16.4 ± 7	15.8 ± 7
Reach full calories	27.9 ± 11	25.2 ± 8	32.0 ± 11	27.8 ± 8
Bronchopulmonary dysplasia	28 (65%)	23 (49%)	23 (92%)	20 (63%)
Retinopathy of prematurity (≥stage 3)	6 (14%)	4 (9%)	5 (21%)	4 (13%)
Inotrope dose (mg/kg)	48.9 ± 41	64.5 ± 43	55.0 ± 45	63.5 ± 41
Duration of inotrope therapy (days)	5.2 ± 4	6.0 ± 4	5.6 ± 4	6.3 ± 4

Note: Values are expressed as occurrence, percentage, or mean value plus or minus standard deviation. The *P* values were not significant for all comparisons.

(Courtesy of Couser RJ, Ferrara B, Wright GB, et al: Prophylactic indomethacin therapy in the first twenty-four hours of life for the prevention of patent ductus arteriosus in preterm infants treated prophylactically with surfactant in the delivery room. *J Pediatr* 128:631–637, 1996.)

tients vs. 93% of placebo-treated patients. Twenty-one percent of infants treated with indomethacin failed to respond to the study dose, whereas 47% of placebo-treated infants were nonresponders. The number of infants undergoing surgical ligation in the indomethacin group was half that in the placebo group. Long-term outcomes were similar between groups, including intraventricular hemorrhage, duration of oxygen therapy, endotracheal intubation, length of stay in the neonatal ICU, time to regain birth weight or achieve full caloric intake, incidence of bronchopulmonary dysplasia, and survival (Table 3). There were no significant differences in the occurrence of adverse events, such as oliguria, elevated plasma creatinine concentration, thrombocytopenia, pulmonary hemorrhage, or necrotizing enterocolitis.

Conclusions.—Low-dose indomethacin therapy, given within 24 hours after birth, can decrease the incidence of hemodynamically significant PDA in low–birth weight infants who receive prophylactic surfactant. This treatment reduces the need for surgical ligation, although it does not produce any differences in other outcome variables. Early low-dose indomethacin treatment may become a useful part of the overall management of very low birth weight infants who receive prophylactic surfactant therapy.

▶ The ductus arteriosus plays a critical role in the fetus, in the transition from intrauterine to extrauterine existence, and in the newborn. In the healthy newborn, it constricts within hours after birth and ultimately undergoes permanent closure through fibrosis. The biochemical basis for closure of the ductus has been the subject of intense study, and Tristani-Firouzi and associates recently appear to have made a major breakthrough in understanding the mechanism whereby oxygen induces ductal constriction.[1, 2]

They ascribe oxygen-induced constriction of the rabbit ductus arteriosus to the inhibition of a 4-aminopyridine-, voltage-sensitive potassium channel. These novel studies on the role of K^+ channels in O_2-induced constriction of the ductus may help clarify mechanisms of oxygen sensing and signal transduction. It will be important to study these same mechanisms in the pulmonary and cerebral circulations. Perhaps that will aid us in controlling blood flow to the various organs.

The standard remedy of taking an aspirin and calling the physician back the next morning will fail when the patient is a premature infant with PDA. The symptomatic or silent ductus is observed in 20% to 60% of preterm infants with respiratory distress. This rate is dependent on patient characteristics and on the vigor with which the ductus is sought by echocardiography. At least 50% of infants with birth weights of less than 750 g will have significant shunting through the ductus arteriosus. The collaborative Belgian-Dutch trial explored for the first time, in a randomized fashion, the efficacy of aspirin versus indomethacin in the treatment of PDA in neonates with respiratory distress syndrome.[3] Although the stated outcome objective was defined as the "need for additional oxygen supply on the 28th postnatal day," the discussion centers on the ductal closure and the side effects of the medication. Indomethacin, the old standby for the treatment of PDA, was superior to aspirin, closing 92% of the PDAs vs. 43% in the aspirin group ($P < 0.0001$). There were remarkably few side effects in both treatment groups. The 43% closure rate in the aspirin group is not different from reports of spontaneous closure of PDA.[4] The authors conclude that "further studies with aspirin, using other treatment schemes, do not seem warranted." Agreed! However, it was disappointing to learn how little is known about the pharmacokinetics of aspirin in the premature infant.

Couser and associates show that the use of prophylactic indomethacin in the first 24 hours of life in low–birth weight infants decreases the incidence of left-to-right shunting at the ductal level. Ment and colleagues,[5] in a trial of indomethacin to reduce intracranial hemorrhage, demonstrated that the indomethacin-treated infants had significantly fewer problems with patency of the ductus arteriosus. There also has been a suggestion that prophylactic indomethacin therapy may reduce the incidence of pulmonary hemorrhage after surfactant therapy.[6] Indomethacin is effective in closing a symptomatic PDA, although repeated courses may be necessary. Many clinicians are concerned about the side effects of indomethacin, including diminished urine output, gastrointestinal hemorrhage and ischemia, and impairment in cerebral blood flow.

Varvarigou and associates[7] tested various doses of IV ibuprofen using normal saline as the test solution. All the infants who received 3 doses of ibuprofen[1, 2] had closure of their PDA, whereas 7 of the 11 saline-treated infants were still patent. A single dose of ibuprofen was not effective. The infants who received 3 doses of ibuprofen tended to tolerate full feeds earlier, required fewer days of assisted ventilation, and had shorter hospital stays. There were no adverse drug reactions. There also is some preliminary evidence that ibuprofen is effective in preventing intracranial hemorrhage. However, there are no approved IV ibuprofen preparations in the United

States, and it is difficult to obtain any drug to carry out the testing. Hence, even if ibuprofen is a more effective agent than indomethacin, there will be substantial delays before it is generally available. (See also Abstract 11–15.)

I will act as if what I do makes a difference.—William James

A.A. Fanaroff, M.B.B.Ch.

References

1. Tristani-Firouzi M, Reeve S, Tolarava EK, et al: Oxygen induced constriction of the rabbit ductus arteriosus occurs via inhibition of a 4-aminopyridine-, voltage-sensitive potassium channel. *J Clin Invest* 98:1959–1965, 1996.
2. Abman S: Oxygen sensing, potassium channels and the ductus arteriosus. *J Clin Invest* 98:1945–1946, 1996.
3. VanOvermeire B, Brus F, Van Acker KJ, et al: Aspirin versus indomethacin treatment of patent ductus arteriosus in preterm infants with respiratory distress syndrome. *Pediatr Res* 38:886–891, 1995.
4. Knight DB: Patent ductus arteriosus: How important to which babies? *Early Hum Dev* 29:287–292, 1992.
5. Ment LR, Oh W, Ehrendranz RA, et al: Low-dose indomethacin and prevention of intraventricular hemorrhage: A multicenter randomized trial. *Pediatrics* 93:543–550, 1990.
6. 1995 Year Book of Neonatal and Perinatal Medicine, p 302.
7. Varvarigou A, Bardin CL, Beharry K, et al: Early ibuprofen administration to prevent ductus arteriosus in premature newborn infants. *JAMA* 275:539–544, 1996.

Influence of Infection on Patent Ductus Arteriosus and Chronic Lung Disease in Premature Infants Weighing 1000 Grams or Less

Gonzalez A, Sosenko IRS, Chandar J, et al (Univ of Miami, Fla)

J Pediatr 128:470–478, 1996 11–15

Objective.—Given the frequency of patent ductus arteriosus (PDA) and infections among preterm infants, a connection between these 2 complications is possible. A previous epidemiologic study linked PDA and infection to chronic lung disease (CLD) in premature infants. One explanation for this interaction may be increased prostaglandin levels promoting persistent ductal patency. The effects of infection on PDA and CLD were investigated in premature infants, including the possible role of prostaglandins and inflammatory mediators.

Methods.—The prospective study included 114 premature infants with birth weights of 500–1,000 g. The infants were monitored for PDA and infections. All patients underwent measurement of serum 6-ketoprostaglandin $F_{1\alpha}$ and tumor necrosis factor-α on a routine basis and whenever PDA or infection was detected. Multivariate analysis was performed to identify risk factors for PDA closure and CLD.

Results.—Infants with infections were more likely to have late episodes of PDA than were those without infections. When the infection and PDA occurred within less than 5 days of each other, the risk that the PDA would

TABLE.—Odds Ratio for Failure of Patent Ductus Arteriosus (PDA) Closure

Variable	OR	95% CI	*P*
Birth weight ≤750 gm	2.84	1.5–5.6	<0.001
Infection temporally related	19.1	4.0–90	<0.001
High fluid intake	4.7	0.8–26.7	0.06
Incomplete or no indomethacin	4.1	0.5–32.5	0.15
PDA at ≥8 days	5.6	1.0–31.9	<0.04

Abbreviations: OR, odds ratio; *CI*, confidence interval.

(Courtesy of Gonzalez A, Sosenko IRS, Chandar J, et al: Influence of infection on patent ductus arteriosus and chronic lung disease in premature infants weighing 1000 grams or less. *J Pediatr* 128:470–478, 1996.)

fail to close was much increased (odds ratio 19.1; Table). Risk factors for CLD were birth weight, initial severity of respiratory failure, PDA (odds ratio 11.7), and infection (odds ratio 3.1). A temporal relation between PDA and infection greatly increased the risk of CLD (odds ratio 29.6). 6-Ketoprostaglandin $F_{1\alpha}$ levels were higher in infants with infection or PDA. Infants with infection and late PDA also had increased levels of tumor necrosis factor-α.

Conclusions.—In premature infants, infection has an adverse effect on the outcomes of PDA. Infants with PDA and infections are at increased risk of late ductal reopening and failure of the PDA to close. These outcomes may be related to increased prostaglandin and tumor necrosis factor-α levels. When PDA and infection occur together, there is a greatly elevated risk of CLD. New approaches to the treatment of PDA in infected infants are needed.

▶ The incidence of PDA is inversely related to birth weight.[1] Infection rates for this group of infants approach 50%.[1] Thus, it is not surprising that the 2 are related. Anecdotal experiences by many clinicians are confirmed in this report from the University of Miami, where the neonatal group has continued their investigations into CLD. Namely, there are more medical treatment failures for infants with PDA when their birth weight is less than 1 kg. Gonzalez and colleagues were able to confirm the drawn-out hypothesis that infection increases ductal dilatory prostaglandins and inflammatory mediators that negatively modify the outcome of PDA therapy, and increases the incidence of late-onset PDA (after 7 days). All these events ultimately increase the risk of CLD. The obvious answer is to reduce the incidence of nosocomial infections (see Abstract 6–2), but this is easier said than done. There also is a Catch-22 (not the microdeletion variety; see Abstract 2–7) in which PDA is associated with infection that does not respond to medical management and the surgeons refuse to operate until the infection has been cleared. This mandates fluid restriction, which translates into caloric restriction, poor growth, and failure to thrive superimposed on all the other problems. It is necessary to close the ductus and eradicate the infection to break the vicious cycle. (For more on PDA, see Abstract 11–14.)

A.A. Fanaroff, M.B.B.Ch.

Reference

1. Fanaroff AA, Wright LL, Stevenson DK, et al: Very low birth weight outcomes of the National Institute of Child Health and Human Development Neonatal Research Network, May 1991 through December 1992. *Am J Obstet Gynecol* 173:1423–1431, 1995.

Incidence of Vocal Fold Paralysis in Infants Undergoing Ligation of Patent Ductus Arteriosus

Zbar RIS, Chen AH, Behrendt DM, et al (Univ of Iowa, Iowa City)
Ann Thorac Surg 61:814–816, 1996 11–16

Background.—Ligation of patent ductus arteriosus (PDA) can be complicated by left-sided iatrogenic vocal fold paralysis (IVFP) caused by recurrent laryngeal nerve injury. The risk factors associated with IVFP were investigated.

Methods.—All 68 infants aged 12 months or younger who had operative PDA closure at 1 center from 1991 through 1994 were included in the analysis. Patent ductus arteriosus ligation had been done using clips in 52.9%, suture ligatures in 41.2%, and both in 5.9%. The patients' medical records were analyzed retrospectively.

Findings.—Iatrogenic vocal fold paralysis occurred in 6 infants. Only infants without IVFP after operation had significant weight gain from birth to operation. Although the overall incidence of IVFP in all infants undergoing PDA closure was 8.8%, 5 of the 6 infants with IVFP had birth weights of only 1 kg or less. The incidence of IVFP among infants with extremely low birth weights undergoing operation was 22.7%. Iatrogenic vocal fold paralysis was associated only with the use of surgical clips. However, it was not possible to determine whether suture ligature was safer, because clips were used in most of the premature infants in this series.

Conclusions.—Infants with IVFP after PDA ligation were smaller at birth, more premature, and smaller and younger at operation than infants without IVFP. Birth weight of less than 1 kg was the most important risk factor for this complication after operation.

▶ There is a tendency to become complacent with the exceptional surgical subspecialty support that is available for even the smallest immature infants. Thus, it is sobering to realize that iatrogenic factors are now the greatest cause of vocal cord paralysis in infants.[1] As more smaller infants survive, the numbers encountered with symptomatic PDA likely will increase. On the other hand, increased use of indomethacin to prevent intracranial hemorrhage also may reduce the number of cases of symptomatic PDA. The risk of iatrogenic vocal cord paralysis after ductal ligation (clipping) in infants with birth weights of less than 1 kg was 22.7%, in contrast to 2.2% for heavier babies. Birth weight emerged as the major identifiable risk factor, although the surgical technique, specifically the use of clips, may have played a role.

The use of clips, as opposed to sutures, may have been important, but there were insufficient premature infants who did not have clips to draw any firm conclusions. Ascertainment, by flexible fiberoptic nasolaryngoscopy, was confined to infants evaluated for hoarseness, stridor, or inability to wean from nasal continuous positive airway pressure. Asymptomatic infants would not have been evaluated; nonetheless, the prevalence is greater than reports of IVFP of 4% from a decade ago.[2, 3]

A.A. Fanaroff, M.B.B.Ch.

References

1. Zbar RI, Smith RJ: Vocal fold paralysis in infants 12 months of age and younger. *Otolaryngol Head Neck Surg* 114:18–21, 1996.
2. Davis JT, Baciewicz FA, Suriyapa S, et al: Vocal cord paralysis in premature infants undergoing ductal closure. *Ann Thorac Surg* 46:214–215, 1988.
3. Fan LL, Campbell DN, Clarke DR, et al: Paralyzed left vocal cord associated with ligation of patent ductus arteriosus. *J Thorac Cardiovasc Surg* 98:611–613, 1989.

Effects of Umbilical Arterial Catheterization on Mesenteric Hemodynamics

Rand T, Weninger M, Kohlhauser C, et al (Univ of Vienna)
Pediatr Radiol 26:435–438, 1996 11–17

Background.—The use of umbilical artery catheters (UACs) can result in mesenteric blood flow impairment, which may increase the risk of necrotizing enterocolitis (NEC) in newborns. Duplex Doppler sonography was used to determine the degree of vessel obstruction resulting from UAC and the effect on visceral hemodynamics.

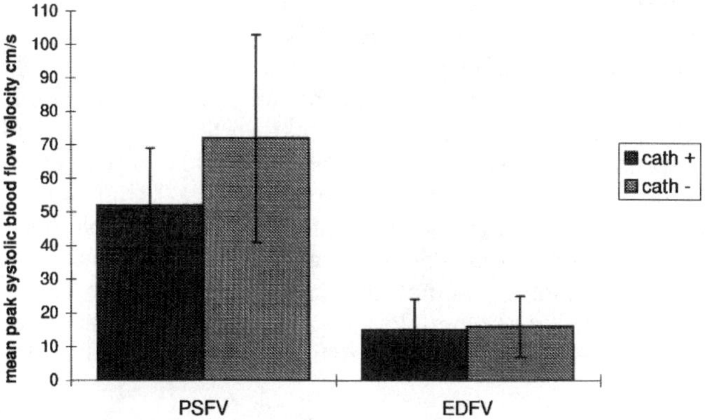

FIGURE 4.—Mean peak systolic blood flow velocity (*PSFV*) and end diastolic blood flow velocity (*EDFV*) measured in the superior mesenteric artery before (*cath* +) and after (*cath* −) removal of the umbilical artery catheter. (Courtesy Rand T, Weninger M, Kohlhauser C, et al: Effects of umbilical arterial catheterization on mesenteric hemodynamics. *Pediatr Radiol* 26:435–438, copyright 1996, Springer-Verlag.)

Methods.—Twelve infants were studied. The UAC was positioned above the ostia of the celiac and superior mesenteric arteries. Ultrasonography was performed before and immediately after UAC removal.

Findings.—Removing the UAC resulted in a significant increase in mean peak systolic blood flow velocity. Pourcelot's resistance index increased from a mean of 0.7 to 0.74 for the celiac trunk and from a mean of 0.73 to 0.76 for the superior mesenteric artery (Fig 4).

Conclusion.—Umbilical artery catheters apparently cause a reduction in mesenteric blood flow. Thus, clinicians must be careful in making the decision to use these catheters in hemodynamically unstable neonates and in newborns with gastrointestinal disease.

▶ We asked Dan Batton, M.D., Chief, Division of Newborn Medicine, William Beaumont Hospital, Royal Oak, Michigan, to comment:

▶ Umbilical arterial catheters have been associated with an increased risk for NEC, which is thought to be, in part, an ischemic bowel disease. Therefore, it is logical to ask the question: Do UACs cause intestinal ischemia? A UAC may decrease intestinal blood flow by 1 of 2 mechanisms: First, it may cause mechanical obstruction of flow to the main intestinal arteries—the celiac trunk and superior mesenteric artery—or, second, it can produce thrombi and emboli.

In this study, there was an increase in blood flow velocity in both the celiac trunk and the superior mesenteric artery immediately after removal of the UAC, suggesting that the catheter was responsible for mechanical obstruction of blood flow to these intestinal arteries. It is not surprising that placement of a UAC in the small aorta of a premature infant will decrease the aortic intraluminal area and lead to a reduction of blood flow to downstream vessels. However, it can be inferred that this is not likely to produce ischemia, as the vast majority of infants who have a UAC have no clinical evidence of having had intestinal ischemia.

In addition, in the randomized trial by Kempley and Gamsu,[1] infants with a high UAC (tip proximal to the origin of the celiac trunk and superior mesenteric artery) had blood flow velocities in these arteries that were identical to those in infants with a low UAC (tip distal to the origin of the celiac trunk and superior mesenteric artery). The presence of a UAC did not significantly reduce intestinal blood flow. A more important question related to UACs is what role they may play in producing clinically significant thromboembolic injury to the intestines of premature infants. Unfortunately, current pulsed-Doppler measurement of blood flow velocity in the proximal intestinal arteries does not provide adequate information for evaluating this question.

D. Batton, M.D.

Reference

1. Kempley ST, Gamsu HR: Randomised trial of umbilical arterial catheter position: Doppler ultrasound findings. *Arch Dis Child* 67:855–859, 1992.

Decreased Cardiac Responses to Auditory Stimulation During Prone Sleep

Franco P, Groswasser J, Sottiaux M, et al (Erasme Univ, Brussels, Belgium; Univ Children's Hosp of Brussels, Belgium)

Pediatrics 97:174–178, 1996 11–18

Background.—Many hypotheses have been advanced to explain the association between prone posture and sudden infant death syndrome (SIDS). Auditory challenges have been shown to induce significant cardiac changes, especially during rapid eye movement (REM) sleep. The relationship between body position during sleep and cardiac responses to auditory stimulation was assessed in healthy infants.

Methods.—Thirty infants, aged a median of 11 weeks, were evaluated by polygraphy for 1 night while sleeping successively in the prone and supine (or vice versa) positions. Behavioral and cardiac responses were documented during REM sleep before and after exposure to 90 dB of white noise.

Findings.—Ten infants woke up during the auditory challenge and were excluded from the analysis. In the remaining infants, there was no significant difference between the prone and supine positions for total sleep time, sleep efficiency, percent REM and non-REM sleep, number of gross body movements, transcutaneous oxygen saturation levels, mean cardiac rate, heart rate variability, number of heart rate drops, mean respiratory rate, and the number or duration of central or obstructive apneas. Auditory challenge in the prone position, compared with the supine position, induced significantly less overall change in heart rate, heart rate drops, and heart rate variability and fewer and shorter central apneas. The findings of autoregressive power spectral analysis of the heart rate were consistent with possible increases in orthosympathetic tone in the prone position.

Conclusion.—In these infants, prone sleeping was associated with a decline in cardiac responses to auditory stimulation and a possible increase in orthosympathetic activity. Prone positioning may be associated with decreased reactivity to danger-signaling stimuli during REM sleep.

► We asked Dr. Carl Hunt, Professor of Pediatrics, Medical College of Ohio, Toledo, to comment:

► Arousal responsiveness is an essential component of the respiratory control system. Impaired arousal responsiveness appears to be the most compelling physiologic explanation for the epidemiologic observation of a threefold to fivefold increase in SIDS rates when infants sleep prone rather than supine.

Because impaired cardiac control may also be an important aspect of the cardiorespiratory control deficit postulated to be important in the pathophysiology of SIDS and prone sleeping, the study by Franco et al. addresses a timely and relevant subject. Based on overnight sleep laboratory recordings in 10 infants who normally slept prone and 10 who slept supine, they report that those who slept prone had decreased cardiac responses to an auditory stimulus.

The study does not have sufficient power to detect differences in sleep characteristics between the 2 sleep positions or to fully characterize the range of normal cardiorespiratory responses to this auditory stimulus. Only REM sleep was studied, and auditory responsiveness was the only arousal stimulus. Most important, in regard to preterm infants, this study design does not address the important question of maturation of this arousal response; the authors studied only full-term infants and only at a mean age of 11 weeks. It will be important to study the maturation of this arousal response as a function of both postconceptional and postnatal age.

These results are important in helping to explain why infants sleeping prone seem to have a better overall quality and duration of sleep. They are consistent with the available epidemiologic data related to sleep position and risk for SIDS. Although we do not yet know how these responses might be qualitatively or quantitatively different in preterm infants, even preterm infants should routinely be sleeping supine at least by the time of neonatal ICU discharge, regardless of postconceptional age.

C. Hunt, M.D.

Randomised Trial of Prophylactic Early Fresh-frozen Plasma or Gelatin or Glucose in Preterm Babies: Outcome at 2 Years

Tin W, for the Northern Neonatal Nursing Initiative Trial Group (South Cleveland Hosp, Middlesbrough, England; et al)

Lancet 348:229–232, 1996 11–19

Background.—Infants born more than 8 weeks premature are at high risk for the development of hemorrhagic and ischemic brain injury. Various methods of preventing these conditions have been tested. One study of early prophylactic treatment with fresh frozen plasma (FFP) showed a lowered risk of intraventricular hemorrhage and suggested that such treatment also may lower the risk of severe hemorrhage. Because the coagulation profile did not change after the infusion of FFP, the benefit may have resulted from circulatory stabilization after intravascular volume expansion. The short- and long-term outcome of early prophylactic treatment with FFP in premature infants was evaluated.

Methods.—Of 776 infants born before 32 weeks' gestation, 257 received treatment with FFP, 261 received treatment with a gelatin-based plasma substitute, and 258 made up a control group given maintenance glucose. The primary outcome measure was survival without major disability at 2 years.

Results.—Follow-up information was obtained for all study infants. Neurologic and developmental assessments were performed at 2 years. The number of infants who died and the number of infants who survived with a severe disability was similar in all groups (Table 6). At 2 years, the surviving children had similar mean developmental quotients.

TABLE 6.—Overall Outcome at Age 2 Years

Outcome	FFP (n=257)	Gelatin (n=261)	Glucose (n=258)
Death before age 2 years			
Neonatal	40	49	43
Postneonatal, perinatally damaged	6	6	5
Postneonatal, other	8	10	5
Alive at age 2 years			
Blind	7	1	3
Deaf	4	5	5
Unable to walk	18	16	26
Total blind, deaf, or unable to walk*	21	20	28
Low DQ† without sensorimotor problems	2	2	0
Other severe disability	0	0	1‡
No severe disability	180	174	176

*Some children had more than 1 sensorimotor disability.
†Less than 3 standard deviations below the mean for the study.
‡Otherwise normal (DQ 95); tube-fed through a gastrostomy for 18 months because of persistent, unexplained food refusal when seen at age 2 years; meets criteria for severe disability.
Abbreviations: DQ, developmental quotient; *FFP,* fresh frozen plasma.
(Courtesy of Tin W, for the Northern Neonatal Nursing Initiative Trial Group: Randomized trial of prophylactic early fresh-frozen plasma or gelatin or glucose in preterm babies: Outcome at 2 years. *Lancet* 348:229–232, 1996. Copyright by The Lancet Ltd. 1996.)

Conclusions.—In these premature infants, the incidence of death and disability was unchanged by early prophylactic treatment with FFP or other methods of intravascular volume expansion. These findings do not support the use of this practice. Future studies should measure their primary outcome at 2 years.

▶ The dogma exceeds the data when the matter of hypotension in low–birth weight infants is the subject of discussion. The stunning and baseless confidence of the proponents of various therapies, despite the fundamental inability to even precisely define hypotension, leaves one breathless. The trial reported here was based on a single prior report suggesting that FFP had reduced the risk of intraventricular hemorrhage (IVH).[1] Because clotting factors did not change, it had been proposed that circulatory stabilization was the mechanism whereby FFP reduced IVH. The trial was planned with this background and the theory that hypovolemia (exacerbated by early cord clamping) might cause cerebral ischemia before there was evidence of hypotension. This was a prospective, multihospital, multidistrict effort with infants enrolled by 2 hours of life. The primary outcome measure was neurologic development at the age of 2 years, and the study was designed to detect an increase in babies surviving without severe disability from 78% to 85%. Amazingly, no child was lost to follow-up. There were the usual number of snafus during the trial, with supply failure, missed second infusion, and delays in thawing the FFP. Sixty-one cases were not approached because the investigators correctly predicted that they would die. All 61 died; is this a remarkable coincidence or not? Seven hundred and seventy-six infants were enrolled. The mortality rate in each group was just over 20%, and when the dust settled and the data had all been massaged, there was no evidence that the routine early use of FFP or some other form of intravascular volume expansion affects the risk of death or disability in infants born more than 8 weeks before term.

So and colleagues[2] from Hong Kong compared colloid vs. crystalloid in a randomized, controlled trial in hypotensive preterm infants. Outcome, as assessed by the number of infants requiring inotropic support and the occurrence of death or chronic lung disease, did not differ between the groups. They concluded from their 63-patient study that isotonic saline was as effective as 5% albumin for treating hypotension in preterm infants.

The search for the optimal management of hypotension in preterm infants has not ended.

A.A. Fanaroff, M.B.B.Ch.

References

1. Beverley DW, Pitts-Tucker TJ, Congdon PJ, et al: Prevention of intraventricular hemorrhage by fresh frozen plasma. *Arch Dis Child* 60:710–713, 1985.
2. So KW, Fok Thai F, Ng Pak C, et al: Randomized controlled trial of colloid or crystalloid in hypotensive preterm infants. *Arch Dis Child* 76:F43–F46, 1997.

12 The Blood

Intravenous Immune Globulin in Neonatal Immune Hemolytic Disease: Does It Reduce Hemolysis?

Hammerman C, Vreman HJ, Kaplan M, et al (Hebrew Univ, Jerusalem; Stanford Univ, Calif)

Acta Paediatr 85:1351–1353, 1996 12–1

Objective.—Intravenous immune globulin (IVIg) has been used successfully to treat some types of Coombs'-positive hemolytic anemia. Although it has been suggested that IVIg exerts its effect by reducing hemolysis, thereby decreasing blood carboxyhemoglobin (COHb), this mechanism has not been proven. The COHb level, corrected for ambient carbon monoxide (COHbc), was compared with serum total bilirubin in term, hyperbilirubinemic, Coombs'-positive infants before and after treatment with IVIg.

Methods.—The COHbc values were determined before and after administration of IVIg to 26 healthy, full-term, direct Coombs'-positive infants. Jaundice was evaluated daily. Exchange transfusion was performed if bilirubin levels reached or exceeded 342 μmol/L.

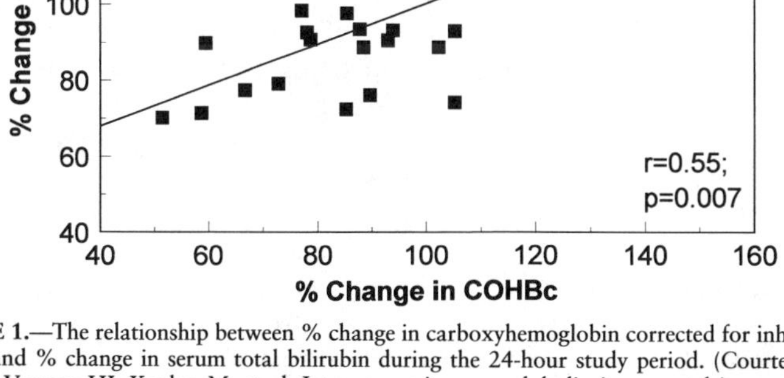

FIGURE 1.—The relationship between % change in carboxyhemoglobin corrected for inhaled carbon monoxide and % change in serum total bilirubin during the 24-hour study period. (Courtesy of Hammerman C, Vreman HJ, Kaplan M, et al: Intravenous immune globulin in neonatal immune hemolytic disease: Does it reduce hemolysis? *Acta Paediatr* 85:1351–1353, 1996).

Results.—Serum bilirubin decreased in 19 infants, 17 of whom were ABO incompatible and 2 of whom were Rh incompatible. None of the responders required a transfusion. The 5 nonresponders who were ABO incompatible and the 2 who were Rh incompatible required exchange transfusions. In responders, but not nonresponders, 24-hour post-IVIg COHbc levels decreased significantly from 1.37 to 1.12% tHb and the decrease was directly correlated with decreased serum levels of bilirubin (Fig 1).

Conclusion.—In IVIg responders, hemolysis, as measured by decreased COHbc levels, was inhibited. The decrease in 24-hour post-IVIg COHbc levels was correlated with decreased serum levels of bilirubin.

▶ Although the association between the use of high-dose IVIG and lowering bilirubin levels in infants with Coombs'-positive hemolytic anemia had been described before, the mechanism had not been proven. Hammerman et al. provide evidence that IVIG inhibits hemolysis in some but not all infants. The latter point should not be missed. The mechanism for the failure to prevent hemolysis is unknown and probably warrants further investigation. This experience also serves to demonstrate that control of bilirubin production can be an effective means of modulating hyperbilirubinemia in a subgroup of infants with increased production as an important contributing cause. Other chemopreventive strategies, like metalloporphyrins, would likely be successful. If combined with a technology to detect increased bilirubin production (e.g., end-tidal CO_2 measurement), then infants with ABO incompatibility and a positive Coombs' test might be targeted for chemoprevention, thus further improving any cost-benefit analysis.

D.K. Stevenson, M.D.

Decreased Fetal Erythropoiesis and Hemolysis in Kell Hemolytic Anemia

Weiner CP, Widness JA (Univ of Iowa, Iowa City)

Am J Obstet Gynecol 174:547–551, 1996 12–2

Purpose.—Previous studies have found lower amniotic fluid changes in optical density measurements (450 nm) in fetuses with anti-Kell vs. anti-D anemia. Anti-Kell hemolytic disease has also been associated with reduced reticulocyte counts, which could result from increased fetal hemolysis or an inadequate fetal response to the anemia. Hemolysis and erythropoiesis were compared in fetuses with anti-Kell and anti-D hemolytic anemia.

Methods.—The study included 93 pregnancies complicated by anti-D or anti-Kell alloimmunization. Initial cordocentesis samples were studied to determine red blood cell antigen type, hemoglobin, hematocrit, reticulocyte count, nucleated red blood cells, total serum bilirubin, umbilical vein respiratory blood gases, serum erythropoietin, and strength of the direct Coombs' test. The same tests were performed in the fetal blood samples used in deciding whether to perform fetal intravascular transfusion, the criterion for which was a hematocrit of less than 30%.

Results.—Eleven fetuses tested positive for the Kell antigen and 54 for RhD. At the initial blood sampling, antigen-positive, nonanemic fetuses were similar in mean gestational age and laboratory values. Hemoglobin concentration was inversely related to reticulocyte count in the infants with anti-D anemia but not those with anti-Kell anemia; this relationship was independent of gestational age. Intravascular transfusion was performed in 73% of fetuses with anti-Kell antibodies and 69% of those with anti-D antibodies. At the time this decision was made, reticulocyte counts and total bilirubin concentrations were both lower in the anti-Kell group. Again, hemoglobin and reticulocyte count were inversely related only in the anti-D group. Both groups of fetuses showed significant increases in erythropoietin from the first to the last blood samples taken. This increase was negatively correlated with hemoglobin and independent of gestational age.

Conclusion.—Fetuses with anti-Kell hemolytic anemia have lower reticulocyte counts and total serum bilirubin levels than do fetuses with anti-D anemia. Thus, fetal blood sampling appears to be a better choice than amniotic fluid analysis for the management of Kell hemolytic anemia. Fetuses with anti-Kell anemia do not have the inverse relationship between hemoglobin and reticulocyte count that is seen in fetuses with anti-D anemia. The findings suggest that anti-Kell anemia may be associated with increased hemolysis of nonhemoglobinized or incompletely hemoglobinized erythroid precursors.

▶ This article is a reminder that not all Coombs'-positive hemolytic anemias are the same with respect to their clinical presentation. It confirms the fact that anti-Kell anemic fetuses have lower reticulocyte counts and total serum bilirubin levels than do comparable anti-D anemic fetuses. The practical outcome of this observation is that fetal blood sampling, rather than amniotic fluid analyses, may be more appropriate for the management of fetal hemolytic disease resulting from Kell antibodies. The authors speculate that, compared with anti-D fetal anemia, the anti-Kell anemia is associated with increased hemolysis of nonhemoglobinized or incompletely hemoglobinized erythroid percursors. If cells are destroyed before hemoglobin is incorporated, there is no heme catabolism and, thus, no bilirubin production. Therefore, the traditional approach to monitoring the fetus needs to be reconsidered in this context.

D.K. Stevenson, M.D.

Blood Transfusion for Haemolytic Disease as a Cause of Leukocytosis in the Fetus

Yankowitz J, Weiner CP (Univ of Iowa, Iowa City)
Prenat Diagn 16:719–722, 1996 12–3

Objective.—Many factors, including the transfusion of packed red blood cells into critically ill adults, can cause leukocytosis. Because fetal intravascular transfusion (IVT) of leukocyte-poor red blood cells is used to treat fetal alloimmune anemia, the effect of IVT on fetal leukocyte count was evaluated.

Methods.—The Weiner method of intrauterine transfusion of leukocyte-poor red blood cells was performed 227 times in 77 pregnancies between 18 and 36 weeks for fetuses with hemolytic disease and a hematocrit of less than 30%. The duration of the transfusion usually was less than 1 hour. Leukocyte count was determined by manual differential counts.

Results.—Leukocyte count increased significantly by 18% during the transfusions, with the increase growing larger with each successive transfusion. Leukocyte count increased by 10.1% during the first transfusion and significantly by 41.8% during the sixth. Expansion of the neutrophil pool was responsible for 42% of the increase in leukocyte count, whereas an increase in monocytes was responsible for 22%. The 29% increase in neutrophil count and the 64.7% increase in monocyte count were significant. Total leukocyte count increased significantly primarily after the middle and final transfusions. Final eosinophil and lymphocyte counts were similar to baseline values. The increase in basophil counts was not significant.

Conclusion.—These findings suggest that the increase in fetal leukocyte count after fetal IVT of leukocyte-poor red blood cells is the result of an immune response and the presence of inflammatory agents.

▶ The differential diagnosis of leukocytosis in the fetus or newborn is dominated by intrauterine acquired infections. Corticosteroid exposure is another potent cause of leukocytosis. Extraordinarily high leukocyte counts also may be stimulated by cytokines such as granulocyte colony-stimulating factor and granulocyte–macrophage colony-stimulating factor, which are being introduced into the neonatal clinical arena.[1] Intrauterine blood transfusion can be added to the list. However, with the widespread use of anti-D globulin, it is only on rare occasions that such transfusions are necessary. The rapid response of the leukocyte count in the fetus, with no evidence of immature forms or a shift to the left, favors demargination as the likely mechanism. Leukocytes, adherent to the vascular endothelium, are released into the circulation, elevating the leukocyte count. Because the leukocytosis increases with each subsequent transfusion, an immune cause is likely. The much-maligned fetal immune system is responding appropriately to the invasive transfusion.

A.A. Fanaroff, M.B.B.Ch.

Reference

1. Cairo, M, Christensen R, Sender L, et al: Results of a phase I/II trial of recombinant human granulocyte-macrophage colony-stimulating factor in very low birth weight neonates; significant induction of circulatory neutrophils, monocytes, platelets, and bone marrow neutrophils. *Blood* 86:2509–2515, 1995.

AS-1 Red Cells for Neonatal Transfusions: A Randomized Trial Assessing Donor Exposure and Safety

Strauss RG, Burmeister LF, Johnson K, et al (Univ of Iowa, Iowa City)
Transfusion 36:873–878, 1996 12–4

Background.—Anemia in premature infants largely results from low erythropoietin levels and the effects of phlebotomy for laboratory tests. Most very low birth weight infants, especially those weighing less than 1 kg, are transfused with red blood cells. Relatively fresh red blood cells often are used because of concerns about increased extracellular potassium concentrations, lowered pH, and decreased red blood cell 2,3-diphosphoglycerate levels in stored blood. Some studies have suggested that red blood cells stored for long periods may be safe for neonates, but these studies did not use red blood cells stored for more than 20 days and did not address AS-1 extended storage preservative. More information is needed on potential toxicity from adenine and mannitol in extended storage solution and on red blood cell 2,3-diphosphoglycerate deficiency from repeated transfusions of stored red blood cells. The feasibility and safety of transfusions with AS-1 red blood cells in very low birth weight infants were evaluated in a randomized, single-blind trial.

Methods.—One group of 21 infants was given AS-1 red blood cells stored for 42 days or less. Another group of 19 infants was given CPDA-1 red blood cells stored for 7 days or less. All infants weighed between 0.6 and 1.3 kg. The clinical and biochemical effects of the AS-1 red blood cells were assessed.

Results.—Infants given transfusions with AS-1 red blood cells were exposed to a mean of 1.6 donors. Infants given transfusions with CPDA-1 red blood cells were exposed to a mean of 3.7 donors. Clinical transfusion reactions and results of multiple laboratory tests were similar for infants given transfusions with AS-1 red blood cells stored for 42 days or less and for infants given transfusions with CPDA-1 red blood cells stored for 7 days or less.

Discussion.—AS-1 red blood cells stored for 42 days or less safely provided all the red blood cells needed by very low birth weight infants. This decreased donor exposure and may have increased the safety of transfusions in this infant population. When 1 infant received 1 entire unit, there was much blood wasted. Newborn infants needing long-term support are assigned to share units, depending on infant weight.

► A major benefit of editing the YEAR BOOK OF NEONATAL AND PERINATAL MEDICINE is the birds' eye view one gets of a broad spectrum of publications.

Each and every journal has its idiosyncratic editor and characteristic style. Some permit rambling discussions, whereas others impose precise, curt contributions. One also gets the flavor of regional practice variations throughout the globe.

Strauss and a talented local cast from the University of Iowa address the safety of administering AS-1 red blood cells, stored for as long as 6 weeks, to infants with birth weights between 600 and 1,300 g. In retrospect, because only 40% of the infants weighing more than 1 kg required a blood transfusion, the data would have been more robust if the study population was confined to infants weighing less than 1,000 g at birth. Nonetheless, these authors do demonstrate no harm from the AS-1 stored cells; biochemical stability in the infants' sera, with even a fall in the serum potassium level; and exposure to fewer donors (albeit more than 1), thus verifying their primary hypothesis. There were no significant adverse outcome differences between the 2 groups. However, in both study groups, systolic blood pressure increased more than 20 mm Hg in one third of the infants, but only 10% to 15% of the transfusions, despite the small volume and slow rate of infusion. Now that the safety of the AS-1 cells has been documented, it will be fascinating to see whether behavior changes.

The erythropoietin era has heralded a major review and change in indications for transfusion. Will this be accompanied by a change in the nature of the transfusions? It makes eminent sense to attempt to use a single donor. Of course, the long-range goal is for a transfusion-free nursery. In the meantime, the use of AS-1 cells should be considered while the role of erythropoietin continues to be investigated (see Abstract 12–8).

A local practice in Iowa, perhaps worthy of broader dissemination, is the packing of the red blood cells by centrifugation to a hematocrit of 85% to 87%, ensuring a consistent volume of red blood cells and maximizing the increase in hematocrit. The packing process requires tight quality control, something we have come to expect and depend on from the transfusion services.

A.A. Fanaroff, M.B.B.Ch.

Serum Erythropoietin Levels During Infancy: Associations With Erythropoiesis

Kling PJ, Schmidt RL, Roberts RA, et al (Univ of Iowa, Iowa City)
J Pediatr 128:791–796, 1996 12–5

Background.—During the physiologic anemia in healthy growing infants, developmentally associated changes that affect tissue oxygenation occur, including increased partial pressure of oxygen in arterial blood. Plasma erythropoietin levels and their association with hemoglobin and reticulocyte counts were determined in healthy term infants.

Methods.—Plasma erythropoietin levels were measured in serial blood samples acquired from 41 normal term fetuses every 4 weeks in the first 6 months of life. These values were compared with one another and with values in the blood of 58 healthy nonsmoking adults.

Findings.—Plasma erythropoietin concentrations were lowest in the first postnatal month and highest in the second postnatal month. This pattern is reciprocal to that observed for hemoglobin during the period of physiologic anemia. The erythopoietin level was associated negatively with hemoglobin and positively with reticulocytes. The slope of the inverse relationship of hemoglobin and plasma erythropoietin in infants was much less steep than that for children and adults with anemia.

Conclusion.—This is the first report of simultaneous patterns of change in plasma erythropoietin, hemoglobin, and reticulocytes during normal infancy. These patterns are consistent with postnatal perturbations in tissue oxygenation. Thus, erythropoietin may play a major role in the regulation of erythropoiesis during normal infancy but at a lower hemoglobin level than for older children and adults with pathologic anemia.

▶ Can we finally claim to understand the physiologic anemia of infancy? This is the first study to show a clear relationship between postnatal plasma erythropoietin levels in full-term infants and the changes in hemoglobin concentration that occur in the first months. The authors also show, for the first time, a direct relationship between erythropoietin levels and reticulocyte counts, thus confirming the key role that erythropoietin plays in the regulation of erythropoiesis in the first 6 months of life.

M.J. Maisels, M.B., B.Ch.

Management of Late Anemia in Rhesus Hemolytic Disease: Use of Recombinant Human Erythropoietin (A Pilot Study)

Ovali F, Samanci N, Dağoğlu T (Istanbul Univ, Turkey)

Pediatr Res 39:831–834, 1996 12–6

Background.—Late anemia in infants with hemolytic disease from Rh incompatibility may be caused by the suppression of erythropoiesis by intrauterine transfusion. Whether recombinant human erythropoietin (rHEPO) treatment reduces the need for erythrocyte transfusion for late anemia associated with Rh isoimmunization was investigated.

Methods.—Twenty infants with Rh isoimmunization diagnosed in utero were studied. All were given IV immunoglobulin, 0.5 mg/kg, within 2 hours of birth. When hemoglobin levels dropped to less than 1.4 mmol/L, hematocrit values declined to less than 0.27, or symptoms apparently related to anemia developed, packed erythrocyte transfusions, 10 mL/kg, were performed. Fourteen days after birth, 10 infants were given rHEPO, 200 units/kg 3 times a week for 6 weeks, and 10 were given placebo. Iron and folate were given concomitantly. Treatment response was defined as a reduction in the need for packed erythrocyte transfusion.

Findings.—Exchange transfusions for hyperbilirubinemia were required in 1 infant in each group. During 4 months of follow-up, the treatment group received a mean of 1.8 erythrocyte transfusions, compared with 4.2 in the control group. In the treatment group, 2 infants did not need

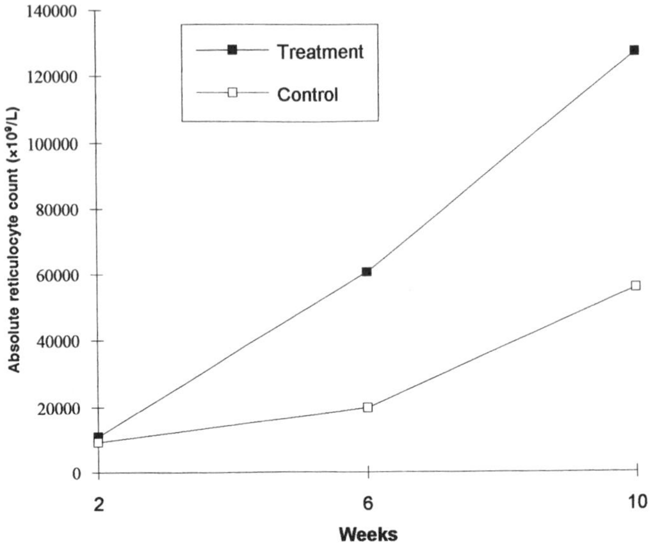

FIGURE 2.—Absolute reticulocyte counts during the study. (Courtesy of Ovali F, Samanci N, Dağoğlu T: Management of late anemia in Rhesus hemolytic disease: Use of recombinant human erythropoietin (A pilot study). *Pediatr Res* 39:831–834, 1996.)

transfusions, and 4 infants needed only 1. In the control group, 1 infant needed 1 transfusion, 1 infant needed 2, and the rest needed 3 or more (Fig 2).

Conclusions.—Recombinant human erythropoietin therapy reduces the need for erythrocyte transfusions for late anemia in infants with Rh isoimmunization. The treatment is worthwhile, considering the risks associated with blood transfusion.

▶ In the days when Rh hemolytic disease was common, pediatricians were quite familiar with the problem of the late anemia that developed in some erythroblastotic infants. A number of mechanisms have been suggested to explain the anemia: anti-D destruction of bone marrow precursors or reticulocytes (in the peripheral circulation) or inappropriately low erythropoietin levels.[1, 2]

The latter mechanism appears to be particularly important in infants who have received intrauterine transfusions and, although there have been previous anecdotal reports of the use of rHEPO in the management of the late anemia that develops in some infants, this is the first randomized controlled trial of this product. These infants appear to have a hyporegenerative state of the bone marrow that probably results from multiple intrauterine transfusions, although it may also occur in those who are treated only with postnatal transfusions or exchange transfusions. The infants have low concentrations of erythropoietin, but their erythroid progenitors remain responsive to erythropoietin.[1] Thus, the use of rHEPO in this situation makes sense.

The infants who received rHEPO had a 50% reduction in the need for blood transfusions and somewhat higher reticulocyte counts (not statistically significant) than those receiving placebo. However, the indications for transfusion were relatively liberal—a hematocrit below 27% or the presence of symptoms such as poor weight gain, lethargy, or feeding difficulties. However, we are not told how many infants met either or both of these criteria. In general, these infants appear to tolerate hemoglobin levels of 5 or 6 g/dL quite well. We don't know what would have happened had the authors withheld intervention (in the absence of clinical signs) until the hematocrit fell below 20% (or even lower), as has been recommended in the past.[3] On the other hand, the authors occasionally encountered abrupt declines in the hematocrit, indicating the need for careful monitoring.

Administering rHEPO is not without cost and inconvenience. In this study, mothers had to bring their infants to a clinic 3 times a week for 6 weeks to receive a subcutaneous injection of rHEPO and, although the number of blood transfusions was significantly reduced, 8 of 10 infants in the treatment group nevertheless required 1 or more transfusions.

M.J. Maisels, M.B., B.Ch.

References

1. Ohls RK, Wirkus PEN, Christensen RD: Recombinant erythropoietin as treatment of the late hyporegenerative anemia of Rh hemolytic disease. *Pediatrics* 90:678–680, 1992.
2. Thorpe JA, O'Connor T, Callenbach J, et al: Hyporegenerative anemia associated with intrauterine transfusion in rhesus hemolytic disease. *Am J Obstet Gynecol* 165:79–81, 1991.
3. Oski FA, Naiman JL: *Hematologic Problems in the Newborn,* ed 3. Philadelphia, WB Saunders, 1982, p 283.

Erythropoietin Course in Newborns With Rh Hemolytic Disease Transfused and Not Transfused *In Utero*

Dallacasa P, Ancora G, Miniero R, et al (Univ of Bologna, Italy; Sant'Orsola Hosp, Bologna, Italy)

Pediatr Res 40:357–360, 1996 12–7

Background.—In most neonates with Rh hemolytic disease, a late anemia develops with a low reticulocyte count, which begins at about 2 weeks after birth. The pathogenic mechanisms of this anemia are not well understood. Three underlying mechanisms have been suggested: anti-D bone marrow precursor destruction, anti-D peripheral reticulocyte destruction, and low erythropoietin (Epo) production.

Purpose.—The purpose of this study was to analyze the pathogenesis of the late anemia of Rh hemolytic disease by examining the relationship between Epo, Hb, and reticulocyte levels in neonates and infants with erythroblastosis fetalis, both those who had received transfusions in utero and those who had not.

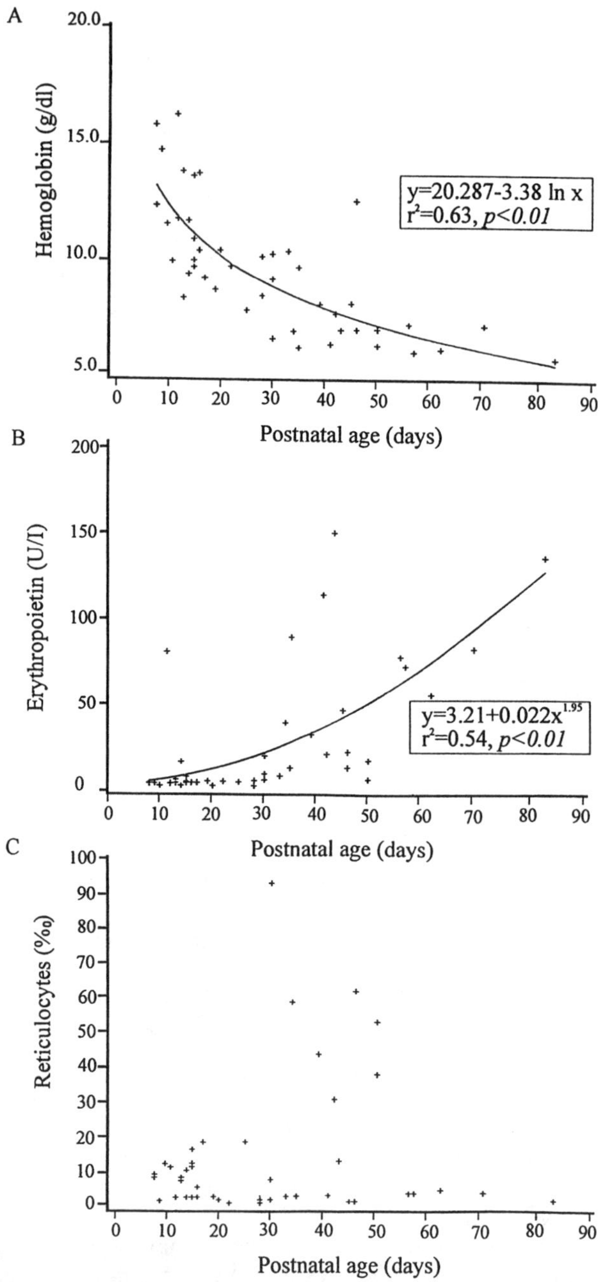

FIGURE 1.—Relation of Hb concentration (g/dL). **A,** erythropoietin levels (units/L); **B,** reticulocyte count (%); **C,** postnatal age for 56 samples from 30 neonates and infants with erythroblastosis fetalis (18 who had intrauterine transfusion and 12 who did not have intrauterine transfusion). (Courtesy of Dallacasa P, Ancora G, Miniero R, et al: Erythropoietin course in newborns with Rh hemolytic disease transfused and not transfused *in utero*. *Pediatr Res* 40:357–360, 1996.)

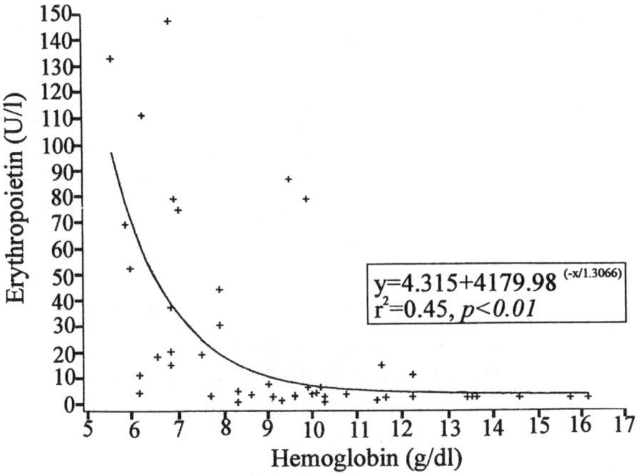

FIGURE 2.—Relation of serum erythropoietin (units/L) and Hb concentration (g/dL) for 56 samples from 30 neonates and infants (aged 8 to 83 days) with erythroblastosis fetalis (18 who had intrauterine transfusion and 12 who did not have intrauterine transfusion). (Courtesy of Dallacasa P, Ancora G, Miniero R, et al: Erythropoietin course in newborns with Rh hemolytic disease transfused and not transfused *in utero*. *Pediatr Res* 40:357–360, 1996.)

Study Population.—The study population consisted of 30 neonates and infants, 3–83 days old, with erythroblastosis fetalis. Of these, 18 had received intrauterine transfusions and 12 had not. Blood samples were collected and analyzed for Hb, Epo, and reticulocyte levels.

Results.—No differences were found between the Epo, Hb, and reticulocyte levels of neonates and infants with and without intrauterine transfusions, so their data were pooled for the purposes of this study. There was an inverse relationship between Epo and Hb levels (Fig 1). There was no relationship between reticulocyte count and Hb levels or between reticulocyte count and Epo levels. The reticulocyte count was low in all but 6 babies. There was an inverse relationship between Epo and Hb levels (Fig 2), but there was no relationship between Hb and reticulocyte levels or between Epo and reticulocyte levels. Anemic neonates had higher levels of serum Epo than did nonanemic neonates, but there were no significant differences in reticulocyte count between these 2 groups. There were no differences in Hb and Epo levels in neonates with or without reticulocytosis. There was a direct relationship between maternal anti-D titer at the last intrauterine transfusion and the number of transfusions required after birth.

Conclusions.—There were no significant differences in the neonates based on whether they had undergone intrauterine transfusions. There was a significant increase in Epo levels in anemic neonates, but there was no corresponding increase in the reticulocyte count. Low Epo production may not be the primary cause of the late anemia of Rh hemolytic disease. It is possible that persisting anti-D antibodies could destroy erythrocyte precursors in the neonate, leading to the characteristic anemia with a low reticulocyte count. The study of anti-D titer in these neonates could assist in the understanding of the pathogenesis of the late anemia of erythroblastosis fetalis.

► These findings appear to contradict those in Abstract 12–6. Evidence that the late anemia of Rh disease does not primarily result from a hyporegenerative state comes from the interesting finding that as the Hb declined between 10 and 80 postnatal days, there was a matching rise in Epo. This rise occurred both in neonates and infants who had received intrauterine transfusions and those who had not. Intrauterine transfusions had been thought to play a particularly important role in suppressing erythropoiesis. Now it appears that this may not be the case. Furthermore, the reticulocyte counts remained persistently low despite rising erythropoietin and falling Hb levels. One possible explanation for this is that circulating anti-D antibodies affect the erythroid precursors in the bone marrow and reticulocytes in the peripheral circulation.

We now have excellent data on normal levels of erythropoietin in the first 7 months and their relationship to Hb levels and reticulocyte counts (see Abstract 12–5). In this study, there was a wide range of erythropoietin levels in the anemic infants, but these levels did increase in response to the anemia, and by 30 days they were well above normal levels and continued to rise thereafter. If this is the case, why would supplemental erythropoietin increase Hb levels in these infants (see Abstract 12–6)? It is apparent that we have not heard the last of this story.

M.J. Maisels, M.B., B.Ch.

Factors Related to Transfusion in Very Low Birthweight Infants Treated With Erythropoietin

Maier RF, for the European Multicentre rhEPO Study Group (Humboldt Universität, Berlin; et al)

Arch Dis Child 74:F182–F186, 1996 12–8

Introduction.—Because of a lack of generally accepted guidelines, transfusion practices vary considerably for very low birth weight (VLBW) infants. Treatment with recombinant human erythropoietin (rhEPO) reduces the need for red blood cell transfusions, but some infants are nonresponders. A group of 120 VLBW infants who were treated with rhEPO were evaluated for factors associated with the need for transfusion and strategies that might improve rhEPO response.

Methods.—Infants were enrolled at 12 centers. Birth weight ranged from 750 to 999 g in 34 infants, from 1,000 to 1,249 g in 43 infants, and from 1,250 to 1,499 g in 43 infants. Participating neonatologists followed red blood cell transfusion guidelines that were derived from their experience. Within these guidelines, the neonatologists in clinical charge made decisions regarding the timing and volume of transfusions. Failure of treatment was defined as transfusion or a venous hematocrit of less than 0.32 during rhEPO treatment.

TABLE 2.—Number (%) of Infants With Blood Transfusions for Various Categorised Prognostic or Time-dependent Factors and Corresponding Odds Ratios With and Without Adjustment for Center Effects (Univariate Analysis)

Factor	*Stratum*	*Infants evaluable (n=)*	*Infants transfused (n (%))*	*Odds ratio unadjusted P value**	*Odds ratio centre adjusted P value†*
Blood loss (ml/kg/day)	≥1·0	61	49 (80·3)	17·45 P<0·001	38·07 P<0·001
	<1·0	58	11 (19·0)		
Birth weight (g)	750–999	34	27 (79·4)	11·22 P<0·001	32·43 P<0·001
	1000–1249	43	23 (51·2)	3·05 P=0·026	5·05 P=0·005
	1250–1499	43	11 (25·6)		
Gestational age (weeks)	≤28	47	33 (70·2)	4·02 P<0·001	4·68 P=0·001
	>28	73	27 (30·0)		
Initial haematocrit	≤0·48	66	40 (60·6)	2·62 P=0·017	2·72 P=0·026
	>0·48	54	20 (37·0)		
Initial reticulocyte count (%)	≤9	67	41 (61·2)	2·73 P=0·017	2·18 P=0·139
	>9	41	15 (36·6)		
Ventilation	Yes	58	35 (60·3)	2·35 P=0·028	3·02 P=0·022
	No	61	24 (39·3)		
Initial serum protein (g/l)	≤45	44	29 (65·9)	2·47 P=0·032	2·00 P=0·157
	>45	66	29 (43·9)		
Iron supplementation (mg/kg/6 weeks)	≤50	52	29 (55·8)	1·09 P=1·0	0·46 P=0·305
	>50	41	22 (53·7)		
Initial serum ferritin (μg/l)	<150	56	30 (53·6)	0·93 P=1·0	0·89 P=0·971
	≥150	47	26 (55.3)		

Note: Homogeneity of odds ratios across centers was not rejected by Zelen's exact test ($P > 0.1$) for any of the analyzed factors, with the exception of initial reticulocyte count.

*Exact *P* value for testing that the odds ratio is 1 for 2 × 2 tables.

†Exact *P* value for testing that the odds ratio is 1 for 2 × 2 tables stratified by center.

(Courtesy of Maier RF, for the European Multicentre rhEPO Study Group: Factors related to transfusion in very low birth weight infants treated with erythropoietin. *Arch Dis Child* 74:F182–F186, 1996.)

Results.—Sixty (50%) infants received at least 1 transfusion during rhEPO therapy. Rates of transfusion at individual centers ranged from 13% to 73%, but the small number of infants treated at 6 of the 12 centers may make interpretation difficult. Median birth weight was significantly greater in untransfused (1,260-g) vs. transfused (1,040-g) infants. Infants with a blood loss of less than 1 mL/kg/day had a significantly lower need for transfusion than those with a loss of 1 mL/kg/day or greater. Other factors associated with the frequency of transfusion were low gestational age (70% for 28 weeks or less), low initial hematocrit (61% for 0.48 or less), and low initial reticulocyte count (9% or less; Table 2).

Discussion.—The need for transfusion in VLBW infants treated with rhEPO depends on the infants' birth weight, gestational age, and initial hematocrit. Additional factors than can be minimized include diagnostic blood loss and iron deficiency. A better rhEPO response might be achieved by reducing diagnostic blood sampling, preventing iron and protein deficiency, and adhering to objective guidelines on transfusion timing and volume.

► Commentary by Richard A. Ehrenkranz, M.D., Professor of Pediatrics and Obstetrics & Gynecology, Yale University School of Medicine:

► Maier and associates evaluated further the rhEPO-treated infants who participated in the second European Multicentre rhEPO trial and sought "to detect prognostic and concomitant factors associated with the decision to transfuse red blood cells during rhEPO treatment, and to assess the impact of centre-specific variations in management and individual problems in 'non-responders.' " They reported that although birth weight, initial hematocrit, and gestational age were the most predictive of transfusion need, "the great heterogeneity of clinical features and management in the participating centres" caused the transfusion rate to vary considerably among the centers. They concluded that to improve rhEPO response in VLBW infants, diagnostic blood loss must be minimized and rational criteria for transfusion in preterm infants must be developed.

Should we be surprised at this conclusion? I am not. I know that rhEPO treatment stimulates erythropoiesis and decreases the need for transfusion. However, without adherence to conservative transfusion guidelines, the decision about when to administer a transfusion to a VLBW infant will vary widely between individual neonatologists within a single neonatal ICU. In addition, without a concerted effort to minimize diagnostic blood loss, blood loss will continue to provide the greatest stimulus associated with the decision to give a transfusion to a VLBW infant. Twenty-eight (23%) of the 120 study patients had been transfused before entry into the study on day 3 of life. Because it takes 7 to 10 days before rhEPO therapy may begin to reduce transfusion needs by producing sufficient red blood cells to keep up with iatrogenic blood loss, we should not expect rhEPO therapy, even if initiated within the first several days of life, to eradicate all transfusion needs. However, the hypothesis that needs to be tested is whether rhEPO treatment initiated within the first several days of life in conjunction with dedicated units of packed red blood cells and conservative transfusion guidelines not only can decrease the number of red blood cell transfusions, but also can decrease blood donor exposure and increase the percentage of transfusion-free infants. Clinical practice patterns might change if that hypothesis were tested and proven.

R.A. Ehrenkranz, M.D.

Recombinant Human Erythropoietin: Possible Role as an Antioxidant in Premature Rabbits

Bany-Mohammed FM, Slivka S, Hallman M (Univ of California, Irvine)

Pediatr Res 40:381–387, 1996 12–9

Background.—Iron is an important catalyst for free oxygen radicals and lipid peroxidation reactions that may be involved in the pathogenesis of several diseases in premature infants. Early in the neonatal period, excessive amounts of extracellular iron are available. The administration of erythropoietin (EPO) may mobilize iron from plasma and inhibit iron-catalyzed reactions.

Methods.—Recombinant human EPO (rhEPO) was given subcutaneously to premature rabbits delivered at 29 days' gestation. One group was kept in room air, and the other was kept in a 100% oxygen environment. The rabbits were randomized within groups to receive rhEPO at 400 or 800 units/kg or placebo just after birth and on day 2 of life.

Findings.—Recombinant human EPO reduced plasma iron and iron saturation of transferrin in the room air and hyperoxia groups. It also increased reticulocytes and erythropoiesis in liver and bone marrow in these groups. With oxygen exposure, nonsedimentable protein (NSP) was increased in bronchoalveolar lavage (BAL). The ability of BAL to inhibit lipid peroxidation was reduced, as measured by malondialdehyde generation, compared with room air exposure. In the animals exposed to 0_2, EPO increased the ability of plasma and BAL to inhibit lipid peroxidation and reduced NSP in BAL. Recombinant human EPO also reduced alveolar thickening and proteinaceous exudate in the hyperoxia group.

Conclusion.—Recombinant human EPO reduces iron-catalyzed oxidant injury and thus may have a therapeutic role as an antioxidant in the early neonatal period. More research is needed to determine whether rhEPO treatment prevents oxidant injury without causing adverse effects.

▶ Here is a new twist on the rationale for the use of rhEPO. Animal data suggest that by stimulating erythropoiesis, rhEPO mobilizes nonheme iron and decreases oxygen injury that depends on the availability of transient metal. Strict transfusion policies have decreased the need for transfusions in premature infants, especially those weighing more than 1,000 g, without the need for rhEPO. Whether rhEPO will become part of our armamentarium for preventing oxidative injury in neonates and avoiding many clinical disease states acquired postnatally by immature individuals exposed to oxygen remains uncertain. Nonetheless, the idea is intriguing and certainly provides another excuse for using rhEPO.

D.K. Stevenson, M.D.

Small Peptides as Potent Mimetics of the Protein Hormone Erythropoietin

Wrighton NC, Farrell FX, Chang R, et al (Affymax Research Inst, Palo Alto, Calif; RW Johnson Pharmaceutical Research Inst, Raritan, NJ)

Science 273:458–463, 1996 12–10

Introduction.—If binding between proteins generally occurs through small epitopes, then there is a good chance of finding small-molecule ligands. Combinatorial procedures to produce diverse molecular shapes testable for binding molecular targets provide new techniques for ligand discovery. Peptides that bind to the extracellular domain of the human erythropoietin (EPO) receptor were sought to derive compounds capable of stimulating erytropoiesis.

Methods and Findings.—Small peptides that bind to and activate the EPO receptor were sought by random phage display peptide libraries and affinity selective techniques. The identified peptides behaved as full agonists in in vitro biological assays, and they stimulated erythropoiesis in mice. The 14–amino acid, disulfide-bonded, cyclic peptide agonists had a minimum consensus sequence YXCXXGPXTWXCXP, where the position represented by X can be occupied by several amino acids. The primary EPO sequence did not include the amino acid sequences of these peptides, which activated signaling pathways identical to those induced by the natural ligand.

Conclusions.—A family of cyclic peptides with erythropoietic activity is identified. The bound structure of these peptides may be useful in designing small-molecule mimetics of EPO with desirable pharmacologic properties. The true value of the techniques used in this study for the discovery of agonists or other cytokine receptors remains to be determined.

▶ Searching for a needle in a haystack is difficult. Looking for the eye of the needle in the same haystack is infinitely more difficult. The odds against finding the designer proteins reported above must have been astronomical. But now that the first wave have been identified and are starting to be put through their paces, the floodgates may open. We can anticipate many more designer peptides to bombard the hormone and cytokine receptors.

It is nothing short of remarkable that the EPO receptor can be activated by this tiny molecule, which bears no resemblance to the usual red blood cell precursor stimulus. One begins to drool at the infinite pharmacologic possibilities and the prospects of manipulating and controlling systems with simple, safe, protein products able to be ingested by even the most immature infants. (See also Abstract 12–8.)

Discovery consists of seeing what everybody has seen and thinking what nobody has thought.—Albert Szent-Gyorgi

A.A. Fanaroff, M.B.B.Ch.

Functional Mimicry of a Protein Hormone by a Peptide Agonist: The EPO Receptor Complex at 2.8 Å

Livnah O, Stura EA, Johnson DL, et al (Skaggs Inst of Chemical Biology, La Jolla, Calif; RW Johnson Pharmaceutical Res Inst, Raritan, NJ; Affymax Research Inst, Palo Alto, Calif)

Science 273:464–471, 1996 12–11

Introduction.—Erythropoietin (EPO) is the main hormone regulating the proliferation and differentiation of immature erythroid cells; its target is EPO receptor (EPOR) on committed progenitor cells in the bone marrow and other hematopoietic tissues. Recent studies have clarified the structure of EPOR. The identification of the EPOR binding site could provide information to be used in the design of a nonpeptide, small-molecule EPOR agonist. Until now, it has been very difficult to make unrelated small molecules mimic the function of a protein. An agonist that mimics the function of EPO was developed.

Findings.—A 20-residue cyclic peptide, unrelated to the natural ligand, was developed that mimicked the function of EPO. A complex of the agonist peptide with the extracellular domain of EPOR had a crystal structure at 2.4-A resolution. It induced nearly perfect dimerization of EPOR. The assembly of the dimer was not the same as that of the human growth hormone receptor complex. This suggested the possibility that signal transduction and cell proliferation could be induced by more than one mode of dimerization. Peptide interaction localized the EPOR binding site, which corresponded to the smaller functional epitope of the human growth hormone receptor.

Conclusions.—A cyclic peptide has been developed, unrelated in sequence and structure to the natural ligand, that produces biologically active dimerization of EPOR, promoting signal transduction and cell proliferation. This EPO mimetic peptide ligand can be considered a "minimal hormone." It may be feasible to design nonpeptidic, small-molecule mimetics for EPO and other cytokines.

► Just the terminology of the title has to pique your interest. "Star Wars" technology and a view of molecular biology in the next century flow through this manuscript. Some paragraphs barely have vowels, there are so many genetic sequences and formulas. Scanning this manuscript, one realizes that traditional physiology now resembles the horse and buggy next to the top-of-the-line Cadillac that is modern molecular biology. It is nothing short of remarkable that a small peptide can mimic EPO. I do not pretend to understand more than the broad concepts of this pioneering research, but I do find it exciting that "a peptide unrelated in sequence and probably in structure to the natural ligand can induce a biologically active dimerization of the EPO receptor that promotes signal transduction and cell proliferation." We are starting to fool Mother Nature, rather than fool *with* Mother Nature.

The possibilities seem endless, and other major pharmacologic breakthroughs are anticipated. (See also Abstract 12–10.)

A.A. Fanaroff, M.B.B.Ch.

Erythrocyte Incorporation of Iron by 56-day-old Infants Fed a ^{58}Fe-labeled Supplement

Fomon SJ, Ziegler EE, Nelson SE, et al (Univ of Iowa, Iowa City; Iowa State Univ, Ames)

Pediatr Res 38:373–378, 1995 12–12

Objective.—Iron supplementation is recommended to prevent iron deficiency in infants. Some authors recommend early iron supplementation in both breast-fed and formula-fed infants. There are few data on iron absorption during the first few months of life. This question was addressed by measuring erythrocyte incorporation of a stable iron isotope in breast- and formula-fed infants.

Methods.—The study included 14 breast-fed and 16 formula-fed 56-day-old infants. Both groups received an iron-58–labeled vitamin-iron supplement, which was given between feedings. The formula-fed infants received a low-iron (about 4-mg/L) formula. Erythrocyte incorporation of ^{58}Fe was measured as a surrogate for iron absorption.

Results.—At 14 days after ^{58}Fe administration, mean erythrocyte incorporation of the isotope was about 8% in the breast-fed infants and 4% in the formula-fed infants. The significant difference was thought to reflect the greater presence of inhibitors of iron absorption in the gastrointestinal tracts of formula-fed infants. Given a mean iron intake of 7.99 mg from the vitamin-iron supplement, infants in the breast-fed group received a

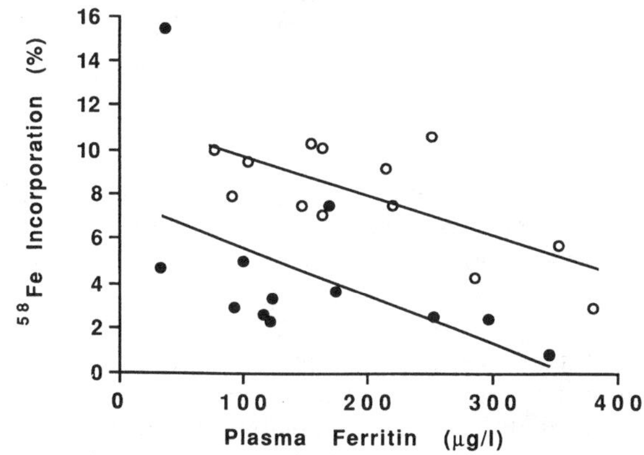

FIGURE 1.—Relation between percentage of iron-58 incorporation 14 days after the administration of ^{58}Fe, and plasma ferritin concentration (average of 56-day and 70-day values) in breast-fed (*open circles*) and formula-fed (*closed circles*) infants. The regression lines are indicated for breast-fed ($y = 11.40 - 0.01758 \cdot x$) and formula-fed ($y = 7.71 - 0.02121 \cdot x$) infants. (Courtesy of Fomon SJ, Ziegler EE, Nelson SE, et al: Erythrocyte incorporation of iron by 56-day-old infants fed a ^{58}fe-labeled supplement. *Pediatr Res* 38:373–378, 1995.)

dose of 0.62 mg, which is in the estimated required range for absorbed iron. There was a significant correlation between ^{58}Fe erythrocyte incorporation and plasma ferritin concentration for the breast-fed infants but not for the formula-fed infants (Fig 1).

Conclusions.—Breast-fed infants can absorb supplemental iron at 2 months of age. Early supplementation will increase body iron stores, decreasing the likelihood of iron deficiency during the first year of life for breast-fed infants. It is unknown whether iron absorption is the same or less before 8 weeks of age.

▶ The neonatologist has long disappeared from the scene by the time the infant is 8 weeks old, healthy, and breast-feeding. Whenever the topic of iron supplementation is raised, particularly for breast-fed infants, neonatologists need to pay attention because the foundation for anemia and learning disability may be laid by simple measures such as failure to provide sufficient iron. Hence, I have included this article from the incredibly productive, if at times provocative, Iowa University nutrition group. The concepts are simple and the evidence clear-cut. Radiolabeled iron can be absorbed by breast-feeding infants in sufficient quantities to replete the iron stores and prevent subsequent iron deficiency. As noted by the authors, "a detailed consideration of the arguments, for and against administration of iron to breast-fed infants before 4 months of age, is beyond the scope of the present communication." I also will avoid the conflict, but emphasize the importance of iron supplementation for preterm infants receiving erythropoietin. Erythropoiesis is limited if iron supplementation is inadequate. Meyer and colleagues reported that IV iron supplementation probably was superior to oral iron supplementation for the preterm population.[1] Ohls and associates have hypothesized that 1 mg/kg/day, given parenterally, would provide an adequate supply of iron for preterm infants receiving erythropoietin.[2] However, too few subjects have been studied to know the optimal iron dose or route of administration for preterm infants. Lest we forget, iron supplementation also can improve verbal learning and memory in iron-deficient adolescent girls.

To improve cognitive functioning, a balanced diet and a good night's sleep are unlikely to go amiss.—Deborah Ashby, Lancet 348:973, 1996.

A.A. Fanaroff, M.B.B.Ch.

References

1. Meyer MP, Haworth C, Meyer JH, et al: A comparison of oral and intravenous iron supplementation in preterm infants receiving recombinant erythropoietin. *J Pediatr* 129:258–263, 1996.
2. Ohls RK, Veerman MW, Christensen RD: Pharmacokinetics and effectiveness of recombinant erythropoietin administered to preterm infants by continuous infusion in parenteral nutrition solution. *J Pediatr* 128:518–523, 1996.

Circulating Megakaryocytes and Their Progenitors in Early Thrombocytopenia in Preterm Neonates

Murray NA, Roberts IAG (Hammersmith Hosp, London)

Pediatr Res 40:112–119, 1996 12–13

Background.—Thrombocytopenia is one of the most important hematologic problems in newborns. It occurs in 22% to 35% of all infants admitted to neonatal ICUs. As many as 72% of sick preterm infants are affected. However, platelet production in such infants has rarely been investigated. Miniaturized assays were developed to study circulating megakaryocyte (MK) progenitors, total cultured MK precursors, and mature MKs.

Methods.—Sixty-three preterm infants, 26 of whom had early thrombocytopenia develop, were prospectively studied. Twenty-one were born to mothers with pregnancy-induced hypertension or were growth retarded. The assays were developed by culturing mononuclear cells purified from 0.5 to 1 mL of preterm peripheral blood. Circulating burst-forming unit (BFU)–MKs and colony-forming unit (CFU)–MKs, total cultured MK precursors, and mature MKs were assessed.

Findings.—At birth, the numbers of all MK precursors were reduced severely in thrombocytopenic infants compared with nonthrombocytopenic infants. Respectively, BFU-MK values were 82 and 663 colonies/mL; CFU-MK values, 596 and 3,267 colonies/mL; total MK precursors, 97 and 301×10^3 cells/mL; and mature MKs, 8 and 37×10^3 cells/mL. By the tenth day, thrombocytopenia resolved in all infants, accompanied or preceded by a recovery to normal numbers of circulating MK progenitors. Sixty-nine percent of the thrombocytopenic infants were also neutropenic. In this group, neutrophil progenitor cells were also severely decreased, compared with the nonthrombocytopenic infants.

Conclusion.—The main cause of thrombocytopenia and neutropenia in these infants appears to be decreased platelet and neutrophil production, a result of reduced numbers of MK and CFU-granulocyte/monocyte progenitors, respectively. The hematologic abnormalities observed in the neonates of mothers with pregnancy-induced hyertension or with intrauterine growth retardation seem to be a consequence of dysregulation of fetal hemopoiesis occurring proximal to committed MK and neutrophil progenitors, probably at the level of the primitive multipotent hemopoietic stem cell.

▶ These authors have broken completely new ground in our understanding of the thrombocytopenia so prevalent in sick preterm infants. They were able to do this by developing a miniaturized assay that allowed them to culture mononuclear cells purified from 0.5–1 mL of neonatal peripheral blood and to quantify precisely the numbers of MK progenitors and the ability of these cells to differentiate in vitro into mature MKs. They were also able to follow the change in MK progenitors during the first week of life in thrombocytopenic and nonthrombocytopenic infants. The magnitude of the differences between the study and control groups was striking, as was the resolution of the thrombocytopenia in all infants by the 10th day. This resolution was accompanied or preceded by a recovery to normal numbers of the circulating MK progenitors. Twenty-one of the 26 thrombocytopenic infants were born to mothers with pregnancy-induced hypertension or were growth retarded.

These findings leave little doubt that in such infants, the thrombocytopenia is a result of decreased platelet production secondary to decreased numbers of MK progenitors and not (as has been suggested in other studies of mothers with pregnancy-induced hypertension) an immune-mediated platelet consumption phenomenon. The authors also emphasize the common association between thrombocytopenia and neutropenia (the neutropenia is also the result of a reduction in circulating primitive granulocyte progenitor cells) and they draw attention to the important association between early thrombocytopenia, neutropenia, and polycythemia that occurs commonly in infants born to mothers with pregnancy-induced hypertension or growth retardation.

In these infants, fetal tissue hypoxia is thought to increase fetal erythropoietin, thus raising hematocrit levels. However, because platelets, neutrophils, and erythrocytes all come from a common multipotent hemopoietic progenitor cell, fetal tissue hypoxia may lead to, to quote the authors, an "erythropoietin-driven disruption of normal hemopoiesis at this primitive progenitor cell level, leading to an imbalance of commitment to lineage restricted progenitor cells ... "We can now better understand the vagaries of the response of the preterm infant's hematopoietic system to a variety of stresses and strains.

M.J. Maisels, M.B., B.Ch.

Nucleated Red Blood Cells: An Update on the Marker for Fetal Asphyxia

Korst LM, Phelan JP, Ahn MO, et al (Pomona Valley Hosp, Pasadena, Calif; Cha Women's Hosp of Seoul, Korea; Queen of the Valley Hosp, Orange, Calif)

Am J Obstet Gynecol 175:843–846, 1996 12–14

Background.—Nucleated red blood cells are commonly observed in the circulating blood of neonates. The most frequent explanations for numbers exceeding 10 are prematurity, rhesus sensitization, maternal diabetes mellitus, and intrauterine growth restriction. Asphyxia may also cause an increase in the number of nucleated red blood cells. In previous work, an association between nucleated red blood cells, hypoxic-ischemic encephalopathy, and long-term neurologic impairment was demonstrated. The use of nucleated red blood cells as a marker for fetal asphyxia was further explored.

Methods.—Data on nucleated red blood cells from 153 singleton, neurologically impaired neonates born at term were compared with data on cord blood nucleated red blood cells of 83 nonasphyxiated neonates born at term. Neurologically impaired neonates were divided into 3 groups: 69 had persistent nonreactive fetal heart rate pattern from addmission to delivery (group 1); 47, reactive fetal heart rate on admission followed by tachycardia with decelerations and absent variability (group 2); and 37, reactive fetal heart rate on admission followed by an acute prolonged deceleration (group 3).

Findings.—The mean number of initial nucleated red blood cells in neurologically impaired neonates was 30.3 per 100 white blood cells, significantly greater than that in the control group (3.4 per 100 white blood cells). Distinct nucleated red blood cell patterns were observed when neurologically impaired neonates were classified according to timing of neurologic impairment. Initial nucleated red blood cells differed significantly among the neurologically impaired groups and the normal group. Values were 48.6 in group 1, 11.4 in group 2, and 12.6 in group 3. At a mean 51.5, maximum nucleated red blood cells values in group 1 were greater than in groups 2 and 3 combined (12.7). Clearance time was also longer in group 1 than in groups 2 and 3 combined—119 hours and 59 hours, respectively.

Conclusions.—Measures of nucleated red blood cells can be used to identify infants with fetal asphyxia. Distinct nucleated red blood cell patterns related to the timing of fetal injury can be observed in fetal asphyxia. Intrapartum injuries are associated with lower nucleated red blood cell values.

▶ Many physicians who care for the fetus and newborn forget to call for examination of the placenta. Pertinent history of the fetus may emerge, and the ratio of nucleated red blood cells (NRBCs) to leukocytes may be examined in fetal vessels. If the ratio exceeds 1:1.5, it is considered excessive and indicative of chronic fetal hypoxia. Other causes of elevated NRBC counts include diabetes mellitus, Rh disease, prematurity, and intrauterine growth retardation. There is an 85% concordance of NRBCs in fetal placental blood vessels with NRBC counts in postdelivery peripheral blood vessels. The NRBC count in the newborn varies inversely with gestational age, which must be taken into account when determining whether a count is elevated or not.

Phelan had shown a relationship between NRBCs, hypoxic-ischemic encephalopathy, and long-term neurologic impairment (see Abstracts 12–15 and 12–16). The above report was designed to extend their series and compare NRBC in asphyxiated infants with a group of normal nonasphyxiated infants. Indeed, regardless of the fetal pathophysiologic mechanism responsible for fetal injury, the NRBC counts were significantly higher among asphyxiated neonates than among their non-asphyxiated peers. They were also able to graphically document the NRBC clearance time suggesting that, if the neonates shows signs of injury and the NRBC count is normal, the injury has occurred further back in time, (i.e. well before delivery). If the infants are born with elevated counts, the insult may have occurred during labor and delivery. The NRBC count may thus be adjunctive evidence of the timing of injury.

In recent years, there has been a trend to attribute most cases of cerebral palsy to events before labor and delivery.[1] The NRBC count may be a piece of evidence supporting such a hypothesis. Naeye[2] has attempted also to use the lymphocyte count to time cerebral injury. He reported a large number of lymphocytes in addition to normoblasts entered the blood of a small group of children after they had begun to experience brain damaging hypoxia-ischemia. The lymphocyte counts returned to normal levels 24 hours later and the normoblasts to normal levels after 24–30 hours.[2] Evidently lymphocytes can enter the circulation in large numbers within 15 minutes and normoblasts within 30 minutes of a severe hypoxic insult.

The blood count of the infant may thus provide circumstantial evidence of asphyxia. Circumstantial evidence has been referred to as Cinderella's ugly sisters, but at times, circumstantial evidence is Cinderella.

A.A. Fanaroff, M.B.B.Ch.

References

1. Naeye RL, Peters EC, Bartholomew M, et al: Origins of cerebral palsy. *Am J Dis Child* 143:1154–1161, 1989.
2. Naeye RL, Localio AR: Determining the time before birth when ischemia and hypoxemia initiated cerebral palsy. *Obstet Gynecol* 86:713–719, 1995.

Nucleated Red Blood Cells: A Marker for Fetal Asphyxia?

Phelan JP, Ahn MO, Korst LM, et al (Pomona Valley Hosp, Pasadena, Calif; Queen of the Valley Hosp, West Covina, Calif; Univ of California, Irvine; et al)

Am J Obstet Gynecol 173:1380–1384, 1995 12–15

Background.—Increased nucleated red blood cells (RBCs) in the circulating blood of neonates is usually associated with prematurity, Rh sensitization, maternal diabetes mellitus, or intrauterine growth retardation. Asphyxia may also increase the number of nucleated RBCs in the circulating blood of newborns. The effect of the presence of nucleated RBCs on hypoxic-ischemic encephalopathy and long-term neonatal neurologic impairment was determined.

Methods.—Data on 46 singleton term neonates with neurologic impairment were compared with data on 83 term newborns without asphyxiation. The neurologically impaired neonates were classified as nonreactive (nonreactive fetal heart rate from admission to delivery), tachycardic (reactive fetal heart rate on admission followed by tachycardia with decelerations), and rupture (uterine rupture).

Findings.—The number of nucleated RBCs per 100 white blood cells was significantly higher in the neurologically impaired than in the intact group, with mean values of 34.5 and 3.4, respectively. Distinct nucleated RBC patterns were found among the different groups of neurologically impaired infants. Nonreactive neonates had the greatest mean nucleated RBC count and longest clearance times.

Conclusions.—Nucleated RBCs were useful for the identification of fetal asphyxia in this limited series. Distinct nucleated RBC patterns were associated with asphyxia consistent with the observed basis for fetal injury. In general, the number of nucleated RNCs decreased the closer the birth was to the asphyxial event. Data on cord blood nucleated RBCs may therefore indicate the timing of fetal neurologic injury.

Relationship Between Neonatal Nucleated Red Blood Cell Counts and Hypoxic-Ischemic Injury

Leikin E, Verma U, Klein S, et al (New York Med College/Westchester County Med Ctr, Valhalla)
Obstet Gynecol 87:439–443, 1996 12–16

Background.—Elevated nucleated red blood cells (RBCs) in umbilical cord blood may be a useful indicator of chronic intrauterine hypoxia. The association between nucleated RBCs in the immediate neonatal period and intraventricular hemorrhage and/or periventricular leukomalacia, two complications of chronic hypoxic ischemia in utero, was investigated.

Methods.—Four hundred forty-one infants who weighed 500–1,750 g were studied. Nucleated RNCs were obtained, and neonatal cranial fontanel sonography was performed on the third and seventh days of life. Nucleated RBCs were compared in infants with normal and abnormal sonographic findings and between weight- and gestational age–matched normal and abnormal groups.

Findings.—Infants with normal and abnormal US findings differed significantly in mean gestational age, birth weight, birth weight percentile, Apgar score, respiratory distress syndrome, and mortality. Nucleated RBCs—40.5 and 41.8 per 100 white blood cells, respectively—were not significantly different. Growth-restricted neonates had a significant increase in nucleated RBCs (Table 3), even after adjustment for gestational age (Table 4).

Conclusions.—Preterm infants with and without intraventricular hemorrhage and periventricular leukomalacia have comparable nucleated

TABLE 3.—Nucleated Red Blood Cell (RBC) Counts by Birth Weight Percentile Subsets

	Mean RBC	*t*	P
≤10th percentile (*n* = 72)	89.7 ± 196.6	2.3	.02
>10th percentile (*n* = 369)	46.4 ± 132.3		
≤25th percentile (*n* = 164)	86.9 ± 229.6	3.8	.000
>25th percentile (*n* = 277)	36.8 ± 38.8		
≤50th percentile (*n* = 283)	65.9 ± 178.5	2.4	.01
>50th percentile (*n* = 158)	31.2 ± 34.8		

(Courtesy of Leikin E, Verma U, Klein S, et al: Relationship between neonatal nucleated red blood cell counts and hypoxic-ischemic injury. *Obstet Gynecol* 87:439–443, 1996. Reprinted with permission from The American College of Obstetricians and Gynecologists.)

TABLE 4.—Nucleated Red Blood Cell Counts by Birth Weight Percentiles Controlled for Gestational Age in Weeks

	Gestational age ≤28 wk	Gestational age >28 wk
≤10th percentile (n = 72)	285 ± 409 (n = 12)	50.6 ± 77.3 (n = 60)
>10th percentile (n = 369)	65.1 ± 182.7 (n = 184)	27.7 ± 32.9 (n = 185)
t	3.6	3.2
P	.000	.001

(Courtesy of Leikin E, Verma U, Klein S, et al: Relationship between neonatal nucleated red blood cell counts and hypoxic-ischemic injury. *Obstet Gynecol* 87:439–443, 1996. Reprinted with permission from The American College of Obstetricians and Gynecologists.)

RBCs. Nucleated RBCs are significantly increased in growth-restricted fetuses. When nucleated RBCs are used as a marker of intrauterine hypoxia, clinicians must consider birth weight percentile.

▶ The relationship between neonatal nucleated RBC counts and neonatal conditions continues to be explored, mainly by cohort comparisons. The most recent report (Abstract 12–16) is based on a retrospective analysis that compared normal and abnormal groups based on US findings. Questionably, grades 1 and 2 intraventricular hemorrhage (IVH) are included as "normal" and, not surprisingly, abnormal findings included grades 3 and 4 IVH and/or periventricular leukomalacia (PVL). A comparison of the mean nucleated RBC levels for the 2 groups showed no difference. Two reasonable conclusions are supported by the data: that elevations in nucleated RBC counts occur in growth restricted fetuses and in infants of lower gestational ages. However, the design of the study does not warrant another conclusion, that "there seems to be no role for [nucleated RBCs] in determining the timing of neurologic injury." The null hypothesis is not so easily accepted, and the statement is too sweeping anyway.

Because the nucleated RBC response is an adaptive one, its relationship to long-term outcome is understandably not well assessed by the identification of surrogates of long-term outcome such as IVH and PVL. The elevation in nucleated RBC is simply a tell-tale sign of chronic intrauterine hypoxic stress (i.e. a stress that must have begun at least 6–10 hours before birth). Thus, the lack of an elevation in the nucleated RBC might be helpful to interpret events at or around the time of labor and delivery. The exact timing of intrauterine events generally remains a matter of speculation, or depedent on postnatal imaging studies that sometimes provide clues as to the time of injury, although not always as to its mechanism. Moreover, the windows of time in which injuries might have occurred prenatally remain relatively large; therefore, exact timing is not possible.

The article on nucleated RBC counts by Phelan et al. (Abstract 12–15), again limited by its design, supports the notion suggested by Leikin et al (3) PN4 that events occurring maybe 6–10 hours before delivery might be reflected in the nucleated RBC count or elevations in erythropoietin. As

Bernischke pointed out in his review,[1] the nucleated RBC response can also continue after birth with a subsequent postnatal elevation in nucleated RBC that occurs in response to an event closer to the time of labor and delivery. Thus, following the nucleated RBC after birth may be helpful to understand the fetal circumstance in and around the time of labor and delivery. However, the fetal response is complex and there may be other factors that influence nucleated RBC counts; therefore, they must be interpreted carefully and in the context of the particular case in question.

D.K. Stevenson, M.D.

Reference

1. Bernischke K: Placenta pathology questions to the perinatologist. *J Perinatol* 371–376, 1994.

Neonatal Purpura Fulminans in Association With Factor V R506Q Mutation

Pipe SW, Schmaier AH, Nichols WC, et al (Univ of Michigan, Ann Arbor)

J Pediatr 128:706–709, 1996 12–17

Objective.—Neonatal purpura fulminans can result in major organ impairment. An infant with neonatal purpura fulminans who had resistance to activated protein C and was heterozygous for the factor V R506Q mutation was seen.

> *Case Report.*—A girl, delivered at 38 weeks of gestation, had purpuric lesions 8 hours after birth. Despite antibiotic treatment, lesion size and number increased. Plasma was administered. Prothrombin time and antithrombin III levels were elevated, whereas activated partial thromboplastin time and fibrinogen levels were low. Antibiotic therapy was discontinued at 72 hours, and the lesions resolved during the next 10 days. Cranial ultrasonography and CT confirmed thrombosis. Plasma administration was discontinued after 12 days, and the patient was released on day 17. Child and mother both showed activated protein C resistance; both were heterozygous for the factor V R506Q mutation. There appear to be no long-term complications.

Conclusion.—Protein C resistance should be checked in infants with rare neonatal purpura fulminans.

▶ Commenting on this article is Louis P. Halamek, M.D., Professor of Pediatrics, Division of Neonatal and Developmental Medicine, Stanford University Medical Center, Palo Alto, California:

▶ Thrombotic complications in neonates are not an uncommon occurrence in a busy level III neonatal ICU. Thrombotic events, especially those occurring in noninstrumented neonates in the first 24 hours of life, should initiate a thorough evaluation including detailed family history and laboratory evaluation for resistance to activated protein C as well as deficiencies in protein C, protein S, and antithrombin III. Variability in clinical presentation is great,[1] as is the potential to prevent or ameliorate long-term sequelae.

L.P. Halamek, M.D.

Reference

1. Greengard JS, Eichinger S, Griffin JH, et al: Variability of thrombosis among homozygous siblings with resistance to activated protein C due to an Arg→Gln mutation in the gene for factor V. *N Engl J Med* 331:1559–1562, 1994.

Changes in Left Thoracic Duct Lymph Flow During Progressive Anemia in the Ovine Fetus

Davis LE, Hohimer AR, Brace RA (Oregon Health Sciences Univ, Portland; Univ of California, San Diego)

Am J Obstet Gynecol 174:1469–1476, 1996 12–18

Introduction.—Anemia in fetal sheep produces a widening of the plasma-interstitial osmotic gradient, as measured in implanted capsules. No previous studies have investigated the effects of anemia on lymph flow. Fetal sheep were studied to determine the effects of anemia on thoracic duct lymph flow and on plasma and lymph protein concentration gradients.

Methods.—Anemia was produced in near-term fetal sheep by withdrawing 60–150 mL of blood over 5 successive days. Changes in thoracic duct lymph flow were measured across a range of outflow pressures. The lymph flow function curve was determined by regression analysis. Analysis of variance for repeated measures was done to compare the protein concentrations in lymph and plasma.

Results.—Bleeding reduced the fetal hematocrit from 35% to 14%. The thoracic duct lymph flow rate increased from 0.12 to 0.28 mL/min/kg at the same time. The protein concentration was unchanged in plasma but decreased from 2.6 to 2.4 g/dL in lymph; the difference between the 2 protein concentrations increased from 1.04 to 1.34 g/dL. The rate of protein return to the circulation increased from 11.5 to 23.7 mg/min. There was no change in central venous pressure, which stayed under the breakpoint pressure. The level at which the lymph flow rate plateaued was unchanged; however, there was no change in the breakpoint or stopflow pressure of the lymph flow function curve.

Conclusions.—Progressive anemia in late-term fetal sheep produces corresponding increases in lymph flow and thus in capillary filtration. Outflow pressure is not a limiting factor on the increase in lymph flow. Chronic fetal anemia is associated with increased thoracic duct lymph

flow, which returns protein to the circulation, helping to limit the expansion of extravascular fluid volume.

► The relation between severe fetal anemia and hydrops is well established. Little time and thought probably are given to the pathophysiologic consequences of progressive anemia. As a result, this report, which addresses such issues, caught my attention. The authors review the physiologic consequences of the anemia, directing our attention to the increase in capillary hydrostatic pressure, which may result from a decrease in the ratio of precapillary-to-postcapillary resistance during vasodilation or from cardiac mechanisms, such as elevated central venous pressure. Initially, there is an increase in myocardial capillary growth and coronary flow with anemia. Ultimately, myocardial function fails and central venous pressure rises.

There are complex relations between capillary hydrostatic pressure, interstitial colloid osmotic pressure, interstitial fluid volume, central venous pressure, and lymph flow. Hence, if hydrostatic pressure is increased, a rise in lymph flow and a fall in interstitial colloid osmotic pressure serve to limit increases in interstitial fluid volume.[1]

Lymph flow is presented artfully as a lymph flow function curve (lymph flow vs. outflow pressure). The study showed a gradual increase in lymph flow and an increase in transcapillary filtration with progressive anemia. When the hematocrit was as low as 14%, lymph flow in the thoracic duct more than doubled; however, in this study, central venous pressure did not increase.

The conclusion that extravascular fluid increases in anemic fetuses because of increased capillary hydrostatic pressure before the onset of congestive heart failure is warranted from the available evidence. Persistence of the anemia eventually will cause the heart to fail, which then will accelerate the accumulation of extracellular fluid.

A.A. Fanaroff, M.B.B.Ch.

Reference

1. Aukland K, Reed RK: Interstitial-lymphatic mechanisms in the control of extracellular fluid. *Physiol Rev* 73:1–78, 1993.

13 Renal Endometabolism

Cerebral Metabolic Rate for Glucose During the First Six Months of Life: An FDG Positron Emission Tomography Study

Kinnala A, Suhonen-Polvi H, Äärimaa T, et al (Univ of Turku, Finland; Åbo Akademi Univ, Turku, Finland)

Arch Dis Child 74:F153–F157, 1996 13–1

Background.—Previous research on the developing brain has revealed a series of changes that affect cerebral glucose utilization. Local cerebral metabolic rate for glucose (LCMRGlc) in neonatal brains during maturation was measured using positron emission tomography (PET) and 2-[fluorine-18] fluoro-2-deoxy-D-glucose (FDG).

Methods.—Twenty infants, postconceptional age 32.7–60.3 weeks, underwent PET in the neonatal period. All were neurodevelopmentally normal and normoglycemic. The infants' development was followed up carefully for 12–36 months.

Findings.—At birth, the LCMRGlc for various cortical brain regions and the basal ganglia was low, ranging from 4 to 16 µmol/100 g/min. The LCMRGlc was highest in the sensorimotor cortex, thalamus, and brain stem in infants 2 months of age and younger. It was increased in the frontal, parietal, temporal, occipital, and cerebellar cortical regions by 5 months of age. Whole-brain LCMRGlc generally was correlated with postconceptional age. The functional maturation of the brain regions was reflected in the change in the glucose metabolic pattern.

Conclusions.—The LCMRGlc in infants increases with maturation. Clinicians must consider postconceptional age when interpreting LCMRGlc measurements.

▶ This commentary was contributed by Satish C. Kalhan, M.D., Professor, Department of Pediatrics, Case Western Reserve University School of Medicine, Cleveland, Ohio:

▶ The introduction of new, noninvasive, and safe methodologies in neonatal-perinatal medicine is allowing us to quantify carefully physiologic parameters that previously have been difficult to obtain. In this context, the study by Kinnala and colleagues is significant because they have quantified regional cerebral metabolic rates of glucose in the neonate and related these to development. The authors aimed to develop normal values for local cerebral metabolic rates for glucose. In some respects, theirs is a retrospective analysis, because the infants originally studied either for the evaluation of hypoxic-ischemic brain injury or after neonatal symptomatic hypoglycemia. The group in the present study (n = 20) was selected from the original cohort of 150 infants because of a normal neurodevelopmental outcome on follow-up at 12–36 months of age. No data regarding their clinical and biochemical status at the time of PET is reported in the manuscript, making it difficult to evaluate the effect of acute illness (i.e., hypoxia, hypoglycemia) or recovery from it on the measured parameters. This is important, because the authors suggest a development-related increase in glucose metabolism by the whole brain, as well as by selected regions of the brain. Is it possible that the lower metabolism of glucose at the earlier postconceptional age was caused by other confounding variables at that time, such as a lower plasma glucose concentration or other systemic metabolic disturbances.

It is worthy of note that several of the newer technologies introduced in medicine are not validated against an established "gold" standard. In this context, the reported rates of glucose metabolism (about 19 μmol/100 g/min) by the brain appear to be significantly lower than those previously reported in infants and children (about 25 μmol/100 g/min) using aterio-venous gradients and blood flow measurements across the brain. Further, previous studies in "healthy" children have not demonstrated an age-dependent change in glucose metabolism of the brain.[1]

Thus, although at first these data suggest a development-related change in cerebral glucose metabolism, they should be accepted with caution. In addition, the present study underscores the need for careful evaluation and validation of new technologies, including an examination of confounding variables before acceptance of the data into physiologic or clinical practice.

S.C. Kalhan, M.D.

Reference

1. Settergren G, Lindblad BS, Persson B: Cerebral blood flow and exchange of oxygen, glucose ketone bodies, lactate, pyruvate and amino acids in anesthetized children. *Acta Paediatr Scand* 69:457–465, 1980.

Renal Bicarbonate Excretion in Extremely Low Birth Weight Infants

Ramiro-Tolentino SB, Markarian K, Kleinman LI (State Univ of New York at Stony Brook)

Pediatrics 98:256–261, 1996 13–2

Background.—Because of kidney immaturity in neonates with extremely low birth weights, large amounts of bicarbonate may be lost in the urine. Renal bicarbonate excretion in such infants was documented.

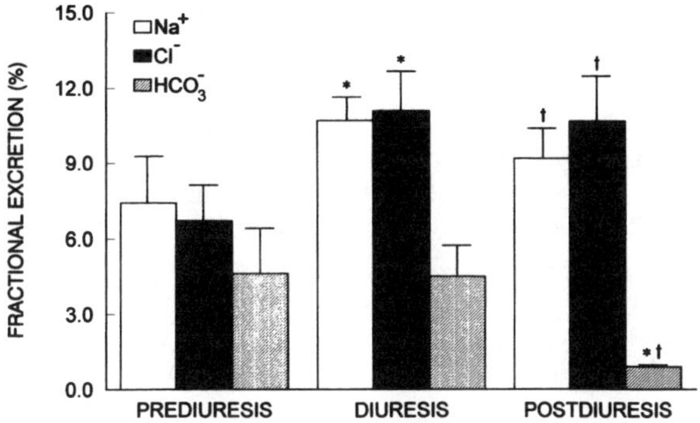

FIGURE 4.—Fractional excretion rates of sodium, chloride, and bicarbonate in the prediuretic, diuretic, and postdiuretic phases. *Asterisk* indicates analysis of variance (*ANOVA*) $P < 0.05$ different from the preceding phase. *Dagger* indicates ANOVA $P < 0.05$ different from the first phase. (Reproduced by permission of *Pediatrics*, courtesy of Ramiro-Tolentino SB, Markarian K, Kleinman LI: Renal bicarbonate excretion in extremely low birth weight infants. *Pediatrics* 98:256–261, copyright 1996.)

Methods.—Twenty-two preterm infants, aged 23–29 weeks' gestation and weighing 540–982 g at birth, were included in the prospective study. Urine and blood samples were collected every 8–12 hours in the first 4 days of life.

Findings.—Three phases of fluid homeostasis (as previously described) were identified: a period of low urine output, of spontaneous diuresis/natriuresis, and of urine output varying according to fluid intake. Urinary excretion of sodium, potassium, chloride, and bicarbonate increased from the prediuretic to the diuretic phase, then declined from the diuretic to the postdiuretic phase. Eighty-eight percent of renal sodium excretion was accompanied by chloride excretion during the diuretic phase. In all 3 phases, the bicarbonate balance was positive. A significant increase occurred in the glomerular filtration rate, filtered load of bicarbonate, and absolute tubular reabsorption of bicarbonate between the prediuretic and diuretic phase (Figs 4 and 5).

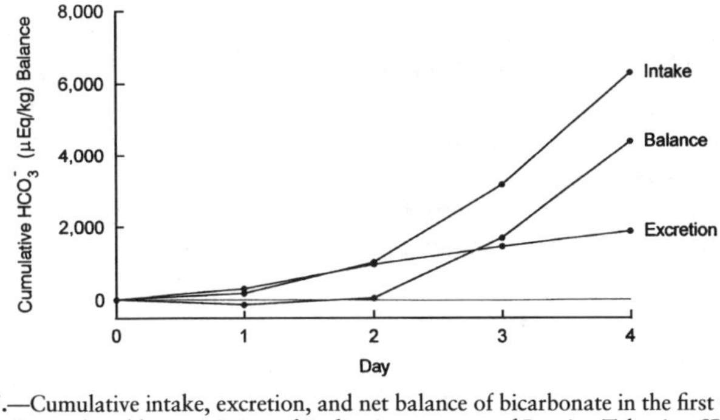

FIGURE 5.—Cumulative intake, excretion, and net balance of bicarbonate in the first 4 days of life of the 22 infants. (Reproduced by permission of *Pediatrics,* courtesy of Ramiro-Tolentino SB, Markarian K, Kleinman LI: Renal bicarbonate excretion in extremely low birth weight infants. *Pediatrics* 98:256–261, copyright 1996.)

Conclusion.—These findings are contrary to the original hypothesis. The total renal bicarbonate excretion of these infants was low in the first 4 days of life, and the net bicarbonate balance was positive. The anion that predominantly accompanied sodium excretion in all 3 phases was chloride, not bicarbonate. The excretion of bicarbonate is apparently independent of sodium excretion in the 3 phases. The increased renal tubular bicarbonate reabsorption in the first week of life may be related to extracellular volume contraction.

▶ We asked Dr. Alan Gruskin, Professor of Pediatrics, Wayne State University School of Medicine, Detroit, Michigan, to comment:

▶ The "kinder, gentler" approach is not limited to phototherapy. This interesting study suggests that managing patients with fluid and electrolyte intake in a gentle fashion without "flooding" the vascular component enables the kidney to do a masterful job of preserving bicarbonate in the extremely low birth weight neonate. The data are consistent with animal studies showing that the bicarbonate excretion is low in the absence of extracellular volume expansion. The low excretion of bicarbonate supports the authors' conclusion that renal bicarbonate loss cannot explain the metabolic acidosis of the extremely low birth weight neonate.

The normally functioning kidney performs 3 critical functions. First, and most important, is maintenance of extracellular volume. Second is maintenance of composition of the internal milieu. Third is the elimination of unnecessary water and solute. Clearly, the kidney operates under a set of priorities that enables extracellular volume to be maintained at the expense of concentration of solute. Also, if infants are to grow normally, there is a need to deposit carbonate in growing bone. Once the kidney takes over from the placenta, it is faced with the combined tasks of decreasing extracellular volume and preserving bicarbonate. The kidney, even in the extremely low birth weight infant, is both wise enough and able to do these 2 things simultaneously—something that many of us are unable to do.

Multiple mechanisms affect the preservation of bicarbonate. They include: factors that control glomerular tubular balance, the time after birth when the mechanisms involved in hydrogen ion secretion are able to lower the urine pH to levels lower than the pK of the bicarbonate buffer system (so that all of the filtered bicarbonate can be absorbed), and changes in the intrinsic resorptive capacity of both proximal and distal tubule. Because blood levels of bicarbonate—even after correcting for any potentially modulating effect of extracellular volume—are substantially lower in neonates and gradually rise to adult levels during the first decade of life, it is clear that the renal threshold, and the factors that influence it, maintain a lower set point for blood levels of bicarbonate in infants than adults. Volume expansion and contraction respectively depress and increase reabsorption of glomerular filtrate with its solutes, thereby modulating the renal threshold. The extracellular contraction after birth can be interpreted as one of many factors that might help to conserve filtered bicarbonate. Its occurrence may be particularly beneficial because it often takes a number of days after birth before urine pH drops below the pK of the bicarbonate buffer system.

As the cellular mechanisms, messengers, and transporters for hydrogen ion and bicarbonate are different from those for sodium, it should not surprise anyone that the reabsorption of the 2 solutes can occur independently. After all, sodium, chloride, and bicarbonate are only married to each other. Unfortunately, as we all know, divorce commonly occurs. Also, because the neonate is more likely after birth to experience acidosis than alkalosis, why should a wise kidney contribute to the process by allowing itself to be a bicarbonate waster?

In short, the neonatal kidney does what it is supposed to do: it allows for extracellular volume to decrease appropriately after birth while enabling maximal conservation of solute necessary for maximal growth to occur. We, as adults, would not be what we are if our kidneys had not done what was necessary while we were growing and if they had not been able to take care of the situation even when we were born prematurely.

A few difficulties in interpreting these data exist. It is not clear what proportion of the subjects needed volume expansion or pressor drugs. Both may alter renal function. Moreover, as pointed out by the authors, it is possible that bicarbonate reabsorption may have been overestimated. It is not clear whether the gas electrodes used had adequate accuracy and linearity in the measurement of the extremely low pCO_2 at the almost negligible urinary bicarbonate concentrations observed. Furthermore, the potential confounding influence of rapid equilibration of urine CO_2 was not determined. It is possible that some degree of CO_2 equilibration occurred during the 36 hours that elapsed between urine collection and laboratory measurement.

Nevertheless, the authors' conclusions and arguments impress me as being accurate and reasonable. This study provides further support to the idea that it is all right to be "kind and gentle" in the management of neonatal fluid and electrolyte requirements. Long live the kidneys!

A. Gruskin, M.D.

Congenital Adrenal Hyperplasia: Neonatal Mass Screening Compared With Clinical Diagnosis Only in the Emilia-Romagna Region of Italy, 1980-1995

Balsamo A, Cacciari E, Piazzi S, et al (Univ of Bologna, Italy; S Orsola Hosp, Bologna, Italy)

Pediatrics 98:362–367, 1996 13–3

Background.—Screening for congenital adrenal hyperplasia resulting from 21-hydroxylase deficiency (21ase-def CAH) has become relatively widespread, although its usefulness remains uncertain. A screening vs. case-survey only was performed in the Emilia-Romagna region of Italy to compare the results of neonatal mass screening with those of clinical diagnosis.

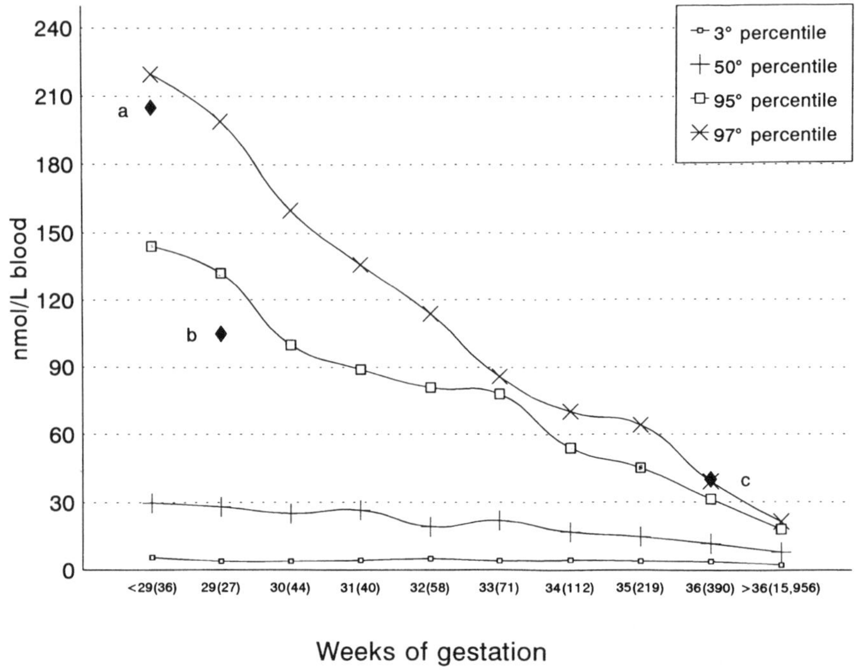

FIGURE 2.—Percentiles of 17α-hydroxyprogesterone values (nanomoles per liter of blood) according to gestational age *(number of patients in parentheses)*. The letters *a, b,* and *c* correspond to the spot value of the preterm congenital adrenal hyperplasia patients. (Reproduced by permission of *Pediatrics*, courtesy of Balsamo A, Cacciari E, Piazzi S, et al: Congenital adrenal hyperplasia: Neonatal mass screening compared with clinical diagnosis only in the Emilia-Romagna region of Italy, 1980–1995. *Pediatrics* 98:362–367, copyright 1996.)

Methods.—Screening for CAH was carried out from March 1980 to September 1983 (period A) and from March 1991 to the present (period C; data processed through August 1995). The neonatal mass screening was suspended from October 1983 to February 1991 (period B; 203,700 newborns). Coverage rates were 95% for period A (88,930 newborns) and 100% for period C (128,330 newborns). During period B, a case-survey program, still operative, was started. Detection of 21ase-def CAH cases was by a questionnaire sent to appropriate centers in the region. Screening used radioimmunoassay for 17α-hydroxyprogesterone (17α-OHP).

Results.—During the combined A and C periods, neonatal screening resulted in the diagnosis of 13 cases of classic 21ase-def CAH. Two false negative cases were found in these periods. Eight newborns with the disorder were identified in period B by case-survey. The overall incidence of classic 21ase-def CAH for the white population was 1:18,302. According to the periods examined, the incidence ranged from 1 in 15,518 newborns by screening to 1 in 25,462 when case-survey alone was used. The sensitivity and specificity of screening for classic CAH were 83% and 99.8%, respectively, for period A and 90% and 99.2%, respectively, for period C. A retrospective analysis of 16,953 consecutive tests performed in period C revealed that cutoff levels relating to gestational age were the best recall criterion for preterm neonates (Fig 2). Compared with case-survey only, the percentage of salt-wasting forms and the male-to-female ratio were higher during the screening period. Both detection methods identified cases of nonclassic 21ase-def CAH.

Discussion.—In many cases of 21ase-def CAH, a delay in diagnosis can be fatal. Eight of the 13 cases of classic CAH diagnosed by screening had not been clinically suspected. Without screening, some male patients may not be identified, and some mildly or even severely virilized female infants may be identified as boys. Even in areas with adequate neonatal services and screening programs, clinical observation for CAH should be continued.

▶ The neonatal metabolic screening programs have been very successful. Early detection prevents disastrous complications, including severe retardation and life-threatening crises. Screening for CAH, a rare disorder, is designed to identify these infants before they experience potentially life-threatening salt-wasting crises. Opinion is divided as to the usefulness of screening. This report by Balsamo and colleagues definitely favors screening. They have reported their extensive experience, including an 8-year period when screening was suspended. Direct assay of 17α-hydroxyprogesterone has made the testing quicker and simpler, with sensitivity and specificity exceeding 90%.

When case ascertainment was used, the incidence of CAH appeared to be 1 in 25,462 live births, but with screening, the incidence is 1 in 18,302 births. It is imperative to realize that even in an area with adequate and dedicated neonatal and endocrinologic services, "clinical diagnosis of classical CAH might be delayed or misinterpreted and salt-wasting crises could cause neonatal deaths." Screening is indispensable for a prompt diagnosis in more than 60% of the cases, particulary in the males. However, for the screening process to be effective, notification of positive results and prompt initiation of therapy are imperative. The neonatal screening programs continue to expand, and are an excellent investment of resources.[1] The optimal timing of initial screening must be documented because many neonates require repeated screening because of shorter hospital stays (see Abstract 15–5).

Believing where we cannot prove.—Tennyson

A.A. Fanaroff, M.B.B.Ch.

Reference

1. Committee on Genetics: Newborn screening fact sheets. *Pediatrics* 98:473–501, 1996.

Influence of Bilirubin on Surface Tension Properties of Lung Surfactant
Amato M, Schürch S, Grunder R, et al (Univ of Berne, Switzerland; Univ of Calgary, Alberta Canada)
Arch Dis Child 75:F191–F196, 1996 13–4

Objective.—Exogenous surfactant therapy can reduce the severity and mortality of neonatal respiratory distress syndrome (RDS). However, this treatment fails in up to 30% of infants. In infants with RDS with hyperbilirubinemia, bilirubin can leak into the alveolar space from capillaries, causing so-called yellow hyaline membrane disease. Little is known about how bilirubin in the lung might affect the surface activity of surfactant. Bilirubin's effects on the surface tension activity of 2 different lung surfactants were investigated in vitro.

Methods.—The surfactants studied were the porcine-derived surfactant Curosurf and the synthetic surfactant Exosurf. A captive bubble surfactometer was used to determine the effects of phospholipid and bilirubin, in varying concentrations, on the surface-tension–lowering properties of these surfactants. The study focused on the compression of film area needed to achieve minimum surface tension.

Results.—In the absence of bilirubin, surface tension activity was higher with Curosurf than with Exosurf. Values for area compression were 30% vs. 76%, respectively, at low surfactant dose, and 25% vs. 85% at high surfactant dose. At the concentrations studied, 0.25–1.0 mg/mL, bilirubin had negligible surface activity. At a phospholipid dose of 0.5 mg of Curosurf per mL, bilirubin increased the film area compression of lipid extract surfactant from 30% to 55% at a bilirubin concentration of 0.25 mg/mL, 59% at a bilirubin concentration of 0.5 mg/mL, and 68% at a bilirubin concentration of 1.0 mg/mL. A similar but less marked adverse effect on film area compression of porcine lipid extract surfactant was noted at a phospholipid dose of 1.0 mg of Curosurf per mL. (25% to 26%, 39%, and 44%, respectively). Bilirubin caused no further reduction of the surface tension properties of Exosurf at any phospholipid dose.

Conclusion.—Bilirubin impairs the surface tension properties of porcine lipid extract surfactant in vitro, this study finds. It has no significant effect on the already low surface activity of synthetic surfactant, however. The findings suggest the need for more aggressive management of hyperbilirubinemia in infants with RDS, including treatment with lipid extract surfactant.

▶ Amato and associates remind us, once again, of the interaction of bilirubin with surface-active materials. Although the observation is not fundamentally new, the authors suggest a vulnerability of extract surfactant compared with synthetic surfactant. Although mechanisms are hypothesized for the adverse effect of bilirubin on extract surfactant, further studies are needed to determine whether surfactant-associated proteins (SP-B or SP-C) interact with bilirubin in ways that affect adsorption, spreading, or squeeze out. This study prudently suggests that a more aggressive approach to neonatal hyperbilirubinemia in the presence of RDS, or a more aggressive approach to RDS in infants with hyperbilirubinemia and treated with lipid extract surfactant, is warranted. Whether any of these observations have a consequence in vivo in the human neonate with yellow hyaline membranes remains a matter of speculation.

D.K. Stevenson, M.D.

Bilirubin Has Widespread Inhibitory Effects on Protein Phosphorylation

Hansen TWR, Mathiesen SBW, Walaas SI (Univ of Oslo, Norway; Univ of Pittsburgh, Pa)

Pediatr Res 39:1072–1077, 1996 13–5

Background.—Bilirubin may produce neurotoxic effects by modulating neuronal protein phosphorylation systems. The mechanism of bilirubin-induced inhibition of protein phosphorylation was studied.

Methods and Findings.—In vitro phosphorylation assays and a variety of protein substrates and purified protein kinases were used. Bilirubin-inhibited cyclic adenosine monophosphate (cAMP)-dependent, cyclic guanosine monophosphate (cGMP)-dependent, Ca^{2+}-calmodulin-dependent, and Ca^{2+}-phospholipid-dependent protein kinases, regardless of substrate properties. Bilirubin concentrations of 20–125 μmol resulted in 50% inhibition. Kinetic analysis was done using the isolated catalytic subunit of cAMP-dependent kinase and a synthetic peptide substrate derived from the protein phospholemman. Bilirubin, 50 μmol, reduced the apparent maximum velocity of the reaction, regardless of whether adenosine triphosphate or peptide concentrations were varied, without significantly changing the apparent K_m value.

Conclusions.—Bilirubin inhibits the phosphorylation of several proteins that are catalyzed by a number of protein kinases. The underlying mechanism may be a general noncompetitive one. Because protein phosphorylation plays a central role in regulating and controlling cellular metabolic processes, some of bilirubin's toxic effects on the cell may be mediated through such protein phosphorylation inhibition.

► That bilirubin can cause brain toxicity should not be disputed further. However, uncertainty exists about the conditions under which the neurotoxic effects of bilirubin occur and what determines the permanence of brain damage or death in the syndrome of kernicterus. Morever, ignorance is not a good companion of confidence, regardless of the opinion held. The experiments by Hansen et al. are intriguing in that they support the hypothesis that the neurotoxic effects of bilirubin may involve modulation of neuronal protein phosphorylation systems. The widespread nature of bilirubin effects indicates that inhibition of protein phosphorylation is consistent with the expectation that a variety of cellular processes might be affected. The clever twist in these experiments is that the inhibitory effects were observed in the absence of respiratory enzymes or organelles, suggesting that the effects are not solely attributable to bilirubin-induced inhibition of oxidative phosphorylation[1] and that a direct effect of bilirubin on protein phosphorylation must be considered.

Unlike previous experiments, the bilirubin concentrations used were within the range found in strongly jaundiced foci in the brains of kernicteric newborns. Although the information is derived from in vitro experimentation, the fact that bilirubin inhibits the phosphorylation of several proteins catalyzed by a number of protein kinases, possibly by a general noncompetitive mechanism, is like a "smoking gun." However, what makes the gun go off in a particularly unlikely instance remains an unsolved mystery. Of course, if one plays with guns, accidents are more likely to happen, even if infrequently. Similarly, not every infant with a high bilirubin concentration will have kernicterus develop; however, if high levels of bilirubin are allowed to occur, then kernicterus will be more likely.

D.K. Stevenson, M.D.

Reference

1. Hansen TWR, Bratlid D, Walaas SI: Bilirubin decreases phosphorylation of synapsin I, a synaptic vesical-associated neuronal phosphoprotein, in intact synaptosomes from rat cerebral cortex. *Pediatr Res* 23:219–223, 1988.

Outcome of Severe Congenital Hypothyroidism: Closing the Developmental Gap With Early High Dose Levothyroxine Treatment

Dubuis J-M, Glorieux J, Richer F, et al (Univ of Montreal; Université Laval, Quebec, Canada)

J Clin Endocrinol Metab 81:222–227, 1996 13–6

Introduction.—Screening for congenital hypothyroidism permits early intervention to prevent mental retardation. However, newborns with severe congenital hypothyroidism still may be left with significant intellectual impairment, even after treatment with levothyroxine at a dosage of 6 µg/kg/day. The effects of earlier treatment with higher doses of levothyroxine were assessed in newborns with severe congenital hypothyroidism.

Methods.—The study included 45 infants with screen-detected, permanent congenital hypothyroidism. The infants started treatment at a median age of 14 days and a median initial levothyroxine dosage of 11.6 µg/kg/day. Ten infants had severe hypothyroidism, defined as an area of the knee epiphyses of less than 0.05 cm^2; the rest were considered to have moderate hypothyroidism. At 18 months of age, psychomotor development was assessed in 8 children from each group. The children were matched for family socioeducational level.

Results.—The infants had above-normal mean plasma free levothyroxine levels during the first few months of life. However, their mean plasma triiodothyronine levels were normal and they had no evidence of hyperthyroidism. Four weeks after the start of treatment, the children's mean plasma thyroid-stimulating hormone level was less than 4.5 mIU/L. Patients with severe hypothyroidism still had delayed bone maturation at 1 year. There was no difference in the mean development quotient at 18 months' follow-up: 107 for the severe group and 110 for the moderate group.

Conclusions.—Earlier treatment with a higher dose of levothyroxine can improve the developmental outcomes for newborns with severe congenital hypothyroidism. With this treatment, the outcomes are the same as for patients with moderate hypothyroidism. Longer follow-up in larger numbers of patients is needed to confirm the results. An initial levothyroxine dosage of 10–15 µg/kg/day causes no apparent problems with iatrogenic hyperthyroidism.

► In the fetus, normal brain development is dependent on adequate thyroid hormone levels. Before the introduction of systematic neonatal screening for congenital hypothyroidism, this condition was a major cause of mental retardation. Screening substantially reduced the associated morbidity and intellectual deficits; however, depending on the severity of the hypothyroidism at the time of diagnosis, the infants may still turn out to be intellectually subpar and 10% may require special education, as compared with 40% of hypothyroid infants before screening.[1] Critical factors in the long-term outcome include age at diagnosis and appropriateness of therapy. Dubuis and colleagues appear to have improved the outcome for infants with severe congenital hypothyroidism through the use of an earlier onset of therapy with higher doses of levothyroxine, verifying the approach suggested by Fisher and Foley.[2] The latter authors previously had documented a 13-point deficit in intelligence quotient for infants with severe hypothyroidism in whom less aggressive therapy was started at 5 weeks of life, in contrast with the current series of infants, who were first treatea at 2 weeks of life.

Whereas there remains little doubt about the benefits of earlier therapy, the debate about the dosage persists. Infants with moderate congenital hypothyroidism may not need higher dosages, and the dosage also is dependent on the underlying etiology. Concerns regarding iatrogenic hyperthyroidism, craniosynotosis, and psychomotor retardation were based on massive (up to 500-mg/day) dosages of levothyroxine but appear to be unwarranted with dosages of 10–15 mg/kg/day.

This encouraging report, wherein the developmental gap between severe and moderate congenital hypothyroidism was narrowed by the combination of earlier onset of therapy and a higher dosage of levothyroxine, needs validation. Disease severity is estimated from bone maturation and/or plasma levothyroxine levels at the time of diagnosis and from etiologic diagnosis or screening. A knee epiphysis of less than 0.05 cm^2 at diagnosis was used to define severe congenital hypothyroidism in the present study.

A.A. Fanaroff, M.B.B.Ch.

References

1. Tillotson SL, Fuggle PW, Smith I, et al: Relation between biochemical severity and intelligence in early treated congenital hypothyroidism: A threshold effect. *BMJ* 309:440–445, 1994.
2. Fisher DA, Foley BL: Early treatment of congenital hypothyroidism. *Pediatrics* 83:785–789, 1989.

Dual-energy X-ray Absorptiometry Studies of Bone Mineral Status in Newborn Infants

Koo WWK, Walters J, Bush AJ, et al (Univ of Tennessee, Memphis)
J Bone Miner Res 11:997–1002, 1996 13–7

Background.—Dual-energy x-ray absorptiometry (DEXA), a generally accepted noninvasive tool for determining bone mineralization in vivo, is being increasingly used in children. This technique has also been successfully adapted for measuring whole-body bone mineral status in neonates. However, the normative data available for neonates are very limited. The total body and regional bone mineralization of human newborns was documented.

Methods.—One hundred fifty singleton newborn infants, weighing 1,002–3,990 g and aged 2–42 weeks' gestation, were assessed using DEXA. Eighty-five infants were preterm, and 79 were of low birth weight. The predictive value of anthropometric measurements, race, and sex on bone mineral status variability was also determined. A whole-body DEXA scanner with a pediatric platform was used.

Findings.—The continuous independent variables, gestational age, birth weight, study weight, study bare weight, and study length, were very significantly correlated. A highly significant correlation was also found between independent and each of the dependent variables, total body bone mineral content, total body area, and total body bone mineral density. Body weight was the best single determinant of bone mineral status. The inclusion of postnatal age (during the first week after birth), race, sex, or season did not further explain bone mineral status.

Conclusion.—Dual-energy x-ray absorptiometry can be performed even in small preterm infants in the newborn period. These findings will be useful in future reasearch on conditions that may affect bone mineralization in infants.

▶ Although we try hard to provide optimal enteral and parenteral nutrition, we still see abnormalities of bone mineralization and their consequences in the extremely premature infants now surviving in our nurseries. It comes as no surprise that the most important predictor of bone mineral status is body weight, but what the technique of DEXA allows us to do is to quantify total body mineralization and thus see how we can influence mineralization. Ultimately, we want to prevent the pathologic demineralization that occurs in tiny infants, and the ability to measure the outcome is an essential step toward realizing this goal.

M.J. Maisels, M.B., B.Ch.

Early Management and Postnatal Investigation of Prenatally Diagnosed Hydronephrosis

Owen RJT, Lamont AC, Brookes J (Leicester Gen Hosp, England)
Clin Radiol 51:173–176, 1996 13–8

Introduction.—Patients with antenatally detected hydronephrosis require close follow-up. The value and ease of implementing an investiga-

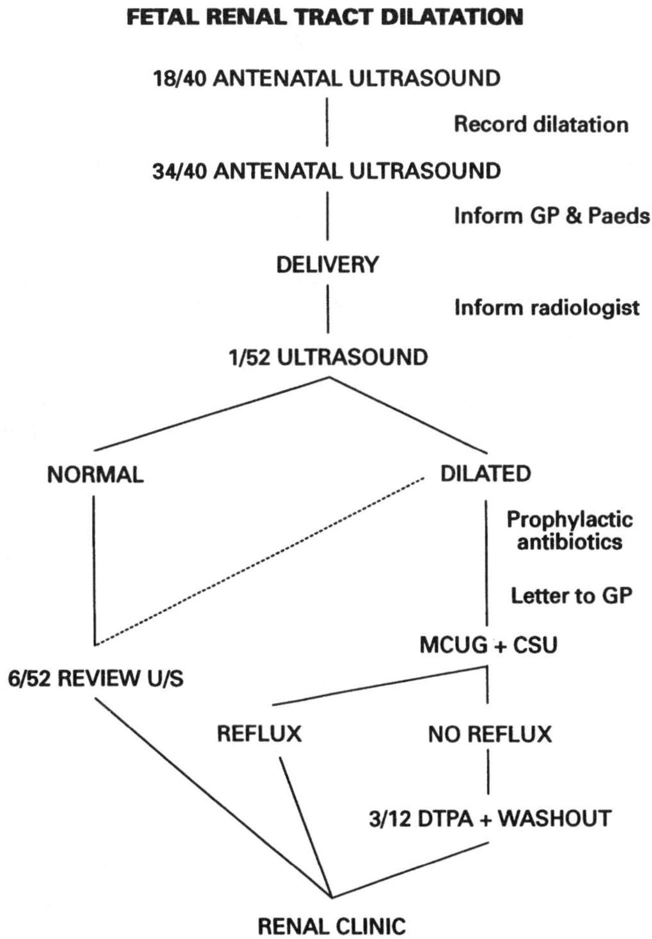

FIGURE 2.—Algorithm for investigation of fetal renal tract dilatation detected in utero. *Abbreviations: CSU,* catheter specimen of urine; *DTPA,* diethylenetriamine pentaacetic acid; *GP,* general practitioner; *MCUG,* micturating cystourethrogram; *Paeds,* pediatrician; *u/s,* ultrasound. (Courtesy of Owen RJT, Lamont AC, Brookes J: Early management and postnatal investigation of prenatally diagnosed hydronephrosis. *Clin Radiol* 51:173–176, 1996.)

TABLE 1.—Results of Screening Program

Pregnancies screened	3809
antenatal hydronephrosis at 18–20 weeks	80
antenatal hydronephrosis at 34 weeks	57
Postnatal hydronephrosis	35
pelvi-ureteric junction obstruction	6
vesico-ureteric reflux	4
multicystic dysplastic kidneys	5
functional assymmetry on renogram	2
large volume nonobstructed systems	14
lost to follow-up	4

(Courtesy of Owen RJT, Lamont AC, Brookes J: Early management and postnatal investigation of prenatally diagnosed hydronephrosis. *Clin Radiol* 51:173–176, 1996.)

tional protocol to reduce hospital visits and increase the efficiency of detection and follow-up of congenital hydronephrosis was evaluated.

Methods.—A detailed investigational protocol was established for antenatal fetal hydronephrosis. For 1 year, all pregnant women with fetal anomaly US examinations or dilatation of the renal pelvis at 18–20 weeks' gestation were reexamined at 34 weeks' gestation. Dilatation was considered to be present if the maximum anteroposterior diameter of the renal pelvis was 5 mm or greater (Fig 2). If the renal pelvis was 8mm or greater at 34-week follow-up, patients were entered into the trial. Fetuses with prenatally diagnosed hydronephrosis underwent US examination within 1 week of birth and at 6 weeks of age.

Results.—Renal pelvis dilatation was identified in 80 (2.1%) of 3,809 pregnancies (3,811 live births) at 18 weeks' gestation. Of these, 23 were normal on US examination at 34 weeks' gestation. Another 23 fetuses had a normal US at 1 week of age. Twenty-two of these 23 findings were normal at 6 weeks of age. The 35 remaining infants underwent further evaluation. Multicystic dysplastic kidneys were identified and confirmed by technetium-99m dimercaptosuccinic acid scintigraphy in 5 infants. Of 30 direct micturating cystograms performed, 4 revealed reflux. The 26 patients without reflux underwent ^{99m}Tc diethylenetriamine pentaacetic acid renography. Of these, 6 had a pelvi-ureteric junction obstruction, 4 had some functional asymmetry, and 14 had large-volume nonobstructed systems (Table 1). Using this protocol, hospital visits were reduced by about 66%.

Conclusions.—Antenatal US screening allows the identification of uropathies that will require further investigation postnatally and can identify potentially lethal urologic abnormalities. Early management of congenital hydronephrosis within the radiology department is a realistic way to avoid unnecessary referrals and produce significant cost savings.

Prognostic Significance of Antenatally Detected Fetal Pyelectasis
Ouzounian JG, Castro MA, Fresquez M, et al (Univ of Southern California, Los Angeles)
Ultrasound Obstet Gynecol 7:424–428, 1996 13–9

Introduction.—Fewer than 25% of infants with congenital hydronephrosis have the condition diagnosed within their first year of life. Ultrasonographic identification of pyelectasis in utero may minimize diagnostic delays and potentially reduce morbidity in fetuses at risk for hydronephrosis. The prognostic implications of ultrasonographically detected fetal pyelectasis were evaluated to establish useful clinical guidelines for perinatal management.

Methods.—Ninety-eight fetal kidneys from 84 patients were evaluated for fetal pyelectasis in a 24-month retrospective record review. Fetal hydronephrosis was defined as ultrasonographically detected fetal calyceal dilatation (pyelectasis) of 5 mm or greater, measured in the anteroposterior diameter of a transverse section through fetal kidneys. This low threshold was used so that minimal, but potentially significant, dilation would not be overlooked.

Results.—Fetal pyelectasis was found more frequently in the left than the right kidney, and in males than in females. Of 84 fetuses, 48 (57.1%) with pyelectasis had hydronephrosis after birth (Table 1). Consistent with prenatal US, neonatal hydronephrosis was more common in the left kidney. Thirteen infants (15.4%) with hydronephrosis underwent surgical pyeloplasty at a mean age of 6 months (range, 3–18 months). Fetal pyelectasis of 8 mm had a sensitivity of 91% and a specificity of 72% in predicting subsequent neonatal hydronephrosis. With a threshold of 5 mm, the sensitivity was 100% and specificity was 28%. Six patients with fetal pyelectasis had unexplained high maternal serum α-fetoprotein (MSAFP) levels, and 3 of these 6 who underwent prenatal amniocentesis had normal amniotic fluid α-fetoprotein levels. Three of 6 patients with high MSAFP levels had pregnancy-induced hypertension. Of these, 2 underwent induction of labor at 37 weeks' gestation for intrauterine growth retardation and oligohydramnios, respectively. None of the infants with high MSAFP levels had subsequent hydronephrosis.

TABLE 1.—Mean (± SD) Values of Ultrasonographically Measured Fetal Pyelectasis Correlated With Gestational Age and the Presence or Absence of Hydronephrosis

	Neonatal hydronephrosis					
		Absent			*Present*	
	n	*< 33 weeks*	*> 33 weeks*	*n*	*< 33 weeks*	*> 33 weeks*
Left pyelectasis (mm)	28	5.7 ± 1.4	7.6 ± 2.4	30	17.0 ± 8.4	16.9 ± 8.5
range		4–8	4–10		5–26	5–34
Right pyelectasis (mm)	8	6.2 ± 1.7	5.5 ± 1.9	18	15.4 ± 3.3	17.1 ± 5.1
range		4–8	4–9		10–24	5–36

(Courtesy of Ouzounian JG, Castro MA, Fresquez M, et al: Prognostic significance of antenatally detected fetal pyelectasis. *Ultrasound Obstet Gynecol* 7:424–428, 1996.)

Conclusions.—A fetal pyelectasis of 5 mm was 100% sensitive in identifying potential hydronephrosis. A finding of fetal pyelectasis of 5 mm at any gestational age is reason for follow-up US examinations and detailed postnatal evaluation.

▶ Abnormalities of the urinary tract are common, accounting for a high percentage of fetal anomalies. There has been a loose consensus that pathologic dilatation of the upper urinary tract should be diagnosed when the renal pelvis is 10 mm or greater. Ouzounian and colleagues (Abstract 13–9) observed that fetal pyelectasis was more common in the left kidney and in males. From their records, when fetal pyelectasis was called at 8 mm, the sensitivity was 91% and the specificity was 72%. Reducing the threshhold to 5 mm yields the ideal sensitivity of 100%, but diminishes the specificity to 24%. Dudley and colleagues[1] reviewed their findings from US on 18,766 patients during a 5-year period commencing in 1990. Antenatal hydronephrosis, defined as an anteroposterior diameter of the renal pelvis greater than 5 mm, was detected in 100 fetuses (0.59%). Sixty-four had postnatal hydronephrosis at 1 week, 6 weeks, or both after delivery; 21 had urologic anomalies. They reported that vesicoureteric reflux was the most common urologic finding and would be missed if the cutoff for investigation of antenatal hydronephrosis is kept at 10 mm. However, setting the threshold for re-investigation at 5 mm will overdiagnose the condition and lead to a lot of unnecessary parental anxiety.

The presence of fetal pyelectasis leaves clinicians with a multitude of options as they wend their way through a complex algorithm such as the one in Figure 2 from the report by Owen and associates (Abstract 13–8). If fetal hydronephrosis is confirmed, then the family history must be reviewed in detail and careful examination of the bladder, other organs, and amniotic fluid undertaken. A karyotype may be indicated. Most situations call for serial US; however, if there is bilateral hydronephrosis and oligohydramnios, early intervention and delivery may be warranted. Postnatal scans, voiding cystourethrograms, and renal scans will dictate the optimal course of management. Bear in mind that US is an unreliable way to diagnose reflux. Renal function may be lost as a result of obstruction, infection, or both. Therefore, chemoprophylaxis is recommended for all infants with postnatal renal dilatation.

Early recognition and intervention (postnatally) will enhance the prospects for preserving renal function. Nobody wants to miss a diagnosis, but overinterpreting US findings provokes anger and anxiety. It is important for perinatal health care providers to use the appropriate consultants and to function as a well-coordinated team with all the team members on the same page, keeping the lines of communication between the providers and with the family wide open.

A.A. Fanaroff, M.B.B.Ch.

Reference

1. Dudley JA, Haworth JM, McGraw ME, et al: Clinical relevance and implications of antenatal hydronephrosis. *Arch Dis Child* 76:F31–F34, 1997.

14 Developmental Pharmacology and Toxicology

Impact on Blood Pressure and Intestinal Perfusion of Dobutamine or Dopamine in Hypotensive Preterm Infants

Hentschel R, Hensel D, Brune T, et al (Univ Children's Hosp, Münster, Germany)

Biol Neonate 68:318–324, 1995 14–1

Background.—Oxygen supply to the gut is critical in hypotensive states. This is thought to play a major role as an ischemic factor in the pathogenesis of necrotizing enterocolitis in high-risk infants. Treatment of hypotension in infants sometimes includes catecholamine infusion with dobutamine or dopamine. The effect of dobutamine and dopamine on blood pressure and intestinal perfusion in hypotensive preterm infants was investigated.

Methods.—Twenty preterm infants with protracted arterial hypotension refractory to volume therapy were studied prospectively. Dobutamine or dopamine, 10 µg/kg/min, was administered. Doppler US of the superior

TABLE 2.—Hemodynamic Variables Before and During Treatment With Dobutamine or Dopamine

	Treatment group			
	dobutamine		dopamine	
	before	during	before	during
MAP, mm Hg	31.0 ± 6.8*	37.7 ± 9.8	27.7 ± 3.6*	36.0 ± 9.3
Heart rate, bpm	133 ± 17*	152 ± 16	141 ± 16	153 ± 20
V_m, cm/s	25.8 ± 13.5*	31.5 ± 16.0	16.3 ± 5.0	19.0 ± 6.0
PI	0.81 ± 0.07*	0.74 ± 0.11	0.89 ± 0.06*	0.79 ± 0.07

Note: Values are given as mean plus or minus standard error of the mean. There were 10 infants in each treatment group.
*Difference before and after treatment was statistically significant for $P < 0.05$.
Abbreviation: MAP, mean arterial pressure.
(Courtesy of Hentschel R, Hensel D, Brune T, et al: Impact on blood pressure and intestinal perfusion of dobutamine or dopamine in hypotensive preterm infants. *Biol Neonate* 68:318–324, 1995, S. Karger AG, Basel.)

mesenteric artery was performed to verify intestinal perfusion. Blood pressure also was recorded.

Findings.—Both groups had significant increases in mean arterial pressure. Mean blood flow velocity increased from 25.8 to 31.5 cm/sec after dobutamine, and from 16.3 to 19 cm/sec after dopamine. (The increase for dobutamine was significant.) The vascular resistance of the superior mesenteric artery declined from a mean of 0.81 to 0.74 for dobutamine and from 0.89 to 0.79 for dopamine, both of which were significant (Table 2)

Conclusions.—Both of these catecholamines in the dosages tested are equally effective in increasing mean arterial pressure. Both significantly increase intestinal perfusion. Thus, these agents probably do not have a negative effect on mesenteric blood supply that predisposes infants to necrotizing enterocolitis.

▶ Comment prepared by M.D. Reed, Pharm.D., Professor of Pediatrica, Case Western Reserve University and Director, Pediatric Clinical Pharmacology and Toxicology, Rainbow Babies and Childrens Hospital, Cleveland, Ohio:

▶ The catecholamines, dopamine and dobutamine, commonly are used in critically ill newborn infants. Although these 2 agents possess different pharmacologic effects as a result of their actions on different adrenergic receptors, in practice, they often are used interchangeably. The vast majority of data that have addressed the different effects of these 2 compounds relative to age and the neonate have been obtained in animals; only very limited data assessing the differential effects of dopamine and dobutamine in human preterm and full-term infants are available. An understanding of the pharmacologic effects of these 2 agents, partilcularly their effects on regional blood flow, would seem to be of paramount importance in determining their use in critically ill, preterm and full-term infants at risk for the development of necrotizing enterocolitis.

In a prospective evaluation, 20 consecutive preterm infants with arterial hypotension were randomly assigned to receive either 10 μg/kg/min of dopamine or dobutamine (median 28 weeks' gestation and 1 day postnatal age at the time of the study, for both groups) by electric infusion pump. All patients received volume infusion (10 mL/kg) and were enrolled in this study if they remained hypotensive 1 hour afterward. With the infants supine, immediately before and 30–45 minutes after starting the catecholamine infusion, Doppler US was performed on the superior mesenteric artery, allowing determination of the study's primary outcome variables of systolic maximum velocity, end-diastolic maximum velocity, mean maximum velocity, and resistance index; the other important hemodynamic outcome variables (systolic, diastolic, and mean arterial pressures, and heart rate) were determined by oscillometry or pressure transducer and by routine measurements of partial pressure of carbon dioxide, partial pressure of oxygen, and pH. The study infants ranged in age from 25 to 36 weeks' gestation and from 2 hours to 17 days postnatal age; no differences were identified between the treatment groups relative to birth weight (range, 830 to 2,610 g), actual body weight, or age. All study infants received artificial ventilatory support throughout the study. Overall, the mean arterial pressure increased significantly for both groups (mean [±SD]), from 31 (±6.8) to 37.7 (±9.8) mm Hg with dobutamine, and from 27.7 (±3.6) to 36 (±9.3) mm Hg with dopamine. The heart rate also increased from 133 (±17) to 152 (±16) beats/min and from 141 (±16) to 153 (±2) beats/min in the dobutamine and dopamine groups, respectively. Further, the mean maximal flow velocity and the resistance index fell in both treatment groups. These findings demonstrate that both drugs administered at a dosage of 10 µg/kg/min were equally effective in raising mean arterial pressure and significantly increasing intestinal perfusion, suggesting that neither drug should have a negative influence on mesenteric blood flow or predispose a patient to the development of necrotizing enterocolitis.

Since their introduction to clinical medicine, both dopamine and dobutamine have been and continue to be used extensively in the neonatal and pediatric ICUs. Despite their widespread use and numerous publications regarding their clinical pharmacology in infants and children, many questions persist as to the comparative attributes of these agents in pediatric patients of all ages. Both drugs are complex-acting pharmacologic agents. The cardiovascular effects of dopamine are mediated by several distinct receptors that vary in their affinity for the drug. At low dosages, dopamine stimulates dopamine-I receptors located in the renal, mesenteric, and coronary beds. At moderate dosages, dopamine exerts a positive inotropic effect as a result of its stimulation of β_1-adrenergic receptors, and at high dosages, dopamine raises systemic vascular resistance by stimulating α_1-adrenergic receptors. In contrast, the dose-related pharmacologic effects of dobutamine result from the drug's complex effects on the α- and β-adrenergic receptors. (Dobutamine is a racemic mixture. The 2 enantiomers have differing receptor effects that can be additive or antagonistic with each other.) The present study attempted to determine the pharmacologic differences between these 2 clinically important catecholamines in a group of hypotensive preterm infants. The authors' finding that there were no differences between the 2 drugs in the important hemodynamic parameters determined must be interpreted relative to the study design. This study used the same dosage, 10 µg/kg/min, for both drugs. To assess for differences between the 2 drugs, a prospective, comparative study incorporating sequentially increasing dosages (i.e., a dose-ranging study) would need to be performed to account for the important dose-dependent effects of each of these complex pharmacologic agents. The results of an ongoing double-blind, comparative, dose-ranging study being performed in our own pediatric ICU hopefully will address these important questions in older infants and children. Such a study needs to be performed in the neonatal ICU. Until then, it would appear that neither dopamine nor dobutamine poses a tremendous risk of predisposing hypotensive preterm infants to the development of necrotizing enterocolitis.

M.D. Reed, Pharm.D.

Ampicillin for Neonatal Group B Streptococcal Prophylaxis: How Rapidly Can Bactericidal Concentrations Be Achieved?

Bloom SL, Cox SM, Bawdon RE, et al (Univ of Texas, Dallas)
Am J Obstet Gynecol 175:974–976, 1996 14–2

Background.—Although several strategies have been proposed to interrupt group B streptococci transmission to the neonate, the prevention of early-onset sepsis is still controversial. It is not known whether ampicillin, given within 1 hour of delivery, reaches significant concentrations in the fetus. How rapidly bactericidal concentrations of ampicillin for group B streptococci are reached in maternal and fetal sera and amniotic fluid was investigated.

Methods.—Ampicillin was given to 40 women at various intervals between 3 and 67 minutes before elective cesarean delivery. Amniotic fluid samples were obtained by amniocentesis just before the uterine incision was made, and umbilical and maternal serum samples were acquired at delivery.

Findings.—The average levels of ampicillin in maternal and umbilical cord sera exceeded the minimum bactericidal concentrations reported for group B streptococci. These levels were achieved as soon as 5 minutes after ampicillin was infused. Bactericidal concentrations of ampicillin in the amniotic fluid were also detectable as early as 5 minutes. However, these amniotic fluid levels were achieved in only 85% of the pregnancies.

Conclusions.—Bactericidal levels of ampicillin in fetal blood and amniotic fluid are usually achieved within 5 minutes after a standard maternal dose of 2 g. Thus, neonatal prophylaxis should not be withheld when delivery is imminent.

► "We must use our time as a tool, not as a couch," according to John F. Kennedy. Ampicillin doesn't waste any time crossing from the mother's circulation to the fetus and into the amniotic fluid. Bactericidal levels (greater than 2 µg per mL of ampicillin), defined as the lowest concentration of antimicrobial that kills more than 99% of the bacterial inoculum, were achieved as soon as 3 minutes after the ampicillin infusion is started. Who needs anything faster? However, for unknown reasons, bactericidal concentrations, easily achieved in maternal and fetal serum within 5 minutes, were achieved in the amniotic fluid in only 85% of pregnancies studied. The clinical relevance of these findings was debated by the authors, who noted that "some strains of group B streptococci are not sterilized until 20 to 24 hours in the presence of 1 or even 10 µg/mL ampicillin." Furthermore, if the streptococci have invaded and injured fetal tissues, the situation is not rapidly reversible. Now that we know the pharmacokinetics of ampicillin, the Centers for Disease Control and Prevention has recommended penicillin for prophylaxis; presumably the time frames would be the same.[1] No doubt this will induce further pharmacodynamic studies. (See Abstracts 3–10 and 5–13).

A.A. Fanaroff, M.B.B.Ch.

Reference

1. Schuchat A, Whitney C, Zangwill K: Prevention of perinatal group B streptococcal disease. A public perspective. *MMWR Morb Mortal Wkly Rep* 45:1–24, 1996.

Effect of Drugs on Chemoreceptor Responsiveness in Fetal Sheep

Boekkooi PF, Baan J Jr, Teitel DF, et al (Univ of California, San Francisco)
Pediatr Res 38:938–943, 1995 14–3

Background.—The drugs used during labor may affect chemoreceptor function, thus altering the heart rate response to hypoxemia. The effects of ketamine, morphine, and pentobarbital and of the β-adrenoreceptor blocker propranolol on chemoreceptor responsiveness were examined in unanesthetized fetal sheep.

Methods and Findings.—Eleven fetal lambs of 125–133 days' gestational age were studied. All were chronically instrumented with a catheter in a hindlimb artery and vein and in a forelimb artery. In 6 fetuses, a carotid arterial oximeter catheter was placed. An inflatable cuff occluder was applied around the maternal hypogastric artery and acute fetal hypoxemia was induced repeatedly by decreasing uterine blood flow. Ketamine and morphine were found to markedly attenuate the chemoreflex response. However, neither pentobarbital nor propranolol affected chemoreflex response.

Conclusion.—Some drugs can blunt the cardiovascular response to hypoxemia. Thus, caution is needed when interpreting heart rate responses to hypoxemia in the fetuses of mothers given these agents.

► Commenting on this article is William E. Benitz, M.D., Associate Professor of Pediatrics, Clinical Director of Intensive Care Nursery, Division of Neonatal and Developmental Medicine, Stanford University School of Medicine, Palo Alto, California:

► This demonstration of drug-induced blunting of fetal chemoreceptor responses to hypoxia should raise concern not only regarding obscuration of such stresses from detection by fetal heart rate monitoring, but also regarding potential sequelae of impairment of fetal and neonatal protective chemoreceptor reflexes during drug exposures. The recent report that halothane accentuates hypocarbia-induced cerebral vasoconstriction in cats indicates that therapeutic agents may also *augment* homeostatic chemoreceptor reflexes. Such altered homeostasis may be hazardous to the health of our patients, and it behooves us to be aware that we often get much more than we desire from the medications we give them.

W.E. Benitz, M.D.

Saliva as a Valid Alternative to Serum in Monitoring Intravenous Caffeine Treatment for Apnea of Prematurity

Lee TC, Charles BG, Steer PA, et al (Univ of Queensland, Australia; Mater Mother's Hosp, Brisbane, Australia)

Ther Drug Monit 18:288–293, 1996 14–4

Objective.—Caffeine, with its low toxicity and long terminal half-life, is a potentially useful alternative to theophylline for the treatment and prevention of apnea of prematurity. There are few data by which to determine the dose-response relationship of caffeine in these patients. Particularly in very ill premature newborns, monitoring of saliva caffeine concentrations would be a less invasive alternative than blood sampling. Serum and saliva caffeine content were compared in premature infants receiving IV caffeine therapy for apnea of prematurity.

Methods.—Fifty-nine premature newborns were studied. They were randomized to receive caffeine citrate in a dose of 3, 15, or 30 mg/kg once daily for 7 days; treatment started with a loading dose of twice the maintenance dose. A total of 131 serum and saliva pairs were collected and tested by high-performance liquid chromatography for caffeine content. The precision and bias of these measurements were statistically analyzed.

Results.—Caffeine concentrations of 0.28 to 93.3 mg/L were measured in serum, compared with 0.35 to 91.5 mg/L in saliva. The mean ratio of the serum caffeine concentrations to the saliva caffeine concentrations was 0.924; the measurements were not significantly different in precision. Mean caffeine concentrations were 29.9 mg/L in serum vs. 27.7 mg/L in saliva.

Conclusion.—Saliva sampling may avoid the need for blood sampling in monitoring caffeine therapy for apnea of prematurity. This noninvasive monitoring technique will be especially valuable in very low birth weight infants.

▶ As research on caffeine treatment for apnea of prematurity continues, an alternative introduced in the 1970s is again becoming popular. This article by Lee et al. suggests that monitoring of caffeine concentrations can be less invasive, contributing further to the ease of this alternative pharmacologic treatment of infants. The article confirms the fact that salivary caffeine concentration monitoring is a satisfactory alternative to blood sampling across a wide range of caffeine doses used to treat apnea.

However, nothing is perfect. The authors point out that, although there is no significant difference in precision between the serum and salivary data, the mean serum caffeine concentration exceeded the corresponding mean salivary concentrations by a small amount. The authors interpreted this as possibly being the difference between measuring the total concentration of the drug in serum and measuring the concentration in saliva which was indicative of only the free concentration in serum. No confirming data were supplied. A few other factors were also considered, such as time of sampling and the practical disadvantage of the time required for sample collection in premature infants (5–30 minutes). Also, be aware of the java-drinking mother for a possible contribution to the caffeine in breast milk. In the meantime, stay awake!

D.K. Stevenson, M.D.

Excretion of Fluoxetine and Its Metabolite, Norfluoxetine, in Human Breast Milk

Taddio A, Ito S, Koren G (Univ of Toronto)

J Clin Pharmacol 36:42–47, 1996 14–5

Background.—Fluoxetine, a common antidepressant, may be taken by women who are breast-feeding. The infants of such women may ingest a pharmacologically significant amount of the agent through nursing. Breast milk concentrations of fluoxetine and norfluoxetine were measured in 1 group of women to estimate infant drug exposure from nursing.

Methods.—Ten women nursing 11 infants were included. The mean dose of fluoxetine was 0.39 mg/kg per day. The women were asked to collect 3–6 milk samples throughout a dosing interval and to report any adverse effects in their infants.

Findings.—Mean infant doses of fluoxetine and norfluoxetine, estimated for an infant breast-fed exclusively and ingesting 1,000 mL of milk per day, were 0.077 mg and 0.084 mg, respectively. The total dose of fluoxetine and norfluoxetine was 0.165 mg, equivalent to 10.8% of the maternal dose and adjusted on a milligram-per-kilogram basis in an infant weighing 4 kg. The mothers observed no adverse effects in their infants.

Conclusion.—Nursing infants receive about one tenth of the adult therapeutic dose of fluoxetine in their mothers' breast milk. Although the women in the current study reported no short-term adverse effects in their infants, the potential long-term consequences need to be studied.

▶ Commenting on this article is Louis P. Halamek, M.D., Professor of Pediatrics, Division of Neonatal and Developmental Medicine, Stanford University Medical Center, Palo Alto, California:

▶ Fluoxetine (Prozac) is one of the most commonly prescribed medications in the United States, especially among women of childbearing age. Mothers receiving this therapy are often faced with a choice between continuing what may be effective therapy for their own health and providing the optimum source of nutrition for their infants. Given the large numbers of potential study subjects, the paucity of data on the safety of fluoxetine in lactating women is both surprising and depressing.

L.P. Halamek, M.D.

Neonatal Withdrawal From Maternal Volatile Substance Abuse

Tenenbein M, Casiro OG, Seshia MMK, et al (Univ of Manitoba, Winnipeg, Canada; Children's Hosp, Winnipeg, Manitoba, Canada)

Arch Dis Child 74:F204–F207, 1996 14–6

Background.—Volatile substance abuse is common worldwide. Although it occurs in 15% to 20% of high school seniors in the United States and results in 100 documented deaths annually in the United Kingdom, its exact incidence is unknown. It is estimated that 12,000 infants are born every year to mothers who are abusers of volatile substances. There are no reports of a neonatal withdrawal syndrome. The incidence of a withdrawal syndrome in neonates born to mothers who have abused volatile substances during their pregnancy was examined, the severity of this syndrome was graded, and the effectiveness of treatment with phenobarbital was reported.

Methods.—During a period of 4 years, all infants who were born to mothers who had abused volatile substances during their pregnancy, or who were born with the distinctive hydrocarbon odor, were studied. The Finnegan Neonatal Abstinence Scoring System was used to grade the severity of withdrawal before and after treatment. Phenobarbital was used to treat withdrawal.

Results.—There were 48 infants studied; 27 were treated with phenobarbital. Typical withdrawal symptoms included excessive and high-pitched crying, sleeplessness, hyperactive Moro reflex, tremor, hypotonia, and poor feeding. Treatment was begun at a mean of 27.1 hours after birth and lasted a mean of 5.8 days. Phenobarbital was effective in 17 of the 27 infants treated, and borderline in 3. No benefit from treatment was seen in the other 7 infants.

Discussion.—Infants born to mothers who have abused volatile substances during their pregnancy experience a withdrawal syndrome. A characteristic hydrocarbon odor is a marker of its occurrence. The Finnegan Neonatal Abstinence Scoring System was useful in grading the severity of withdrawal. Phenobarbital was generally effective in treating the withdrawal syndrome.

▶ My mental image of Winnipeg is that it was very cold, clear, and inhabited by model citizens. I wondered what the population did for kicks when they were not playing or watching hockey. I anticipated that hard drug use (opiates and cocaine) would be uncommon but was surprised by the number of pregnant women who abused the solvents used in paint, lacquers, and glue. These women are exposed to a variety of chemicals, including toluene, a substance implicated in congential heart defects, which is common to these products. They now have the distinction of forming the basis for the initial report of an abstinence syndrome in noenates born to mothers who have abused volatile substances.

The evidence for a specific neonatal withdrawal syndrome from maternal volatile substance abuse is presented in a simple but logical fashion. The sentinel features are the characteristic odor (in both the mother and baby) and the presence of a metabolic acidosis. The hyrdocarbon odor evidently is difficult to miss, but the neurologic features given were nonspecific. The latter included a high-pitched cry, excessive crying, sleeplessness, tremors, hypotonia, and poor feeding. Other features, such as nasal stuffiness, sneezing, yawning, sweating, and diarrhea or vomiting, which typify opiate withdrawal, were not observed. The Finnegan Scoring system was helpful in identifying infants who were withdrawing from volatile substances, and for monitoring their response to therapy.

Difficulties with ascertainment of all women exposed to volatile substances during pregnancy reduces to estimates the frequency of the problem. The National Institute on Drug Abuse estimated that 12,000 infants are born each year to mothers who have abused volatile substances during pregnancy. Why have we been so slow to recognize the syndrome? Perhaps it was blended into the general drug withdrawal category and, in the United States, it may be compounded by the use of other substances, including alcohol. However, the odor and the presence of metabolic acidosis should have raised a red flag somewhere. We all should be on the lookout for these infants so that they may receive appropriate intervention.

A.A. Fanaroff, M.B.B.Ch.

15 Miscellaneous Topics

A Controlled Trial of Nurse Practitioners in Neonatal Intensive Care
Mitchell-DiCenso A, Guyatt G, Marrin M, et al (McMaster Univ, Hamilton, Ont, Canada)
Pediatrics 98:1143–1148, 1996 15–1

Background.—Nurse practitioners are well-established members of primary care delivery teams, but few randomized, controlled trials have evaluated the effectiveness of nurse practitioners in the tertiary care setting. In the first trial to consider the safety, effectiveness, and efficiency of clinical nurse specialists/neonatal practitioners (CNS/NPs), neonatal outcome was compared for infants randomized to care by the CNS/NP team or by the pediatric resident team.

Methods.—The trial enrolled neonates admitted during a 1-year period to the study institution's neonatal ICU (NICU), a 33-bed tertiary-level unit. On the NICU staff at the time were 7 neonatologists, 3 neonatal trainees, 15 residents, and 4.5 CNS/NPs. The CNS/NP team provided care during the day and the pediatric residents provided care from 4 PM to 8 AM. During the trial, infants assigned to the pediatric resident team were cared for around the clock by pediatric residents. Both teams were supervised by neonatologists. Of the 821 infants enrolled during the study, 414 were randomly assigned to the CNS/NP team and 407 to the pediatric resident team.

Results.—The 2 groups of neonates were similar in sex distribution, percentage of vaginal deliveries, birth weight distribution, number of multiple births, mean gestational age, and mean Apgar scores. There were 19 infant deaths (4.6%) in the CNS/NP group and 25 (5.9%) in the resident group; complications occurred in 55.6% and 54.1%, respectively, of infants in the 2 groups. The average length of hospital stay was greater, but not significantly so, in the CNS/NP group (12.5 vs. 11.7 days). On the various indicator conditions, performance was comparable except for jaundice and charting, which favored the CNS/NP group. The Neonatal Index of Parent Satisfaction, administered on the fifth day after NICU admission, yielded a mean score of 139 in the resident group and 140 in the CNS/NP group. The Minnesota Infant Development Inventory (MIDI) was completed when the infant was 8 months of age. Of the 450 infants whose parents returned the MIDI, 2.6% in the CNS/NP group and 0.9% in the resident group performed 30% or more below their age level. The cost of care per infant, based on medical expenses and family expenses, was $978 greater in the CNS/NP group ($14,245 vs. $13,267).

Discussion.—This study of neonates randomized to CNS/NP and pediatric resident care during their NICU stay found the 2 teams to be comparable in all tested measures of performance and outcome. Findings support the use of CNS/NPs in the NICU setting, in which fewer pediatric residents are available and increasing numbers of surviving infants are receiving care.

▶ Commenting on this article is Michele Walsh-Sukys, M.D., Associate Professor of Pediatrics, Case Western Reserve University, and Co-director, Newborn Intensive Care Unit, Rainbow Babies & Childrens Hospital, Cleveland, Ohio:

▶ The authors are to be congratulated for having conducted a randomized, controlled trial of a complicated intervention: care of neonates by neonatal nurse practitioners vs. pediatric residents. The use of the randomized, clinical trial for the assessment of the impact of drug treatments is well worked out and relatively easy to contreol with the use of an identical placebo. However, the study of technologies and other treatments is much more daunting. The methodologic obstacles are considerable, yet the authors have vaulted many of these. A large sample of neonates was randomly assigned to the care of a practitioner team or a resident team. Outcome measures were selected to measure the quality of care, cost of care, and parent satisfaction. The authors acknowledge that some of these outcome tools were new and not validated. This is the only methodologic weakness in an otherwise sophisticated study.

When assessed at 8 months corrected age, mortality, resource utilization, costs of care, and parent satisfaction were similar between the resident and practitioner teams. The authors correctly conclude that care given by practitioners and residents is equivalent. On the face of it, this is a reassuring finding. But closer inspection raises some questions. Why is the care given by fully trained specialized professionals only equivalent to, not superior to, that given by a group that is still in training?

The real difference between practitioners and residents lies in the hours worked. The practitioner group worked from 8 AM to 4 PM 7 days a week, whereas the resident team worked 24 hours a day 7 days a week. When the NPs were off, the residents cared for their patients. Thus, the practitioners were present only 33% of the time. Perhaps what the study is really measuring is an inherently superior style of care whose impact is diluted by cross-coverage 66% of the time. The authors argue that this reflects the "real world." Again, this is certainly true; practitioners work fewer hours than residents because residents are in training, and practitioners are full-time professionals. Yet, the "real world" dynamic arises from 2 imperatives: there are insufficient practitioners to staff NICUs around the clock, and the salaries of practitioners are substantially higher than those of residents. Indeed, in the United States, because most teaching hospitals receive a subsidy for the education of primary care residents such as those in pediatrics, there is an inherent financial disincentive to pursue replacing residents with practitioners. Thus, unless the funding equation changes, or the residency review committee further limits the time residents may spend in the NICU, we are unlikely to see NICUs fully staffed by NPs.

M. Walsh-Sukys, M.D.

A Randomized Controlled Trial of Early Physiotherapy for High-risk Infants

Weindling AM, Hallam P, Gregg J, et al (Univ of Liverpool, England)

Acta Paediatr 85:1107–1111, 1996 15–2

Objective.—Children at risk for cerebral palsy (CP) have been treated conservatively, receiving physiotherapy only if abnormal muscle or motor function developed. Clinical studies have failed to show any differences between these children and untreated children. The results of early introduction of physiotherapy targeted at infants at risk for CP were compared with the results of conservative treatment in similar infants.

Methods.—Infants aged 35–40 weeks with abnormal cranial US findings and with either cystic periventricular leukomalacia (PVL), porencephaly, parenchymal involvement by an intraventricular hemorrhage, periventricular echodensities for more than 2 weeks, persistent ventricular enlargement, or hydrocephaly requiring shunting were randomly assigned to receive early physiotherapy (30 boys and 21 girls) or standard treatment (29 boys and 25 girls). Patients were given motor, developmental, and neurologic assessments at 12 and 30 months. The early group (EP) began physiotherapy at an average of 39 weeks, whereas the standard treatment group (ST) began physiotherapy at an average of 76 weeks.

Results.—By 12 months, 9 infants had died, 9 were lost to follow-up, and 5 (1 EP and 4 ST) were impaired. By 30 months, 10 infants had died, 12 were lost to follow-up, and 2 more ST infants were impaired. Seventeen EP and 19 ST children were walking independently, but 45% showed significant neurologic impairment. There were no differences between treatment groups. The positive predictive value of cranial US was only 54%. Cystic PVL was the best predictor of impairment.

Conclusion.—Cranial US was not an accurate predictor of the development of CP in infants at risk, possibly because of the variety of disabilities affecting these children.

▶ There is a huge difference between doing good for the patient and feeling as if you are doing good. Physiotherapy has been used for a host of muscular, neurologic, respiratory, orthopedic, and spinal disorders. Physiotherapy has been a standard component and integral part of therapy for the neurologically handicapped infant with hypertonia, hypotonia, spasticity, and CP. Previous studies of early physiotherapy, done about a decade ago, failed to show any substantial differences between early treatment and control groups.[1, 2] Weindling and colleagues hoped that, with the advent of more sophisticated radiologic and imaging techniques, infants at risk for CP could be better identified and selected for intervention. They must join the ranks of the disappointed, however, because they failed to demonstrate beneficial outcome differences in the early physiotherapy group. Furthermore, despite the high-technology approach, CP was predicted correctly in only just over half the infants. The group was very heterogeneous in terms of their abilities and disabilities, which may account for the failure to demonstrate benefit from the intervention.

Other approaches to proving benefits have been suggested,[3] including a series of controlled single case studies in which the intervention is randomized, as is done in behavioral and cognitive physiology. This means we should look for further trials. In the meantime, we will continue to collaborate with our physiotherapists, who provide a valuable assessment service. Although there was no concrete evidence that physiotherapy was beneficial, there was no evidence that it was harmful.

We would accomplish many more things if we did not think of them as impossible.—C. Maleshbes

A.A. Fanaroff, M.B.B.Ch.

References

1. Goodman M, Rothberg A, Houston-McMillan JE, et al: Effect of early neurodevelopmental therapy in normal and at risk survivors of neonatal intensive care. *Lancet* 2:1327–1330, 1985.
2. Piper MC, Kunos VI, Willis DM, et al: Early physical therapy effects on the high risk infant: A randomized controlled trial. *Pediatrics* 78:216–224, 1986.
3. Bower E, McLellan DL: Evaluating therapy in cerebral palsy. *Child Care Health Dev* 20:409–419, 1994.

Non-invasive Perinatal Necropsy by Magnetic Resonance Imaging

Brookes JAS, Hall-Craggs MA, Sams VR, et al (Middlesex Hosp, London; Univ College, London)
Lancet 348:1139–1141, 1996 15–3

Introduction.—Perinatal necropsy often provides valuable information about the cause of fetal death, but there may be resistance to the procedure among parents, clinicians, and pathologists. When there is reluctance to perform internal necropsy or a perinatal pathologist is not available, examination by MRI might provide similar information by noninvasive means. Twenty fetuses were examined by both MRI and necropsy to compare the extent of diagnostic information obtained by each technique.

Findings.—The stillborn, miscarried, or aborted fetuses ranged from 15 to 39 weeks' gestational age. Ten were delivered in the second trimester and 10 in the third trimester. Diagnostic findings showed broad agreement between MRI and necropsy, and findings were the same in 8 cases. Necropsy yielded more detailed information than MRI in 8 cases, and MRI provided more extensive information in 4 cases. Overall, MRI had equivalent or better diagnostic sensitivity than internal necropsy examination in 60% of cases. Whereas MRI was sensitive in the detection of CNS macroscopic abnormalities and produced high-resolution images of the musculoskeletal system, it was less successful in depicting cardiovascular anomalies.

Discussion.—Stillborn, miscarried, or aborted fetuses can be examined by MRI when consent for internal necropsy is denied or as a supplement to information obtained at necropsy. In these 20 cases, MRI-derived diagnostic information was judged equivalent in overall clinical significance to that obtained at necropsy.

► Although there is conclusive evidence of the value of the perinatal necropsy with new important information uncovered in 44% of cases, consent for necropsy is neither given nor sought in at least 40% of perinatal deaths.[1, 2] Regional surveys in the United Kingdom revealed that minimal standards (44% to 50%) are often not achieved.[3] It is almost fair to say that getting permission for a necropsy has become a lost, if not a dying, art. An anonymous source remarked that "if it's worth not doing, it's worth not doing well." Brookes and colleagues present coercive evidence for MRI examination when permission for a perinatal necropsy has not been obtained. There was close agreement between MRI-derived information and that obtained by pathologic internal necropsy. Magnetic resonance imaging is particularly useful for the examination of the brain, eliminating the need for prolonged formalin preservation before dissection. The combination of MRI and internal necropsy would be the most sensitive method to detect lesions of all varieties and descriptions.

A.A. Fanaroff, M.B.B.Ch.

References

1. Cartlidge PH, Dawson AT, Stewart JH, et al: Value and quality of perinatal and infant post mortem examinations: Cohort analysis of 400 consecutive deaths. *BMJ* 310:155–158, 1995.
2. Hussain AN, O'Connor GT: The perinatal autopsy: A neglected source of discovery. *IARC Sci Publ* 112:151–162, 1991.
3. Chiswick M: Perinatal and infant postmortem examination. *BMJ* 310:141–142, 1995.

A Complex Retinoic Acid Response Element in the Uncoupling Protein Gene Defines a Novel Role for Retinoids in Thermogenesis

Rabelo R, Reyes C, Schifman A, et al (McGill Univ, Montreal)
Endocrinology 137:3488–3496, 1996 15–4

Introduction.—Retinoids are involved in a large spectrum of physiologic activities, including control of cell proliferation and differentiation. There is recent evidence that retinoids may stimulate the expression of the uncoupling protein (UCP), a key element in brown adipose tissue (BAT) thermogenesis. The molecular bases for a metabolic role of retinoic acid (RA) in UCP gene expression were reported.

Methods.—Plasmids, cell culture, transfections, DNA binding assays, brown adipocyte isolation, and Northern blot analysis were performed using freshly isolated brown adipocytes from rat BAT.

Results.—All-*trans*-RA and 9-*cis*-RA powerfully increased UCP messenger RNA levels in isolated rat brown adipocytes. The sequence -2399/-2490 (called R90) was identified as the RA-responsive sequence in the rat UCP gene using transient transfection experiments in HIB-1B cells, a BAT-derived cell line. With maximal concentrations of all-*trans*-RA or 9-*cis*-RA, R90 mediated a 20- to 70-fold stimulation of the chloramphenicol acetyltransferase reporter gene. The non-BAT cells were significantly less responsive and the RA effect was less when the chloramphenicol acetyltransferase gene was driven by a heterologous promoter rather than the UCP minimal promoter. Three discrete sequences were identified as being essential for the RA response within R90 by footprinting and site-directed mutagenesis. This defined the complex RA response element of this gene. It is known that critical bases in these sequences are arranged in pairs of putative half-sites. Using electrophoretic mobility shift assays with in vitro translated receptors and HIB-1B nuclear extracts with anti-RARγ or anti-RXR antibodies, RARγ-RXR heterodimers can bind to the R90. Transient transfection experiments overexpressing selected receptors and dose-response analyses of RA isomers and analogues further support the participation of RARγ-RXR heterodimers in RA stimulation.

Conclusions.—Retinoids strongly stimulate the rat UCP gene expression through a complex RARE. The RARE is comprised of 3 pairs of half-sites and defines a novel role for retinoids in the regulation of facultative thermogenesis and energy expenditure.

▶ Understanding thermal regulation helped build the foundation for the modern era of neonatology. A critical element in thermal regulation and the major site of nonshivering thermogenesis in mammals is the brown adipose fat. The highly vascular, mitochondrial, rich brown fat is responsive to cold exposure and diet. The metabolic pathways and controls of the brown fat gradually have been elucidated. Uncoupling protein or thermogenin, located in the inner membrane of the mitochondria, stimulates heat production. For many years, this was thought to be induced by norepinephrine acting through cyclic adenosine monophosphate. Silva, the senior author of this paper, previously had demonstrated that thyroid hormone also is essential for the response to cold and that thriiodothyronine (T_3) and norephinephrine act in concert.[1] In this article, a novel role for retinoids in the regulation of nonshivering or facultative thermogenesis and energy balance is presented in a series of elegant experiments. Retinoids have a broad spectrum of activity, including control of embryonic development and maintenance of the immune system. They may play a critical role in lung development and the prevention of lung injury (see Abstract 10–15). One can only speculate as to how a deficiency of retinoids in extremely immature infants may not only alter the thermal regulatory capability but also increase the risks for sepsis and oxidant lung injury.

A.A. Fanaroff, M.B.B.Ch.

Reference

1. Silva JE: Full expression of uncoupling protein gene requires the concurrence of norephinephrine and triodothyronine. *Mol Endocrinol* 12:706–713, 1988.

The Effect of Early Discharge and Other Factors on Readmission Rates of Newborns

Soskolne EI, Schumacher R, Fyock C, et al (St Joseph Mercy Hosp, Ann Arbor, Mich; Univ of Michigan, Ann Arbor)

Arch Pediatr Adolesc Med 150:373–379, 1996 15–5

Introduction.—A great financial emphasis has been placed on hospitals recently to discharge mothers and infants as soon as possible. A mother usually stays in a hospital for 24 hours after a vaginal delivery. Under early or very early discharge (by 24 or 48 hours of age) programs, readmission may be more common. The relation between early discharge, breast-feeding, and other factors and hospital readmission of newborns was assessed.

Methods.—There were 117 newborns who were readmitted to the hospital within the first 3 weeks of life; they were compared with a control group of 147 newborns born during the same period who were not readmitted. A review was done of the medical records of all readmitted infants and their birth records. Medical records were reviewed for length of stay, birth weight, size relative to gestational age, Apgar score at 5 minutes, sex, delivery method, method of feeding, complete blood cell count, weight at discharge, and frequency of elimination.

Results.—Readmission did not seem to be affected by early discharge, defined as discharge before 24, 36, or 48 hours of age. There was a signficantly lower risk of readmission for newborns whose initial stay was longer than 72 hours. Vaginal delivery and length of stay less than 72 hours were factors in the initial hospitalization that were associated with readmission. Other factors included need for performance of a complete blood count, presence of jaundice, gestational age of 37 weeks or less, and discharge weight of less than 3 kg. Trends were observed between breast-feeding and readmission and between breast-feeding and jaundice or dehydration.

Conclusions.—Hospital readmission within the first 3 weeks of life is not associated with early discharge before 48 hours of age. As a potentially significant cost-saving measure that will help reduce the nation's total health care bill, it is recommended that pediatricians and obstetricians continue to strive for early discharge of newborns and their mothers. To define the risks and probabilities of readmission more clearly, further studies are necessary.

▶ Seldom does a perinatal issue feature in the presidential elections, but such was the case in the 1996 presidential debates. Both President Clinton and Senator Dole frequently referred to their respective roles in preventing short hospital stays for mothers and their newborns. Each, in turn, alluded to the elimination of "drive-by deliveries." Indeed, it was both rewarding and somewhat reassuring to see the U.S. Congress responding favorably to the statement from the American Academy of Pediatrics Committee on the Fetus and Newborn regarding the criteria for a short stay and promptly passing the Bradley Bill, which mandates a 48-hour hospital stay for the mother-infant dyad.[1]

This case-controlled analysis of hospital readmission for newborns identifies the well-known risk factors for readmission, including short hospital stay, breast-feeding, jaundice, gestational age of 37 weeks or less, discharge weight of less than 3 kg, and vaginal delivery. Presumably, if a baby is delivered by cesarean section and goes home with its mother, a short stay is automatically avoided. Jaundice and preterm infants between 35 and 37 weeks' gestation who masquerade as full-term infants were featured in an article in the 1996 YEAR BOOK OF NEONATAL AND PERINATAL MEDICINE.[2] If the Academy guidelines are followed, the families and health care providers are appropriately educated, and the postdischarge care is closely supervised, the problems of a short stay can be minimized. Catherine DeAngelis, the editor of *Archives of Pediatrics and Adolescent Medicine,* observed that "readmission is a valuable variable for managed cost, but there might be equally bad or worse things than their child's being readmitted to a hospital." There certainly are, and failure to recognize that the child has a problem requiring attention or readmission tops the list.

A.A. Fanaroff, M.B.B.Ch.

References

1. Committee on the Fetus and Newborn: Hospital stay for healthy term newborns. *Pediatrics* 96:788–790, 1995.
2. Brown AK, Johnson L: Loss of concern about jaundice and the reemergence of kernicterus in full-term infants in the era of managed care. YEAR BOOK OF NEONATAL AND PERINATAL MEDICINE, pp xvii–xxviii, 1996.

Topical Ointment Therapy Benefits Premature Infants

Nopper AJ, Horii KA, Sookdeo-Drost S, et al (Stanford Univ, California)
J Pediatr 128:660–669, 1996 15–6

Background.—Premature infants are born with immature skin that has an ineffective epidermal barrier. The epidermal barrier function is found in the stratum corneum. At 32–34 weeks' gestation, the stratum corneum becomes functionally mature. In premature infants, this maturation process is accelerated, and by 2 weeks after birth, even very premature infants will have a functionally mature stratum corneum. The maturity and effectiveness of the epidermal barrier can be determined by measuring transepidermal water loss. In premature infants, this water loss can be 10–15 times greater than in infants carried to term. Such tremendous water loss is associated with significant morbidity, and the rate of nosocomial infection in the neonatal ICU can be 30%. Topical therapy may improve epidermal barrier function. The cutaneous and systemic effects of topical therapy in premature infants were evaluated in a prospective, randomized study.

Methods.—There were 60 infants born at less than 33 weeks' gestation. Treated infants had a preservative-free petroleum ointment applied every 12 hours for 2 weeks. Control infants received routine skin care but did not receive the ointment. Transdermal water loss, fluid intake, weight gain, skin condition, fungal and bacterial cultures, and blood, urine, and CSF cultures positive for microorganisms were monitored.

Results.—Transepidermal water loss was significantly lower in the first 6 hours after the initial application of ointment in treated infants. Thirty minutes after application, transepidermal water loss was decreased by 67%, and 4–6 hours after application, it was decreased by 34% (Table 2). Decreases in transepidermal water loss were significant on day 14 (Table 3). Treated infants had significantly higher skin condition scores on days 7 and 14. Treated infants also had significantly less colonization of the axilla on days 2, 3, or 4, and on day 14. Treated infants had a 3.3% rate of positive blood or CSF cultures, compared with 26.7% in control infants. Fluid intake and weight gain or loss were similar in both groups.

Conclusions.—Topical therapy with this preservative-free ointment decreased transepidermal water loss and the degree of dermatitis and bacterial colonization of the axillary skin. The skin of premature infants may be an entry point for invasive bacteria. In premature infants, the use of a preservative-free ointment during the first weeks of life may lower the risk of nosocomial infection. More frequent and extended treatment with the ointment also may be beneficial. Future studies should evaluate the effects of such treatment on electrolyte balance, intraventricular hemorrhage and

TABLE 2.—Transepidermal Water Loss on Day 0 Before and After Topical Ointment Therapy

	Time 0	At 30 min	At 60 min	At 4–6 hr
Treated side	15.1 ± 9.2 (27)	4.9 ± 3.1 (26)	6.4 ± 3.9 (26)	9.9 ± 7.0 (26)
Control side	14.9 ± 10.5 (27)	13.2 ± 8.6 (26)	12.8 ± 7.0 (26)	13.9 ± 8.1 (26)
Difference (mean ± SE)	0.2 ± 0.5	8.4 ± 1.5	6.4 ± 0.9	4.0 ± 0.8
p value	0.95	0.0001	0.0001	0.0001

Note: The transepidermal water loss values of the treated and untreated side of the infant represent mean ± SD in g/m^2/hr before (time 0) and after topical ointment application. The sample size (*n*) is represented in *parentheses*. The *P* values compare the transepidermal water loss values of the infants' treated and control sides at various time intervals.

(Courtesy of Nopper AJ, Horii KA, Sookdeo-Drost S, et al: Topical ointment therapy benefits premature infants. *J Pediatr* 128:660–669, 1996.)

TABLE 3.—Transepidermal Water Loss of the Treatment and Control Groups on Days 0–14

	Day 0	Day 2, 3, or 4	Day 7	Day 14
Treatment	15.6 ± 9.9 (28)	10.3 ± 5.1 (28)	7.7 ± 3.5 (24)	5.9 ± 2.6 (17)
Control	17.7 ± 10.9 (28)	12.5 ± 6.7 (28)	9.4 ± 3.5 (26)	8.1 ± 3.7 (20)
Difference (mean ± SE)	2.1 ± 2.8	2.2 ± 1.6	1.7 ± 1.0	2.2 ± 1.1
p value	0.45	0.61	0.08	0.04

Note: The treatment and control group values represent mean transepidermal water loss ± SD in g/m^2/hr. Transepidermal water loss measurements were made before the first application (day 0) and 10–12 hours after the previous application of ointment (day 2, 3, or 4, and days 7 and 14) in the treated group. The sample size (*n*) is represented in *parentheses*. The *P* values compare the treated and control groups' mean transepidermal water loss values on different days.

(Courtesy of Nopper AJ, Horii KA, Sookdeo-Drost S, et al: Topical ointment therapy benefits premature infants. *J Pediatr* 128:660–669, 1996.)

patent ductus arteriosus, caloric requirements, and length of hospital stay in premature infants.

▶ Lack of integrity of the skin in the extremely immature infant has been the source of much frustration for neonatal clinicians. Although the birth process rapidly accelerates skin maturation, paucity of keratinization of the stratum corneum results in a host of problems, including impaired barrier functions, increased evaporative water losses, difficulties with thermal regulation, and a greater tendency to break down from routine handling for procedures such as venipunctures, heel sticks, and probe or electrode placement.

Efforts to correct these defects have been episodic, and the skin of the newborn has not received the attention it deserves. It is encouraging to note the excellent results generated by Nopper and associates with the application of a bland, nontoxic, preservative-free agent. Skin integrity was sustained; there was a substantial reduction in insensible water loss, although this did not translate to significant changes in water balance. Also, there were fewer infections in the treated infants. The therapy was universally applauded by the neonatal ICU nurses, which is not something that can be taken for granted with most interventions. The nurses liked what they saw and, apart from some technical problems with slippery IVs and sliding electrodes, which have since been solved, the study was completed without a hitch. It is interesting to note that the application of Aquafor has become the standard of care in the Stanford nursery, despite the authors' standard disclaimer that "additional investigations are needed for further evaluation of topical ointment therapy..." The optimal time for the initial application remains to be determined; should it commence in the delivery room? How frequently should the topical ointment be applied? Further, will this become the standard of care for all nurseries?

The evidence is strong, but not overwhelming, that we should embark on such a routine. The treatment is benign and the consequences of skin breakdown are severe.

A.A. Fanaroff, M.B.B.Ch.

Dermal Injury Following the Use of Fiberoptic Phototherapy in an Extremely Premature Infant

Hussain K, Sharief N (Basildon Hosp, England)

Clin Pediatr (Phila) 35:421–422, 1996 15–7

Introduction.—The fragile skin of infants born at less than 28 weeks' gestation is highly vulnerable to injury. Skin injuries caused by thermal agents, chemical agents, and adhesive tapes have been reported in these very premature patients. However, this is the first reported case of skin injury caused by fiberoptic phototherapy for jaundice of prematurity.

Case Report.—Infant, born at 25 weeks' gestation, was electively intubated and stabilized. Initial respiratory requirements were moderate. After management of low blood pressure, the infant was transferred to a closed incubator and given natural surfactant. At 48 hours, the infant was noted to have jaundice, with a serum bilirubin level of 88 μmol/L. A fiberoptic phototherapy blanket system was used to deliver phototherapy. The blanket was changed as part of full nursing care every 6 hours. At 78 hours, the patient's blood pressure began to decline again. There was an extensive, erythematous, denuded area of skin on the back (which had been in contact with the biliblanket) that looked like a partial thickness burn. Hypotension could not be controlled, even with intensive colloid and inotropic support. The patient died at 85 hours, shortly after signs of disseminated intravascular coagulation and severe metabolic acidosis appeared.

Discussion.—This premature newborn had thermal injury resulting from the use of a fiberoptic phototherapy system, (i.e., a biliblanket). This burn is difficult to explain because fiberoptic systems should not transfer heat; there was no evidence of chemical or other thermal injury. Malfunction of the biliblanket system in the closed incubator environment is one possibility.

▶ This comment was co-authored by Rena Gale, M.D., Head, Department of Neonatology, Bikur Cholim University; Head, Department of Neonatology, Bikur Cholim Hospital, Jerusalem, Israel:

▶ It is of interest that the first report of dermal injury after fiberoptic phototherapy should come from Britain, where the technique began 42 years ago. Since the use of the fiberoptic technique for phototherapy in the neonate was first described 6 years ago,[1, 2] no documentation of skin injury has been reported, even in tiny premature infants in whom phototherapy with biliblankets seems most effective,[3] alone or in combination with conventional phototherapy.[4]

However, the possibility of a photosensitivity reaction should be considered. Although an inherited predisposition to photosensitivity is a possibility, the presence of exogenous photosensitizers, such as riboflavin,[5] which are routinely added to the alimentation solution in large quantities (1.4 mg/5 mL of multivitamin infusion, pediatric solution), also need to be excluded as possible causes. The use of fiberoptic phototherapy appears to be safe, but prudence dictates that close observation of all patients under phototherapy is desirable.

R. Gale, M.D.
D.K. Stevenson, M.D.

References

1. Gale R, Dranitzki Z, Dollberg S, et al: A randomized, controlled application of the Wallaby phototherapy system compared with standard phototherapy. *J Perinatol* 10:239–242, 1990.
2. Rosenfeld W, Twist P, Concepcion L: A new device for phototherapy treatment of jaundiced infants. *J Perinatol* 10:243–248, 1990.
3. Tan KL: Comparison of the efficacy of fiberoptic and conventional phototherapy for neonatal hyperbilirubinemia. *J Pediatr* 125:607–612, 1994.
4. Holtrop PC, Ruedisueli K, Maisels MJ: Double versus single phototherapy in low birth weight newborns. *Pediatrics* 90:674–677, 1992.
5. Vreman HJ, Stevenson DK: Metalloporphyrin-enhanced photodegradation of bilirubin in vitro. *Am J Dis Child* 144:590–594, 1990.

Defects in the Determination of Left-Right Asymmetry

Splitt MP, Burn J, Goodship J (Univ of Newcastle upon Tyne, England)
J Med Genet 33:498–503, 1996 15–8

Introduction.—Situs solitus refers to the normal orientation of the heart and abdominal organs. A perfect reversal of situs solitus with a left heart loop is known as situs inversus. This reversal of organs occurs in about 1 in 10,000 individuals. Any arrangement of internal organs other than situs solitus or situs inversus is called heterotaxy or situs ambiguous. The incidence of cardiac abnormalities is 3% to 9% in individuals with situs inversus. Most individuals with heterotaxy have complex cardiovascular malformation, splenic anomalies, and a variety of gastrointestinal anomalies. Defects in laterality are described on the basis of ciliary function.

Laterality Defects With Normal Cilia.—Most individuals with situs inversus or heterotaxy have no symptoms of ciliary dyskinesia. A notable group of individuals with lateral defects are those who have a complete absence of visceral asymmetry with evidence for either bilateral left-sidedness or bilateral right-sidedness. This anomaly is known as isomerism sequence, Ivemark syndrome, asplenia/polysplenia syndrome, or laterality sequence. Both right and left isomerism sequence are correlated with a wide spectrum of severe heart malformations. Individuals with right isomerism sequence usually have asplenia, and patients with left isomerism sequence may have multiple spleens. Individuals with isomerism sequence frequently have intestinal rotation and fixational abnormalities. There is evidence that a recessive gene is responsible for these anomalies, but there is also evidence that this form of inheritance is autosomal dominant. This reinforces the need for taking a careful pedigree in families with affected children and for evaluation of the parents for situs inversus. So far, the only locus for heterotaxy has been mapped on the X chromosome at Xq24-q27.1. Genetic counseling is also important because children with complex heart lesions are surviving to reproductive age (Fig 2).

Laterality Defects With Abnormal Cilia.—Nearly 25% of individuals with complete situs inversus have primary ciliary dyskinesia (PCD) (1 in 30,000–40,000). Individuals with PCD have immotile or dyskinetic cilia of the respiratory epithelium with secondary chronic respiratory tract infections. Clinical features occur in about 90% of affected children and include chronic rhinitis, sinusitis, opacity of the frontal sinuses, nasal polyps, recurrent lower respiratory tract infections, and middle ear infections. Diagnosis is best made by ciliary biopsy. Some reports indicate that affected men may be infertile because of immotile sperm flagellae. The spermatozoa of men with PCD are normal and could be fused with oocytes during in vitro fertilization. Women with PCD may have reduced fertility because of decreased ciliary movement in the fallopian tubes. Because patients with complex congenital heart disease do not routinely have ciliary biopsies, it may be that ciliary dyskinesia is overlooked in some patients. There is an autosomal recessive inheritance pattern in individuals with PCD. No genes for PCD have been mapped, but X-linked inheritance is probable.

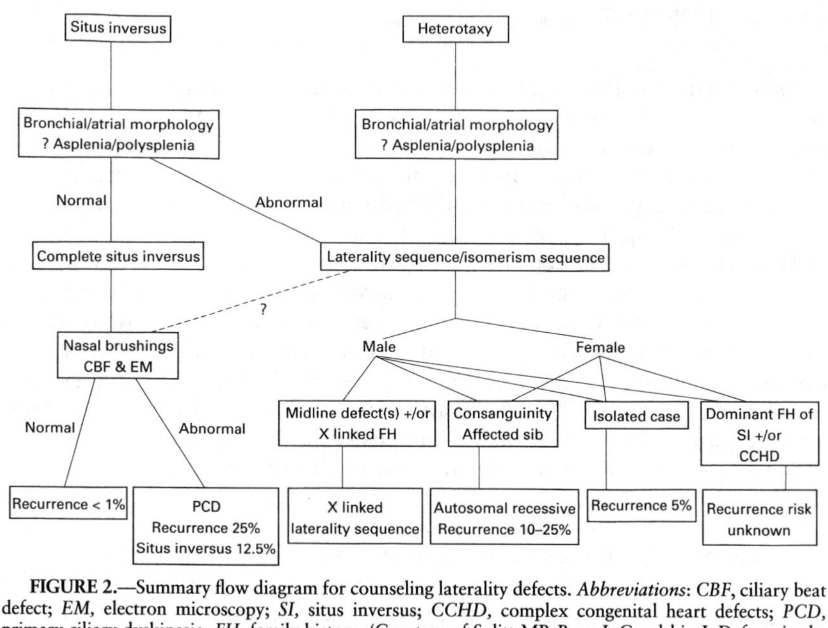

FIGURE 2.—Summary flow diagram for counseling laterality defects. *Abbreviations*: *CBF*, ciliary beat defect; *EM*, electron microscopy; *SI*, situs inversus; *CCHD*, complex congenital heart defects; *PCD*, primary ciliary dyskinesia; *FH*, family history. (Courtesy of Splitt MP, Burn J, Goodship J: Defects in the determination of left-right asymmetry. *J Med Genet* 33:498–503, 1996.)

Conclusion.—Many questions remain concerning laterality disturbances in humans. The study of animal models is the most likely avenue for new information concerning the genetic basis of left-right asymmetry.

▶ Here is an article reviewing everything you ever wanted to know about "sidedness" and the spectrum of malformations, ranging from complete reversals to the various failures to establish asymmetry. The symmetry in biology is fascinating in itself; however, when one realizes that asymmetry is what has to be established in the midst of symmetry, the potential for mistakes in development seem considerable. Complete reversal or situs inversus occurs with a prevalence of about 1 in 10,000. The incidence of heterotaxy is generally much lower and is almost invariably associated with complex cardiovascular malformations. The other wrinkle, of course, with laterality defects is whether cilia are normal or abnormal. The summary flow diagram (see Fig 2) tells the story at a glance. The article makes one of the great mysteries of development a little less mysterious but no less fascinating.

D.K. Stevenson, M.D.

Three-dimensional Ultrasound: Accuracy of Distance and Volume Measurements

Riccabona M, Nelson TR, Pretorius DH (Univ Hosp, LKH Graz, Austria; Univ of California, San Diego)

Ultrasound Obstet Gynecol 7:429–434, 1996 15–9

Introduction.—Two-dimensional US imaging is sufficiently accurate to be used routinely for distance measurement. Its use in volume measurement is not accurate, particularly with irregularly shaped objects. Three-dimensional devices are available and require validation before clinical use. The accuracy of 3-dimensional US distance and volume measurements was evaluated using a commercially available 3-dimensional US scanner.

Methods.—Three-dimensional distance measurements were obtained with the transducer directly on a standard tissue-mimicking US phantom by itself in a water bath of 36.8°C and were compared with actual distances in the phantom. Three-dimensional volume measurements were obtained by scanning 21 balloons of varying shapes and volumes in a water bath of about 37°C (Fig 3) and were compared with actual balloon volumes and with conventional 2-dimensional US calculations.

Results.—Distance measurements made with the transducer directly on the phantom surface had a mean absolute error of 1.9% and 6.1%, respectively, for measurement in the plane of acquisition and in other orientations. With the phantom immersed in a water bath and the transducer on the water surface, there was a mean absolute error of 1% in the plane of acquisition and 1% in all other planes for distance measurements. The conventional 2-dimensional US volume estimates had a mean absolute error of 12.6%, compared with a mean absolute error of 6.4% for 3-di-

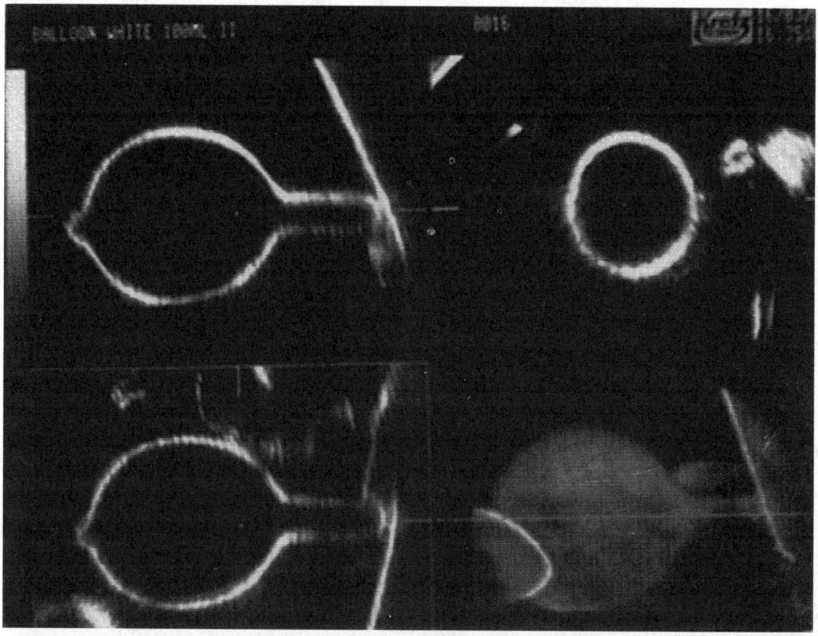

FIGURE 3.—Images of a balloon used for volume measurement showing simultaneous display of 3 orthogonal sectional planes of a balloon together with a surface-weighted rendered image. (Courtesy of Riccabona M, Nelson TR, Pretorius DH: Three-dimensional ultrasound: Accuracy of distance and volume measurements. *Ultrasound Obstet Gynecol* 7:429–434, 1996.)

mensional volume estimates. The primary source of error was identification of the mask boundary for 3-dimensional US volume measurements. Accuracy was greatest for 2-dimensional US volume measurements for regular ellipsoidal objects and least for irregular objects.

Conclusions.—For irregularly shaped objects, 2-dimensional volume measurements were far less accurate than 3-dimensional volume measurements. Two-dimensional and 3-dimensional scanners provide similar results for both distance and volume measurements of ellipsoid objects. Further investigation is needed before 3-dimensional US can be used in routine patient management.

► Diagnostic US has become an integral component of fetal evaluation. Aberrations in fetal grouwth or volume of amniotic fluid trigger a series of responses with potentially profound consequences for the mother, fetus, or both. Accurate measurements are mandatory to avoid incorrect diagnoses, unnecessary responses, and much anguish and grief. Distance measurements are surprisingly accurate (± 2%) with the conventional 2-dimensional US imaging used routinely. Two-dimensional imaging is not accurate enough for volume measurements (± 10% to 20%), particularly if irregularly shaped organs are evaluated. Three-dimensional US devices are undergoing clinical investigation in the United States. Under defined conditions, 3-dimensional US precisely measures a range of balloon volumes and geometrics in different orientations in a manner superior to that of 2-dimensional US. Three-dimensional US also provides a variety of planes that enhance anatomical viewing of organs. Clinical experience is now necessary to confirm these mathematical model findings, but that should be just a formality.

Creativity is allowing yourself to make mistakes. Art is knowing which ones to keep.—Scott Adams

A.A. Fanaroff, M.B.B.Ch.

Congenital Hemangioma: Evidence of Accelerated Involution

Boon LM, Enjolras O, Mulliken JB (Children's Hosp, Boston; Harvard Med School, Boston; Hôpital Tarnier-Cochin, Paris)

J Pediatr 128:329–335, 1996 15–10

Background.—Although hemangiomas usually appear in the first 4 weeks of life, some are fully grown at birth. The course of hemangiomas that proliferate in utero, are fully developed at birth, and begin to regress in early infancy was documented.

Methods.—Thirty-one infants with congenital hemangioma seen at 2 centers were analyzed retrospectively. Diagnoses were established clinically and radiologically as well as by biopsy when necessary.

Findings.—Only 3 of 23 congenital hemangiomas were diagnosed on ultrasonography antenatally (Fig 5). The most common morphologic fea-

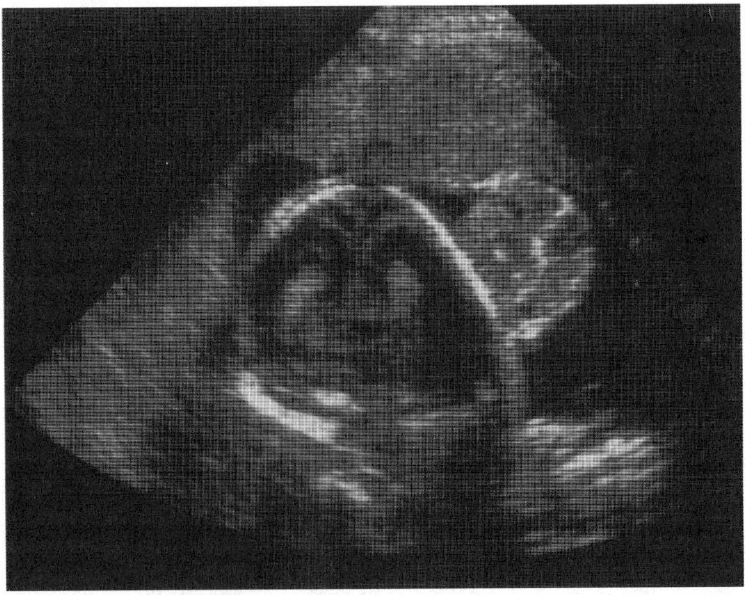

FIGURE 5.—Antenatal sonogram showing large exophytic, inhomogeneous soft-tissue mass arising from a 20-week fetal cranium. Note flattened left parietal bone. (Courtesy of Boon LM, Enjolras O, Mulliken JB: Congenital hemangioma: Evidence of accelerated involution. *J Pediatr* 128:329–335, 1996.)

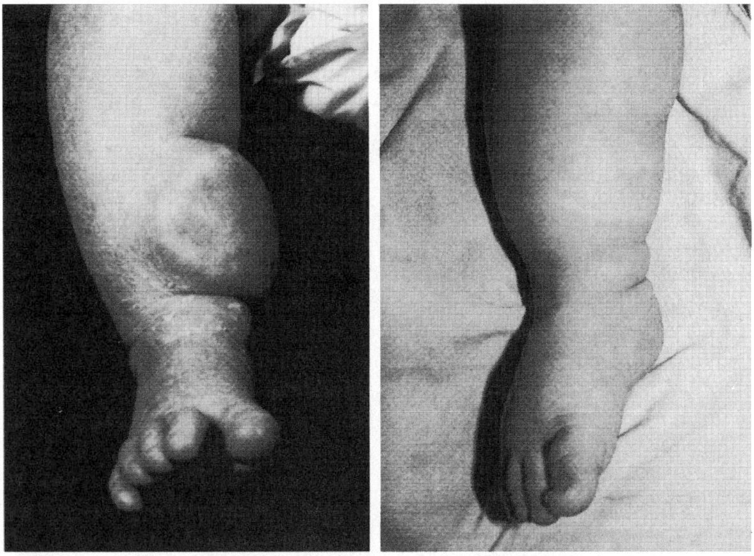

FIGURE 2.—Raised congenital hemangioma of calf, with central telangiectases and pale peripheral halo (**left**). Note dermal atrophy 8 months later (**right**). (Courtesy of Boon LM, Enjolras O, Mulliken JB: Congenital hemangioma: Evidence of accelerated involution. *J Pediatr* 128:329–335, 1996.)

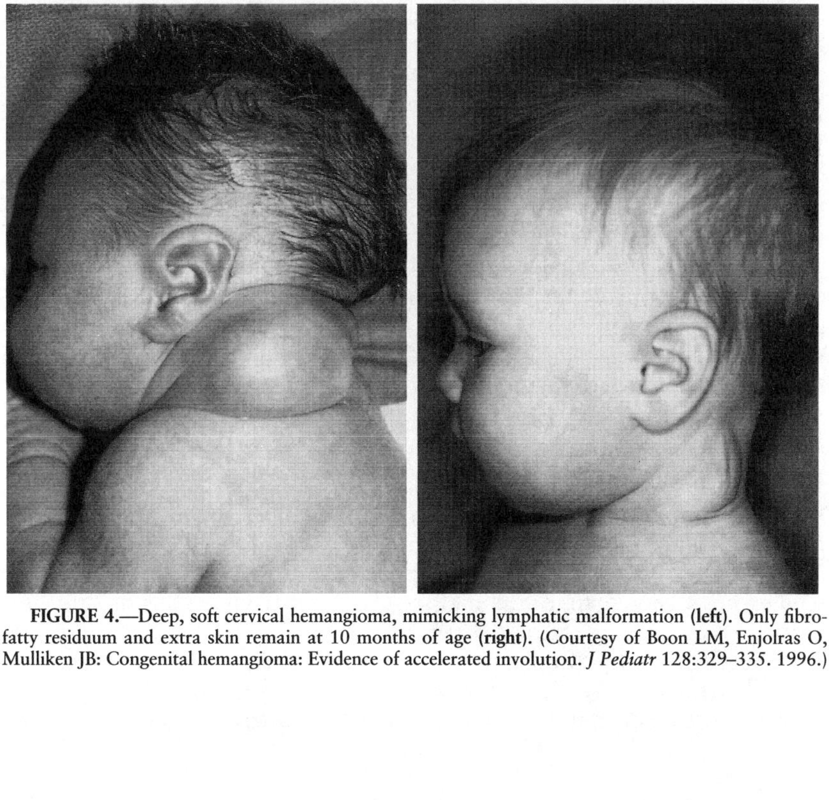

FIGURE 4.—Deep, soft cervical hemangioma, mimicking lymphatic malformation (**left**). Only fibrofatty residuum and extra skin remain at 10 months of age (**right**). (Courtesy of Boon LM, Enjolras O, Mulliken JB: Congenital hemangioma: Evidence of accelerated involution. *J Pediatr* 128:329–335. 1996.)

tures were raised violaceous tumor with ectatic veins, occurring in 8 patients; raised grayish tumor with multiple tiny telangiectasias surrounded by a pale halo, seen in 8; and flat infiltrative tumor with violaceous overlying skin, observed in 5. In 2 patients, hemangiomas were associated with thrombocytopenic coagulopathy. All 24 untreated hemangiomas had regressed by 14 months of age (Figs 2 and 4). Seven patients needed treatment for complications. Three of these tumors responded to systemic corticosteroid therapy, and 4 were resected.

Conclusion.—In some cases, hemangiomas proliferate in utero and are fully developed at birth. These tumors can regress rapidly, which raises new questions regarding the pathogenesis of congenital hemangiomas.

▶ I have seen 1 or 2 of these congenital hemangiomas but was blissfully ignorant of their natural history until enlightened by Boon and colleagues. Most of us are used to seeing what the authors describe as "nascent hemangiomas," which appear in the first days or weeks as small macules before taking on the appearance of the typical strawberry hemangioma during the next few weeks. We usually advise parents that these lesions will grow rapidly for the first 6 months, reach their quiescent stage at 6–12 months, and then regress between 12 and 18 months. As reported here, however, there will be some that are "in full bloom" at birth, and the majority of these will regress spontaneously by age 14 months.

Some of these lesions can be seen on fetal US images as early as the first trimester, suggesting that angiogenic stimulators are at work in utero. If treatment is necessary (for a coagulopathy or deformation of an ear or eye) corticosteroids seem quite effective. A recent series from Israel documented the exceptional efficacy of high-dose oral prednisone in the management of hemangiomas that require intervention.[1]

M.J. Maisels, M.B., B.Ch.

Reference

1. Sadan N, Wolach B: Treatment of hemangiomas of infants with high doses of prednisone. *J Pediatr* 128:141–146, 1996.

Neonatal Circumcision: An End to the Controversy?

Roberts JA (Tulane Univ, Covington, La)
South Med J 89:167–171, 1996 15–11

Introduction.—Circumcision dates back to 4,000 B.C., and according to proponents, it prevents venereal disease, penile cancer, and infection. Others say that good hygienic standards prevent these penile problems. Recent studies have shown that circumcision prevents balanoposthitis and phimosis, as well as cancer of the penis. Uncircumcised men are more susceptible to sexually transmitted diseases. In the 1970s, the American Academy of Pediatrics Task Force on Circumcision decided that there was "no absolute medical indication for routine circumcision of the newborn."

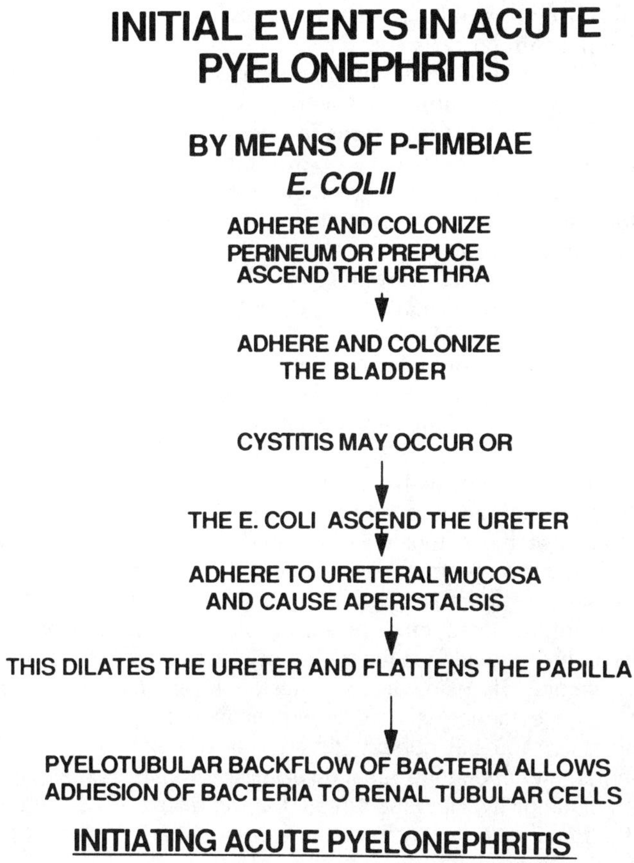

FIGURE 2.—Pathogenesis of pyelonephritis. (Courtesy of Roberts JA: Neonatal circumcision: An end to the controversy? *South Med J* 89:167–171, 1996. Reprinted by permission.)

However, another study showed that 95% of the male infants with neonatal pyelonephritis were uncircumcised.

Bacterial Adherence.—Urinary tract infection has been more common in uncircumcised infants, perhaps because the presence of a foreskin allows bacterial adherence and meatal colonization. In Army hospitals, the total number of urinary tract infections was lower in the late 1970s but increased in the 1980s, coincident with a decrease in circumcision procedures. In foreskins removed by circumcision, studies found that bacteria, such as P-fimbriated *Escherichia coli* (*E. Coli*), which are associated with acute pyelonephritis, adhered to the inner mucosal surface. A study of the monkey shows that initial events leading to acute pyelonephritis involves P-fimbriated *E. coli* that adhere to and colonize the urethra and the bladder, and cause cystitis. Acute pyelonephritis is initiated by the dilatation of the ureter and the flattening of the renal papilla, which allows pyelotubular backflow of bacteria at low pressure so that the same bacteria adhere to renal tubular cells (Fig 2).

End-stage Renal Disease.—Significant renal damage can occur in those infants who have infections in the first years of life. There is a 1% frequency of urinary tract infections in uncircumcised male infants. Renal scarring occurred in 10% to 15% of all infants with acute pyelonephritis. Up to 3% of infants with scarring will have renal insufficiency. There could be 20,000 cases of acute pyelonephritis annually if circumcisions were discontinued in this country.

Conclusions.—Neonatal circumcision is an important prophylactic operation. The American Academy of Pediatrics now states that "newborn circumcision has potential medical benefits and risks." This simple prophylactic procedure should be continued if it is associated with a low incidence of complications, can prevent disease, and is done under local anesthesia so that the infant feels no pain.

▶ Selecting a manuscript with a single author that reflects an opinion rather than a research product is a deviation from the usual YEAR BOOK policy. However, because the author was bold enough to suggest that his manuscript would end the controversy on neonatal circumcision, I thought it fair game to share his optimism, whether founded or not, with subscribers. Roberts presents a perspective on neonatal circumcision, concluding that "the overwhelming evidence leads to my conclusion that the common American practice of neonatal circumcision is an important prophylactic operation." The evidence is that circumcision prevents carcinoma of the penis, phimosis, and balanoposthitis. It reduces urinary tract infections, pyelonephritis, and end-stage renal disease, as well as sexually transmitted diseases, including HIV. He does stress that the risks and benefits should be explained to families, truly informed consent should be obtained, and a local anesthetic should be used.[1-3]

Not everyone interprets the evidence in the same way. There is a vociferous group constantly bombarding the Committee on the Fetus and Newborn with literature and letters demanding the cessation of this barbaric procedure. This includes the national organization of circumcision information resource centers (NOHARMM is the National Organization to Halt Abuse and Routine Mutilation of Males). They would argue vehemently with Winberg and colleagues, who irreverently queried whether "the prepuce was a mistake of nature." Whether to rectify this "mistake" by circumcision will remain a controversial topic, despite Roberts' whimsical title. However, more sophisticated and humane ways of performing neonatal circumcision are being practiced.

A large number of men never feel whole after realizing that a part of their body has been cut off.—J. Bigelow

I think I could have accepted a deformity that was an accident in nature, but I can't accept that somebody did that to me.–J. Bigelow

A.A.Fanaroff, M.B.B.Ch.

References

1. Wiswell TE: Circumcision and update. *Curr Prob Pediatr* 22:424–431, 1992.
2. Schoen EJ: Circumcision updated—indicated? *Pediatrics* 92:860–864, 1993.
3. Winberg J, Bollgren I, Gothefors L, et al: The prepuce: A mistake of nature? *Lancet* 1:598–599, 1989.

Circumcision: Successful Glanular Reconstruction and Survival Following Traumatic Amputation

Sherman J, Borer JG, Horowitz M, et al (State Univ of New York, Brooklyn)
J Urol 156:842–844, 1996 15–12

Background.—Although routine circumcision in newborns is associated with a small risk of complications, such complications can be tragic. Traumatic glans amputations with and without urethral amputations in 7 infants were reported.

Patients and Outcomes.—The infants were 6 white boys, aged 8 days, and 1 black boy, aged 5 months. Circumcision was performed freehand in 1 patient and with a Mogen clamp in another patient. In the remainder, circumcision was done with a protective shield. Excised glanular tissue remained viable for up to 8 hours after accidental amputation. After 8.5–108 months of follow-up, all boys had an acceptable cosmetic result. None of the 8-day-old infants had long-term complications. However, a distal urethral fistula formed in the 5-month-old patient (Figs 3, 4, and 5).

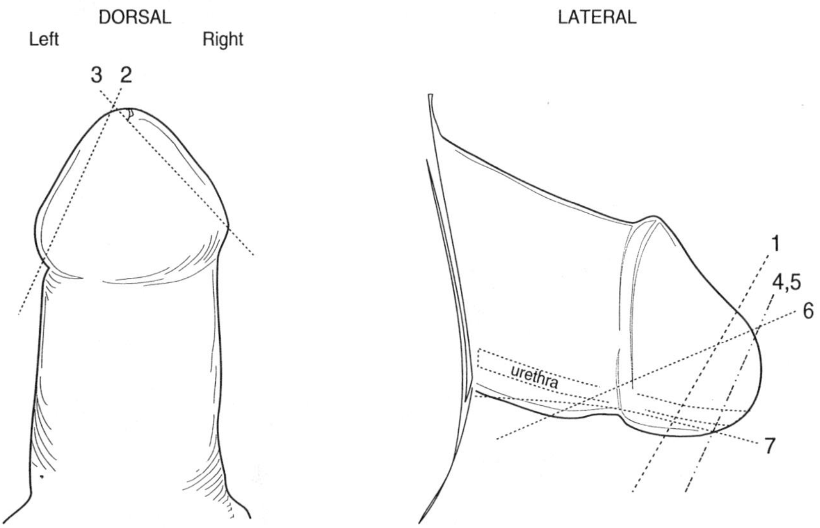

FIGURE 3.—Amputation injuries. *Numbers* and *dotted lines* represent patients and corresponding injuries. (Courtesy of Sherman J, Borer JG, Horowitz M, et al: Circumcision: Successful glanular reconstruction and survival following traumatic amputation. *J Urol* 156:842–844, 1996.)

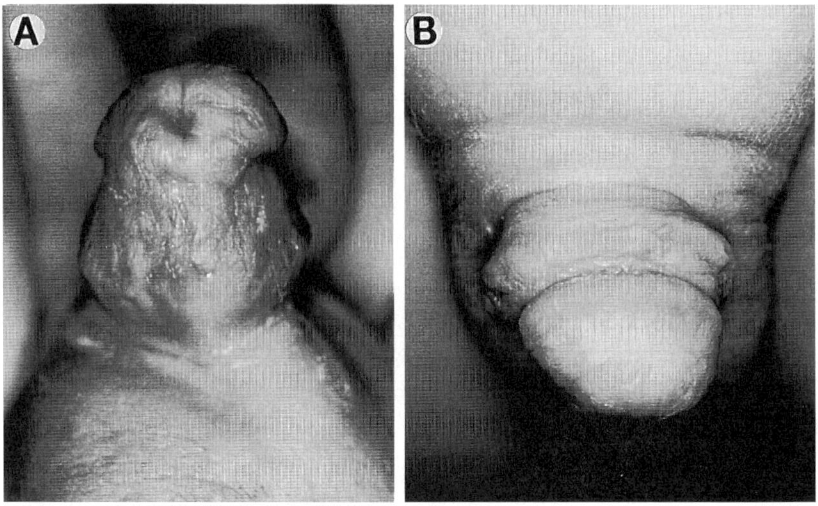

FIGURE 4.—Result of glanular reconstruction at 10 months postoperatively in 1 patient. **A**, ventral aspect of penis. **B**, dorsal aspect of penis. (Courtesy of Sherman J, Borer JG, Horowitz M, et al: Circumcision: Successful glanular reconstruction and survival following traumatic amputation. *J Urol* 156:842–844, 1996.)

Conclusion.—Some traditional mohels excise the skin on the distal side of the shield or excise the foreskin with no shield, compressing the foreskin between the fingers just beyond the tip of the glans before excision. If the ventral foreskin is advanced too far distally, it can pull up on the frenulum, which also brings the urethral meatus and ventral glans forward, possibly

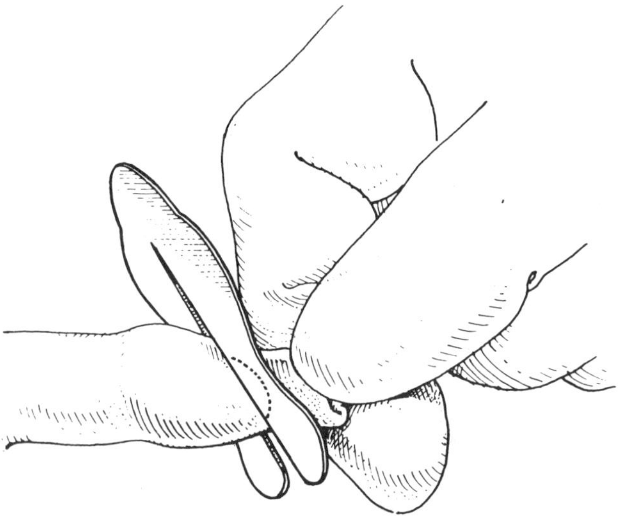

FIGURE 5.—Protective shield at oblique orientation angled parallel to corona with foreskin pulled distally. (Courtesy of Sherman J, Borer JG, Horowitz M, et al: Circumcision: Successful glanular reconstruction and survival following traumatic amputation. *J Urol* 156:842–844, 1996.)

resulting in excision of a portion of the glans with the ventral penile and frenular skin attached to it. In most of the patients described above, this appeared to be the mechanism of injury. When distal amputation occurs, the glans and/or urethra should be reanastomosed, even when surgical repair is delayed for as long as 8 hours.

▶ I was profoundly relieved to read this report. Not only is the most dreaded complication of circumcision correctable, but the resurrected organ is cosmetically acceptable. As about 65% of all male infants in the United States are circumcised, about 1.3 million circumcisions are performed annually. We have no idea of the size of the population from which these cases were selected, nor are we told over what period these complications occurred, so we cannot calculate the risk of this rare complication. Considering the millions of infants who have been circumcised, the number of significant complications is minimal; the most common complication is bleeding.

In 6 of the 7 reported cases, the circumcision was performed by a mohel, an individual specially trained in the performance of Jewish ritual circumcision. Most mohels are well trained and highly experienced. However, as the authors point out, a rigorously orthodox mohel will not use the Mogen clamp because it crushes the tissue before the foreskin is excised with a scalpel just distal to the clamp. The traditional mohel uses a simple protective shield that does not crush the foreskin before it is excised but does increase the possibility of amputation of part of the glans. As a teacher of mine once wisely counseled, "When the mohel is finished, make sure he doesn't throw away the wrong piece." This report makes such advice even more prescient.

M.J. Maisels, M.B., B.Ch.

Developmental Dysplasia of the Hip. A Population-based Comparison of Ultrasound and Clinical Findings

Rosendahl K, Markestad T, Lie RT (Univ Hosp, Bergen, Norway; Med Birth Registry of Norway)

Acta Paediatr 85:64–69, 1996 15–13

Background.—The prevalence of developmental dysplasia of the hip (DDH) appearing after 1 month of age and the need for surgery have not changed substantially in recent decades. Currently, there is no generally accepted method for determining which hips will stabilize with time and which will progress to dislocation if untreated. Agreement between clinical and US examinations in the assessment of hip abnormalities in an unselected, healthy newborn population was investigated, and the effects of adding US to routine clinical screening in the management and understanding of DDH were determined.

Methods.—A total of 3,613 newborns were examined for DDH within 48 hours of delivery. Clinical and US hip stability were classified as stable, borderline unstable, dislocatable, or dislocated. Morphology on US was classified as normal, immature, or dysplastic. Early treatment was indicated by persistent clinical or sonographic dislocatability or dislocation,

TABLE 1.—Classification of Hip Morphology and Stability by US

Morphology	
Normal	Well-formed bony acetabular roof with an angular lateral margin and a narrow cartilaginous rim (Graf type 1b, $\alpha \geq 60°$)
Immature	Adequately formed bony acetabular roof with a rounded lateral margin and a wide cartilaginous rim, i.e., a physiological retardation of the acetabular ossification (Graf type IIa, $50° \leq \alpha < 60°$)
Dysplastic	Minor: deficiently formed bony acetabular roof with a rounded to flattened lateral margin and a wide cartilaginous rim, i.e. a maturational deficit (Graf type IIc/D, $43° \leq \alpha < 50°$, and IIa—)
	Major: poorly formed bony acetabular roof with a flattened lateral margin and a wide cartilaginous rim (Graf type IIIa/b and IV, $\alpha < 43°$)
Stability	
1. Stable hip	
2. Borderline unstable hip	A gap can be visualized between the femoral head and the acetabulum
3. Dislocatable hip	The femoral head can be dislocated lateral to the baseline, followed by a concentric reduction into the acetabulum
4. Dislocated	The femoral head is seen constantly lateral to the baseline

Note: Table has been modified from Graf R: Sonographie der Säuglingshüfte. Ein kompendium. 4. Auft. Stuttgart: Enke, 98:71–72, 1993.
(Courtesy of Rosendahl K, Markestad T, Lie RT: Developmental dysplasia of the hip: A population-based comparison of ultrasound and clinical findings. *Acta Paediatr* 85:64–69, 1996.)

TABLE 4.—Agreement Between Sonographically and Clinically Determined Hip Stability in 3,613 Infants (Left Hips)

	Ultrasound stability		
	Stable	Borderline unstable	Dislocatable /dislocated
Clinical stability			
Stable*	3463	45	23
Borderline unstable	1	9	13
Dislocatable/dislocated	6	5	48

Note: The clinical findings are based on the reexamination when applicable.
*Not reexamined if US morphology and stability were normal
(Courtesy of Rosendahl K, Markestad T, Lie RT: Developmental dysplasia of the hip: A population-based comparison of ultrasound and clinical findings. *Acta Paediatr* 85:64–69, 1996.)

major dysplasia, or minor dysplasia combined with an unstable femoral head.

Findings.—One hundred twenty-three infants (3.4%) underwent early treatment. Forty-five percent of these patients met both US and clinical criteria for treatment. Forty-two percent were treated on the basis of US findings alone, and 13% were treated on the basis of clinical findings alone. At the first clinical assessment, 30% of the infants with clinically dislocated or dislocatable hips were judged to have stable or just borderline unstable hips. Ninety-seven percent of the 486 patients with immature or minor dysplastic but stable hips on US had spontaneous normalization. No sonographic improvement was seen in 3% of this group at 1–3 months of age, and treatment was begun. During the 3-year observation period, late DDH was seen in only 1 infant (Tables 1, 4, 5, and 6).

Conclusion.—The addition of sonographic dysplasia as an indication for early splinting may double the treatment rate for DDH in infants. However, late dislocation may be virtually eliminated through this strategy.

▶ From past studies, we know that about 2% of newborns have some degree of hip instability but only 2 in 1,000 progress to dislocation if left

TABLE 5.—Association Between Sonographic Hip Morphology and Clinical Stability in 3,613 Infants (Left Hips)

	Ultrasound morphology			
			Dysplastic	
	Normal	Immature	Minor	Major
Clinical stability				
Stable*	3055	425	45	4
Borderline unstable	3	2	16	3
Dislocatable	3	11	27	7
Dislocated	0	0	5	7

Note: The clinical findings are based on reexamination when applicable.
*Not reexamined if US and first clinical findings were normal
(Courtesy of Rosendahl K, Markestad T, Lie RT: Developmental dysplasia of the hip: A population-based comparison of ultrasound and clinical findings. *Acta Paediatr* 85:64–69, 1996.)

TABLE 6.—Agreement Between US and Clinical Findings Based on a Classification Into Normal, Borderline, or Pathologic Hips (3,613 Left Hips)

	Ultrasound findings (morphology and stability)		
	Normal*	Borderline†	Pathological‡
Clinical findings			
Stable	3403	46	23
Borderline unstable	2	9	13
Dislocatable/dislocated	6	6	48

Note: The clinical findings are based on the reexamination when applicable.
*Normal/immature and stable.
†Minor dysplasia and/or borderline unstable.
‡Major dysplasia and/or dislocatable/dislocated.
(Courtesy of Rosendahl K, Markestad T, Lie RT: Developmental dysplasia of the hip: A population-based comparison of ultrasound and clinical findings. *Acta Paediatr* 85:64–69, 1996.)

untreated. In this analysis, the combination of clinical and US examinations led to treatment of 3.4% of infants, about 40% of whom were treated on the basis of US findings alone. It is disconcerting to learn that 4 infants, shown to have major dysplasia of the hip by US, were considered normal on clinical examination, even when the examination was repeated by an experienced pediatrician *who knew the ultrasound findings!* On US, these hips had a poorly formed bony acetabular roof with a flattened lateral margin and a wide cartilaginous rim but appeared normal on examination. Furthermore, 23 hips that were judged stable by clinical examination were revealed to have major dysplasia or were dislocatable or dislocated on US.

It seems clear that if US were to become a routine part of newborn evaluation, it would lead to the treatment of many more infants; but is this necessarily a good idea? In their previous, randomized trial,[1] the same authors found a prevalence of late subluxation or dislocation of 0.3 in 1,000 when all infants were screened by US, compared with an incidence of 0.7 in 1,000 in those who received US screening only in the presence of risk factors (abnormal physical examination, breech position, or family history of developmental dysplasia of the hip). In those who were screened only by a physical examination, the incidence was 1.3 in 1,000. These differences were not statistically significant.

Given the current fiscal climate and length of stay for the average newborn, there is no possibility of routine US screening before discharge ever becoming a reality in the United States. In addition, these authors and others have shown that even though hips are clinically unstable or show dysplasia on sonograms, most will develop normally without treatment.[2] However, there is no doubt that ultrasound will reveal a significant number of false negative clinical findings. What to do? I would opt for a middle road, using a US examination if risk factors are present or if clinical examination produces abnormal results. As a large number of these infants improve spontaneously, the best time to do this US evaluation is at 2 weeks.

M.J. Maisels, M.B., B.Ch.

References

1. Rosendahl K, Markestad T, Lie RT: Ultrasound screening for developmental dysplasia of the hip in the neonate. The effect on treatment rate and prevalence of late cases. *Pediatrics* 94:47–52, 1994.
2. Terjesen T, Holen KJ, Tegnander A: Hip abnormalities detected by ultrasound in clinically normal newborn infants. *J Bone Joint Surg (Br)* 78B:636–640, 1996.

16 Postnatal Growth and Development

Randomized Outcome Trial of Human Milk Fortification and Developmental Outcome in Preterm Infants

Lucas A, Fewtrell MS, Morley R, et al (Inst of Child Health, London; Univ Dept of Pediatrics, Cambridge, England; Norwich Hosp, England)

Am J Clin Nutr 64:142–151, 1996 16–1

Background.—Studies have shown that the method of preterm infant feeding in the weeks just after birth has a major effect on long-term outcomes. Human milk may not meet the nutrient needs of such infants. The value of fortified breast milk, given alone or with preterm formula, in improving neurodevelopment and growth at 18 months was investigated.

Methods.—The study included 275 preterm infants whose mothers chose to provide breast milk. By random assignment, a multinutrient fortifier or control supplement with phosphate and vitamins was given for a mean of 39 days. Breast milk comprised 47.6% and 46.4% of enteral intake in the 2 respective groups. When sufficient breast milk was unavailable, preterm formula supplements were used.

Findings.—Overall, no significant growth advantages were noted in the fortified group. However, when breast milk exceeded 50% of intake, the infants receiving fortification gained weight faster. Compared with the control group, the fortified infants had higher plasma urea levels beginning in week 2, greater plasma calcium levels, and a higher increase in alkaline phosphatase by week 6. The fortified group also had more clinical infections, a nonsignificant increase in necrotizing enterocolitis incidence, and higher white blood cell and platelet counts. At 18 months, developmental scores were slightly, nonsignificantly greater in the fortified infants.

Conclusions.—Although breast milk fortifiers can improve short-term growth in preterm infants, their beneficial effects on long-term development are still unproven. Potential adverse consequences and better fortification strategies need to be investigated.

► This comment has been provided by William D. Rhine, M.D., Assistant Professor of Pediatrics, Stanford University School of Medicine, Co-director of ECMO, Lucile Salter Packard Children's Hospital at Stanford, Palo Alto, California:

▶ We again have Dr. Lucas and colleagues to thank for trying to answer at least one of the very important but almost too routine questions of neonatology, "What should we feed premature infants?" This well-planned, prospective, randomized trial even includes an appropriate control arm of "sham" fortifier, which is clearly more than nothing. Many neonatologists either don't know, don't agree with, or don't act on the underlying premise that breast milk alone has inadequate phosphate and other vitamins. Indeed, these authors considered it unethical to not supplement with such compounds at minimum. The fact that there were any detectable differences in any metabolic outcome is remarkable considering that during the 5–6 weeks of the study, breast milk accounted for less than 50% of the average enteral intake. As the authors caution, not too much should be read into small differences near a *P* value of 0.05 when so many variables are observed. One of the strongest findings is that if most intake comes from breast milk, then fortifier will likely improve growth. Perhaps because of lack of size and power, this study did not find any long-term neurodevelopmental effects of breast milk fortification. However, this does not mean we can ignore the potential effects of diet on development of the premature infant. Instead, we must acknowledge both our ignorance and the need for further studies in this matter.

W.D. Rhine, M.D.

Neurodevelopmental Outcome at 36 Months' Corrected Age of Preterm Infants in the Multicenter Indomethacin Intraventricular Hemorrhage Prevention Trial

Ment LR, Vohr B, Oh W, et al (Yale Univ, New Haven, Conn; Brown Univ, Providence, RI; Univ of Washington, Seattle; et al)

Pediatrics 98:714–718, 1996 16–2

Introduction.—Low-dose indomethacin has been found to decrease the incidence of intraventricular hemorrhage, a cause of neurodevelopmental handicaps, in very low birth weight preterm infants. A prospective trial conducted at 3 institutions confirmed this finding, but other studies suggested that treatment with indomethacin reduces cerebral blood flow, increasing the risk of developmental handicaps. Neonates who received indomethacin were followed up and evaluated at 36 months' corrected age for neurodevelopmental outcome.

Methods.—The randomized, placebo-controlled trial enrolled 431 neonates weighing 600–1,250 g at birth. None had evidence of intraventricular hemorrhage at cranial echoencephalography, performed between 5 and 11 hours after birth. After randomization, 209 infants received IV indomethacin (0.1 mg/kg 6–12 hours after birth and every 24 hours for 2 more doses) and 222 were given placebo. Each child was tested at 36

TABLE 2.—Neurologic Data for Children at 36 Months' Corrected Age: Primary Indomethacin Intraventricular Hemorrhage Prevention Trial

Characteristic	Indomethacin	Placebo	*P*
n	173	170	
Blind*	1/85 (1%)	1/73 (1%)	1.0
Deaf*	1/69 (1.5%)	1/66 (1.5%)	1.0
Cerebral palsy	13/166 (8%)	14/167 (8%)	1.0

*Numbers of children who underwent either vision or hearing screens in the past 18 months.

(Courtesy of Ment LR, Vohr B, Oh W, et al: Neurodevelopmental outcome at 36 months' corrected age of preterm infants in the multicenter indomethacin intraventricular hemorrhage prevention trial. *Pediatrics* 98:714–718, 1996. Reproduced by permission of *Pediatrics*, copyright 1996.)

months' corrected age with the Stanford-Binet Intelligence Scale and the Peabody Picture Vocabulary Test-Revised (PPVT-R). Routine neurologic examination also was part of the follow-up evaluation.

Results.—There were 384 survivors, including 192 (92%) of the indomethacin group and 192 (86%) of the placebo group. Neurodevelopmental assessment was conducted in 173 infants randomly assigned to receive indomethacin and 170 assigned to receive placebo. One child from each group was blind and 1 from each group was deaf; 8% of children in each group had evidence of cerebral palsy (Table 2). In the group of 248 children with intelligence quotient (IQ) data, those treated with indomethacin had a significantly younger mean gestational age than those given placebo; ventriculomegaly was found on cranial US at term in 5 of 110 infants in the placebo group and in none of the 115 infants given indomethacin. Mean Stanford-Binet IQ scores at 36 months' corrected age were 89.6 for the indomethacin group and 85.0 for the placebo group (Table 4). The PPVT-R scores yielded similar findings.

Conclusions.—Indomethacin decreases cerebral blood flow velocity in preterm very low birth weight infants, reducing the incidence and severity of neonatal intraventricular hemorrhage. In this series of infants, early low-dose indomethacin also improved survival at 36 months' corrected

TABLE 4.—Influence of Low-dose Prophylactic Indomethacin and IVH on Stanford-Binet IQ Scores at 36 Months' Corrected Age

Treatment	No IVH	Any IVH	All Infants
Indomethacin	90.5 ± 18.53* n = 114	81.1 ± 21.22 n = 12	89.6 ± 18.922 n = 126
Placebo	86.1 ± 20.65 n = 102	79.7 ± 21.19 n = 20	85.0 ± 20.79 n = 122
P	.10	.86	.074

*Values are mean plus or minus standard deviation.

Abbreviations: IVH, intraventricular hemorrhage; *IQ*, intelligence quotient.

(Courtesy of Ment LR, Vohr B, Oh W, et al: Neurodevelopmental outcome at 36 months' corrected age of preterm infants in the multicenter indomethacin intraventricular hemorrhage prevention trial. *Pediatrics* 98:714–718, 1996. Reproduced by permission of *Pediatrics*, copyright 1996.)

age, decreased the incidence of ventriculomegaly, and was not associated with adverse cognitive or motor outcome.

▶ This commentary was contributed by Maureen Hack, M.D., Professor of Pediatrics, Director of Neonatal High Risk Follow-up Program, Case Western Reserve University School of Medicine, Cleveland, Ohio:

▶ Ment and associates reassure us that indomethacin given to prevent intraventricular hemorrhage has no detrimental effect on 3-year outcomes. However, indomethacin did not decrease the incidence of cerebral palsy. The common pathway to cerebral palsy, although it includes periventricular hemorrhage, probably is multifactorial. Thus, we should not be surprised that a single drug such as indomethacin, which had an effect solely on periventricular hemorrhage but not periventricular leukomalacia or chronic lung disease, did not influence the rate of cerebral palsy. I am concerned about the widespread use of prophylactic indomethacin therapy because of its potential side effects. Among other findings, there have been reports that indomethacin might increase the rate of retinopathy of prematurity.[1] This was not examined by Ment and associates.

Because the proof of the pudding is in the eating, we will need further studies to evaluate the long-term effects of indomethacin. A major confounding factor is the diagnosis of "cerebral palsy." More specific neurologic sequelae need to be identified and described to elucidate whether indomethacin has any beneficial effect on 3-year outcomes, which would justify any neonatal and possibly later side effects. Also see reference 2 for more on the use of indomethacin.

M. Hack, M.D.

References

1. Darlow BAW, Jorwood LJ, Clemett RS: Retinopathy of prematurity: Risk factors in a prospective population-based study. *Paediatr Perinat Epidemiol* 6:62–80, 1992.
2. Lindemann R, Blystad W, Egge K: Retrolental fibroplasia in premature infants with patent ductus arteriosus treated with indomethacin. *Eur J Pediatr* 138:56–58, 1982.

Quality of Life Among Young Adults Born With Very Low Birthweights

Bjerager M, Steensberg J, Greisen G (State Univ Hosp, Copenhagen)

Acta Paediatr 84:1339–1343, 1995 16–3

Purpose.—As survival improves for very low birth weight (VLBW) infants, there is concern as to whether they enjoy the same quality of life as normal birth weight (NBW) infants as they grow to adulthood. Quality of life (QoL) was compared in young adults who were VLBW vs. NBW at birth.

Methods.—The study included 85 subjects, 18–20 years of age, who weighed less than 1,500 g at birth. In telephone interviews, the subjects responded to a QoL questionnaire. The questionnaire was based on the well-defined QoL model of Aggernæs, which encompasses the issue of the person's subjective QoL. Objective and subjective QoL scores were calculated for each of the 4 "universal human needs" defined by Aggernæs: elementary biological needs, warm human relations, meaningful occupations, and diverse and exciting experiences. A group of 85 young adults with birth weights of greater than 2,500 g were studied for comparison.

Results.—The VLBW and NBW groups showed very few differences in QoL scores, either objective or subjective. The exception was a subgroup of 19 VLBW subjects with self-reported handicaps or chronic diseases who had lower objective and subjective QoL scores. In this group, the subjective scores were only slightly higher than the objective scores.

Conclusion.—Young adults born with VLBW appear to have a level of QoL similar to that of their NBW peers, provided they are free of handicaps. The VLBW children lag behind their peers during childhood, but this problem might be addressed by extra resources to meet the special needs of these children. Quality of life is adversely affected for VLBW infants who grow up with handicaps or chronic diseases.

▶ Dr. Ernest Krug, Director, Developmental Pediatrics, William Beaumont Hospital, Royal Oak, Michigan, comments:

▶ Twenty-year follow-ups of VLBW infants are rare, as are studies examining QoL. We also need to remember that these are outcomes for infants treated in the early 1970s, before the full flowering of neonatal intensive care (only 4 infants who weighed < 1,000 g survived). It is not particularly surprising that the authors found that VLBW subjects who were *free of handicaps* had subjective and objective QoL scores fully comparable to those of NBW control group. Summarizing a quotation by Isabell Rapin, which concludes the paper, those with reasonably good social skills and a "niche in the marketplace" have a reasonable life in spite of early insults to their well-being. In the neonatal ICU, it is difficult to decide which infant will likely have a poor QoL, and we should be careful about making assumptions regarding the QoL of another person that are based on inadequate data and personal preference.

E. Krug, M.D.

Extremely Low-birth-weight Children and Their Peers: A Comparison of School-age Outcomes

Halsey CL, Collin MF, Anderson CL (Loyola Univ, Maywood, Ill; MetroHealth Med Ctr, Cleveland, Ohio)

Arch Pediatr Adolesc Med 150:790–794, 1996 16–4

Backgound.—Some researchers suggest that children born prematurely may "grow into" intellectual and educational deficits as demands increase. Seven-year developmental and educational outcomes in 1 cohort of mostly middle-class, very low birth weight (VLBW) children were investigated to determine the incidence of developmental disability and the need for special educational services.

Methods.—Fifty-four of a cohort of 104 VLBW survivors of presurfactant treatment were studied. The cohort was born between 1984 and 1986 at 1 center. The control group consisted of 58 children matched for race, sex, and socioeconomic status. Thirty of these children had low birth weights (1,500 to 2,500 g), and 28 had birth weights exceeding 2,500. Teacher reports of classroom placement and special educational services were obtained, and tests of cognitive, motor, language, and visual-motor integration abilities were performed.

Findings.—Fifty percent of the VLBW children were in regular classrooms and needed no special services, compared with 70% of the low–birth weight control group and 93% of the full-term group. This trend toward increasing need for special services with decreasing birth weight was significant. The test scores of the VLBW group were significantly lower than those of the control groups, although these scores generally fell in the average range. In 79% of the VLBW children, cognitive scores were average but were a mean of 14 to 17 points lower than the scores of the control groups. Significant disabilities were noted in 20% of the VLBW children, including cerebral palsy, mental retardation, autism, and low intelligence with severe learning problems.

Conclusion.—Even in optimal socioeconomic environments, half of all children surviving VLBW need special educational services. One fifth of these children have significant disabilities. Compared with matched peer groups, these children had weaknesses on all objective measures.

► As neonatologists, we vacillate between elation at our ongoing successes in keeping VLBW infants alive and the sobering realities of subsequent developmental and educational problems. These authors previously reported that evaluation before age 18 months of surviving VLBW infants provides a misleadingly optimistic picture. When retested later, the same children performed significantly worse, suggesting that intellectual and educational deficits will appear as demands increase.[1] Here, the authors show that at age 7 years, 50% of a cohort of VLBW infants (birth weight less than 1,000 g) born between 1984 and 1986 required special services in school and—although most of the group had test results that were within the average range—they averaged 14–17 points lower than the 2 comparison groups.

When compared with larger, population-based studies,[2] this study suffers from the weakness of having a single, hospital-based cohort and an apparent lack of blinding of the principal author, who did the developmental testing. Nevertheless, in addition to the 20% incidence of significant disabilities (cerebral palsy, mental retardation, autism, low intelligence, and severe learning problems), the finding that 1 out of every 2 VLBW children required special educational services is even more striking given that this population was predominantly white and middle class. Of those who were lost to follow-up, significantly more were black, uninsured, and sicker during their hospital stay. Thus, the reported outcomes are almost certainly more optimistic than would have occurred if the entire cohort had been studied. It is also sobering to note that 30% of children who weighed 1,500–2,500 g at birth subsequently required special school services. In contrast to the findings of Hack et al.,[2] the performance of the subgroup of children with birth weights less than 750 g was no different from those with birth weights of 750–1,000 g.

To provide a 7-year follow-up, we generally require a cohort born 10 years or more before publication and, inevitably, this leads to the view (the hope?) that because of the advances in care that have taken place during the past decade (antenatal steroids, surfactant, etc), similar children born today might do considerably better. Currently, there is no evidence to support this belief. In this study, grade 3 or 4 intracranial hemorrhage occurred in 12 of 54 children (22%) in the VLBW group—a rate that would be considered high by today's standards. Nevertheless, 8 of these 12 children were in regular classrooms with no special needs; thus, the study outcomes cannot be blamed on intracranial hemorrhage.

The authors provide no information regarding periventricular leukomalacia, which, if extensive, is universally associated with significant neurologic handicap. For infants weighing less than 1,500 g, however, the presence of severe periventricular leukomalacia is not related to gestational age and is unlikely to have contributed significantly to these findings. In 1991, Saigal et al. demonstrated the profound impact that social class has on the cognitive abilities and school performance of surviving VLBW children,[3] and it is disappointing to find that even with socioeconomic advantages, 20% of VLBW children are significantly disabled, and 50% require special educational services. This population will place an increasing burden on an already widely criticized national educational system.

M.J. Maisels, M.B., B.Ch.

References

1. Collin M, Halsey C, Anderson C: Emerging developmental sequelae in the "normal" extremely low birthweight infant. *Pediatrics* 88:115–120, 1991.
2. Hack M, Taylor G, Klein N, et al: School-age outcomes in children with birthweights under 750 g. *N Engl J Med* 331:753–759, 1994.
3. Saigal S, Szatmari P, Rosenbaum P, et al: Cognitive abilities and school performance of extremely low birth weight children and matched term control children at age 8 years: A regional study. *J Pediatr* 118:751–760, 1991.

Cognitive and Neurologic Development of the Premature, Small for Gestational Age Infant Through Age 6: Comparison by Birth Weight and Gestational Age

McCarton CM, Wallace IF, Divon M, et al (Albert Einstein College of Medicine, Bronx, NY; Research Triangle Inst, Research Triangle Park, NC; Univ of North Carolina at Chapel Hill)

Pediatrics 98:1167–1178, 1996 16–5

Background.—Premature infants who are small for gestational age (SGA) are thought to be at increased risk for adverse outcomes because of the shortened gestational period compounded by intrauterine growth retardation (IUGR). However, the direct effects of IUGR in premature infants have not been established. The neurologic and cognitive outcomes of premature SGA infants were compared with those of premature infants of appropriate gestational age (AGA).

Methods.—One hundred twenty-nine premature SGA infants and 300 premature AGA infants were compared. Cognitive and neurologic outcomes were determined at 1, 2, 3, and 5 and/or 6 years, with the children stratified by gestational age in 2-week intervals or by 500-g birth weight increments.

Findings.—At each age, SGA children had significantly lower cognitive scores than did the AGA children of comparable gestational ages. Also, neurologic status was more likely to be normal at all assessments in the AGA than in the SGA infants of similar gestational age. The SGA and AGA children did not differ at any age when grouped by birth weight. Cognitive impairment was strongly correlated with neurologic abnormality in both groups. However, SGA had a significant effect on cognitive outcome independent of neurologic status at all ages except 3 years.

Conclusions.—Infants who are SGA have a higher risk for neurodevelopmental impairment than comparably premature AGA infants, regardless of degree of prematurity. Cognitive impairment may be largely, though not completely, attributed to a greater incidence of neurologic abnormalities in SGA infants at each gestational age.

Cost of Care for a Geographically Determined Population of Low Birthweight Infants to Age 8–9 Years: I. Children Without Disability

Stevenson RC, McCabe CJ, Pharoah POD, et al (Univ of Liverpool, England; Univ of Sheffield, England)

Arch Dis Child 74:F114–F117, 1996 16–6

Background.—The cost of neonatal intensive care treatment for low–birth weight infants is a concern in many countries. Little is known about the medium- and long-range costs of care for such infants as they progress through childhood and adulthood. A geographically defined population was studied in 5 health districts that comprise Merseyside, England.

Methods.—The cohort included all children weighing 1,500 g or less at birth and a 10% random sample of children weighing 1,501–2,000 g without clinical deficits born in 1980 and 1981 to Merseyside mothers. These children and their age-matched, sex-matched, and school class–matched controls were followed up to 8 or 9 years of age.

Findings.—Overall, 641 children survived without disability, and 227 did not survive. The average cost of neonatal care per low–birth weight child was 13 times higher than that of a control subject. Neonatal costs for children weighing 1,000 g or less at birth were 55 times greater than for control children. Through childhood, the children with low birth weights continued to use more hospital and family practitioner services than their matched controls.

Conclusions.—The mean cost of medical care for low–birth weight children with no disability was $4,142—4.7 times higher than the cost of care for control children at $896. Among low–birth weight children, the demand for medical services was increased until at least 8–9 years of age.

▶ Many studies have detailed the increased cost of care for low–birth weight infants, but few have included the cost of subsequent hospitalization and care by the primary care physician. Almost none have used a geographically based sample. In this study, children born to mothers in 5 health districts were included in the sample and assessed at ages 3–4 years and 8–9 years. Such regional samples, rather than hospital-based samples, provide a much more reliable estimate of what is happening in the real world. Now, more than ever, we ignore the cost of care at our peril. It is not surprising, but sobering, to note that the costs for children weighing less than 1,000 g at birth are 55 times greater than for control infants in a study that *excluded those children with "clinical disabilities."* On the other hand, children who weigh less than 1,000 g represent only 0.5% of the population, so their overall impact on health care is quite modest.

M.J. Maisels, M.B., B.Ch.

Catch-up Growth During Childhood Among Very Low-birth-weight Children

Hack M, Weissman B, Borawski-Clark E (Case Western Reserve Univ, Cleveland, Ohio; Emory Univ, Atlanta, Ga)

Arch Pediatr Adolesc Med 150:1122–1129, 1996 16–7

Background.—Very low birth weight (VLBW) children have poor growth attainment as a result of intrauterine, neonatal, or postnatal growth failure. In the past, authorities believed that catch-up growth in such children did not occur after 2–3 years of age. Recent research, however, has shown that catch-up (or compensatory) growth can occur up to 8 years of age in children born with VLBWs. Growth attainment and the correlates of catch-up growth at 8 years of age in 1 cohort of children with birth weights of less than 1,500 g were investigated.

Methods.—Two hundred forty-nine children born between 1977 and 1979 were included in the 8-year longitudinal study. One hundred ninety-nine were appropriate for gestational age at birth, and 50 were small for gestational age. Three hundred sixty-three children with normal birth weights also were studied.

Findings.—Among the VLBW children, catch-up growth to above the 3rd percentile occurred between 40 weeks and 8 months, between 8 and 20 months, and up to 8 years of age. Fifty-four percent of these children were subnormal in weight and 60% were subnormal height at 40 weeks. At 8 months, these proportions were 33% and 22%, respectively. At 8 years, 8% were subnormal in both height and weight. Children who were small for their gestational age had lower rates of catch-up growth. In a multivariate analysis, factors predicting percentile distribution of height were maternal height, race, birth weight, and neurologic abnormality. Subnormal height was predicted by maternal height, small-for-gestational-age status, and neurologic abnormality.

Conclusions.—Catch-up of height and weight to above the third percentile can occur among children who have had earlier growth failure. Although most catch-up growth occurs in infancy, it can continue throughout childhood, to 8 years of age. However, the mean growth measures of the VLBW children in this series continued to be significantly lower than those of the children with normal birth weights.

▶ My colleague, Maureen Hack, stands tall among those dedicated, talented few who have managed to combine research and clinical service in their follow-up developmental programs. She now informs us that more of the low–birth weight infants, graduates from the neonatal ICU, are standing as tall as their full-term peers. As a group, they remain smaller, with many exceptions. It is fascinating to follow up the growth patterns of these low–birth weight infants and recognize the interrelations between growth and neurologic development. The exercise of predicting growth for the group as a whole is relatively simple; the growth of each individual child is much less predictable unless he or she has cerebral palsy, in which case you can bet against catch-up growth. Much more growth is anticipated during adolescence, so it is important to keep tabs on this distinctive cohort. Indeed, they presently are being summoned back for a series of evaluations. Many of them are in college, some are married, and some are parents themselves, and I am pleased to report that Dr. Hack will share their progress with us as soon as it is available.

In reviewing the continued catch-up of the appropriately grown infants, the haunting question is why they grew so poorly during their sojourn in the nursery. How well will they catch up developmentally?[1] What interventions can be initiated to accelerate catch-up growth? More attention to energy balance in the neonatal ICU, measures to prevent the development of chronic lung disease, and avoidance of cerebral catastrophes are a good start. Close monitoring of all growth parameters and caloric enhancement during infancy all may contribute to a larger, healthier child.

A.A. Fanaroff, M.B.B.Ch.

Reference

1. Hack M, Breslau N, Weissman B, et al: Effects of very low birthweight and subnormal head size on cognitive abilities at school age. *N Engl J Med* 325:231–237, 1991.

Do Growth-retarded Premature Infants Have Different Rates of Perinatal Morbidity and Mortality Than Appropriately Grown Premature Infants?

Piper JM, Xenakis EM-J, McFarland M, et al (Univ of Texas, San Antonio)
Obstet Gynecol 87:169–174, 1996 16–8

Introduction.—It is commonly believed that the stress of the intrauterine environment induces accelerated maturation in growth-retarded fetuses, which suggests that growth-retarded fetuses could benefit from preterm delivery to prevent fetal death. However, there is conflicting evidence regarding these assumptions. Perinatal morbidity and mortality were compared in growth-retarded and appropriately grown preterm infants at the same gestational age.

Methods.—Data on all infants delivered during a 15-year period were reviewed to identify singleton infants delivered at 24–36 weeks' gestation. Of these infants, those with a birth weight at or lower than the 10th

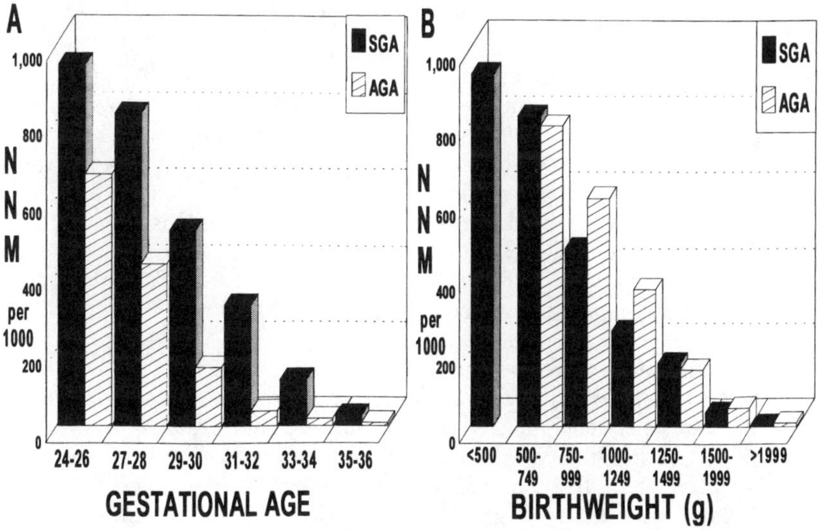

FIGURE 1.—Neonatal mortality (*NNM*) rates in small-for-gestational-age (*SGA*) and appropriate-for-gestational-age (*AGA*) pregnancies compared by gestational age (**A**) and birth weight (**B**). Neonatal death rates in SGA pregnancies were significantly higher by gestational age ($P < 0.05$) but not by birth rate. (Courtesy of Piper JM, Xenakis EM-J, McFarland M, et al: Do growth-retarded premature infants have different rates of perinatal morbidity and mortality than appropriately grown premature infants? *Obstet Gynecol* 87:169–174, 1996. With permission of the American College of Obstetricians and Gynecologists.)

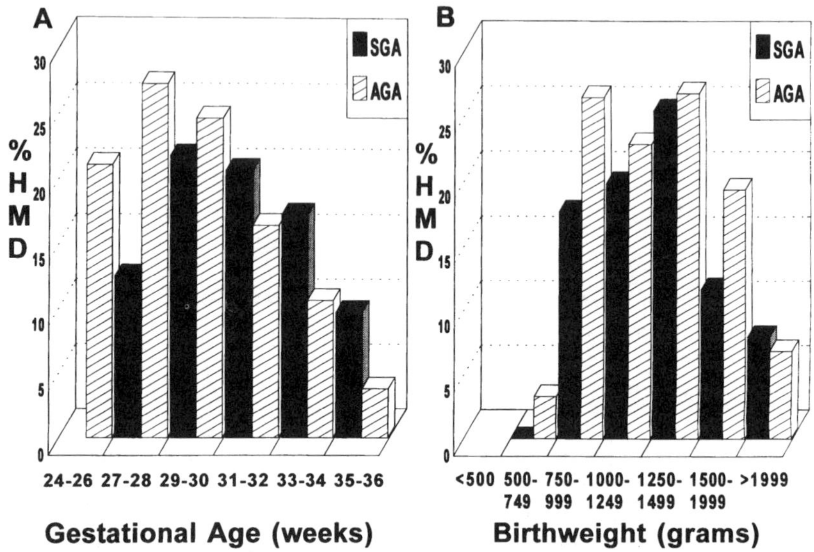

FIGURE 2.—Hyaline membrane disease (*HMD*) rates in small-for-gestational-age (*SGA*) and appropriate-for-gestational-age (*AGA*) pregnancies compared by gestational age (**A**) and birth weight (**B**). Comparison by gestational age revealed an overall significantly higher rate of HMD in the SGA pregnancies compared with the AGA pregnancies ($P < 0.05$). In contrast, when compared by birth weight categories, the rate of HMD was lower in the SGA than in the AGA pregnancies ($P < 0.05$). (Courtesy of Piper JM, Xenakis EM-J, McFarland M, et al: Do growth-retarded premature infants have different rates of perinatal morbidity and mortality than appropriately grown premature infants? *Obstet Gynecol* 87:169–174, 1996. With permission of the American College of Obstetricians and Gynecologists.)

percentile were identified as small for gestational age (SGA), and those with a birth weight between the 11th and 89th percentiles were identified as appropriate for gestational age (AGA). These 2 groups were compared for perinatal mortality, congenital anomaly, and perinatal morbidity rates.

Results.—The study population included 1,012 SGA and 3,171 AGA infants born before 37 weeks' gestation. In the SGA pregnancies, 72% of the infants survived and 17% of the fetuses and 11% of the neonates died. In the AGA pregnancies, 83% of the infants survived and 7% of the fetuses and 10% of the neneonates died. Compared with the AGA pregnancies, perinatal death rates were significantly higher in the SGA pregnancies at every gestational age but did not differ significantly in the 2 groups when stratified by birth weight (Fig 1). There was no significant difference in anomaly rates between the 2 groups. Compared with the AGA pregnancies, the SGA pregnancies had more frequent indications for cesarean delivery and of fetal heart rate abnormalities, but there were no significant differences between the 2 groups for Apgar score at 5 minutes, birth trauma, and neonatal sepsis. Compared with the AGA infants, the SGA infants had a significantly higher rate of hyaline membrane disease when matched by gestational age but a significantly lower rate when matched by birth weight (Fig 2).

Conclusions.—Growth retardation is a significant and independent predictor of perinatal mortality and morbidity. Therefore, elective preterm delivery of SGA fetuses is not justified.

▶ A question is posed in the title of this article, and an unequivocal response is provided in the conclusion. This should satisfy even the most ardent critic. Piper and colleagues used a 15-year cohort to compare the outcomes of SGA (10th percentile or below) with AGA (11th to 89th percentile) infants delivered before 37 weeks' gestation. Gestational age was based on maternal history and rarely modified by US findings. Significantly higher fetal and neonatal mortality was observed in the SGA group in each gestational age category. Higher rates of hyaline membrane disease were present in the SGA infants. This confirms the findings of Tyson and associates,[1] who reported a higher incidence of respiratory distress syndrome in SGA than AGA infants.

A new dimension was that this population had a very high rate of congenital malformations (13% to 14%), far in excess of the anticipated 2% to 4%, irrespective of the growth pattern. This warrants further explanation. Twenty-four percent of this cohort were SGA, and even accounting for the exclusion of infants above the 90th percentile, this cohort appears to be skewed to the small side, with an excessive rate of malformation. Which came first? The burning question is whether these data are generalizable. It is imperative to probe the large databases, such as the Oxford Vermont and the NICHD Neonatal Research Network, to find out whether these groups come up with similar answers. However, the way in which those databases are being collected, with constriction by birth weight, may preclude any answers except for infants with gestational ages in the lower ranges.

A.A. Fanaroff, M.B.B.Ch.

Reference

1. Tyson JE, Kennedy K, Broils S, et al: The small for gestational age infant accelerated with delayed pulmonary maturation? Increased or decreased survival? *Pediatrics* 534–538, 1995.

Neonatal Cranial Ultrasound Abnormalities in Low Birth Weight Infants: Relation to Cognitive Outcomes at Six Years of Age

Whitaker AH, Feldman JF, van Rossem R, et al (Columbia Univ, New York; City College of New York; Univ of Pennsylvania, Philadelphia; et al)
Pediatrics 98:719–729, 1996 16–9

Objective.—Cognitive impairments in low–birth weight (LBW), very low birth weight, and extremely low birth weight infants range from mental retardation to more subtle learning deficits. The most common perinatal brain injuries observed on brain imaging include isolated germinal matrix/intraventricular hemorrhage (GM/IVH) and parenchymal lesions/ventricular enlargement (PL/VE). The relation of these abnormalities

TABLE 2.—Global Cognitive Functioning by Ultrasound Status*

Global Cognitive Outcomes†	All, n (%) (n = 597)	Ultrasound Group, n (%)			Comparisons, Odds Ratio (95% Confidence Interval)	
		NA (n = 468)	GM/IVH (n = 83)	PL/VE (n = 46)	GM/IVH vs NA	PL/VE vs NA
Normal intelligence‡	529 (88.6)	436 (93.2)	73 (88.0)	20 (43.5)	…§	…§
Borderline intelligence†	38 (6.4)	26 (5.6)	5 (6.0)	7 (15.2)	1.1 (0.4–3.1)	5.9 (2.3–15.2)‡
MR‡	30 (5.0)	6 (1.3)	5 (6.0)	19 (41.3)	5.0 (1.5–16.8)‖	69.0 (24.8 –192.1)‡
Mild MR¶	5 (0.8)	2 (0.4)	0 (0.0)	3 (6.5)	…¶	…¶
Moderate to profound MR¶	25 (4.2)	4 (0.9)	5 (6.0)	16 (34.8)	…¶	…¶

*See Table 1 for definitions of outcomes. Significance levels for the χ^2 tests of differences among all 3 groups are indicated beside the variable label in the first column. Multinomial logistic regressions were used to compare each US abnormality group to the no abnormality group on the prevalence of borderline intelligence and mental retardation, with the log odds of borderline intelligence vs. normal intelligence and mental retardation vs. normal intelligence as dependent variables. The significance level for each comparison, as determined by the *t* statistic associated with the log odds ratio, is indicated immediately beside the confidence interval.

†$P < 0.050$.

‡$P < 0.001$.

§Reference category.

‖$P < 0.010$.

¶Odds ratio not calculated because of small number of cases for this category.

Abbreviations: GM/IVH, germinal matrix/intraventricular hemorrhage; *MR*, mental retardation; *NA*, no abnormalities; *PL/VE*, parenchymal lesions/ventricular enlargement.

(Courtesy of Whitaker AH, Feldman JF, van Rossem R, et al: Neonatal cranial ultrasound abnormalities in low birth weight infants: Relation to cognitive outcomes at six years of age. *Pediatrics* 98:719–729, 1996. Reproduced by permission of *Pediatrics*, copyright 1996.)

to cognitive outcomes in school-aged children was investigated prospectively in a large, regionally defined LBW cohort studied since the age of 2 years.

Methods.—Mental retardation, borderline intelligence, and normal intelligence were assessed in 685 children at home by a pediatric nurse and a psychologist using a variety of instruments. Multivariate analysis was performed to evaluate the independent predictive effects of US and perinatal and neonatal risk factors on cognitive status.

Results.—Whereas general intellectual functioning and adaptive functioning were normal, there were significantly more children with mental retardation and significantly fewer children with borderline intelligence, with rates of mental retardation and borderline intelligence varying considerably among groups (Table 2). Children with PL/VE were more likely to have mental retardation (odds ratio, 65.8) and were born on average 2.5 weeks earlier than children of normal intelligence. Children with borderline intelligence were born an average of 1.2 weeks earlier. Whereas children with GM/IVH were more likely to have mental retardation (odds ratio, 4.6), GM/IVH was not related to borderline intelligence. The sole cause of mental retardation in half the children was PL/VE, and children

TABLE 6.—Specific Cognitive Outcomes in Children With Normal Intelligence in Relation to Ultrasound Status*

Outcome	Ultrasound Groups NA	GM/IVH	PL/VE
Language			
	n = 429	n = 73	n = 17
Overall (TOLD SLQ)	95.6 ± 16.1	94.6 ± 18.4	91.9 ± 17.8
	n = 428	n = 73	n = 19
Receptive (TOLD LIQ)	97.2 ± 13.7	95.5 ± 15.2	93.4 ± 14.4
	n = 432	n = 73	n = 17
Expressive (TOLD SPQ)	94.7 ± 17.1	94.5 ± 19.6	91.8 ± 19.3
	n = 436	n = 73	n = 20
Verbal reasoning (SB area score)	104.3 ± 10.9	102.9 ± 10.5	98.9 ± 10.8†
Short-term memory (SB area score)	101.4 ± 11.4	99.2 ± 11.0	102.0 ± 12.7
Quantitative reasoning (SB area score)	108.8 ± 10.0	107.2 ± 9.1	104.5 ± 10.9
Visual perceptual organization			
Abstract visual reasoning (SB area score)†	102.1 ± 13.0	101.2 ± 10.4	94.0 ± 10.0‡
	n = 431	n = 73	n = 20
Visual-motor integration (VMI standard score)†	93.1 ± 10.7	92.2 ± 10.7	86.2 ± 13.2§
	n = 421	n = 71	n = 18
Visual perceptual skills (TVPS perceptual quotient)†	106.9 ± 19.7	105.7 ± 20.6	93.8 ± 21.6‡

*All data are expressed as mean plus or minus standard deviations. Significance levels for tests of differences among the 3 US status groups (*F*) are indicaed beside the name of each outcome; significance levels for tests of differences between each of the US abnormality groups and the no abnormality group (*t*) are given in the columns for germinal matrix/intraventricular hemorrhage and parenchymal lesions/ventricular enlargement.

†$P < 0.050$.

‡$P < 0.010$.

§$P < 0.005$.

Abbreviations: GM/IVH, germinal matrix/intraventricular hemorrhage: *LIQ*, listening quotient; *NA*, no abnormality; *PL/VE*, parenchymal lesions/ventricular enlargement; *SB*, Stanford-Binet scale; *SLQ*, speaking quotient; *TVPS*, Test of Visual Perceptual Skills; *VUI*, Developmental Test of Visual Motor Integration.

(Courtesy of Whitaker AH, Feldman JF, van Rossem R, et al: Neonatal cranial ultrasound abnormalities in low birth weight infants: Relation to cognitive outcomes at six years of age. *Pediatrics* 98:719–729, 1996. Reproduced by permission of *Pediatrics*, copyright 1996.)

with PL/VE scored significantly lower on tests of visual perceptual organization than did children with no US abnormalities (Table 6). Cognitive abilities such as language, short-term memory, and quantitative skills did not differ significantly between groups. The number of days on mechanical ventilation increased the risk of mental retardation. Maternal social disadvantage and fetal growth rate increased the risk of borderline intelligence but not mental retardation.

Conclusions.—Days on mechanical ventilation was the only non-US measure that was independently predictive of mental retardation. Because PL/VE contributes significantly to cognitive impairments in LBW infants, prevention of white matter injuries could improve cognitive outcomes in these children.

▶ Brain injury in the premature infant is a major problem. Preventing brain injury and predicting the long-term outcome of the most vulnerable, extremely LBW children is a daunting challenge. Society, the families, and third-party payers are putting increased pressure on the neonatal community to distinguish extremely low birth weight infants with a good prognosis from those with a significant probability of neurodevelopmental impairment. The ethics, economics, epidemiology, legal issues, and logistics of addressing this problem provide fuel for many graduate courses. Factors such as birth weight, gestational age, chorioamnionitis, type of delivery, Apgar scores, neonatal sepsis, chronic lung disease, and levels of thyroid hormones may be helpful in defining group outcomes but are of limited value in predicting the potential of the individual infant.

This report is a significant contribution to predicting long-term outcome. It is a well-conducted, population-based study of LBW infants. Because ultrasonographic assessment had been performed during the neonatal period, the authors were able to correlate cranial US abnormalities with cognitive abilities at school age. Evidence of white matter injury was the most important determinant of long-term function. The imaging studies were indubitably of significant benefit in predicting outcome.

Indeed, techniques for cerebral assessment and imaging have now become a routine part of neonatal intensive care. Cerebral US, CT, and MRI, complemented by electroencephalography, positron emission tomography scanning, near-infrared spectroscopy, and, in some centers, continuous cerebral function monitoring, are all part of the package used to determine immediate care and predict outcomes. Ultrasound is the cheapest, most convenient, and least invasive technique, so it is reassuring to find that it is of predictive value.

Stewart and colleagues[1] were the first to estimate the probability of neurodevelopmental disorders on the basis of the US appearance of the brain at the time of hospital discharge. Ventricular dilatation, hydrocephalus, and cerebral atrophy carried significant probabilities for adverse outcomes. These data held true through 8 years of age.[2] Whitaker and associates add their data to the expanding pool, correlating neonatal US abnormalities with neurologic and neurodevelopmental problems.[3, 4]

Under the bludgeonings of chance my head is bloody, but unbowed.—W.E. Henley

A.A. Fanaroff, M.B.B.Ch.

References

1. Stewart AL, Reynolds EOR, Hope PL, et al: Probability of neurodevelopmental disorders estimated from ultrasound appearance of brains of very preterm infants. *Dev Med Child Neurol* 29:3–11, 1987.
2. Roth SC, Baudin J, McCormick DC, et al: Relation between the ultrasound appearance of the brain in very preterm infants and neurodevelopmental impairment at eight years. *Dev Med Child Neurol* 35:755–768, 1993.
3. De Vries LS, Eken P, Groenendaal F, et al: Correlation between the degree of periventricular leukomalacia diagnosed using cranial ultrasound and MRI later in infancy in children with cerebral palsy. *Neuropediatrics* 24:263–268, 1993.
4. Van de Bor M, den Ouden L, Guit GL: Value of cranial ultrasound and magnetic resonance imaging in predicting neurodevelopmental outcome in preterm infants. *Pediatrics* 90:196–199, 1992.

Prediction of Early Outcome in Resolving Chronic Lung Disease of Prematurity After Discharge From Hospital

Iles R, Edmunds AT (Royal Hosp for Sick Children, Edinburgh, Scotland)
Arch Dis Child 74:304–308, 1996 16–10

Background.—Chronic lung disease (CLD) of prematurity, characterized by chronic respiratory disease and a persistent oxygen requirement, is associated with high levels of morbidity and mortality. Infants with CLD have high admission rates in the first year. More discriminatory, quantitative measures are needed to identify infants at risk of unexpected episodes of hypoxemia with or without apnea, especially among infants with resolving lung disease. It was hypothesized that recordings of mean individual arterial oxygen saturation and its variability could be used to determine the risk of morbidity and mortality in infants with significant lung disease of prematurity.

TABLE.—Sensitivity and Specificity of Oxygen Saturation Measurements in Predicting Hospital Readmission and SIDS/ALTE

	Hospital readmission		*SIDS/ALTE*	
	Sensitivity	*Specificity*	*Sensitivity*	*Specificity*
(A) $MSaO_2$ <90%	0·8	0·73	1	0·57
(B) $MSaO_2$ <90%	1	0·76	1	0·75
(A) $\delta MSaO_2$ >6%	0·05	0·86	0	0·84
(B) $\delta MSaO_2$ >6%	0·52	0·13	0·88	1

Note: (*A*), data without exclusion of artifact; (*B*), data following exclusion of artifact.
Abbreviations: SIDS, sudden infant death syndrome; *ALTE*, apparent life-threatening event; $MSaO_2$, mean arterial oxygen saturation; $\delta MSaO_2$, change in mean arterial oxygen saturation.
(Courtesy of Iles R, Edmunds AT: Prediction of early outcome in resolving chronic lung disease of prematurity after discharge from hospital. *Arch Dis Child* 74:304–308, 1996.)

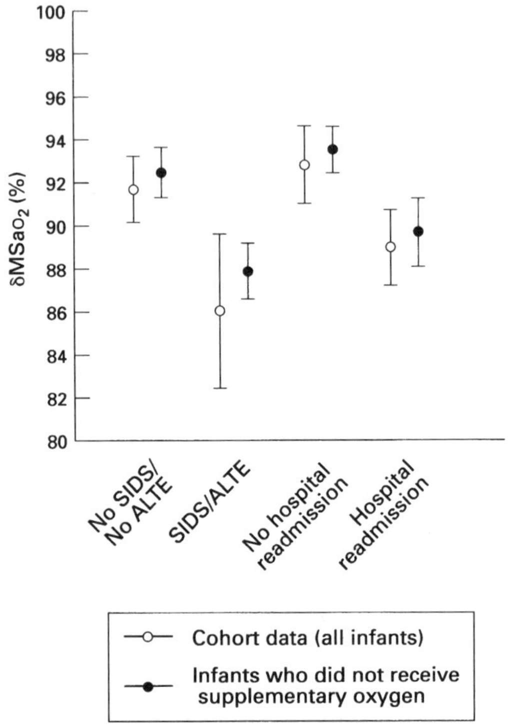

FIGURE 3.—Mean arterial oxygen saturation (*MSaO$_2$*) and 95% confidence intervals for clinical outcome groups. Sudden infant death syndrome/acute life-threatening event (*SIDS/ALTE*) vs. no SIDS/no ALTE: whole cohort, $P = 0.04$; infants not receiving supplemental oxygen, $P = 0.0001$. Hospital readmission vs. no hospital readmission: whole cohort, $P = 0.001$; infants not receiving supplemental oxygen, $P = 0.0002$. (Courtesy of Iles R, Edmunds AT: Prediction of early outcome in resolving chronic lung disease of prematurity after discharge from hospital. *Arch Dis Child* 74:304–308, 1996.)

Methods.—Recordings of arterial oxygen saturation were obtained for 35 infants breathing room air before discharge from the neonatal unit. The data were analyzed to provide the mean individual arterial oxygen saturation and the variability of mean individual oxygen saturation. Clinicians not involved in the study decided infants' suitability for discharge with or without home oxygen prescription. This decision was based on overall clinical perceptions and visual analysis of oxygen saturation data.

Findings.—Hospitalization within 3 months of discharge was predicted by a mean individual arterial oxygen saturation of less than 90% with a sensitivity of 1.0 and a specificity of 0.76. Mean individual arterial saturation of less than 90% also predicted sudden infant death syndrome (SIDS) or acute life-threatening event (ALTE) with a sensitivity and specificity of 1.0 and 0.75, respectively. A variability of the mean individual oxygen saturation exceeding 6% predicted SIDS or ALTE with a 0.88 sensitivity and a 1.0 specificity (Table; Fig 3).

Conclusions.—Infants with mean individual arterial oxygen saturation levels of less than 90% should be prescribed supplemental oxygen to protect them from increased morbidity and even mortality. Infants with arterial oxygen saturation values of greater than 92% or less than 90% on "spot" oximetry need not be assessed further. When values fall between 90% and 92%, more detailed analysis is needed before deciding whether to continue oxygen.

► Newer monitoring equipment in neonatal ICUs should make it relatively simple to collect and store simultaneously obtained heart rate and pulse oximeter monitoring data and allow a calculation of mean arterial oxygen saturation and the variability in arterial oxygen saturation during a 6-hour period, as was done by these authors. When artifacts were excluded, these measurements showed a high degree of sensitivity and specificity in relation to the risk for SIDS/ALTE or readmission to the hospital. The differences in mean arterial oxygen saturation between the infants subsequently readmitted because of SIDS/ALTE and those who were not are striking, with no overlap of the 95% confidence intervals.

Some will wonder, however, why infants with oxygen saturations below 90% were discharged without supplemental oxygen. (Decisions regarding discharge were made by clinicians not involved in the study but who did have access to previous pulse oximetry readings). I would also like to see the positive and negative predictive values of these measurements. If we are to use mean oxygen saturation and variability in oxygen saturation as screening tests for infants who are at risk for subsequent morbidity and mortality, then we need to know more than just the sensitivity and specificity. A sensitivity of 1 for the SIDS/ALTE group means that every infant who was admitted with a diagnosis of SIDS/ALTE had, at the time of discharge from the nursery, a mean arterial oxygen saturation of less than 90%. A specificity of 0.57 tells us that 57% of infants who were not readmitted with SIDS/ALTE had a mean arterial oxygen saturation of greater than 90%. What we would like to know, however, is what proportion of infants who had a mean arterial oxygen saturation of less than 90% were readmitted (the positive predictive value), and the proportion who had a mean arterial oxygen saturation of 90% or greater who were not readmitted (the negative predictive value). Unfortunately, the authors do not provide us with the raw data to permit us to calculate these values. They do say that an arterial saturation of greater than 92% obtained by "spot" oximetry indicates that the infant can safely be discharged without supplemental oxygen. However, this was a relatively small cohort, and we need to remember that the normal range for arterial oxygen saturation in *nondistressed, growing premature infants* is 95% to 100%.[1]

M.J. Maisels, M.B., B.Ch.

Reference

1. Poets CF, Southall DP: Noninvasive monitoring of oxygenation in infants and children: Practical considerations and areas of concern. *Pediatrics* 93:737–746, 1994.

Low Triiodothyronine Concentration in Preterm Infants and Subsequent Intelligence Quotient (IQ) at 8 Year Follow Up

Lucas A, Morley R, Fewtrell MS (Med Research Council Dunn Nutrition Unit, Cambridge, England)

BMJ 312:1132–1133, 1996 16–11

Background.—Premature infants have clinically important changes in endocrine physiology. Previous research has demonstrated that plasma levels of many hormones are reduced in premature infants compared with full-term ones. Thyroid hormones that are critical signals for brain development—prolactin, testosterone, and triiodothyronine—are affected. Low triiodothyronine levels in preterm infants and subsequent intelligence quotient (IQ) scores 8 years later were reported.

Methods and Findings.—Plasma triiodothyronine levels were measured longitudinally in 279 infants at 1–3 days of life, 4–7 days of life, and then weekly until infants were discharged from the hospital or weighed 2,000 g. In 236 children (representing 94% of the survivors), IQ was tested at 7.5–8 years. Children with minimum triiodothyronine levels below 0.3 $nmol/L^3$ had substantial IQ deficits, even after adjustment for birth weight, gestation, sex, and 5-minute Apgar score. The adjusted deficit in IQ with low triiodothyronine levels was 6.6 points. The deficit on the verbal scale was 8.5 points.

Conclusions.—The magnitude of the association between triiodothyronine concentration and IQ score deficits, the persistence of this association after adjustment for confounding factors, and the known relationship between neonatal hypothyroidism and impaired brain development suggest that this association is causal. The causes of low triiodothyronine levels in preterm infants remain unclear.

▶ This comment has been provided by Phyllis A. Dennery, M.D., Assistant Professor of Pediatrics, Stanford University School of Medicine; Lucile Salter Packard Children's Hospital at Stanford, Palo Alto, California:

▶ In this article, Lucas et al. demonstrate a persistent cognitive deficit at 7.5–8 years in preterm infants with low triiodothyronine (T_3). Hypothyroidism has often been implicated in abnormal brain development in the past. In a recent study in *The New England Journal of Medicine,*[1] infants with severe hypothyroxinemia had a risk of disabling cerebral palsy that was nearly 11 times that of infants without this condition, even after adjustment for gestational age and multiple prenatal, perinatal, and early neonatal variables. That study further suggested equally that severe hypothyroxinemia in preterm infants may be an important cause of neurologic abnormality at 2 years of age. This study by Lucas et al. extends these findings using follow-up into the school years and shows that hypothyroxinemia has clinically important, long-lasting sequelae. A commentary accompanying the *British Medical Journal* article asks the question, "Do preterm infants need thyroxine replacement?"[2] Perhaps we should consider administering thyroxine at appropriate doses to all preterm infants to prevent the possible cognitive deficits observed in the Lucas study. It is nonetheless discouraging that another publication suggests that thyroxine administration to infants at less than 30 weeks' gestation did not appear to increase plasma T_3 levels but did alter thyroxine levels, suggesting a maturation process in the deiodination of thyroxine.[2] A better understanding of thyroid metabolism will allow us to suggest appropriate strategies for ensuring euthyroid states in the premature patient.

P.A. Dennery, M.D.

References

1. Vulsma T, Kok JH: Prematurity-associated neurologic and developmental abnormalities and neonatal thyroid function [editorial; comment]. *N Engl J Med* 334:857–858, 1996.
2. Brook CGD: Commentary: Do preterm infants need thyrotine replacement? *BMJ* 312:1133–1134, 1996.

The Relation Between Neonatal Thyroxine Levels and Neurodevelopmental Outcome at Age 5 and 9 Years in a National Cohort of Very Preterm and/or Very Low Birth Weight Infants

den Ouden AL, Kok JH, Verkerk PH, et al (TNO Prevention and Health, Leiden, The Netherlands; Academic Med Centre, Amsterdam; Univ of Leiden, The Netherlands)

Pediatr Res 39:142–145, 1996 16–12

Background.—Preterm infants commonly have transient hypothyroxinemia. The effects of this condition, however, have not been established definitively. Studies of large numbers of patients with long-term follow-up are not available. The relationship between thyroxine levels in the first week of life and outcomes at 5 and 9 years of age was investigated

TABLE 1.—Mean Thyroxine Level and Percentage of Hypothyroxinemia [Thyroxine (T4) ≤3 SD] by Gestational Age

Gestational age	Total (*n*)	Mean T_4 SD	Mean T_4 Calculated *	≤3 SD† (%)
<26	6	−3.4	33	83.3
$26–27^{+6}$	79	−3.3	43	70.8
$28–29^{+6}$	177	−2.8	71	44.1
$30–31^{+6}$	253	−2.4	93	24.1
≥32	202	−1.9	117	15.3

*For comparison with other published studies, T4 values were calculated with a regression equation [T4 (SD) = −4.064 + 0.0184 × T4 nmol/L], based on a correlation of simultaneously obtained blood spot T4 and serum T4 in 115 low birth weight on seventh day of life, determined in the same laboratory.

†Less than 60 nmol/L.

(Courtesy of den Ouden AL, Kok JH, Verkerk PH, et al: The relation between neonatal thyroxine levels and neurodevelopmental outcome at age 5 and 9 years in a national cohort of very preterm and/or very low birth weight infants. *Pediatr Res* 39:142–145, 1996.)

TABLE 3.—Unadjusted and Adjusted Odds Ratio (95% Confidence Interval) for Thyroxine (Standard Deviation) on Different Outcome Measures at Ages 5 and 9 Years

	OR		
Outcome	Unadjusted	Adjusted for gestational age	Adjusted for all perinatal factors
Handicap*	1.3 (1.1–1.5)	1.4 (1.1–1.7)	1.3 (1.0–1.6)
Disability and handicap*	1.1 (0.9–1.1)	1.2 (0.9–1.5)	1.0 (0.8–1.2)
Neurological dysfunction*	1.2 (1.1–1.5)	1.4 (1.1–1.7)	1.3 (1.1–1.6)
Speech language dysfunction*	1.0 (0.8–1.1)	1.0 (0.8–1.2)	0.9 (0.8–1.2)
Mental retardation*	1.1 (0.9–1.5)	1.0 (0.9–1.6)	1.1 (0.8–1.6)
School failure†	1.3 (1.1–1.5)	1.3 (1.1–1.5)	1.3 (1.1–1.6)

*Age 5 years.
†Age 9 years.
Abbreviation: OR, odds ratio.
(Courtesy of den Ouden AL, Kok JH, Verkerk PH, et al: The relation between neonatal thyroxine levels and neurodevelopmental outcome at age 5 and 9 years in a national cohort of very preterm and/or very low birth weight infants. *Pediatr Res* 39:142–145, 1996.)

prospectively in a cohort of very preterm and/or very low birth weight infants in The Netherlands.

Methods.—Seven hundred seventeen such infants born in 1983 were included. Neurodevelopmental outcomes were assessed when the children were 5 years old, and school performance was documented at 9 years of age. Neonatal thyroxine concentrations were determined from filter paper eluates.

Findings.—Thirty-two percent of the infants had thyroxine levels of more than 3 SDs below the mean. The proportion of infants with such low levels increased as gestational age decreased. Ninety-six percent of the surviving children underwent extensive neurodevelopmental evaluation at 5 years of age. Thirteen percent had a disability, and 14% had a handicap. Eighty-three percent of survivors were available at 9 years for further evaluation. Fifty-four percent of these children were in mainstream educational settings in a grade appropriate for their age. Twenty-seven percent were in mainstream educational settings but had been held back in a lower grade. Eighteen percent of the children were in special education. School failure at 9 years as well as neurologic dysfunction at 5 years were significantly associated with decreased neonatal thyroxine levels, even after adjustment for other perinatal factors (Tables 1 and 3).

Conclusions.—In this cohort, long-term school performance and neurologic problems were associated with lower neonatal thyroxine concentrations. However, whether this relationship is causal remains unclear. If it is causal, substitution treatment may be helpful in preventing some neurologic and learning deficits.

▶ Once again, our Dutch colleagues provide us with important data from their nationwide prospective follow-up study of low–birth weight infants born in 1983 in The Netherlands. They evaluated the neurodevelopmental outcome of these children at age 5 years and their school performance at age 9. This study compliments that of Ruess et al.,[1] also a population-based study, in 3 counties of central New Jersey. Ruess et al. had the advantage of a cranial US image of every infant, but their length of follow-up was only 2 years. Both studies demonstrated an association between hypothyroxinemia and decreasing gestation.

In this study by den Ouden et al., the magnitude of the observed effect on handicap, neurologic dysfunction, and school failure was modest, the adjusted odds ratio being only 1.3 with 95% confidence limits of 1.0–1.6. In contrast, Reuss et al. found a relative risk of disabling cerebral palsy, adjusted for other variables, of 4.4 with 95% confidence intervals of 1.0–18.6 and a reduction of nearly 7 points in the mental development score. Perhaps if this population had been followed to ages 5 or 9 years, as in the Dutch study, the magnitude of these risks might have decreased.

Vulsma and Kok[2] point out that hypothyroxinemia in low–birth weight infants may be the result of some type of nonthyroidal illness, a metabolic adaptation of the preterm infant to extrauterine life, or incomplete maturation of the hypothalamic-pituitary-thyroid access. They argue that the low serum thyroxine concentrations seen in preterm infants should more appropriately be termed "hypothyroidism" rather than "hypothyroxinemia" because there is good evidence that, contrary to popular belief, the human fetus both requires thyroid hormone during development and receives it from the mother. Maternal thyroxine crosses the placenta as early as the second month of pregnancy and, even late in gestation, a significant amount of thyroxine in the fetal circulation still originates in the mother. They suggest that thyroid hormone "which is indispensable for cerebral development, is supplied by the mother until the fetus is completely self supporting in the production of this hormone."[2] Is the hypothyroxinemia found in low–birth weight infants a cause of cerebral palsy and mental retardation, or is it simply a related finding in small sick infants? These questions can only be answered by an appropriately designed, randomized, controlled trial in which the developmental outcome of 2 groups of very low birth weight infants are compared—one that receives supplemental thyroxine and one that does not.

M.J. Maisels, M.B., B.Ch.

References

1. Reuss ML, Paneth N, Pinto-Martin JA, et al: The relation of transient hypothyroxinemia in preterm infants to neurologic development at two years of age. *N Engl J Med* 334:821–827, 1996.
2. Vulsma T, Kok JH: Prematurity-associated neurologic and developmental abnormalities and neonatal thyroid function. *N Engl J Med* 334:857–858, 1996.

The Effects of *In Utero* Diagnostic X-Irradiation on the Development of Preschool-age Children

Ornoy A, Patlas N, Schwartz L (Hebrew Univ, Jerusalem; Jerusalem Inst for Child Development)

Isr J Med Sci 32:112–115, 1996 16–13

Introduction.—Most reports agree that the developing embryo and fetus may be affected by ionizing irradiation only after being exposed to doses above a threshold of 5–10 rads. There is no proof that such a threshold exists concerning long-term developmental sequelae. The possible effects of diagnostic X-irradiation on the development of preschool-age children was evaluated in children born to mothers who were exposed during pregnancy to diagnostic X-irradiation, either to the abdomen and pelvis or to other areas. A group of nonexposed children of similar socioeconomic status acted as controls.

Methods.—Fifty-two children born to women who had been exposed to diagnostic X-irradiation to the abdomen, pelvis, or both; 60 children born to mothers exposed during pregnancy to X-irradiation in areas other than the abdomen or pelvis; and 62 normal children whose mothers were not exposed were evaluated at 1–5 years of age. The examination included: physical, medical and neurologic examination by a developmental pediatrician; psychological evaluation using the Bayley Developmental Scales for children 1–2.5 years; psychological evaluation using the McCarthy Developmental Scales for children 3–5 years; and completion of a detailed questionnaire regarding the time, type, and location of the X-irradiation, course of pregnancy and delivery, and child's behavior and medical history.

Results.—Twenty women underwent radiographic examination of the stomach and upper gastrointestinal tract. Most women also underwent fluoroscopic examinations for 2–8 minutes (total irradiation exposure of 1–10 rads). The total exposure for all other radiographic examinations ranged from 0.5 to 4.0 rads. All X-irradiation exposure occurred in the first trimester. In the X-irradiation group, 1 child had microcephaly and 1 had hydrocele, which disappeared spontaneously. All except 2 women who underwent radiographs of the skull, teeth, chest, or neck were exposed in the first trimester of pregnancy. The maternal exposure dose of these radiographs was 0.2–2.0 rads and the fetal exposure was a small fraction of this dose. Of 60 children from this maternal group, 2 had very mild developmental delay, 1 of whom had microcephaly. No children in the control group had anomalies or developmental retardation. There were no between-group differences in the motor or cognitive scores and all children scored above 80 on the Bayley or McCarthy Developmental Scales. It appears that the in utero exposure of the human embryo at early gestation to diagnostic X-irradiation had no significant deleterious effects on any of the developmental parameters evaluated.

Conclusion.—First trimester exposure to diagnostic X-irradiation does not seem to have deleterious effects on childhood development. Exposure during later pregnancy may be more deleterious to the developing brain, but second- and third-trimester exposure is rare.

▶ Deanne Wilson-Costello, M.D., is a Senior Fellow in the Division of Rainbow Babies & Childrens Hospital, Cleveland, Ohio. She provides the commentary below:

▶ In an era when public fear is heightened by announcements of newly discovered carcinogenic or embryotoxic exposures, it is refreshing to reaffirm the apparent safety of diagnostic radiography. The typical diagnostic radiation doses of 20–5,000 mrad not only fall well below the threshold for structural or genetic damage,[1] but also, as shown in this study, pose no apparent threat to the more subtle aspects of brain development and function.

In a study examining radiation doses to extremely low birth weight infants from diagnostic radiographs, we found total body doses between 40 and 150 mrad per infant with the largest doses to infants with chronic lung disease and necrotizing enterocolitis. Maximum organ doses for the sickest infants were 330 mrad to the breast, 240 mrad to the thyroid, and 230 mrad to the testes, with the similar conclusion that the doses obtained from diagnostic radiography are small in comparison to the doses that form the basis for cancer risk estimates.[2]

We must humbly recognize, however, that the complete impact of radiation exposures, even at large doses, may be difficult to assess in small populations. Certain effects are time dependent and take many years to manifest. More than 40 years ago, The Oxford Study of Childhood Cancers suggested an association between the risk of childhood leukemia and in utero exposure to diagnostic radiographs.[3] Although the initial analysis of prenatally irradiated atomic bomb survivors failed to demonstrate any increased risk, the long-term follow-up data 40 years after the radiation exposure demonstrated an increased cancer-related mortality.[4]

The authors of this paper appropriately note that the failure to detect any measurable increase in developmental delay or behavioral problems among children exposed to low-dose diagnostic radiography in utero may be related, not only to the low radiation dose, but also to the early timing of the exposures, typically before 8 weeks' gestation. In the studies of in utero exposed atomic bomb survivors, significant harmful effects of radiation on the developing brain were observed only for those exposed between 8 and 15 weeks post conception (the period of neuronal proliferation and migration) and to a lesser extent, between 16 and 25 weeks' gestation (the period of differentiation and synaptogenesis). No subjects exposed at less than 8 weeks or greater than 26 weeks' gestation had mental retardation.[5]

The apparent differences in radiosensitivity among cells at different times in development make it difficult for any measurable damage to be detected in small numbers of atomic bomb survivors, critically ill preterm infants, or in utero exposed children.

One picture is worth a thousand words.—A Chinese proverb

D. Wilson-Costello, M.D.

References

1. Brent R: *Semin Oncol* 16:347–368, 1989.
2. Wilson-Costello D, et al: *Pediatrics* 97:369–374, 199
3. Steward A, et al: *Lancet* 1956:447–448, ii.
4. Yoshimoto Y, et al: *RERF Tech Rep* 4–88, 1988.
5. Otake M, et al: *RERF Tech Rep* 16–87, 1987.

Moderate Prenatal Alcohol Exposure and Psychomotor Development at Preschool Age

Larroque B, Kaminski M, Dehaene P, et al (INSERM, Villejuif, France; Roubaix Hosp, France; Calmette Hosp, Lille, France)
Am J Public Health 85:1654–1661, 1995 16–14

Background.—Consumption of high amounts of alcohol during pregnancy have been associated with fetal alcohol syndrome, with particular CNS dysfunction. It was hypothesized that moderate alcohol consumption during pregnancy also would have CNS effects that would last into childhood. The hypothesis was examined in a longitudinal study by investigating the psychomotor development of preschool-aged children of mothers who drank moderate amounts of alcohol during pregnancy.

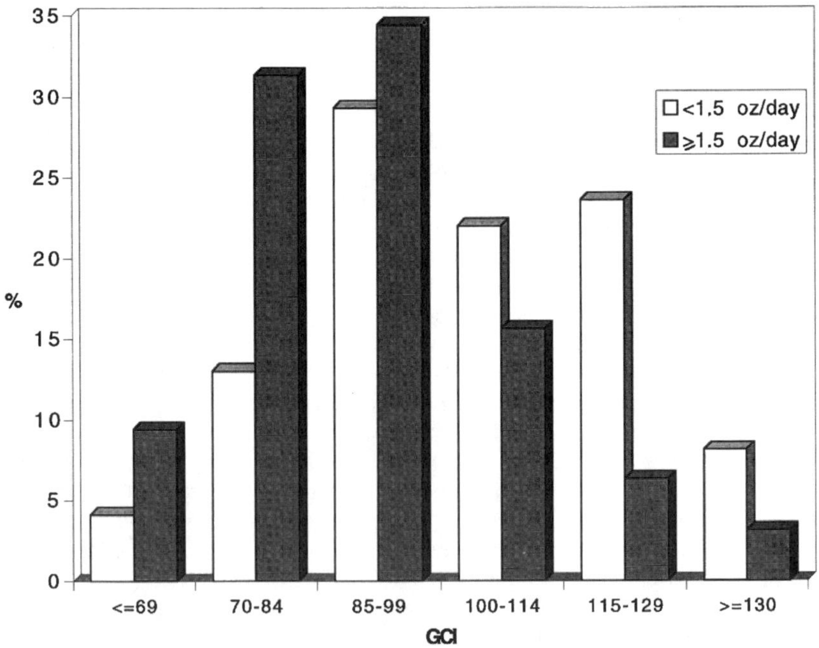

FIGURE 1.—Distribution of general cognitive index (*GCI*) scores among children of mothers drinking less than 1.5 oz/day of absolute alcohol during pregnancy and among children of mothers drinking 1.5 oz/day or more of absolute alcohol during pregnancy. (Courtesy of Larroque B, Kaminski M, Dehaene P, et al: Moderate prenatal alcohol exposure and psychomotor development at preschool age. *Am J Public Health* 85:1654–1661. Copyright 1995 by the American Public Health Association.)

Methods.—Psychomotor development was assessed, using the McCarthy scales of children's abilities, in 160 children at approximately 4.5 years of age. Alcohol consumption had been determined for the first trimester of the pregnancy and for the period before pregnancy, using a structured questionnaire in interviews with the mothers. A dose-response relationship between prenatal alcohol exposure and psychomotor deficiencies was investigated, using multiple regression analysis to control for the following confounders: birth order, maternal educational level, maternal employment, family status, family stimulation score, sex, tobacco consumption during pregnancy, and birth weight.

Results.—Alcohol consumption during pregnancy was significantly related to general cognitive index, verbal, performance, and quantitative scale scores, but not memory or motor scales. After controlling for confounding factors, the children of mothers who drank at least 1.5 oz of absolute alcohol had a mean general cognitive index score 7 points lower than did the children of mothers who were light drinkers during pregnancy (Fig 1).

Conclusion.—Prenatal exposure to moderate alcohol consumption significantly affects the psychomotor development of preschool-aged children. Therefore, interventions for reducing alcohol consumption should not be reserved for alcoholic mothers.

▶ Mitchell DeJonge, M.D., neonatologist, William Beaumont Hospital, Royal Oak, Michigan, comments:

▶ Ever since Jones and Smith coined the expression "fetal alcohol syndrome" more than 20 years ago, the impact and long-term consequences of drinking during pregnancy have been the focus of extensive research.[1] It is now clear that infants who show physical signs consistent with fetal alcohol syndrome will have some degree of mental impairment ranging from subtle to severe mental retardation. However, what remains unclear is the effect on infants born to mothers who drink "moderately" or "lightly" during pregnancy.

It seems intuitive that there would be a direct relationship between the amount of alcohol consumed during pregnancy and the effects, both physical and cognitive, on the infant. However, dating back to the mid 1970s, studies evaluating the effect of moderate drinking (defined as 1.5 oz of absolute alcohol per day) have resulted in conflicting conclusions, some studies showing significant effects of moderate drinking and others showing little to no effect.

This study hypothesized that moderate alcohol consumption in pregnancy will have effects on the CNS of the child, as demonstrated by a decrease in the psychomotor portion of a well-recognized developmental test. Maternal drinking history was assessed at the first prenatal visit by a standard questionnaire—a method fraught with error but the best research tool available at the present time. After multiple confounders were controlled for—including birth order, maternal education, maternal employment at the time of infant evaluation, family status, family stimulation score, sex, and age of the child at examination—it was found that 3 drinks or more per day during pregnancy caused a 7-point reduction in the mean score of the general cognitive index of the McCarthy scales.

This is not the first study to document the potential effects of moderate alcohol consumption during pregnancy, but it does underscore the notion that children who are born to mothers who drank during pregnancy—even in the absence of the typical physical findings of fetal alcohol syndrome—may have subtle to significant cognitive and psychomotor deficits. Unfortunately, Larroque et al. do not shed light on many of the more subtle questions regarding drinking during pregnancy. These questions include the importance of gestational age at exposure to alcohol, pattern of exposure (binge vs. chronic drinking), and magnitude of the exposure to alcohol, which may ultimately lead to development concerns.

M. DeJonge, M.D.

Reference

1. Jones KL, Smith AW: Recognition of the fetal alcohol syndrome in early infancy. *Lancet* 2:999–1001, 1973.

Survivors of Extracorporeal Membrane Oxygenation at 1 Year of Age: The Relationship of Primary Diagnosis With Health and Neurodevelopmental Sequelae

Bernbaum J, Schwartz IP, Gerdes M, et al (Children's Hosp of Philadelphia; Children's Seashore House, Philadelphia)

Pediatrics 96:907–913, 1995 16–15

Background.—Concerns have been raised regarding the health of infants with cardiorespiratory failure able to survive with the aid of extracorporeal membrane oxygenation (ECMO). To date, most studies of ECMO outcomes have simply reported outcomes in entire populations, without considering the original nature of the infant's illness. The type and extent of health problems and neurodevelopmental sequelae in infants needing ECMO treatment and the association of these findings with primary diagnoses were investigated.

Methods.—Eighty-two neonates treated with ECMO between May 1990 and December 1993 were included. Indications for ECMO were meconium aspiration syndrome in 26%, congenital diaphragmatic hernia (CDH) in 34%, persistence of fetal circulation in 16%, and sepsis in 9%. The infants were assessed at 6 and 12 months of age.

Findings.—Seventy-nine percent of the infants survived. Survival varied significantly, depending on the primary diagnosis. Infants with CDH had the worst outcomes, with an overall survival of 68% and a more complicated hospital course and longer ECMO duration. At discharge, the infants with CDH had a greater incidence of bronchopulmonary dysplasia, gastroesophageal reflux, feeding dysfunction, and hypotonia. Overall, this ECMO population scored in the normal range developmentally. However,

TABLE 3.—Discharge Morbidity

	Total Discharge Population (n = 65)	MAS (n = 21)	CDH (n = 19)	Sepsis (n = 7)	PFC (n = 10)	*P* Value
Neurologic morbidity						
Neurologic insults (IVH, infarct, PVL)	10 (15%)	4 (19%)	5 (26%)	1 (14%)	0	NS
Extra-axial fluid collection	30 (46%)	7 (35%)	12 (63%)	3 (43%)	4 (40%)	NS
Seizures (clinical or by EEG)	18 (28%)	7 (33%)	1 (5%)	3 (43%)	3 (30%)	NS
BPD	26 (40%)	7 (33%)	12 (63%)	1 (14%)	2 (20%)	.053
GER	26 (40%)	3 (14%)	15 (79%)	2 (29%)	3 (30%)	<.001
Need for tube feeding	39 (60%)	13 (62%)	15 (79%)	4 (57%)	4 (40%)	NS
Hypotonia	43 (66%)	12 (57%)	17 (89%)	6 (86%)	4 (40%)	.023
Abnormal BAERs	2 (3%)	0	2 (11%)	0	0	NS

Abbreviations: MAS, meconium aspiration syndrome; *CDH,* congenital diaphragmatic hernia; *PFC,* persistence of fetal circulation; *IVH,* intraventricular hemorrhage; *PVL,* periventricular leukomalacia; *NS,* not significant; *EEG,* electroencephalogram; *BPD,* bronchopulmonary dysplasia; *GER,* gastroesophageal reflux; *BAER,* brain stem auditory evoked response.

(Reproduced by permission of *Pediatrics,* courtesy of Bernbaum J, Schwartz IP, Gerdes M, et al: Survivors of extracorporeal membrane oxygenation at 1 year of age: The relationship of primary diagnosis with health and neurodevelopmental sequalae. *Pediatrics* 96:907–913, copyright 1995.)

infants with CDH had significantly lower motor and slightly lower cognitive scores at 1 year of age. At 1 year, 75% of the infants with CDH continued to have some degree of hypotonicity affecting the acquisition and quality of gross motor skills (Tables 3 and 4).

Conclusion.—An accurate assessment of the efficacy of ECMO requires an analysis of the extent and morbidity in the surviving population. Infants with CDH have more neurodevelopmental, respiratory, and feeding abnormalities in the first year of life. Stratifying outcomes by primary diag-

TABLE 4.—Outcome at 6- and 12-month Visits

	6-Month Visit		12-Month Visit	
	MAS (n = 16)	CDH (n = 17)	MAS (n = 12)	CDH (n = 14)
Weight, g	7124 ± 1143	7253 ± 1241	9215 ± 1391	9311 ± 1575
Head circumference, cm	43 ± 2	44 ± 2	46 ± 2	47 ± 3
BPD	4 (25%)	6 (35%)	2 (17%)	7 (50%)
GER	3 (19%)	9 (53%)	0	6 (43%)*
Remains on tube feeding	1 (6%)	6 (35%)	0	5 (36%)†
Hypotonic	6 (38%)	13 (76%)†	1 (8%)	11 (79%)‡
MDI	100.2 ± 16.6	88.3 ± 26.1	97.5 ± 22.6	87.0 ± 22.3
PDI	108.1 ± 14.7	81.0 ± 20.6‡	99.3 ± 26.6	75.3 ± 23.0†

**P* < 0.01.
†*P* < 0.05.
‡*P* < 0.001.

Abbreviations: MAS, meconium aspiration syndrome; *CDM,* congenital diaphragmetic hernia; *BPD,* bronchopulmonary dysplasia; *GER,* gastroesophageal reflux; *MDI,* Mental Developmental Index; *PDI,* Psychomotor Developmental Index.

(Reproduced by permission of *Pediatrics,* courtesy of Bernbaum J, Schwartz IP, Gerdes M, et al: Survivors of extracorporeal membrane oxygenation at 1 year of age: The relationship of primary diagnosis with health and neurodevelopmental sequalae. *Pediatrics* 96:907–913, copyright 1995.)

nosis provides more information for improving intervention methods and counseling parents.

▶ We asked Dr. Robert Schumacher, Associate Professor of Pediatrics, University of Michigan Medical Center, Ann Arbor, Michigan, to comment:

▶ When counseling the parents of potential neonatal ECMO candidates, I am often tempted to say, "I've got good news and bad news: ECMO works." The use of ECMO has resulted in high survival rates (80% of 11,182 infants reported to the Neonatal Pulmonary Registry of ECMO by July 1996) in a group of infants who were, presumably, at high risk for dying. If this is true, then nationwide the use of ECMO is responsible for hundreds of extra neonatal survivors (both normal and handicapped) per year. ECMO follow-up studies report a "handicapping" rate of anywhere from 10% to 20%, a value similar to rates seen in similar groups of "non-ECMO" infants.

If the rate of survival without ECMO was 20% (arguable), then over the life of the ECMO registry there has been a net gain of about 6,000 neonatal "survivors." However, among these survivors will be nearly 1,000 additional handicapped infants. When looked at from an individual or family perspective, these numbers are equally disconcerting. The use of ECMO increases the chance of parents going home with a handicapped child from approximately 1 in 25 to 1 in 7. As Bernbaum and colleagues point out, stratification of outcome by primary diagnosis provides a more meaningful estimate of outcome probability. On an individual basis, "...parents may be better informed about what may lie ahead in their child's future." From a public health perspective, such information can be useful if rationing of health care resources becomes a reality.

I wholeheartedly agree that infants who require ECMO should not be assessed simply as "ECMO patients." Labels such as these could be helpful to parents who identify with other "ECMO parents." However, the label ignores the fact that these are parents of infants who had severe respiratory failure (and often multiorgan system failure) from a variety of causes.

R. Schumacher, M.D.

In Utero Exposure to Phenobarbital and Intelligence Deficits in Adult Men

Reinisch JM, Sander SA, Mortensen EL, et al (Indiana Univ, Bloomington; Inst of Preventive Med, Copenhagen; Harvard Univ, Cambridge, Mass)
JAMA 274:1518–1525, 1995 16–16

Background.—Behavioral problems, learning disabilities, and deficits in intelligence may be more common among individuals exposed to barbiturates prenatally. The association between phenobarbital exposure in utero and intelligence score deficits in men was investigated. Whether exposure variables and/or postnatal environmental factors mediate the magnitude of the postnatal effect was also studied.

Methods.—Two double-blind studies were conducted. Subjects were men born at the largest hospital in Copenhagen between 1959 and 1961. Exposed and unexposed members of this birth cohort were matched on a variety of maternal variables. The former group was exposed to phenobarbital during gestation through maternal medical therapy. Their mothers had no history of a CNS disorder and no other psychopharmacologic treatment during pregnancy. The first study included 33 exposed men and 52 controls, and the second study included 81 exposed men and 101 controls.

Findings.—Verbal intelligence scores were significantly lower than predicted among men exposed prenatally to phenobarbital. The magnitude of these negative effects was increased by lower socioecomonic status and being the product of an unwanted pregnancy. Exposure in the last trimester of pregnancy was most harmful.

Conclusions.—Exposure to phenobarbital during prenatal development can adversely affect long-term cognitive performance. Poor outcomes are magnified by detrimental environmental conditions that interact with the prenatal biological insult. The timing of drug use appears to play an important role in the seriousness of the consequences.

▶ This study bothers me. Phenobarbital has been used for many years for a variety of maternal indications, to prevent neonatal hyperbilirubinemia, and, most recently, to prevent intraventricular or periventricular hemorrhage in the preterm infant.[1] It is sobering to discover that between 1950 and the late 1970s, more than 22 million children were born in the United States to women who were taking prescribed barbiturates during pregnancy. There are solid data documenting adverse behavioral and cognitive side effects in children treated with phenobarbital for seizure disorders, but in such cases exposure to phenobarbital has usually lasted for 1 or more years.

In this study, the duration of exposure averaged 90 days in the first study and 32 days in the second and, in some cases, was as short as 5–10 days. The mothers who were treated did not have seizure disorders or other neurologic problems. The major indications for treatment included pregnancy-induced hypertension, preeclampsia, eclampsia, hyperemesis, and use as a sedative or hypnotic. The adult men who had been exposed to phenobarbital in utero had verbal intelligence scores that were approximately 0.5 of a standard deviation (8 points) lower than predicted.

The potential impact of these findings is staggering given that millions of children throughout the world have been exposed to these drugs both in utero and in early childhood. The known and potential effects of phenobarbital are protean and include abnormalities in endocrine, neural, and behavioral function in laboratory animals.

The magnitude of the negative effects found in this study was exaggerated in those from lower socioeconomic groups and in the offspring of "unwanted" pregnancies. Premature infants are more likely be born to single mothers and those of lower socioeconomic status. Thus, it appears that detrimental environmental conditions can interact with a prenatal, biological insult to magnify the negative outcome.

Given these observations, one would be concerned about the recent controlled trial by Shankaran et al.[1] showing that antenatally administered phenobarbital decreases the incidence of periventricular/intraventricular hemorrhage in low–birth weight infants. This should be good, but did any harm come to those who received phenobarbital but did not have an intraventricular/periventricular hemorrhage? In a 3-year follow-up, no adverse consequences of phenobarbital exposure were detected.[2] If anything, the phenobarbital-exposed infants did slightly better than the controls. Another 5–7 year follow-up of children exposed to phenobarbital in utero also showed slightly better cognitive scores in the phenobarbital-exposed children,[3] although there was some delay in puberty.[4]

We don't have 20 years of follow-up for these cohorts, and it is unlikely that we will get them. What to do? This retrospective cohort study by Reinisch et al. reports an association between an intervention and an outcome 20 years later. Although the subjects were matched with controls, there are numerous opportunities for bias. In 2 randomized controlled studies (the gold standard), there was a small cognitive *benefit* to those exposed to phenobarbital. But the issue is probably no longer relevant. We can control jaundice easily in low–birth weight infants with phototherapy. During the past decade, the incidence of severe intraventricular hemorrhage has declined significantly and should decline even further with increasing use of antenatal steroids. I look forward (with some nervous anticipation) to the first 20-year follow-up of infants exposed to antenatal steroids.

M.J. Maisels, M.B., B.Ch.

References

1. Shankaran S, Cepeda E, Muran G, et al: Antenatal phenobarbital therapy and neonatal outcome. I: Effect on intracranial hemorrhage. *Pediatrics* 97:644–648, 1996.
2. Shankaran S, Woldt E, Nelson J, et al: Antenatal phenobarbital therapy and neonatal outcome. II: Neurodevelopmental outcome at 30 months. *Pediatrics* 97:649–652, 1996.
3. Valaes T, Kipouros K, Petmezaki S, et al: Effectiveness and safety of prenatal phenobarbital for the prevention of neonatal jaundice. *Pediatr Res* 14:947–952, 1980.
4. Yaffe SJ, Dorn LD: Effects of prenatal treatment with phenobarbital. *Dev Pharmacol Ther* 15:215–223, 1990.

17 Epidemiology

Very-low-birth-weight Outcomes of the National Institute of Child Health and Human Development Neonatal Research Network, May 1991 Through December 1992

Fanaroff AA, Wright LL, Stevenson DK, et al (Case Western Reserve Univ, Cleveland, Ohio; Natl Inst of Child Health, Bethesda, Md; Stanford Univ, Palo Alto, Calif; et al)

Am J Obstet Gynecol 173:1423–1431, 1995 17–1

Background.—Although outcomes among very low birth weight (VLBW) infants continue to improve, the shifting limits of viability for VLBW immature infants continue to present a challenge to the perinatal team. The risk of death for infants weighing 501–1,500 g was determined according to gestational age, birth weight, and sex. In addition, birth

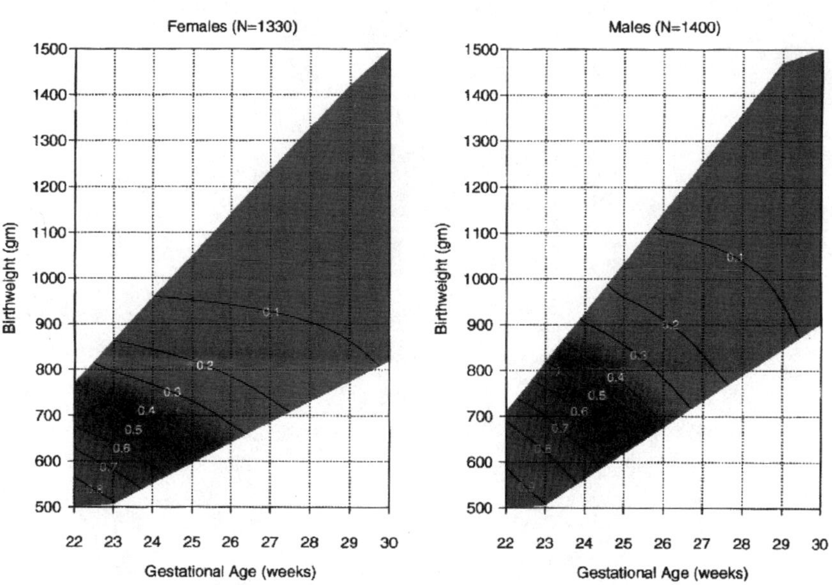

FIGURE 1.—Estimated mortality by birth weight, gestational age, and sex. (Courtesy of Fanaroff AA, Wright LL, Stevenson DK, et al: Very-low-birth-weight outcomes of the National Institute of Child Health and Human Development Neonatal Research Network, May 1991 through December 1992. *Am J Obstet Gynecol* 173:1423–1431, 1995.)

TABLE 2.—Morbidity, Mortality, and Length of Stay for Infants Born Between May 1, 1991 and Dec. 31, 1992

	501-750 gm (n = 869)	*751–1000 gm (n = 982)*	*1001–1250 gm (n = 1153)*	*1251–1500 gm (n = 1275)*	*All infants, 501–1500 gm (N = 4279)*
Morbidity*					
Respiratory distress syndrome	89 (68–95)	83 (71–93)	58 (40–79)	39 (29–53)	64 (51–76)
Surfactant therapy	59 (33–73)	64 (46–88)	44 (30–63)	26 (21–37)	46 (38–58)
Oxygen at 28 days	42 (24–58)	52 (37–73)	27 (6–60)	8 (1–26)	30 (17–47)
Postnatal corticosteroids	25 (12–55)	21 (6–37)	6 (0–11)	1 (0–5)	12 (4–20)
Chronic lung disease†	23 (5–50)	26 (8–62)	16 (0–56)	8 (1–31)	18 (3–45)
Intraventricular hemorrhage‡					
Grade I	15 (5–42)	15 (10–27)	18 (6–41)	18 (2–37)	17 (8–35)
Grade II	9 (3–17)	9 (2–14)	6 (1–11)	4 (0–8)	6 (2–12)
Grade III	11 (0–18)	9 (4–19)	5 (1–17)	2 (0–4)	6 (3–10)
Grade IV	14 (0–26)	7 (0–15)	3 (0–6)	1 (0–4)	5 (1–9)
Periventricular leukomalacia§	10 (3–29)	10 (0–20)	8 (2–36)	5 (0–18)	8 (4–22)
Necrotizing enterocolitis ≥ Stage II	6 (0–13)	6 (0–10)	5 (1–7)	4 (0–7)	5 (2–9)
Late septicemia	31 (19–45)	31 (10–50)	22 (5–34)	9 (3–13)	22 (10–30)
Indomethacin for patent ductus arteriosus	45 (14–94)	48 (25–89)	30 (12–83)	17 (4–78)	34 (14–85)
Surgery for patent ductus arteriosus	17 (2–34)	11 (0–33)	6 (0–30)	1 (0–14)	8 (1–27)
Length of stay (days, mean)					
Survival	123 (101–171)	89 (77–106)	64 (52–74)	44 (34–57)	69 (61–82)
Death	14 (3–36)	25 (8–58)	20 (2–61)	21 (1–80)	18 (5–37)
Mortality*					
By day 3	37 (17–55)	9 (2–25)	4 (1–7)	2 (0–8)	11 (6–17)
By day 7	41 (23–59)	11 (3–30)	5 (2–11)	3 (1–10)	13 (8–20)
By day 14	45 (28–59)	13 (3–31)	5 (2–13)	4 (1–10)	15 (10–22)
By day 28	50 (34–72)	15 (6–36)	6 (2–16)	4 (1–10)	17 (13–26)
By day 120	55 (34–74)	18 (7–41)	7 (3–18)	5 (2–10)	19 (15–27)
Before discharge	56 (34–74)	19 (7–42)	8 (3–18)	5 (2–10)	19 (15–28)

*All data are expressed as percentages with center ranges in parentheses.
†Oxygen at 36 weeks after conception.
‡Most severe grade in infants who had ultrasonography (n = 3,667).
§Of infants who had ultrasonography after age 2 weeks (n = 2,605).
(Courtesy of Fanaroff AA, Wright LL, Stevenson DK, et al: Very-low-birth-weight outcomes of the National Institute of Child Health and Human Development Neonatal Research Network, May 1991 through December 1992. *Am J Obstet Gynecol* 173:1423–1431, 1995.)

weight–related changes in mortality and morbidity during a 5-year period were documented.

Methods and Findings.—Perinatal data were collected prospectively by 12 centers from May 1991 through December 1992 and compared with data from 1987 through 1990. The more recent cohort consisted of 4,276 infants. Ten percent of the mothers of these infants were younger than 18 years. Fifty-five percent were black; 31%, white; and 11%, Hispanic. Fourteen percent had received no prenatal care. Twenty percent had been given antenatal corticosteroids. Half of the infants were born by cesarean delivery. Overall survival in this cohort was 81%, compared with 74% in the earlier cohort. Survival in the later cohort was 44% among infants weighing 501–750 g at birth, 81% among those weighing 751–1,000 g, 92% among those weighing 1,001–1,250 g, and 95% among those weighing 1,251–1,500 g. Girls had a significantly increased chance of survival than boys at similar birth weights and gestational ages (Fig 1). In all birth weight categories, survival increased between 1987 and 1992, with no accompanying increase in morbidity. The occurrence of major morbidity, which increased with decreasing birth weight, included late-onset septicemia in 22%, chronic lung disease in 18%, severe intraventricular bleeding in 11%, and necrotizing enterocolitis in 5%. Corticosteroids were given for chronic lung disease in 12% of the infants, including 36% of those who were oxygen dependent at 28 days (Table 2).

Conclusions.—Infant mortality associated with VLBW has decreased in the past 5 years. Birth weight, gestational age, sex, and survival rate interact. Increased survival is unassociated with a higher medical morbidity.

► It is no surprise to hear that survival for the smallest infants continues to improve with each advancing year, and this large, hospital-based cohort from 12 participating centers confirms this. It is also nice to hear that although major morbidity increases with decreasing birth weight, improved survival produced no increase in the proportion of infants surviving with significant morbidity (chronic lung disease, intracranial hemorrhage, or necrotizing enterocolitis).

These data are useful because they provide a benchmark against which other centers can measure their own outcome data. The only depressing finding from this study is that even in major university centers, which are distinguished for their quality of perinatal and neonatal care, antenatal corticosteroids were given to only 21% of the mothers. One hopes that the publication of the National Institutes of Health consensus conference on this subject[1] will lead to a dramatic increase in steroid use throughout the country as well as in the National Institute of Child Health and Human Development Neonatal Research Network. I look forward to their next report documenting outcomes after 80% of their mothers have received antenatal steroids.

M.J. Maisels, M.B., B.Ch.

Reference

1. NIH Consensus Development Conference on the Effect of Corticosteroids for Fetal Maturation on Perinatal Outcomes: Effect of corticosteroids for fetal maturation on perinatal outcomes. *JAMA* 273:413–418, 1995.

Rating Authors' Contributions to Collaborative Research: The PICNIC Survey of University Departments

Davies HD, for PICNIC (Univ of Calgary, Alta, Canada; Dalhousie Univ, Halifax, NS, Canada; Univ of British Columbia, Vancouver, BC, Canada; et al)

Can Med Assoc J 155:877–882, 1996 17–2

Objective.—All individuals listed as authors on a scientific paper should be authors. An author is defined as one who makes a substantial contribution to concept and design or to analysis and interpretation, to writing or critical revision, and final approval. A standard for attributing credit to multiple authors is lacking. Chairs of all pediatric departments in Canada were surveyed to determine the value they placed on faculty participation in multicenter studies and the relationship between authorship and promotion and tenure.

Methods.—A questionnaire asking whether research roles should be indicated on curricula vitae, how faculty members' contributions to published research papers should be related to authorship position, which of 3 options for listing authors is preferred, and how participation in single-center vs. multicenter studies affects authorship position was sent to 16 department chairs. A telephone survey was used to ascertain whether faculty deans' offices had written criteria for evaluating research papers in conjunction with promotion and tenure decisions. Responses were analyzed statistically.

Results.—Fifteen department chairs responded, and 12 responses were complete. Two department chairs detailed institutional policies. Eleven permitted faculty members to indicate their role in a research project on curricula vitae. Eleven believed that all collaborators should be listed as authors, 10 considered the principal investigator to be first author and the individual or individuals who made the greatest contribution, and most did not like the idea of listing a research group as the collective author. Seven respondents believed that participation in multicenter studies was more valuable than participation in single-center studies and that contributions of investigators in multicenter studies were valued more highly. One dean's office had written criteria for evaluating authorship of research papers for considerations of promotion or tenure.

Conclusion.—Most pediatrics departments and medical school deans' offices have no criteria, written or otherwise, for evaluating authorship and contribution to published studies. Most place a higher value on participation in multicenter than in single-center studies. Formal guidelines are needed to objectively rate the contributions of investigators to research publications.

► For all investigators who contribute time and effort to large collaborative trials, this review brings home the reality that no universal criteria exist for assessing the type of contribution made by individuals to published collaborative research. This is disconcerting, considering the increasing number of young clinical investigators who have chosen career pathways engaging them in large collaborative trials. How to deal with order of authorship, authorship in industry-initiated and industry-sponsored research, and acknowledgment in the boilerplate of a manuscript are all issues that remain unresolved. Although the article is Canadian, the problem is not foreign, and the academic community in the United States has also offered no solutions. A lot of careers hang in the balance!

D.K. Stevenson, M.D.

Viability, Morbidity, and Resource Use Among Newborns of 501- to 800-g Birth Weight

Tyson JE, for the National Institute of Child Health and Human Development Neonatal Research Network (Univ of Texas, Dallas; George Washington Univ, Washington, DC; Natl Inst of Child Health and Human Development, Bethesda, Md)

JAMA 276:1645–1651, 1996 17–3

Background.—The decision to use mechanical ventilation in extremely premature infants can be difficult. A better understanding of prognostic factors in these infants would help clinicians make treatment decisions. Uncertainty of resource requirements makes it difficult to ensure that infants who would benefit from mechanical ventilation receive proper treatment, and difficult to compare the cost-effectiveness of mechanical ventilation and other therapies. The prognostic value of various risk factors on viability and the effect of mechanical ventilation on neonatal outcome in extremely premature infants were evaluated.

Methods.—All infants weighing 501–800 g who were born during a 2-year period in the 12 centers of the National Institute of Child Health and Human Development Neonatal Research Network were evaluated. The information analyzed included the relation of risk factors to the use of mechanical ventilation and to survival, the use of mechanical ventilation in different risk categories, the use of resources, viability and maximum survival rates, hospital stay, and morbidity.

Results.—There were 1,126 infants assessed. The overall mortality rate was 43%; 15% of all the infants died without mechanical ventilation. Among infants without mechanical ventilation, the mortality rate was 93%. There was an increase in the likelihood of survival with mechanical ventilation equivalent to an increase in birth weight between 57 and 90 g for girls, small-for-gestational-age infants, and infants whose mothers received antenatal steroids. In these same groups of infants, the advantage in survival without severe brain injury was equivalent to an increase in birth weight between 64 and 107 g. Girls in the lowest birth weight group had higher mortality without mechanical ventilation than larger boys with a similar likelihood of survival with mechanical ventilation. The mean hospital stay was 115 days; this is much greater than the 18-day standard for survivors under the diagnosis-related group reimbursement system. Resource investment was high, but varied substantially between risk categories. If mechanical ventilation had been used for all infants who died, the resource use would have increased significantly, and an additional 8 infants would have survived (a maximum of 6 infants without severe brain injury per 100 infants in the 501- to 800-g birth weight category).

Conclusions.—Various factors, including birth weight, sex, maturity, and use of antenatal steroids, affect survival, morbidity, and use of resources in extremely premature infants with mechanical ventilation. The use of mechanical ventilation for girls weighing 100 g less than boys is supported, other factors being equal. The diagnosis-related group reimbursement system may compromise the use of resources for these infants who would benefit from mechanical ventilation. These findings may improve treatment decision-making and help the debate about the benefits and burdens of intensive care for these infants.

▶ Because our center is an active participant in the National Institute of Child Health and Human Development Neonatal Research Network, it would be somewhat incestuous for me to comment critically on this manuscript. I wish, however, to draw your attention to this thoughtful and provocative analysis from the network database. Careful prospective collection of data in a uniform manner, with standardized definition for all morbidities, strengthens the conclusions. The concept of translating sex, growth retardation, and the use of antenatal steroids to birth weight equivalents is food for thought that, personally, I found very palatable. Discussion of treatment decisions for low–birth weight, immature infants usually is hampered by the inability to apply group outcome data to the individual patient under consideration. It is important to bring to the forefront the issues of "relative benefits and burdens of care," ethics, and the extent to which informed consent is necessary as these infants are subjected to an array of unproven therapies. It is, perhaps, unrealistic for the authors to expect that the "treatment decisions for marginally viable patients will be enhanced if these decisions are explicitly described, empirically evaluated and openly discussed." However, it is a worthwhile goal. (See also reference 1 and Abstract 17–1.)

The ultimate measure of a man is not where he stands in moments of comfort and convenience, but where he stands during challenge and controversy.—Martin Luther King, Jr.

A.A. Fanaroff, M.B.B.Ch.

Reference

1. Tyson J: Evidence-based ethics and the care of extremely premature infants. *Future Child* 5:197–213, 1995.

Score for Neonatal Acute Physiology: Validation in Three Kaiser Permanente Neonatal Intensive Care Units

Escobar GJ, Fischer A, Li DK, et al (Kaiser Permanente Med Care Program, Oakland, Calif; Kaiser Permanente Med Ctr, Walnut Creek, Calif; Kaiser Permanente Med Ctr, Sacramento, Calif; et al)

Pediatrics 96:918–922, 1995 17–4

Background.—Most measures of illness severity have been developed in tertiary care settings, and their applicability in community neonatal ICUs is untested. The operational characteristics of the score for neonatal acute physiology (SNAP) were assessed.

Methods.—Scores were assigned prospectively to all 1,251 NICU admissions at 3 community centers during 11 months. Other variables were also documented.

Findings.—The SNAP perinatal extension was found to be a reliable predictor of newborn inhospital mortality. The area under the receiver operator characteristic curve was 0.95. The SNAP was also found to be a good predictor of total length of stay, by itself and combined with other variables. Its predictive ability among infants of low birth weight was better than among those of normal birth weight, being most limited among infants admitted to exclude sepsis. Including the major diagnostic categories of congenital heart disease or complex illness in a model containing birth weight, SNAP and transport status did not improve the predictive ability of this model.

Conclusions.—Although the SNAP has limitations when used in infants weighing 2,500 g or more, this tool is generally very useful for outcomes research. A multifunctional scale suitable for use with all birth weights may be created by modifying some of the SNAP parameters.

► Commenting on this article is William E. Benitz, M.D., Associate Professor of Pediatrics, Clinical Director of Intensive Care Nursery, Divisions of Neonatal and Developmental Medicine, Stanford University School of Medicine, Palo Alto, California:

► Validation of the SNAP and SNAP–perinatal extension scores in this more heterogenous population is an important extension of prior work on these acuity scoring tools, which appear to be useful in predicting mortality and length of stay for infants admitted to intensive care nurseries. As these authors point out, the SNAP is too complex for routine clinical use, requiring scoring of 26 different items. Their advocacy for development of a simpler scoring system and for coalescence rather than proliferation of scoring systems should be applauded, but it remains to be seen whether this objective is achievable. Finally, as Richardson and colleagues[1] have noted, the system most suitable for risk adjustments in outcomes research and that most useful at the bedside may not be the same.

W.E. Benitz, M.D.

Reference

1. Richardson DK, Phibbs CS, Gray JE, et al: Birth weight and illness severity: Independent predictors of neonatal mortality. *Pediatrics* 91:969–975, 1993.

The Effects of Patient Volume and Level of Care at the Hospital of Birth on Neonatal Mortality

Phibbs CS, Bronstein JM, Buxton E, et al (Veterans Affairs, Palo Alto, Calif; Stanford Univ, Calif; Univ of Alabama, Birmingham; et al)

JAMA 276:1054–1059, 1996 17–5

Introduction.—Because the sickest neonates usually are treated in level III tertiary neonatal ICUs (NICUs), the crude mortality rates often are higher for these centers, compared with the rates for level I or II NICUs. With risk adjustments made for major risk factors and infant birth weight, the NICU patient volume and the level of NICU care available at the hospital of birth were examined for their effects on neonatal mortality.

Methods.—All births in nonfederal hospitals in California with maternity services were reviewed for 1990. Of 472,209 singleton births, 53,229 were classified as likely NICU admissions. Birth certificates, death certificates, and infant discharge abstracts were reviewed. Neonatal-related mortality was defined as any mortality within the first 28 days of life or any other mortality occurring in the first year of life if the infant had remained hospitalized continuously since birth.

Results.—Significant effects on mortality were observed for both patient volume and level of NICU care at the hospital of birth. A significantly lower risk-adjusted neonatal mortality rate was observed in infants born in hospitals with a level III NICU with an average census of at least 15 patients per day than in those born in a hospital without an NICU. The risk-adjusted neonatal mortality rate for infants born in smaller level III NICUs and level II and II+ NICUs, regardless of size, was similar to that of hospitals without an NICU and was significantly greater than that of hospitals with large level III NICUs.

Conclusions.—The risk-adjusted neonatal mortality rate was significantly lower for births in hospitals with level III NICUs with an average daily census of 15 patients per day, compared with smaller level III NICUs, level II+ NICUs, and level II NICUs. The cost of birth of infants at hospitals with large level III NICUs was not different from that of infants born at other hospitals. It may be time to consider concentrating high-risk deliveries in urban areas in a smaller number of hospitals with level III NICUs to keep infant mortality as low as possible without increasing costs.

▶ When the history of neonatal-perinatal medicine is recounted, there will be a series of triumphs, punctuated by the tragedy of defragmentation or deregionalization of perinatal care. Commencing with a few centers of excellence in the late 1960s and the organization of neonatal transport services, regionalization emerged as an official concept and term in the early 1970s. Impetus for the melding of high-risk obstetric services and neonatal intensive care came from the Robert Wood Johnson Foundation, which funded a demonstration project and the March of Dimes–sponsored publication entitled *Towards Improving the Outcome of Pregnancy.*[1, 2] The concept was based on the premise that all pregnant women would have uniform access to high-quality care. Risk assessment would be carried out throughout pregnancy and identified high-risk women would be referred for childbirth at tertiary care centers. Outreach education was a major component of all regional perinatal centers. The system worked, and it worked well. It was good for mothers and it was good for babies, and the outcomes continued to show improvement. The model was adopted throughout the United States and in many other parts of the world.

However, for several reasons, including shifting market forces, failure to constrain costs, and the emergence of managed care, the availability of trained specialists to establish higher levels of care in the community hospitals and changing hospital affiliations and partnerships have disrupted regionalization. Powell and associates commented that, "the spirit of cooperative planning and referral that made possible the development of effective regionalized perinatal care networks appears to be eroding."[3] They documented that in Washington State, the overall percentage of low–birth weight infants born at tertiary centers rose from 1980 to 1982 through 1986 to 1988 but then declined significantly. They demonstrated that among infants weighing less than 2,000 g, nontertiary delivery was associated with greater, potentially preventable mortality.

The evidence, as presented by Phibbs and colleagues, continues to reveal the benefits of regionalization. Infants delivered in tertiary centers (soon to be referred to as subspecialty centers) as opposed to specialty or basic centers have the best outcomes. These authors showed that among infants in California who needed neonatal intensive care, the highest rates of survival were seen only in the high-volume level III units. Survival rates were lower for HMO and Medicaid patients compared with patients who had private insurance. These data have to be widely disseminated. Regionalization is still endorsed by the March of Dimes.[4] The informed consumer, who has a choice, will continue to use the subspecialty centers. As providers, we must monitor our outcomes closely, be willing to compare our outcomes with those of similar units, and strive for adequate financing of perinatal services. Every effort has to be made to attract the top pediatric and obstetric residents into the field of neonatal-perinatal medicine.

We do have an enemy. The enemy of our time is inaction.—William J. Clinton

A.A. Fanaroff, M.B.B.Ch.

References

1. March of Dimes Birth Defects Foundation, Committee on Perinatal Health: *Towards Improving the Outcome of Pregnancy: Recommendations for the Regional Development of Maternal and Perinatal Health Services.* White Plains, NY, March of Dimes Birth Defects Foundation, 1977.
2. McCormick MC, Shapiro S, Starfield BH: The regionalization of perinatal services: Summary of the evaluation of a national demonstration program. *JAMA* 253:799–804, 1985.
3. Powell S, Holt V, Hickok D, et al: Recent change in delivery site of low birth weight infants in Washington: Impact on birth weight specific mortality. *Am J Obstet Gynecol* 173:1585–1592, 1995.
4. March of Dimes Birth Defects Foundation, Committee on Perinatal Health: *Towards Improving the Outcome of Pregnancy: The 90s and Beyond.* White Plains, NY, March of Dimes Birth Defects Foundation, 1993.

Prenatal Magnesium Sulfate Exposure and the Risk for Cerebral Palsy or Mental Retardation Among Very Low-birth-weight Children Aged 3 to 5 Years

Schendel DE, Berg CJ, Yeargin-Allsopp M, et al (Ctrs for Disease Control and Prevention, Atlanta, Ga)
JAMA 276:1805–1810, 1996 17–6

Background.—Recent research suggests that prenatal exposure to magnesium sulfate may greatly reduce the risk of cerebral palsy (CP) in infants with very low birth weight (VLBW). This relationship was further investigated.

Methods.—All 1,097 infants born with VLBW between 1986 and 1988 in 29 Georgia counties were included in the study. Follow-up data were obtained on all 519 VLBW infants born in the Atlanta metropolitan area who survived infancy. This latter group was assessed for the development of CP or mental retardation (MR) by 3–5 years of age.

Findings.—In the whole cohort, prenatal magnesium sulfate exposure was not associated with infant mortality. Among the Atlanta-born survivors, those exposed to magnesium sulfate had a lower prevalence of CP or MR than those who were not exposed. The odds ratios for CP and MR were not affected by multivariate adjustment.

Conclusions.—Prenatal exposure to magnesium sulfate reduces the risk of CP and possibly MR among infants with VLBW. This decreased risk is apparently not the consequence of selective mortality of infants exposed to magnesium sulfate.

▶ Are there no limits to the actions and benefits of this venerable and relatively prosaic drug? This is the third study to demonstrate a significant association between prenatal exposure to magnesium sulfate ($MgSO_4$) in VLBW infants (less than 1,500 g) and a reduction in CP.[1, 2] The authors also provide us with important new information—the absence of any association between prenatal $MgSO_4$ exposure and infant mortality. This is important because $MgSO_4$ administration might increase mortality among those susceptible to CP development, thus reducing the number of available susceptible subjects. There are other possible confounders. Magnesium sulfate is often given to women with preeclampsia. Infants of preeclamptic women are often small for dates and are more mature for a given birth weight and might therefore be less likely to have CP. Preeclamptic women also have higher levels of corticotropins and vasoactive intestinal peptides, which might be neuroprotective.[3] However, when a subgroup analysis was performed on children of women without preeclampsia/eclampsia, a similar beneficial effect of prenatal $MgSO_4$ was found. Among children of women without preeclampsia/eclampsia, none who were exposed prenatally to $MgSO_4$ had CP, compared with 7.9% of those who were not exposed. For the whole population, the magnitude of the effect of $MgSO_4$ exposure was striking—a 90% reduction in the risk of CP and a 70% reduction in the risk of MR.

A neuroprotective effect of magnesium has been demonstrated in neonatal animal models, and in her editorial comment on this article,[3] Karen Nelson discusses the possible mechanisms for this effect. Magnesium is anti-excitotoxic, an antioxidant, and alters the production of nitric oxide. Among other things, it has been shown to prevent eclamptic convulsions and traumatic hearing loss and has been used for cardiac arrhythmias, the treatment of migraine, neurotrauma, and persistent pulmonary hypertension of the newborn. It reduces bacterial invasiveness and toxin release. It has beneficial effects in myocardial infarction including reduction of reperfusion injury, improvement in energy metabolism, and a decrease in platelet adhesiveness, all of which might contribute to its beneficial effect on the brain.

As all studies to date have been observational, we cannot conclude that the association between prenatal $MgSO_4$ exposure and a decreased risk for cerebral palsy and mental retardation is causal. Nevertheless, the fact that this has been observed in 3 separate studies and that these associations are unusually strong, makes it likely that the association is causal. If so, should magnesium be added to prenatal vitamin and mineral supplements? Karen Nelson concludes that "too little is known about the causes of prenatal or perinatal brain injury in very premature infants, and about what constitutes optimal levels of magnesium for fetal development, to justify intervention outside of randomized trials at present." Nevertheless, given what we know about the magnesium content of green leafy vegetables, nuts, whole grain cereals and beans, her advice to pregnant women is "eat your veggies."

We must also remember that all of these studies deal with VLBW infants (less than 1,500 g). They represent about 1% of all live births, although their rates of CP are 50–60 times higher than those weighing more than 2,500 g.[4] But infants weighing 1,500 g or more are responsible for about 70% of all CP. None of these studies have addressed the possible protective effects of $MgSO_4$ on infants weighing more than 1,500 g and, as the prevalence of CP in these infants is so much lower (than in those below 1,500 g), such studies will be more difficult to perform but are, nevertheless, essential.

Apparently several randomized trials are planned or under way and, if they can confirm the findings of the observational studies, we will have a simple, safe, and inexpensive intervention with a drug, familiar to all American obstetricians, that can reduce the risk of CP.

M.J. Maisels, M.B., B.Ch.

References

1. Nelson KB, Grether JK: Can magnesium sulfate reduce the risk of cerebral palsy in very low birthweight infants? *Pediatrics* 95:262–269, 1995.
2. Hauth JC, Goldenberg RL, Nelson KG, et al: Reduction of cerebral palsy with maternal $MgSO_4$ treatment in newborns weighing 500-1000g. *Am J Obstet Gynecol* 172(part 2):419, 1995.
3. Nelson KB: Magnesium sulfate and risk of cerebral palsy in very low birthweight infants. *JAMA* 276:1843–1844, 1996.
4. Cummins SK, Nelson KB, Grether JK, et al: Cerebral palsy in four northern California counties, births 1983 through 1985. *J Pediatr* 123:230–237, 1993.

The Feasibility of a Randomized Clinical Perinatal Trial: Maternal Magnesium Sulfate for the Prevention of Cerebral Palsy

Rouse DJ, Hauth JC, Nelson KG, et al (Univ of Alabama, Birmingham)

Am J Obstet Gynecol 175:701–705,1996 17–7

Background.—Recent epidemiologic data suggest that the maternal use of magnesium sulfate is associated with a reduced risk of cerebral palsy in infants surviving preterm birth. The feasibility of performing a randomized study of magnesium sulfate given to mothers intrapartum to prevent cerebral palsy in infants born preterm was investigated.

Methods and Findings.—From a literature review, the cumulative rates of delivery, neonatal survival, and cerebral palsy for progressively longer gestational age intervals beginning at 24 weeks' gestation were calculated. A minimum of 1,189 neonates at a gestation of between 24 weeks 0 days and 27 weeks 6 days would be needed for a randomized trial. The number of gravid women who delivered in the 4-week interval would need to be greatly increased to compensate for neonate loss to follow-up, maternal ineligibility, and failure of enrollment. One million pregnancies would be needed to produce the number of eligible gravid women. Shorter gestational age intervals would require fewer neonates but more pregnancies. Because of the declining prevalence of cerebral palsy at more advanced gestational ages, extending the gestational age interval would substantially increase the minimum number of neonates to 1,982 but decrease the necessary number of pregnancies only slightly.

Conclusion.—Conducting a prospective, randomized study of the efficacy of administering magnesium sulfate to women to prevent cerebral palsy in infants surviving preterm birth would be very difficult. Another possibility would be to use severe neonatal cranial abnormalities as the primary end point in a study of the neuroprotective effects of maternal magnesium sulfate in preterm birth survivors.

▶ Retrospective analyses have titillated investigators with the consideration of a randomized, clinical, perinatal trial evaluating maternal magnesium sulfate for the prevention of cerebral palsy. Although the temptation exists to design a smaller trial focused on a surrogate for cerebral palsy, a definitive trial would be necessary and, indeed, would be formidable, requiring a concerted, multicentered effort because of the sample size requirement for generating the necessary number of eligible gravid women. Shortening or extending the gestational age interval would have little effect on the size of the trial in practical terms. Nonetheless, a randomized, controlled trial would probably be the only way to resolve the issue, as women treated with magnesium sulfate are exposed to the drug for so many disparate reasons.

Most importantly, any trial designed for this purpose should involve the collaboration of neonatologists and perinatologists, as the primary outcome would be directly impacted by follow-up compliance and the definition of cerebral palsy as the primary outcome. Whether the maternal magnesium sulfate administration has a benefit for the fetus—and, if so, under what conditions the full benefit would be realized—remain unclear issues. Neonatologists should caution their colleagues, based on their own collective history, that certain perceived advantages for therapies, based on retrospective experience, turn out not to be advantageous and are sometimes harmful.

D.K. Stevenson, M.D.

Prevalence of Cerebral Palsy in Twins, Triplets and Quadruplets

Yokoyama Y, Shimizu T, Hayakawa K (Kinki Univ, Osaka, Japan; Osaka Univ, Japan)

Int J Epidemiol 24:943–948, 1995 17–8

Background.—Cerebral palsy is more frequent in twins and triplets than in singletons. Risk is presumably greater for quadruplets as well. The frequency of cerebral palsy in multiple births was investigated, including an attempt to identify associated risk factors.

Methods and Findings.—A Japanese registry of multiple births was used to identify 705 sets of twins, 96 sets of triplets, and 7 sets of quadruplets, all born after 1977. Cerebral palsy was present in 0.9% of the twins, 3.1% of the triplets, and 11.1% of the quadruplets. The risks of at least 1 child per multiple birth having cerebral palsy were 1.5% for twins, 8.0% for triplets, and 42.9% for quadruplets. On logistic regression analysis, significant risk factors for cerebral palsy were decreased gestational age and asphyxia. Cerebral palsy was 20 times more likely to occur in infants with gestational ages of less than 32 weeks, compared with 36 weeks or greater.

Conclusion.—Triplets and quadruplets are at greater risk of cerebral palsy than twins. This risk is strongly related to decreasing gestational age at birth. As the proportion of multiple births increases, prospective parents need counseling on the associated risks of cerebral palsy and other complications.

▶ This article reminds us again that the risk of producing at least 1 child with cerebral palsy increases dramatically in twin, triplet, and quadruplet pregnancies, exceeding 40% in the last circumstance. Not surprisingly, the major factor contributing to this phenomenon is lower gestational age in the multiple-gestation pregnancies. More is definitely not better in neonatology.

D.K. Stevenson, M.D.

18 Ethics

End-of-Life Decisions for Surgical Neonates: Experience in The Netherlands and United States

Caniano DA, Hazebroek FWJ, DenBesten KE, et al (Ohio State Univ, Columbus; Children's Hosp, Columbus, Ohio; Erasmus Univ, Rotterdam, The Netherlands)

J Pediatr Surg 30:1420–1424, 1995 18–1

Background.—For critically ill neonates unlikely to recover, decisions must be made about limiting medical intervention and the manner in which the dying process will occur. End-of-life decision-making for neonates in 2 surgical ICUs (SICUs)—one in The Netherlands and one in the United States—was compared.

Methods.—Data were obtained on all the neonatal deaths occurring in the 2 children's hospitals. Between January 1990 and July 1993, 362 neonates were admitted to Sophia Children's Hospital (SCH) in The Netherlands and 125 to the Columbus Children's Hospital (CCH) in the United States. The neonates who died were classified as having a poor prognosis and expected to die (group 1) or having a good prognosis and expected to survive (group 2).

Findings.—The death rates were comparable in the SCH and CCH SICUs—12% and 14%, respectively. Mean survival was only 1.5 days in group 1, compared with 26.5 days in group 2. The criteria for assigning neonates to group 1 differed between SICUs. At SCH, the criterion was "expected poor quality of life," and at CCH, it was "futility." Criteria for assigning neonates to group 2 were similar, including significant postoperative complications. The percentages of neonates with a do-not-resuscitate (DNR) order were comparable in the 2 SICUs, but the application of the DNR order differed. For most neonates at SCH, life support was either withheld or withdrawn. At CCH, infants with a DNR order were not offered further escalation in treatment. Mean length of survival after the DNR order was 4 days at SCH and 7 days at CCH.

Conclusions.—In these 2 SICUs, DNR orders were specified for more than half the critically ill neonates. The criteria for DNR status and treatment implementation after DNR orders differed between the SICUs.

▶ Jonathan Hellman, M.B.B.Ch., F.C.P.(SA), F.R.C.P.(C), Associate Professor of Paediatrics, University of Toronto, and Clinical Director, Neonatal Intensive

Care Unit, The Hospital for Sick Children, Toronto, Canada, contributed the following commentary:

► The manner in which end-of-life decisions are made, by whom, on what basis, and how these decisions are implemented is now the subject of much discussion among caregivers of the critically ill neonate. The authors of this report from 2 individual pediatric surgical ICUs, one in the US and one in The Netherlands, have uncovered some important differences in their criteria for DNR status and the implementation of patient care after the DNR, despite fairly similar patient populations and overall mortality rates. In characterizing their criteria for DNR orders, the American surgeons clearly favored use of the term futility over quality-of-life terminology frequently used by the Dutch surgeons. The impact of the DNR was the withdrawal of mechanical ventilation in the majority of the SCH infants, whereas the CCH unit used a narrower interpretation of DNR as no CPR with other treatment measures being maintained. The differences in this approach may explain a longer average survival of 7 days in the CCH than the 4 days seen in the SCH.

The reasons for these differences are difficult to determine. Is it different societal expectations of medical technology, a greater expression of the parental role in demanding continued aggressive support, fear of litigation unless medical futility can be determined? Reports such as this raise a number of questions: how much "transparency" is there in the communication in each unit?[1] how reflective are these particular surgical units of other units in their respective countries or of the neonatal intensive care units in their respective institutions?; has this analysis led to the development of guidelines (or paradigms à la Benitz[2]) in the CCH? Despite this desire for more texture to the data provided, the study represents the start of the process that must be undertaken if caregivers are to reflect critically on end-of-life decision-making in critically ill newborn infants. Such reviews of practice and comparison among physicians in different social contexts brings with it the hope that we can reach an understanding of the values implicit in the technical process of withdrawal of life-sustaining care and possibly construct and defend a moral theory of practice for future decisions in this difficult area. As Brody[3] suggests, compassionate withdrawal of treatment requires moving from a "tactical approach (focusing on each intervention)," such as we have here, to a "strategic approach (aiming at defined goals)," e.g., promoting the comfort of the patient and the family, withdrawing burdensome interventions, etc.

J. Hellman, M.B.B.Ch.

References

1. King NMP: Transparency in neonatal intensive care. *Hastings Cent Rep* May/June:18–25, 1992.
2. Benitz WE: A paradigm for making difficult choices in the intensive care nursery. *Camb Q Healthc Ethics* 2:281–294, 1993.
3. Brody H, Campbell ML, Faber-Langendoen K, et al: Withdrawing intensive life-sustaining treatment—Recommendations for compassionate clinical management. *N Engl J Med* 326:652–657, 1997.

Foregoing Intensive Care Treatment in Newborn Infants With Extremely Poor Prognoses

de Leeuw R, de Beaufort AJ, de Kleine MJK, et al (Univ of Amsterdam; Univ Hosp, Leiden, The Netherlands; St Joseph Hosp, Veldhoven, The Netherlands; et al)

J Pediatr 129:661–666, 1996 18–2

Background.—Few quantifiable data are available on how neonatologists deal with ethical dilemmas in daily practice. A multicenter study in 4 Dutch neonatal ICUs (NICUs) was reported.

Methods.—Data were obtained on all 181 infants dying in these NICUs during 1993. Excluding patients for whom foregoing treatment was not under discussion, the neonates for whom death appeared inevitable were labeled "A cases," and those for whom treatment was foregoing because of extremely poor prognosis were labeled "B cases."

Findings.—Thirty-five neonates died despite full continuation of treatment. In 98 A cases and 48 B cases, representing 81% of all deaths, treatment was foregone because of no chance of survival or a very poor prognosis. The medical team eventually reached a consensus of opinion about these neonates, although several sessions were required for some. The parents of 3 neonates disagreed with the team's advice. Treatment was continued for 2 of these infants. In a large majority of B cases, the decision to forego treatment was based on the finding of severe cerebral damage. For B cases, the neonatologists had to decide whether continuing treatment was justifiable or treatment withdrawal was preferred in view of the extremely poor prognosis.

Conclusions.—Intentional, active termination of a neonate's life is rare in Dutch NICUs. More often, intensive therapy is withheld or withdrawn after consideration of the neonate's expected quality of life. The decision to introduce and/or sustain aggressive treatment for such neonates should be viewed as carrying a responsibility of at least equal weight. An ethical and legal framework is needed to ensure that patients receive the maximum benefit from technology without being subjected to pointless suffering.

▶ This description of the criteria and process for discontinuing intensive care in The Netherlands provides a yardstick against which neonatologists in other countries may wish to assess the benefits or pitfalls of this practice. The present study clearly reflects that quality-of-life criteria are used routinely in decision-making and are considered justifiable medical practice. It also demonstrates that active euthanasia was not practiced (based on the distinction that actions that hasten death in the terminal phase are not considered euthanasia).

The authors acknowledge that this 1993 study, when compared with similar data from 1990, suggests a liberalization of discontinuation procedures. This raises a question as to the extent to which practice in NICUs in The Netherlands has been influenced by the broader social context, which is tolerant of euthanasia and assisted suicide (despite the fact that the act of intentionally ending a patient's life is still under criminal classification in The Netherlands' penal code). I believe the findings in this study should quell any fears that euthanasia is prevalent in critically ill newborn infants in Dutch NICUs and should dispel the specter of the "slippery slope" argument that acceptance of physician discretion in making quality-of-life judgments may encourage active euthanasia.

As we all struggle to navigate the legal and ethical pathways in our attempts to find the most compassionate way to ameliorate the suffering of newborn infants and their families, the Dutch are to be commended for their openness in attempting to promote discourse on this sensitive subject. For some contrasting approaches to the moral aspects of neonatal care see a report by Versluys and de Leeuw,[1] the AAP Committee on Bioethics statement,[2] and Campbell and McHaffie's view on the British scene.[3]

J. Hellman, M.B.B.Ch.

References

1. Versluys Z, de Leeuw R: A Dutch report on the ethics of neonatal care. *J Med Ethics* 21:14–16, 1995.
2. Committee on Bioethics: Ethics and the care of critically ill infants and children. *Pediatrics* 98:149–152, 1996.
3. Campbell AGM, McHaffie HE: Prolonging life and allowing death: Infants. *J Med Ethics* 21:339–344, 1995.

Birth Weight-specific Mortality for Extremely Low Birth Weight Infants Vanishes by Four Days of Life: Epidemiology and Ethics in the Neonatal Intensive Care Unit

Meadow W, Reimshisel T, Lantos J (Univ of Chicago)

Pediatrics 97:636–643, 1996 18–3

Background.—The value of aggressive resuscitative measures for many very low birth weight (VLBW) infants has been intensely debated. The current authors' impression is that most of the VLBW infants who die do so rapidly. If this is true, then discussions of the appropriateness of treatment that consider only survival rates may be misguided.

Methods and Findings.—The outcomes of 429 VLBW infants admitted to one neonatal ICU (NICU) during 3 years were analyzed. Forty-seven percent of the 429 VLBW infants alive on day of life (DOL) 1 survived to be discharged. Birth weight and illness severity both independently predicted likelihood of survival on DOL 1. About 80% of the deaths occurred in the first 3 days of life. Thus, once an infant had survived to DOL 4, the likelihood of survival was enhanced markedly. Although survival after DOL 4 continued to depend on illness severity, it did not depend on birth weight. Overall, although 53% of VLBW infants who were admitted died, only about 13% of all NICU bed-days were devoted to infants who died, a figure that did not vary as a function of birth weight.

Conclusions.—Predictions of survival of VLBW infants should be corrected by including DOL. When DOL is considered, the prognostic value of birth weight declined rapidly. Furthermore, birth weight–specific mortality and day of death for nonsurvivors were correlated inversely. Consequently, medical resources allocated to nonsurvivors remained low and were independent of birth weight.

► This paper confirms that birth weight is a significant predictor of survival in VLBW infants but that its predictive value becomes diminished by 72 hours. Early medical intervention in this group of infants born between 1989 and 1991 did not unduly prolong the dying, extend the suffering, or use inordinate resources for those infants who died. (The study addresses only the issue of survival and does not pretend to inform the issue of morbidity in survivors.) The authors believe that their findings lend weight both to the reasonableness of physicians in offering such care and of parents in requesting/assenting to it. They also question how this information should reframe the debate about whether intensive care should be offered or initiated for such infants.

Certainly, problematic early decisions based solely on birth weight can be refined by 72 hours of neonatal intensive care as a type of "diagnostic test"; this may help parents and physicians believe that death occurred despite everything having been done and avoid some of the anguish of early decision-making. (This study did not examine the effect of decisions to withhold or withdraw life-sustaining treatment; the authors acknowledge that very few infants in their NICU are removed from mechanical ventilation for quality-of-life concerns.) Conversely, generating a momentum of care in the first few days of life and overcoming the first "critical period," may create not only a false expectation of survival for parents (in about 20% of cases), but also the expectation of a good-quality survival. Furthermore, with improvements in managing the medical problems of the first 72 hours, survival rates will increase and may lead to a greater incidence of late deaths with the potential for more prolonged suffering. In Hack's report on the change in delivery room practice in infants weighing less than 750 g during two time periods (1990–1992 compared with 1982–1988); with a significant increase in delivery room endotracheal intubation and the use of surfactant, fewer infants died at less than 24 hours and more deaths occurred after 28 days.[1]

There is no question that individualized decision-making can be better informed by more accurate prognostic information, and there are a number of positive elements to the practice of initiating treatment in VLBW infants and allowing a "natural selection" process to occur. However, unless we are solely fixated on survival, as long as early aggressive treatment has the potential to exacerbate the extent of human suffering and utilization of resources, the advisability of initiating such care at birth will remain a hotly contested issue.

J. Hellman, M.B.B.Ch.

Reference

1. Hack M, Friedman H, Fanaroff AA: Outcomes of extremely low birth weight infants. *Pediatrics* 98:931–937, 1996.

Resolving the Clinical and Ethical Dilemma Involved in Fetal-Maternal Conflicts

Pinkerton JV, Finnerty JJ (Univ of Virginia, Charlottesville)
Am J Obstet Gynecol 175:289–295, 1996 18–4

Background.—The moral acceptability of court-ordered treatment for pregnant women refusing recommended interventions has attracted much debate. Some authorities argue that such treatment is never justifiable, as a woman's autonomy must be respected, even if there is a risk of harm to the fetus. Other authorities argue that state intervention is justified to promote fetal well-being in certain circumstances. However, the proponents of the latter view disagree as to the circumstances in which state intervention is warranted. A set of guidelines for managing maternal-fetal dilemmas was developed by a subcommittee of the Hospital Ethics Committee at the University of Virginia Health Sciences Center after studying the issue for nearly 1 year.

Clinical and Ethical Dilemmas Involved in Fetal-Maternal Conflicts.—The subcommittee reviewed the recent medical literature and relevant court cases. Views on the management of maternal-fetal conflicts range from absolute respect for a woman's autonomy with no tolerance for state intervention, to respect for autonomy with gentle persuasion, to recourse to the courts if needed, overriding a woman's autonomy to promote fetal well-being. Over time, the decisions in court cases have progressed from the routine subordination of a woman's autonomy and bodily integrity to the interests of the fetus to respect for a woman's autonomy.

Conclusions.—When a competent pregnant woman and her care providers disagree about interventions such as fetal blood transfusions, fetal surgery, and cesarean section, providers should respect the informed choice of the woman. Although education and respectful persuasion may be used to encourage a woman to change her mind, her autonomous decision must ultimately be heeded. Ethics consultation services may be involved when a satisfactory resolution cannot be reached. Subsequently, the issue may be referred to the Ethics Committee, which may involve administrative and legal personnel. Court intervention should be sought only in extreme cases and after all other avenues have been exhausted.

► This comment has been provided by Françoise Baylis, Ph.D., Associate Professor, Faculty of Medicine, Bioethics Education and Research, and Department of Philosophy, Dalhousie University, Halifax, Nova Scotia, Canada:

► When a pregnant woman is not competent, attempts should be made to determine what her wishes would have been were she capable of participating in the decision-making process. These wishes, presuming they can be known with the assistance of a surrogate decision-maker, should be respected. When the patient's previous wishes cannot be known, a decision should be made by the surrogate on the basis of the patient's best interests. The authors add, however, that the surrogate's decision should be critically evaluated by the caregivers to ensure that it is being made in the best interests of the mother and her fetus. This statement contradicts the earlier claim, which focused on the woman's best interests, so the reader cannot be sure of the final conclusion regarding decision-making by incapable patients.

F. Baylis, Ph.D.

Common Ethical Dilemmas Encountered in the Management of HIV-infected Women and Newborns

Chervenak FA, McCullough LB (New York Hosp/Cornell Med Ctr; Baylor College of Medicine, Houston)

Clin Obstet Gynecol 39:411–419, 1996 18–5

Background.—The medical literature stresses patient autonomy in the management of HIV-infected individuals, especially the issues of informed choice in HIV testing and respect for patient confidentiality in disclosing seropositivity. The current authors object to this narrow focus and believe that an excessive attention to the rights of those with HIV has eclipsed the ethical consideration of the obligations of infected patients and health care providers to prevent the transmission of dangerous infectious diseases. They have urged a rethinking of the "clinical and public health ethics of HIV infection," with particular attention to HIV-infected mothers and newborns.

Ethical Dilemmas in the Management of HIV-infected Women and Newborns.—The authors call for a more balanced ethical approach that addresses both the rights and obligations of HIV-infected women. Using traditional ethical language, they state that physicians must recognize both the autonomy of an HIV-infected woman and her beneficence-based obligations to her sexual and needle-sharing partners, to her fetus, and to the newborn and child the fetus may become. Physicians must determine when to respect patient autonomy and when to intervene to enforce certain beneficence-based obligations to others, a dilemma that is especially difficult when a woman is pregnant and her behavior and choices do not seem to be in the best interest of fetal well-being. An example is an at-risk woman who refuses HIV testing and thus, lacking important information on which to base decisions about zidovudine (ZDV) treatment, may be placing her fetus at increased risk for vertical transmission.

Conclusions.—It is believed that all pregnant women should be offered HIV testing and that those testing positive should have access to ZDV.

Aggressive directive counseling is advocated to ensure a woman's consent to testing and treatment, suggesting that merely offering HIV testing and ensuring the availability of ZDV is not satisfatory from a public policy perspective.

▶ This comment has been provided by Françoise Baylis, Ph.D., Associate Professor, Faculty of Medicine, Bioethics Education and Research, and Department of Philosophy, Dalhousie University, Halifax, Nova Scotia, Canada:

▶ When pregnant women's occupational, lifestyle, or health care behaviors and choices potentially place the developing fetus at risk, there is often talk of the need for state intervention to preclude or curtail these behaviors or choices. In the realm of health care, this issue typically arises when a pregnant woman refuses an intervention recommended by her physician, such as a cessation of excessive alcohol consumption or illegal drugs, HIV testing, and delivery by cesarean section. The ethical dilemma for the physician is whether to respect the woman's reproductive autonomy or to invoke state authority and override her autonomy in pursuit of the fetus' best interests.

Pinkerton and Finnerty (Abstract 18–4) advocate respect for the patient's autonomy, but they recognize education and respectful persuasion as legitimate means to encourage women to alter their behaviors and choices. This view is consonant with that of the American College of Obstetricians and Gynecologists, which states that a woman's right to refuse an intervention should be respected and that court intervention should almost never be used.[1] In contrast, Chervenak and McCullough maintain that state intervention and overriding of the woman's autonomy are appropriate because some women need to be strongly "persuaded" (e.g., presented with a court order) to meet their beneficence-based obligations to their fetuses.[2] As concerns the issue of HIV testing, there is every reason to believe that they would support state intervention and so presumably would support the American Medical Association's endorsement of mandatory HIV-testing for pregnant women.[3, 4]

As these two articles clearly show, there is much disagreement regarding the appropriate management of maternal-fetal dilemmas. In many respects, this is surprising. It is widely accepted that health care providers should respect their competent patients' choices. Why should this standard not apply equally to pregnant women? In response some, including Chervenak and McCullough, will point to the complex and nuanced moral relationships in obstetrics, where physicians perceive that they have obligations to two patients in one body. However, although it may be true that physicians (and patients) have certain obligations to the developing fetus, it is not evident that these obligations justify overriding the choices of competent women. In no other situation are competent individuals deemed to have an obligation to provide medically for another person, so why is this expected of pregnant women with regard to their fetuses, whose personhood is widely contested?

F. Baylis, Ph.D.

References

1. American College of Obstetricians and Gynecologists: Patient choice: Maternal-fetal conflict. American College of Obstetricians and Gynecologists policy statement. Washington, DC, ACOG, Committee Opinion No. 55, Oct. 1987.
2. Chervenak F, McCullough L: *Ethics in Obstetrics and Gynecology.* New York, Oxford University Press, 1994.
3. Shelton DL: Delegates push mandatory HIV testing for pregnant women. *American Medical News* 39.26:1, 93, 1996.
4. Kent C: AMA reaffirms mandatory HIV testing in pregnancy. *American Medical News* 39.48:8, 1996.

Supplemental Reading List

Abad F, Diaz NM, Domenech E, et al: Oral sweet solution reduces pain-related behaviour in preterm infants. *Acta Paediatr* 85:854–858, 1996.

Adair CD, Ernest JM, Sanchez-Ramos L, et al: Meconium-stained amniotic fluid-associated infectious morbidity: A randomized, double-blind trial of ampicillin-felbactam prophylaxis. *Obstet Gynecol* 88:216–220, 1996.

Anandakumar C, Biswas A, Wong YC, et al: Management of non-immune hydrops: 8 years' experience. *Ultrasound Obstet Gynecol* 9:196–200, 1996.

Ansell P, Bull D, Roman E: Childhood leukemia and intramuscular vitamin K: Findings from a case-control study. *BMJ* 313:204–205, 1996.

Baethmann M, Kahn T, Lenard H-G, et al: Fetal CNS damage after exposure to maternal trauma during pregnancy. *Acta Paediatr* 85:1331–1338, 1996.

Coniglio SJ, Anderson SM, Ferguson JE: Functional motor outcome in children with myelomeningocele: Correlation with anatomic level on prenatal ultrasound. *Dev Med Child Neurol* 38:675–680, 1996.

de la Hunt MN, Madden N, Scott JES, et al: Is delayed surgery really better for congenital diaphragmatic hernia?: A prospective randomized clinical trial. *J Pediatr Surg* 31:1554–1556, 1996.

Evans MI, Hume RF Jr, Johnson MP: Integration of genetics and ultrasonography in prenatal diagnosis: Just looking is not enough. *Am J Obstet Gynecol* 174:1925–1933, 1996.

Gunn AJ, Gunn TR, Rabone DL, et al: Growth hormone increases breast milk volumes in mothers of preterm infants. *Pediatrics* 98:279–282, 1996.

Hakulinen AL, Järvenpää A-L, Turpeinen M, et al: Diffusing capacity of the lung in school-aged children born very preterm, with and without bronchopulmonary dysplasia. *Pediatr Pulmonol* 21:353–360, 1996.

Helwig JT, Parer JT, Kilpatrick SJ, et al: Umbilical cord blood acid-base state: What is normal? Am J Obstet Gynecol 174:1807–1814, 1996.

Iannucci TA, Tomich PG, Gianopoulos JG: Etiology and outcome of extremely low-birth-weight infants. *Am J Obstet Gynecol* 174:1896–1900, 1996.

Jiang ZD: Long-term effect of perinatal and postnatal asphyxia on developing human auditory brainstem responses: Peripheral hearing loss. *Int J Pediatr Otorhinolaryngol* 33:225–238, 1995.

Kari MA, Raivio KO, Stenman U-H: Serum cortisol, dehydroepiandrosterone sulfate, and steroid-binding globulins in preterm neonates: Effect of gestational age and dexamethasone therapy. *Pediatr Res* 40:319–324, 1996.

Leth H, Toft PB, Peitersen B, et al: Use of brain lactate levels to predict outcome after perinatal asphyxia. *Acta Paediatr* 85:859–864, 1996.

McCarton CM, Brooks-Gunn J, Wallace IF, et al: Results at age 8 years of early intervention for low-birth-weight premature infants. *JAMA* 277:126–132, 1997.

McClure RJ, Newell SJ: Effect of fortifying breast milk on gastric emptying. *Arch Dis Child* 74:F60–F62, 1996.

Pharoah POD, Cooke T: Cerebral palsy and multiple births. *Arch Dis Child* 75:F174–F177, 1996.

Pierce EA, Foley ED, Smith LEH: Regulation of vascular endothelial growth factor by oxygen in a model of retinopathy of prematurity. *Arch Ophthalmol* 114:1218–1228, 1996.

Suguihara C, Hehre D, Huang J, et al: Decreased ventilatory response to hypoxia in sedated newborn piglets prenatally exposed to cocaine. *J Pediatr* 128:389–395, 1996.

Sumits T, Bennett R, Gould J: Maternal risks for very low birth weight infant mortality. *Pediatrics* 98:236–241, 1996.

Taylor MJ, Saliba E, Laugier J: Use of evoked potentials in preterm neonates. *Arch Dis Child* 74:F70–F76, 1996.

Turjesen T, Holen KJ, Tegnander A: Hip abnormalities detected by ultrasound in clinically normal newborn infants. *J Bone Joint Surg (Br)* 78-B:636–640, 1996.

Valayer J: Conventional treatment of biliary atresia: Long-term results. *J Pediatr Surg* 31:1546–1551, 1996.

von Kries R, Göbel U, Hachmeister A: Vitamin K in childhood cancer: A population based case-control study in lower Saxony, Germany. *BMJ* 313:199–203, 1996.

Wheeler W, Kurachek S, McNamara J, et al: Consequences of hypogammaglobulinemia and steroid therapy in severe bronchopulmonary dysplasia. *Pediatr Pulmonol* 22:96–100, 1996.

Williams K, Hennessy E, Alberman E: Cerebral palsy: Effects of twinning, birthweight, and gestational age. *Arch Dis Child* 75:F178–F182, 1996.

Subject Index*

* *All entries refer to the year and page number(s) for data appearing in this and previous editions of the* Year Book.

D

E

F

G

M

N

S

T

U

W

X

Z

Author Index

A

B

C

D

L

M

N

O

P

Q

R

S

T

U

V